Harold Hillman

SELECTED WRITINGS OF
SIR CHARLES SHERRINGTON

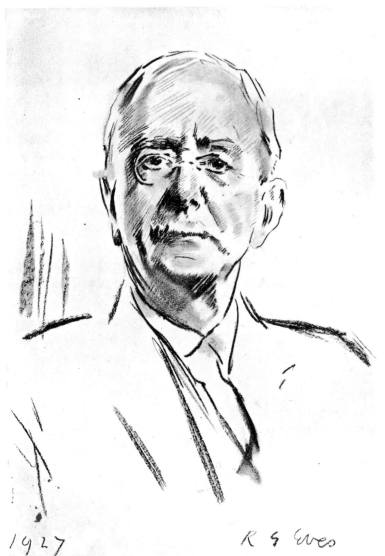

1927   R & Eves

SELECTED WRITINGS OF SIR CHARLES SHERRINGTON

A TESTIMONIAL PRESENTED BY THE
NEUROLOGISTS FORMING THE
GUARANTORS OF THE JOURNAL *BRAIN*

Compiled and Edited by
D. DENNY-BROWN

OXFORD UNIVERSITY PRESS
1979

Oxford University Press, Walton Street, Oxford OX2 6DP

OXFORD LONDON GLASGOW
NEW YORK TORONTO MELBOURNE WELLINGTON
KUALA LUMPUR SINGAPORE JAKARTA HONG KONG TOKYO
DELHI BOMBAY CALCUTTA MADRAS KARACHI
IBADAN NAIROBI DAR ES SALAAM CAPE TOWN

ISBN 0 19 920104 8

FIRST PUBLISHED IN 1939
BY HAMISH HAMILTON MEDICAL BOOKS

REPRINTED 1979

*Reproduced and printed by photolithography and bound in
Great Britain at The Pitman Press, Bath*

A TRIBUTE

TO

SIR CHARLES SCOTT SHERRINGTON
O.M. 1924, G.B.E. 1922

Fellow and Past President of the Royal Society.
M.A., M.D., D.Sc. Cantab.
F.R.C.P., F.R.C.S.
Hon. D.Sc. Oxford, Paris, Manchester, Strasbourg, Louvain, Upsala, Budapest, Athens.
Hon. LL.D. London, Toronto, Harvard, Dublin, Edinburgh, Montreal, Liverpool,
   Brussels, Sheffield, Berne, Birmingham, Wales, and Glasgow.

Fellow of Magdalen College, Oxford.
Waynflete Professor of Physiology in the University of Oxford, 1913-1935.
Holt Professor of Physiology in the University of Liverpool, 1895-1913.
Brown Professor of Pathology in the University of London, and
Lecturer in Physiology, St. Thomas's Hospital, London, 1887-1895.

Nobel Laureate for Medicine, 1932.
Royal and Copley Medal, Royal Society.
Hughlings Jackson Medal, Royal Society of Medicine.
Retzius Gold Medal, Swedish Royal Academy.
Baly Gold Medal, Royal College of Physicians.

President, British Association for the Advancement of Science, 1922.

Hon. Fellow, Caius College, Cambridge.
Hon. Fellow, Royal Society, Edinburgh.
Hon. Member, Royal Irish Academy.
Hon. Member, Société de Neurologie, Paris.
Corresponding Member of l'Institut de France, etc., etc.

" Celui qui, à Cambridge,[1] a été témoin de l'expérience de Sherrington, montrant l'effet relaxant qu'accompagne l'excitation du muscle antagoniste, a enrichi sa connaissance pour toujours.   Je sens encore le triceps du singe se fondre pour ainsi dire entre les doigts, au moment que le biceps se contracte."

Discours d'Ouverture par le Président, H. J. HAMBURGER,
Ninth International Congress of Physiology,
Groningen, September, 1912.

[1] At Fourth International Congress of Physiologists, Cambridge.   See Suppl., *J. Physiol.*, 1898-9, **23**, 26, 31.

PREFACE

The published papers of Sir Charles Sherrington are scattered through many journals over a considerable period of time. Many are now difficult to consult. In them a mass of systematic observation, faithfully recorded, forms both a classical example of scientific method and a monumental contribution to the literature of the nervous system. There is no need to enlarge here upon the importance of this work and the conceptions of its author, to general biological and to physiological science, or to clinical medicine. The guarantors of the journal *Brain*, themselves neurologists and physiologists, wish, by making some reprints and extracts of his published papers more readily available, to pay humble tribute and compliment to the greatness of Sherrington.

All those who have been his pupils and colleagues know full well his generosity and selflessness, his wisdom and breadth of mind, and his stimulus to all who worked with him. Modest to a degree, he is shy of speaking of his own contribution. It is difficult, therefore, to convey to those who lacked the opportunity of personal contact the principles of his method. They were never enunciated as such. We believe, however, that in one sense the soundness of his work, and its ever close touch with reality, arise primarily in the cultivation of the art of simple observation. Such detailed observation of a reaction always preceded an attempted graphic analysis. Thus direct vision and palpation served always to control the caprice and artifice of delicate apparatus. The method is that of clinical medicine, and in rendering more available many of these classical studies in " clinical physiology " we hope further to stimulate clinical neurology.

Perusal of the bibliography here appended will give the reader an impression of the breadth and scope of Sherrington's writings. The method of selection for this volume makes no attempt to give them all adequate representation. Indeed, it is much beyond this compilation to indicate sufficiently all the fruitful observations and contributions which have so abundantly flowed from one pen for over fifty-five years, and still continue. Fortunately comprehensive accounts of some aspects are readily available. The extracts and reprints selected here are designed primarily to present in brief form many of the descriptions of clinical physiology of greatest interest to neurologists. These include the original descriptions of the spinal animal, the experimental isolation of skin and muscle segmentation, the more general observations on reflexes and their interaction, the motor representation in the primate cortex, and the fundamental proof of reciprocal innervation and of postural reflexes. Particular care has been taken to include a discussion of double reciprocal innervation, to make it clear that, contrary to misrepresentations appearing in the literature from time to time, the principle of reciprocal innervation does not require that one member of an antagonistic pair of muscles should be necessarily *completely* relaxed when the other is active. The development of the conception of central inhibition is sketched. Detailed consideration of the more theoretical aspects are omitted, though pains have been taken to indicate where they may be found.

In this way the present selection of writings is designed as an introduction to the subject through the works of the great master, and as a source book for the neurologist, general physiologist, and psychologist.

Those aspects of the subject which have been dealt with at length in the *Integrative Action of the Nervous System* have been omitted, in particular all reference to the investigations of binocular flicker and sensual fusion, and the studies on the scratch-reflex and successive induction. No attempt has been made to include the classical reviews of muscle sense (whose proof comes from Sherrington's work), and of general sensation, to be found in his contributions to Vol. II. of Schäfer's *Physiology*, or to the advances introduced in the teaching and practice of mammalian physiology, also published elsewhere. We should have liked to include some of his published verse. To all these the present collection stands complementary.

Little space could be found for the many observations on the physiological anatomy of the tracts of the spinal cord, the classical description of the mammalian muscle spindle and the proof of the sensory nature of its nerve ending, the investigation of the reflexes of deglutition, of pilomotor reactions, of cholera and tetanus, and the reaction of the white cells of the blood to inflammation, and many others. Many extracts had to be sadly clipped to enable them to have representation at all. If the reader is stimulated to consult the original, the purpose of the volume will have been served.

Nor was there space for more than passing comment on his own advances in laboratory method and technique. Today the decerebrate and decapitate mammalian preparations are a commonplace in laboratory method. It is difficult to assess the enormous impetus to experimental medicine in general due to these advances in standard technique made by Sherrington in 1898 and 1909. Suffice to quote here the words of Professor Camis (*The Physiology of the Vestibular Apparatus*, trans. by Creed, Oxford, 1930, p. 124), who, in commenting on the revolution of ideas concerning the physiology of the labyrinth which took place in 1910-1925, wrote: " . . . but the important factor is that the more recent investigators have been able to take advantage of the vast and comprehensive work that had meanwhile been accomplished in connexion with the physiology of the nervous system and particularly of reflexes. There the work of Sherrington, characterised by tenacity and patience no less than by genius, had prepared the ground and at the same time found the proper methods of procedure, with the result that physiologists who set themselves to work under such circumstances

found ready to their hand not only a theoretical basis to facilitate the prospering of ideas, but also the assistance of a remarkably flexible technique."
Thus, gradually, over a considerable period of time, the work and ideas of one man entered into the whole structure of the physiology of the nervous system to a degree that this volume cannot pretend to evaluate precisely.

The appended Prologue gives a glimpse of the physiologist and a remark which needed saying in 1898, at the time of his earlier studies, more than it does now. It is of interest to speculate how much the change of viewpoint in the present day, certainly as regards neurology, arises from his own achievements.

Since the appended bibliography makes mention only of those others who collaborated directly with him in published work, it is fitting here to indicate briefly the work of many directly associated with and stimulated by him, but *not* in actual collaboration. The enormous bulk of such investigations carried on in his laboratories can only in part be indicated by the mention of names such as those of Warrington, Hofmann, Weed, Camis, Magnus, Viets, Bazett, Penfield, Cobb, Carleton, Bremer, McCouch, Florey, Granit, Ruch, Hoff, Phillips, and Matthes.

The decision to make extracts from many papers, to avoid recapitulation and give wider representation had the approval of Sir Charles, and great care has been taken to keep sufficient context to avoid misrepresentation of his views or argument. I am deeply grateful for the trust and free hand which he has so cordially allowed me in this responsibility. I wish to express my thanks to the Royal Society for kind permission to reprint and extract from many papers in the *Proceedings* and *Philosophical Transactions*, and to the Editorial Board of the *Journal of Physiology* and the Editor of *Nature* for the right to reprint from their journals. I wish to acknowledge with thanks the permission granted by Sir Edward Sharpey-Schafer's trustees and by Miss Schafer to reprint from the *Quarterly Journal of Experimental Physiology*. The Royal Society of Medicine has kindly given permission to quote extracts from a paper in the *Medico-Chirurgical Transactions*. I am much indebted to Mr. Reginald Eves, R.A., for his kind permission to reproduce the frontispiece, and to the Librarian of the Royal Society of Medicine for assistance in compiling a bibliography. I am particularly indebted to Professor John Fulton for a very complete bibliography, especially of published letters and poems, to which I could add very little; to Drs. F. M. R. Walshe and Gordon Holmes for their advice, criticism, and encouragement, and to Dr. M. Newfield, of Messrs. Hamish Hamilton, for the care he has given the production of the volume.

D. D.-B.

London, 1939.

PREFACE TO THE 1979 REPRINTING

THE *Selected Writings* appeared in September 1939, and though it was well received it rapidly became unavailable owing to the loss of storage facilities during the Second World War. Sir Charles continued to publish in the years following, first his famous Gifford Lectures, *Man on his Nature* (1940), The Deneke Lecture *Goethe on Nature and on Science* (1942), *The Endeavour of Jean Fernel* (1946) and finally a brief autobiographical contribution "Marginalia", to a volume in honour of Charles Singer, edited by A. Underwood (1947). He died on 4 March, 1952 at the age of 95, mentally clear and alert to the end. Of the many obituary notices, that by E. G. T. Liddell in *Obit. Not. Roy. Soc.*, Vol. 8, p. 241, 1952 is especially recommended. Professor Liddell was also the author of a remarkable tribute *The Discovery of Reflexes*, Clarendon Press 1960, which describes the very gradual, halting evolution of physiology of the nervous system preceding the extraordinary discoveries of Sherrington.

Enormous advances in neurophysiology have been made in the years since the publication of the *Selected Writings*, but the pattern of organization of the spinal reflexes elucidated by Sherrington is still essential to our understanding of the nervous system. We feel confident that this book and the *Integrative Action of the Nervous System* will remain vital source material for the neurophysiologist. We are greatly indebted to the generosity of the Guarantors of the journal *Brain* for their decision to undertake this reprinting.

D. DENNY-BROWN

CONTENTS

Variability of Innervation: The Lumbo-sacral Plexus in the Monkey (Macacus): The Muscular Ray, or Myotome: The Motor Root-Filaments: The Disposition of Motoneurones for a Muscle has no Segmental (Root) Boundary: The Motor Innervation from the Brachial Plexus: The Pattern of Supply of the Brachial Limb: The Overlapping of Motor Function in the Grey Matter of the Cord: Conclusion.

Methods of Observation: Root Constitution of the Peripheral Nerves of the Lower Limb: Samples of Skin-Fields supplied by Roots entering into the Lumbo-sacral Plexus: Conclusions as to the Segmental Architecture of the Hind-Limb: Samples of Skin-Fields supplied by Roots entering into the Brachial Plexus: Comparison of Segmental Anatomy of Macacus and Man: Variation in the Extent of Overlapping of Skin-Fields in Different Regions: Individual Variation: The Axial Lines and Torsion of the Limbs: The Skin-Field of the Fifth Cranial (Trigeminal) Nerve: The Loss of Sensation following Section of One Dorsal Nerve-Root.

The Afferent Fibres from Limb Muscles: Sensory Fibres in the Nerves to Muscle: The Sensory Innervation of the Eye Muscles; The Proprioceptive Function of the Extrinsic Ocular Muscles: The Influence of Sensory Nerves upon the Movement and Nutrition of the Limbs.

On Spinal Shock: On the Recovery of Spinal Reflexes: The Failure of Regulation of Temperature: Segmental Reflex Effects: The Reflex is not limited by Segmentation: Reflex Discharge Selects Certain Groups of Muscles: The Uniformity of Response despite Spatial Variety of Provocation: Crossed Spinal Reflexes: Reflexes elicited by Percussion: Alternating Reflexes: Inhibition in Spinal Reflexes: Phasic Variation in Reflex Activity of the Cord.

CONTENTS

CONTENTS

PROLOGUE

Morphology has as its object the study of the form of living things, and comparative anatomy it pursues as one of its best and most valuable methods. Of biological studies, those in comparative anatomy are amongst the oldest. The old masters, in pursuing them, delighted to indulge in speculations concerning the use of the structures they described. As the various parts of the mechanisms whose form they examined became known to them, they often had cause to note the suitability of the instrument to its purpose in the life of the creature. They frequently digressed from the immediate object of their treatises to discourse upon the evidences of design in creation of which their observations gave them proof. The Bridgewater Treatises were founded in part to illustrate the beneficent design testified to by the mechanism and vital endowments of the animal body. One of the most famous of these well-known essays was, and has remained, Sir Charles Bell's treatise " On the Hand." Its stately language and wealth of illustration will long preserve it as a masterpiece of popular exposition of science. Yet every chapter seems far from us as a bygone age ; its pages are alive no longer. How has this come about? The facts are true, and therefore living as ever ; the style is classical, and therefore never dying. It is the point of view that has suffered change. The question asked throughout is the question that it was the fashion at that time for biologists, and especially anatomists, to ask and to attempt to answer. It was of a phase that was passed through by such students at the period of the " encyclopædists " and of Rousseau, and lingered for a generation longer. The question asked was one beyond the limit of regions accessible by the means of enquiry that obtains in natural philosophy. It is now generally acknowledged that this kind of teleology lies beyond the province of biology. We desire not to trespass across that limit. We are content to struggle with a humbler problem. The question why ? is not answered by positive science, but only the question how ? and sometimes the question how much ? The physiologist cannot say why a muscle contracts, nor define " life." To dogmatise concerning the " why " of a bird's flight implies the knowing the " why " of the bird's existence. We may be able to see how *things have happened, or how* they will happen ; *and it is a first step in the acquisition of positive knowledge to know that the* ratio rei *is not the " reason why."*

[From Inaugural Address on "The Relation between Structure and Function as Examined in the Arm," *Trans. L'pool. Biol. Soc.*, 1899, **13**, 1.]

SELECTED WRITINGS OF
SIR CHARLES SHERRINGTON

I

ON THE DISTRIBUTION OF THE MOTOR NERVE-ROOTS

[A first step in the analysis of nervous function is to consider the plan on which the motor nerve-fibres are distributed to the muscles. Stimulation of any motor nerve-root was known to produce a complex movement. This movement is shown not to be of any particular functional significance, as some had previously thought, but to be the result of the fusion of the original anatomical myotome of that segment with its neighbours. The myotome exists as a series of parts of many muscles, so that its contraction as a whole produces a bizarre movement. A muscle and its motoneurones in the grey matter of the spinal cord form the true functional unit, and in the limbs the original anatomical segmentation becomes less and less distinct as one passes from nerve-roots distally. Nevertheless, the musculature, treated as a whole, is seen to be made up of a series of laminæ, or rays, parallel with the circular series of muscle segments which make up the trunk musculature.—Ed.]

HISTORICAL INTRODUCTION[1]

AT the commencement of some observations on the reflex mechanisms of the spinal cord in *Macacus rhesus*, difficulties were encountered which made it desirable to attempt for that animal a somewhat particular examination of the distribution of the efferent and afferent spinal nerve-roots belonging to the lumbo-sacral plexus. The present communication has reference to the distribution of the efferent fibres of the roots.

Reil,[2] Scarpa,[3] A. Monro,[4] and Soemmering[5] all paid considerable attention to the arrangement of the root-bundles in the limb plexuses, but physiological work upon the subject commenced with Van Deen,[6] J. Müller,[7] and Panizza.[8] The former two gave an anatomical significance

---

[1] Extract from *Proc. roy. Soc.*, 1892, **51**, 67-78. [2] *De Nervorum Structura*, p. 14.
[3] *De Gangliis et Plexibus.*
[4] *Observations on the Structure and Functions of the Nervous System*, p. 34.
[5] *Anatom, Pars Vta.* [6] *De Differentia et Nexu inter Nervos Vitæ Anim. et Organ.*, Leyden, 1834.
[7] *Physiol. des Menschen*, vol. 2, p. 586. [8] *Annali Universali di Medicina.*

to the plexus, the last a physiological.[1] At Müller's suggestion renewed research was undertaken by H. Kronenberg[2] in 1835. Kronenberg confirmed Müller's observations as to the individual inconstancy of the contribution made by any spinal root to the nerve-cords of the plexus; he also concluded that the excitation of a single nerve-root before its entrance into the plexus produces contraction of almost all the muscles of the limb; and that the arrangement is intended to protect against fatigue. Later, Eckhardt,[3] working in Ludwig's laboratory, arrived at somewhat similar conclusions. He stated that a great number of muscles obtain nerve-fibres each of them from several nerve-roots; that there is a good deal of individual variation; that when a nerve-root is unusually thick the additional fibres in it are not all of them, perhaps none of them, used to supply altogether other muscles not usually supplied by the root; that the distribution of the fibres of a root is not to one group of muscles, but is to several groups, which are often not related to each other in function; that antagonistic groups are often supplied by one and the same root.

Three years after the experiments by Eckhardt, and also under Ludwig, Peyer's[4] experiments on the brachial plexus of the rabbit were made. As Krause,[5] in 1861, repeated Peyer's work on the same limb and the same species, the results of both may be here referred to together. The muscles of the limb each receive nerve-fibres from two, in some cases three, spinal roots; usually the contraction of a muscle on excitation of the spinal roots innervating it is obviously different in degree for each root; the same spinal root does not always supply in different individuals the same muscles; the further the position of a spinal root from the head, the nearer the muscles it supplies to the distal end of the limb; the peripheral trunks of the limb plexus are themselves plexuses of root-bundles. In 1881 Ferrier and Yeo[6] confirmed the above results in experiments on the spinal roots of the monkey. In addition to their experiments on the brachial plexus, they performed four complete experiments on the lumbo-sacral roots. Unlike Kronenberg, Eckhardt, and others, they do not seem to have met with any variation in the results obtained. They revived the view that the efferent distribution of each spinal nerve is based on its physiological function, and that the movement resulting from the excitation of a root is that of a highly co-ordinated functional synergism. Some months later Paul Bert and Marcacci[7] published experiments on the lumbar roots of the cat and dog. They concluded that (i) each root produces a co-ordinate movement, and consists of fibres functionally associated; (ii) when a muscle is functionally divisible its root-supply is multiple.

In 1883 Forgue and Lannegrace[8] published a research on the limb

[1] ". . . the assurance of alternative accessory paths in case of injury," *J. Physiol.*, 1892, **13**, 623. [2] Essay (*De Struct. et Virtut. Plexuum Nervorum*), Berlin, 1836.
[3] *Z. rat. Med.*, 1849, **7**, 306. [4] *Ibid.*, 1854, n.f. **4**, 67.
[5] *Beitrage zur Anat. der Oberen Extremität*, 1861. [6] *Proc. roy. Soc.*, 1881, **32**, 12.
[7] *C. R. Soc. Biol.*, Paris, 1881, 267.
[8] *Gaz. hebd. Sci. méd. Montpel.*, 1883, **5**, 253, 279, 329, 388.

plexuses of the dog, cat, and monkey. The *Comptes Rendus*[1] of the following year contain their reports. As to the lower limb, their account is prefaced by a remark that the highest lumbar root of man is tripled in the dog and monkey. What species of monkey was used is not mentioned in the *Comptes Rendus*. In Macacus the 5th lumbar root is analogous not to the 3rd of man, but to the 4th, and to the 6th of the dog. The chief of their conclusions, drawn from examination of both limbs, are: The majority of muscles are innervated by several roots. Excitation of a root determines in the muscles which it supplies a total, not a partial, contraction. The tributary fibres of the root are disseminated through the muscle supplied by it, and not " cantonnées " in a special zone of it. Each root has a muscular distribution almost absolutely constant in the animals of its own species. The functions of analogous roots differ very little in different mammalian species. Each root supplies muscles of very various, often of antagonistic, action. Excitation of a root gives a combined movement, but an artificial, not a functional. The roots that pass furthest into the member occupy the lowest position in the cord. The innervation of the two planes of flexors and extensors is not always symmetrical. The superficial layers are supplied before the deep.

Herringham,[2] by minute dissection of the human brachial plexus, and, therefore, under disadvantage from inability to distinguish clearly between afferent and efferent fibres, arrived nevertheless at facts and conclusions of great importance. He found much individual variation, but evidence of certain " laws." Thus: any given root-fibre may alter its position relative to the vertebral column, but will maintain its position relative to other fibres; of two muscles, or two parts of a muscle, that which is nearer the head end of the body tends to be supplied by the higher, that nearer the tail end by the lower, root; of two muscles, that nearer the long axis of the body tends to be supplied by the higher, that nearer the periphery by the lower, root; of two muscles, that nearer the surface tends to be supplied by the higher, that further from it by the lower, root.

Recently Langley,[3] in the course of a paper on the sweat nerves to the foot of the cat, refers to the movements of the limb produced by excitation of roots of the sciatic plexus in that animal. He desired to ascertain whether the variation, which he finds considerable in the distribution of the sweat nerves (sympathetic system), has a correlative in the distribution of the nerves to the limb muscles. Like Kronenberg, Eckhardt, and Peyer, he finds that the movements resulting from stimulation of the same nerve-roots are not uniform, and that the want of uniformity goes hand in hand with want of uniformity in the root composition of the plexus, just such as displayed in Herringham's dissections.

---

[1] *C. R. Acad. Sci.*, Paris, 1884, **98**, 685, 829, 1068.
[2] *Proc. roy. Soc.*, 1886, **41**, 423.
[3] *J. Physiol.*, 1891, **12**, 347.

Method

My own observations have been made, during the past three years, chiefly on the lumbo-sacral roots of *Macacus rhesus*; also on the frog, rat, rabbit, cat, and dog, chiefly for the sake of comparing those types with Macacus. The animals have been deeply anæsthetised with chloroform and ether. The excitations of the roots have been made in the spinal canal; the single root, or a component filament from it, has been isolated in the case of the lower roots of the cat and monkey, to a length 5, 6 or 7 cm., and lifted up by a silk ligature on to small platinum electrodes sheathed almost to the points. Series of weak induced currents have been used for excitation, one pint Daniell being in the primary of the ordinary physiological inductorium (R. Ewald's pattern). The secondary coil has usually been at a distance from the primary somewhat more than twice that at which a current was detectable by the tongue. Use has also been made of absolutely minimal stimuli, and largely of mechanical stimuli. For certain purposes, stimulation by quite strong electrical excitation has been used.

VARIABILITY OF INNERVATION

In the course of the experiments[1] it became clear that frequency of individual variation, as regards the anatomical and physiological constitution of the efferent roots of the lumbo-sacral region, is sufficiently great to demand the recognition of a forward and a hindward class innervation for each muscle and for each movement. There is a *forward* class of individuals in which the roots connected with the muscles and the movements lie further forward (headward) than do the roots connected with the same muscles and the same movements in a *hindward* type of innervation. Since reference to this distinction must constantly recur in this paper and is of fundamental importance for appreciation of the problems involved, it seems well to avoid periphrasis and misunderstanding by using in reference to it special terms. A plexus and its trunks and branches will therefore be referred to as *prefixed*[2] if containing spinal root-filaments attached to the cord further forward (headward) than are the root-filaments entering the corresponding trunks and branches of a converse class of plexus which will be referred to conversely as *postfixed*.[3]

Thus, in the frog there is a *prefixed* class of plexus for the hind limb,

---

[1] Extract from the full paper, "Notes on the Arrangement of some Motor Fibres in the Lumbo-sacral Plexus," *J. Physiol.*, 1892, **13**, 635 *et seq.*, which is accompanied by drawings of the different types of plexus, and many examples of variation.—ED.

[2] In the first paper, quoted up to this point, the terms " pre-axial " and " post-axial " were used. These were later abandoned on account of ambiguity (see *J. Physiol.*, 1892, **13**, 636, footnote).—ED.

[3] Langley (*J. Physiol.*, 1891, **12**, 366) had independently found variation in the plexus of the cat in the course of experiments on the sweat nerves to the foot, and considered Sherrington's prefixed and postfixed classes to belong to his Classes III. and I. respectively.

in which, for instance, the 7th root, as well as supplying the antero-internal thigh muscles, supplies muscles in the leg (tibialis anticus). There is a *postfixed* class in which the leg muscles are supplied by the 8th and 9th roots only. The *postfixed* class as measured by this standard is the more usual. The preponderance of the one type may be merely because the above criterion, found convenient for distinguishing in any individual case the direction which variation has taken in it, headward or tailward, does not coincide with the mid-point about which individual variation is in the species really oscillating. Indeed, we have not as yet evidence to show that in this instance variation is oscillating about a single *mean* or maximum of frequency of individual examples. If a Curve of Error, to follow the term employed by Galton, were constructed it might here exhibit two maxima, one on either side of the mean point.

By *prefixed* and *postfixed* classes it is not intended to imply that in the range of individual variation no one type is more frequently exemplified than the others; it is only meant that so frequent is the variation and so few are the data at present before us that it is not certain that any one type is sufficiently predominant to warrant the selection of it as the " normal " one, and that therefore it is better to treat the composition of the plexus of the species as multiple and for convenience divide it into two classes. I have thought two classes, prefixed and postfixed, distinction sufficient to observe in the present description.

In the monkey, as in the frog and cat,[1] the distribution of the same spinal root of the plexus is not in all individuals the same. The fact is evidenced not only by excitation experiments, but also by severance experiments. When one motor spinal root of the limb plexus has been isolated by section of the adjacent ones the degree of movement left is not always the same for the same root in different individuals. For instance, in two young Rhesi in which the 7th cervical root to the brachial plexus had been isolated in the same way (by section of the 4th, 5th, 6th, and 8th cervical and the highest two thoracic roots) the power of grip of the hand was strikingly different in the two individuals; the power of folding the thumb especially was dissimilar in the two; dissection revealed no difference in the extent of the experimental lesion. In the cat the prefixed and postfixed classes of innervation of the limb seemed to be pretty evenly balanced in frequency of occurrence, the prefixed class being rather the less usual of the two. In *Macacus rhesus*, again, there seems to be, judging from sixty-six experiments, a slight preponderance of postfixed type over prefixed. The upper lumbar roots do not appear to vary so much as do the lower and the sacral.

---

[1] Extract, *loc. cit.*, pp. 647 *et seq.* The types of plexus in the frog and cat are described earlier in the paper. The anatomy of the limb in the monkey is considered, and the exceptions from its very close resemblance to that of man are described (p. 643).

THE LUMBOSACRAL PLEXUS IN THE MONKEY (MACACUS)

I will state briefly the arrangement evidenced in the larger number (thirty-seven) of the experiments.

Postfixed Class of Plexus : Spinal Roots and Muscles.

1st sub-thoracic (1st lumbar) root.   Quadratus lumborum, psoas parvus, psoas magnus, external oblique, internal oblique, transversalis.

2nd sub-thoracic.   Quadratus lumborum, psoas magnus, psoas parvus, cremaster, external oblique, internal oblique, transversalis.

3rd sub-thoracic.   Psoas magnus, psoas parvus, cremaster, iliacus, external oblique, transversalis (the lower part only of the three latter), pectineus, adductor longus, sartorius.

4th sub-thoracic.   Psoas magnus, iliacus, pectineus, adductor longus, gracilis (probably the rest of the adductor mass), sartorius, vastus internus, vastus externus, crureus, rectus femoris (slight), obturator externus.

5th sub-thoracic.   Psoas magnus (small prevertebral part of), gracilis, adductor longus (slight), tensor vaginæ femoris, rectus femoris, vastus internus, vastus externus, crureus, sartorius (slight), tibialis anticus (only slightly), extensor hallucis (very slight), extensor longus digitorum (very slight), peroneus longus (very slightly).

6th sub-thoracic.   Part of adductor magnus, tibialis anticus, extensor longus digitorum, extensor hallucis, peroneus longus, peroneus brevis, extensor brevis digitorum, abductor minimi digiti, gastrocnemius (both heads, but slight), popliteus, tibialis posticus, flexor longus digitorum, flexor longus hallucis, soleus (slight), semimembranosus, semitendinosus, plantaris, biceps, upper part of pyriformis, quadriceps (rarely), gracilis (near knee, rarely).

7th sub-thoracic.   Adductor magnus, semitendinosus, semimembranosus, tibialis anticus, extensor longus digitorum, extensor proprius hallucis, peroneus brevis, peroneus longus, plantaris, popliteus, gastrocnemius (both heads), tibialis posticus, flexor longus digitorum, soleus, flexor longus hallucis, flexor brevis digitorum, flexor brevis hallucis, flexor brevis minimi digiti, extensor brevis digitorum, abductor hallucis, abductor minimi digiti, adductor hallucis, large part of pyriformis, interossei and lumbricales, flexor accessorius, obturator internus, quadratus femoris and both gemelli, gluteus medius, gluteus maximus.

8th sub-thoracic.   Biceps, semimembranosus, semitendinosus, gluteus maximus, gastrocnemius (both heads), soleus, tibialis posticus, flexor longus digitorum (slight), flexor longus hallucis, abductor hallucis, flexor brevis hallucis, flexor brevis minimi digiti, flexor brevis digitorum, flexor accessorius, abductor minimi digiti, adductor hallucis, interossei and lumbricales, small part of pyriformis, obturator internus, quadratus femoris and the two gemelli, bladder (slight), sphincter vaginæ, sphincter ani.

9th sub-thoracic.   Flexor brevis digitorum, flexor brevis hallucis, interossei and lumbricales, sphincter vaginæ, obturator internus, sphincter ani, bladder (strongly).

For reasons already given the individuals (twenty-nine out of my series) not conforming fairly to the plexal arrangement just described I have considered it well to treat *en bloc* as forming another class, and to place together as a second experimental series (prefixed).[1]

---

[1] *Loc. cit.*, p. 653.   The muscles in the lists have been rearranged to facilitate comparison with the postfixed class.   Muscles supplied by a root in this series which do not derive supply from that root in the other series are shown in italics.   8th sub-thoracic = 2nd sacral of man.   See p. 38.—ED.

Prefixed Class of Plexus : Spinal Roots and Muscles.

1st sub-thoracic. Quadratus lumborum, psoas parvus, psoas magnus, external oblique, internal oblique, transversalis.

2nd sub-thoracic. Quadratus lumborum, psoas magnus, psoas parvus, cremaster, external oblique, internal oblique, transversalis.

3rd sub-thoracic. Psoas, cremaster, iliacus, external oblique, *internal oblique* (lower part only), transversalis, pectineus, adductor longus, sartorius (upper part especially), *vastus internus, rectus femoris* (upper part especially), *vastus internus, rectus femoris* (upper part, slight), *obturator externus* (slightly).

4th sub-thoracic. Psoas, iliacus, pectineus, adductor longus, gracilis, sartorius (lower part especially), vastus internus, vastus externus, crureus, rectus femoris, obturator externus, *adductor brevis, adductor magnus.*

5th sub-thoracic. Gracilis, tensor vaginæ femoris, rectus femoris, vastus internus, vastus externus, crureus, *adductor magnus, semimembranosus* (slight), tibialis anticus, extensor hallucis, *flexor longus hallucis* (occasionally strongly), *flexor longus digitorum* (occasionally strongly), tibialis posticus (occasionally strongly), extensor longus digitorum, peroneus longus (slight).

6th sub-thoracic. Tibialis anticus, extensor longus digitorum, extensor hallucis, peroneus longus, peroneus brevis, extensor brevis digitorum, abductor minimi digiti, gastrocnemius (both heads, external more than internal head), popliteus, tibialis posticus, flexor longus digitorum, flexor longus hallucis, soleus (slight), semimembranosus, semitendinosus, plantaris, biceps (slight, chiefly deep portion), pyriformis, *abductor hallucis, flexor brevis digitorum, abductor hallucis* (slight), *gluteus medius and minimus, quadratus femoris, the gemelli.*

7th sub-thoracic. Adductor magnus (part of), semitendinosus, semimembranosus, tibialis anticus, extensor longus digitorum, extensor proprius hallucis, peroneus longus (slight), peroneus brevis, plantaris, popliteus, gastrocnemius (both heads), tibialis posticus, flexor longus digitorum, soleus, flexor longus hallucis, flexor brevis digitorum, flexor brevis hallucis and minimi digiti, extensor brevis digitorum, abductor hallucis, abductor minimi digiti, adductor hallucis, pyriformis (especially lateral part), interossei and lumbricales, flexor accessorius, obturator internus, quadratus femoris and the gemelli, *biceps*, gluteus *minimus*, medius and maximus, *sphincter ani* (deeper part).

8th sub-thoracic. Biceps, semimembranosus, semitendinosus, gluteus maximus, gastrocnemius (both heads, internal more than external), soleus, abductor hallucis, flexor brevis hallucis, flexor brevis minimi digiti, flexor brevis digitorum, flexor accessorius, abductor minimi digiti, adductor hallucis, interossei and lumbricales, pyriformis (small part, chiefly medial), obturator internus, quadratus femoris and the two gemelli, bladder[1] (strong), sphincter vaginæ, sphincter ani.

9th[2] sub-thoracic. Sphincter vaginæ, sphincter ani,[3] bladder[1] (strong).

[1] The nervous supply of the sphincter ani, sphincter vaginæ, bladder (both via the sympathetic, hypogastric nerves, and by the sacral nerve roots), cremaster, round ligament of the uterus, vas deferens, nervi erigentes, and the pilomotor nerves to the buttock and tail, is discussed in detail in this paper (*J. Physiol.*, 1892, **13**, 672-686).—ED.

[2] See p. 678, and diagram fig. 9, same paper.

[3] The most obvious difference between prefixed and postfixed types is seen in the distribution of the 9th sub-thoracic (second sacral) nerve in the two. The difference is perhaps more obvious if the root composition of various nerves is studied—*e.g.*, the anterior crural and sciatic nerves in *Macacus rhesus*:

				Anterior Crural.	Sciatic.
Prefixed type ..	..	..	..	3 **4** 5	**5 6 7** 8
Postfixed type ..	..	..	..	3 **4** 5 (6)	5 **6 7** 8 9

(In each case the nerve-root which contributes the main share to the nerve is shown by its number being in thick type. *J. Physiol.*, 1892, **13**, 763.)

These differences are in *normal* animals, and the exceptional cases where suppression or addi-

[1]The distribution of the peripheral nerve trunks is not obviously different, whether by its root-formation the plexus belong to the prefixed or to the postfixed class. The peripheral nerve-trunks are, as regards their muscles, relatively stable in comparison with the spinal roots. When the innervation of the limb-muscles is of the prefixed class, so also is that of the anus, vagina, and bladder; and conversely.

As regards[2] the posterior limit of the region of outflow of motor-fibres to the skeletal muscles of the lower limb it will be seen that according to my own experiments the limit is reached at the same place in the rabbit, the cat, the dog, the Rhesus and the Bonnet monkey—namely, usually in the 9th, less frequently at the lowest edge of the 8th sub-thoracic root, a variation the extreme limits of which lie about 3 millimetres apart on the surface of the cord. As to the relative frequency of occurrence of the post-fixed and prefixed types, that can in result of this variation be distinguished, in the rabbit and dog my experiments are not numerous enough to afford basis for a conclusion; in the cat the extension into the 9th seems about equally common with its absence. In Macacus the two forms seem to be about equally frequent.[3] In Rhesus I have noted thirty-seven examples of the postfixed plexus, twenty-nine examples of the prefixed; in Bonnet three examples of the postfixed and five examples of the prefixed. It is of interest that in several instances the type of brachial and crural plexus was co-incidently examined and ascertained in one and the same individual, and four times a prefixed type of sacral plexus was found accompanying a post-fixed type of brachial plexus. By far the most usual place for the posterior limit of the outflow of motor fibres to the fore-limb has been in my own experience on the rabbit, rat, and macaque at the 2nd thoracic root, but not so in the cat and dog, in which animals the limit usually lies at the 1st thoracic.

As to the downward limit of the motor outflow for the lower limb my experiments indicate that both Forgue and Lannegrace,[4] and also Ferrier and Yeo,[5] are right in the positions they assign to it; that is to say, the limit may fall at the place given by each pair of observers, but it may be that in Macacus the limit found by Ferrier and Yeo is somewhat more usual than that found by Forgue and Lannegrace.

---

tion of a segment has occurred do not enter into this question. " Even in the case of complete suppression together of a lumbar vertebra and of a spinal root, as already described, dissection revealed no obvious difference in the branching or distribution of the very nerve trunks that were most affected by the absence of the absent root. The vertebra and root suppressed were either the sixth or the seventh lumbar, that is to say, the lowest root of the lumbar series did duty for both; though large, it was not extraordinarily so " (p. 761). The afferent nerve-trunks and the mixed sensori-motor appear in mammalian types to undergo variation in their root composition in the same sense. In the frog, the afferent trunks may be of prefixed composition in the same plexus in which the efferent are postfixed (*loc. cit.* p. 761).—ED.

[1] From *Proc. roy. Soc.*, 1892, **51**, 76.

[2] From *J. Physiol.*, 1892, **13**, 739.

[3] In man the anatomical variations of the plexus are similar. See P. Eisler, *Der Plexus lumbo-sacralis des Menschen*, Halle, 1892, and Quain's *Anatomy*, 1895, **3**, Pt. 2, p. 313.—ED.

[4] *Loc. cit.*, 9th post-thoracic.   [5] *Loc. cit.*, 8th post-thoracic.—ED.

THE MUSCULAR RAY, OR MYOTOME

[1]The significance of the distribution of the efferent fibres of a spinal root is, as J. Müller suggested, anatomical (based on metamerism, etc.) rather than functional (based on co-ordinate action, etc.). Excitation of an entire efferent root produces a combined movement due to the action of many muscles, but there is no safe ground for believing that the combination is of a functional character; the weight of evidence is against this.

As to the question whether a muscle, when supplied by several nerve-roots, is supplied by them in such a way that one piece of the muscle is supplied by one root, another by another, although there is certainly great interlapping of regions belonging to the individual roots, I cannot agree with Forgue and Lannegrace when they say, "Excitation of a spinal root determines in the muscles which it supplies a total, not a partial, contraction." Simple inspection is enough to convince one that in the case of some of the larger muscles—e.g., in the thigh and spinal regions—the nerve supply from the individual roots is distinctly partial, that a district of the muscle belongs to this root, another district to that, although always with a large mutual overlap; striking examples are given by the sartorius, 3rd and 4th (Macacus) sacro-coccygeus superior, 7th, 8th, 9th (cat), etc. On the other hand, as the distal end of the limb is approached, the intermingling of the root-districts in the several muscles becomes more intimate, and in the muscles of the sole the intermingling of the muscle-fibres belonging to individual nerve-roots is so complete as to baffle analysis, except by the degeneration method. In the sphincter muscle of the anus there is an overlap of the motor distributions of the right and left halves of the body. The sphincter ani is supplied by four nerve-roots, two right-hand, two left-hand. Any three of these may usually be cut through without the anus becoming patulous, or exhibiting asymmetry. Conversely, excitation of any one of the efferent roots supplying it causes contraction of both right and left halves of it. The innervation of the bladder from its right- and left-hand roots is, on the other hand, neither in the case of its sympathetic nor its direct spinal supply of a bilateral character.

[2]The above observations confirm, therefore, the facts first clearly stated by Eckhardt.[3] Eckhardt wrote concerning the frog's plexus, "A great number of muscles in the limb obtain nerve-fibres each of them from several nerve-roots. Most of the thigh muscles almost always, some of the leg muscles frequently, are supplied by three, the latter more often by two nerve-roots." In Rhesus there seems but one muscle of the lower limb that receives its nerve-supply from a single root—viz., the tensor vaginæ femoris, from the 5th lumbar; and sometimes one finds that muscle distinctly obtaining fibres from the 4th as well.

---

[1] From *Proc. roy. Soc.*, 1892, **51**, 77.

[2] Extracted from the large paper on " Notes on the Arrangement of some Motor Fibres in the Lumbo-sacral Plexus," *J. Physiol.*, 1892, **13**, 736.   [3] *Z. rat. Med.*, 1849, **7**, 306.

When a muscle is supplied by three nerve-roots it is noticeable that the middle root of the three usually causes the most powerful contraction. This is well exemplified by the tibialis anticus and the 5th, 6th, and 7th roots. Many other examples could be cited illustrating the point, and it may be accepted as a general rule.[1]

In the lower limb one finds for each muscle the outflow of efferent fibres to it spread unbrokenly over a certain considerable longitudinal region of the cord. I mention this because a different arrangement holds for the bladder and iris muscles, and because Peyer and Krause for the pronator radii teres of the rabbit found an outflow of fibres in the 7th cervical root and in the 1st thoracic root, but not in the intervening root of the 8th cervical nerve. This observation appeared curious enough to demand repetition, and I have repeated it twice and found on each occasion that the pronator in the rabbit is no exception to the general rule because it may be innervated from the 8th cervical as well as from the 7th, and 1st thoracic.

In the great majority of instances *muscles innervated by the same nerve-root lie adjacent to one another, so that a continuous sheet, or band, or ray of muscular tissue is supplied by the same nerve-root.* Among the sacral nerve-roots an exception to this rule for distribution is certainly met with not infrequently in the case of the lowest filaments of the 8th subthoracic root, or the entire 9th subthoracic root. These are then distributed to the sacro-coccygeal muscles on the one hand and on the other to intrinsic muscles of the sole, far distant from the sacro-coccygeal muscles. It must not be thought that this is merely a separation between the regions of distribution of the *dorsal* division of the nerve-trunk on the one hand and of the *ventral* division of the nerve-trunk on the other. When the dorsal division of the 9th nerve has been cut through, on exciting the anterior root a considerable portion of the sacro-coccygeal muscles still act, and the sphincter ani still acts, together with short muscles in the foot.[2]

If by a ray[3] be meant a continuous band of muscle passing from the body axis to the periphery it is not difficult to trace in the limb the rays belonging to the 3rd, 4th, 5th, 6th, 7th, and 8th subthoracic segments, and to see that of these the 7th and 8th penetrate to the free apex of the limb. The ray of the 9th segment is less easily traced in its continuity. The distal part of it is obvious enough, namely the intrinsic plantar muscles, but in the thigh and leg its traces are often obscure, sometimes, I think, not demonstrable.

It is clear that, broadly described, the musculature of the limb is built up by successive contributions of segments, which, reviewed in series passing from the segmentally headward to the segmentally hinder, first extend stepwise down the antero-internal muscle-mass of the thigh, occupying its whole width from the adductor magnus internally to the vastus externus

---

[1] Some detailed figures of the amount of isotonic " lift " from tibialis anticus from 5th, 6th, and 7th roots is given here in the original paper.—ED.

[2] Further notes on the root innervation of the peronei are given here in the original.—ED.

[3] From *J. Physiol.*, 1892, **13**, 767, 769.

externally, and including the whole of the latter muscle; that after composing this region of the thigh they extend stepwise down the leg, occupying the front of it from the inner surface of the tibia internally to behind the peroneal muscles externally so as to include the latter group, and in Rhesus more than half the circumference of the limb. The next step is on to the dorsum of the foot, occupying its whole width, and forming the short extensor but not the dorsal interossei. The length of the limb having thus been reached and occupied by, in both Macacus and the cat and rabbit, the successively longer and longer out-thrusts of four segments, a number of other segments, usually two in the cat and rabbit, usually three in Macacus, thrust out each a process which extends along the back of the process of the segment immediately anterior (*i.e.*, headward) to it and throughout the whole length of the limb. These segments are so intimately fused in the plantar region that it is difficult to pick out from the rest any one muscle which shows more of this or that constituent. But in the leg and thigh it is less difficult to demonstrate, for in them it can be shown that the more superficial muscles—the gastrocnemius, the soleus, the semitendinosus and the surface portion of the biceps—belong to spinal segments more posterior than do the long flexors of the digits, the semimembranosus and the deeper part of the biceps. And the former groups are posterior to the latter. The gastrocnemius and soleus are supplied mainly from 7th and 8th roots, but the flexor perforans mainly from the 6th and 7th. The inner hamstrings in the cat are each supplied by the 8th, 7th, and 6th roots, but the supply of the semitendinosus (the more superficial) is more from the 8th than is the supply of the semimembranosus, while the supply of the semimembranosus is more from the 6th than is the supply of the semitendinosus.

It is curious to notice[1] that the external head of the gastrocnemius seems to be innervated from a set of root-filaments lying more anterior than do those for the internal head. The outflow to the external head is represented less in the rootlets of the 8th than is the outflow to the internal head; in the rootlets of the 6th it is more abundant than is the outflow to the internal head. After division of the 6th and 7th roots it atrophies much more than does the internal head. After section of the 6th and 8th roots it does not suffer atrophy obviously more than the internal head, excitation of the muscular nerves to each giving a fairly good contraction.

The innervation of the inner head of the gastrocnemius appears to be extremely similar to that of the soleus. The external head has an outflow which extends further forward (upward) than that of either the internal head or of the soleus. The plantaris receives less fibres from the 5th than does the outer head of gastrocnemius, and approximates towards inner head and soleus. The peronei, judged from their root supply, belong to the anterior rather than to the posterior nomenclature of the leg, although they are extensors of the ankle-joint.

[1] Extract from *J. Physiol.*, 1892, **13**, 728.

The remarkable fact that the external or short saphenous nerve, a nerve described as purely sensory by all authorities without exception as far as I have found, does in *Macacus rhesus* contain motor fibres for the plantar muscles of all the pedal digits has been already mentioned.[1] I have not yet fully analysed the root constitution of the branch. As regards afferent fibres it contains constituents from the 7th root more abundantly than from the 6th, from the 6th more abundantly than from the 8th (1st sacral). It appears to contain motor fibres from the 7th and 8th and often 9th roots, so that whether the nerve-trunk to the plantar muscles descends in front of the mass of the great sural triceps or behind it, the final connections of muscle-fibre and nerve-root remain the same whichever route is taken. Despite the extraordinary amount of individual variation already discussed above, the connection between the position of the central starting-point (the nerve-root) and the peripheral end-station (the muscle-fibre) is therefore, for the same parts in the same individual, definite and fixed enough.

THE MOTOR ROOT FILAMENTS[2]

[*The outflow of emerging motor fibres to a muscle from the spinal cord is spread evenly through the individual filaments of a motor root, even for such small muscles as the separate intrinsic muscles of the digits.*]

A glance at the form of the well-developed mammalian limb suffices to awaken the idea that the pollex and the hallux belong to the anterior or preaxial edge of the appendage, and the fifth digit to the posterior or postaxial edge. This idea is suggested by numerous facts of which it is unnecessary to attempt a recapitulation here. The dissections of Herringham afforded striking exemplification of the degree to which careful examination of the parts can be made to reveal evidence of the mutual anterior and posterior, preaxial and postaxial relationships of the small individual parts comprised in even the distal segment itself. Experiments confirmatory of Herringham's observations had shown me that both in Rhesus and in cat the cutaneous nerves display in a striking manner the preaxial and postaxial relationships of one digit to another.[3] But from the nerve-supply of the muscular elements of the limb, I have sought almost in vain for evidence of a similar arrangement. I expected that in the hand and foot of the monkey such evidence might be well obtained because of the fine divisions of the musculature in them and because of the series of intrinsic muscles being in them arranged parallel with the axis of the limb, and therefore ranging from the preaxial to the postaxial borders. In *Macacus rhesus* the movements of the foot, hallux, and digits are particularly free, more so than in the Bonnet and in many monkeys; there could not seem a better subject for analysis of the problem. Excitation of the 6th, the 7th, the 8th, or the 9th subthoracic roots each causes contraction of the intrinsic

[1] Earlier in the same paper.—ED.   [2] Extract from *J. Physiol.*, 1892, **13**, 743.
[3] *Cf.* p. 56 of this volume, and also Langley on Sweat Nerves, *J. Physiol.*, 1891, **12**, 347.

muscles of the foot. The upper three of these nerve-roots are very large, and their component fibre-bundles, the rootlets of the root, spread like the ribs of a half-closed fan from their point of common investment by the dura to the line of their attachment to the spinal cord. The rootlets can easily be used for isolated excitation as in experiments described above. Will excitation of the most anterior filaments have an effect upon the muscles of the foot different from excitation of the most posterior?

Experiment.—March 13, 1890. *Macacus rhesus.* Strong female. A.C.E. mixture. Right side. At the ankle the following tendons divided: *Tibialis anticus, extensor digitorum et hallucis, peronei, tendo Achillis, flexor longus digitalis et hallucis, tibialis posticus.* The plantar nerves cut, the musculo-cutaneous and anterior tibial nerves remaining. Left side tendons divided as on right. The anterior tibial nerve and the musculo-cutaneous nerves cut. The bloodvessels not interfered with, nor the external and internal plantar nerves. The spinal cord is exposed at the level of the crests of the ilia and above and below that level for a short distance. The dura mater is then slit at the roots of the 9th and 8th subthoracic nerves right and left, and the posterior roots of those nerves cut through near the ganglion, followed upward, and excised. The anterior roots of the nerves are exposed, consisting as usual of a considerable number of fine rootlets; these can be even further subdivided by dissection, but at the risk of damage to the nerve fibres. In the right 7th nerve ten natural bundles are taken, in the right 9th three natural bundles; each of these is ligated close to its exit from the spinal cord, and has a length of about 5 centimetres; can be lifted well up in the wound.

Time, 3.50. Stimulation with minimal efficient currents, the secondary coil is at 29 cm. from the primary, the currents are just perceptible to the tongue when the secondary is at 16·6 cm.

3.54. Highest filament of 7th root; abduction and extension of hallux; extension of all the digits; the movement of the minimal digit seems as sharp and evident as that of the hallux.

    3.57. 2nd filament: same effect.

    3.58. 3rd filament: same effect.

    3.59. 4th filament: same effect.

    4.1. 5th filament: same effect.

    4.3. 6th filament: same effect.

    4.4. 7th filament: same effect.

    4.8. 8th filament: same effect.

    4.9. 9th filament: same effect.

    4.12. 10th filament: same effect; no difference between action of minimus and hallux.

4.15—4.21. The effect of the highest and lowest filaments of the 8th compared in their effect upon the hallux, and no difference discovered. The minimal current for movement of the hallux is with the secondary at 29 for the highest filament, with the secondary at 29·5 for the lowest filament.

4.22—4.26. Compared as to effect on the minimal digit, the same numbers obtained as for the hallux.

4.28. No movement of the toes or hallux obtained from any of the three filaments of the 9th nerve.

Left side: Of the filaments of the anterior roots of the 7th and 8th subthoracic nerves, nine natural bundles taken, ligated and isolated in the same way as on the right side; the rootlets of the 9th taken as four filaments. Secondary coil at 29 cm.

4.44. Highest filament of 7th gives adduction and flexion of hallux, with flexion of all the digits of minimus as much as of rest, and hollowing of the sole.

    4.47. 2nd filament: same effect.

    4.48. 3rd filament: same effect.

4.48.   4th filament: same effect.
4.50.   5th filament: same effect.
4.51.   6th filament: same effect.
4.53.   7th filament: same effect.
4.54.   8th filament: same effect.
4.56.   9th filament: same effect.
4.58.   1st filament of 9th root: same effect.
5.0.   2nd filament of 9th root: same effect.
5.1.   3rd filament of 9th root: same effect.
5.2.   The highest filament of the 8th is then compared for its effect on the hallux with the lowest of the 9th and no difference detected.   Same result on comparing their action on the minimal digit.

I had not anticipated that the experiment would yield the above result. It is, however, similar to three others made with the same object in view; the same result was yielded by all made.   Two of the experiments included the anterior roots of the 7th and the 8th in a series of eighteen filaments examined.   No experiments have been made in the cat and rabbit because of the lesser mutual independence of the digits in those forms.   The above observations are, however, strengthened by similar on other nerve-roots, although not on roots so suitable for minute analysis of the functions of the root-filaments as are the 2nd and 3rd sacral.   The highest and lowest rootlets of the 6th lumbar have given several times, when isolated and excited, an apparently identical effect.   It would therefore appear that with certain limitations[1] the stimulation of a rootlet of an anterior root gives the same qualitative results as does stimulation of the entire root; all the muscles which excitation of the entire root causes to contract are made to contract also by excitation of any one of the rootlets into which the entire root is naturally subdivided.   In other words, *the commingling of the motor fibres to various muscles is great even at their very exit from the cord, and each of the natural rootlets of the root consists of an aggregate of fibres often representing as far as the skeletal muscles are concerned all the groups of nerve-fibres contained in the entire root.*   " The individual bundles of the anterior root are in miniature the entire root itself and give results in quality broadly the same as does it, although not in quantity."[2] This commingling of different nerve-fibres at their very exit from the cord points to a probability of their sources of origin within the cord being also commingled in the transverse plane of the cord, if not in the longitudinal.

THE DISPOSITION OF MOTONEURONES FOR A MUSCLE HAS NO SEGMENTAL (ROOT) BOUNDARY

[*The outflow of motor fibres reflects their origin from longitudinal columns of motor cells in the grey matter of the spinal cord, each column representing a muscle.*]

Although the commingling which thus occurs affects each constituent rootlet of the spinal root, and appears to make each filament to a great

---

[1] Sherrington, *Proc. Physiol. Soc.*, p. viii; *J. Physiol.*, 1892, **13**, and below.
[2] Sherrington, *Proc. Physiol. Soc.*, *loc. cit.*

extent a miniature of the entire root itself, in certain segments of the cord the existence of marked individual differences in the functions and distribution of the root filaments are easily discoverable.

In six of the experiments dealing with analysis of the filaments composing the anterior root of the 6th nerve the following results occurred. The series of filaments composing the root had been in each case parted into the small natural bundles. These may be numbered from above downwards, 1, 2, 3, 4, 5, 6. In one case 6, 5, 4, and 3 were found to give contraction of the intrinsic muscles of the foot, the flexors predominating in the action upon the digits, whereas bundles 1 and 2 supplied no intrinsic muscle of the foot. In the other 6 and 5 gave contraction of the intrinsics of the foot, while 4, 3, 2, and 1 did not. Each result was repeated many times on the occasion and precautions taken to avoid escape of current, the whole intradural length of the 5th, 7th, and 8th roots in each case being completely excised. Under all the precaution taken the same result recurred unfailingly on these two occasions. Very frequently the 6th anterior root contains no fibres to the intrinsic flexors of the foot, and the three exceptions above occurred in individuals in which the plexus was certainly not so low as in the typical conformation of the *postfixed* pattern.

Again, on two occasions in which the intrinsic flexors of the digits were not represented in the 9th anterior root, the 8th anterior root on being split into five filaments gave evidence that the short flexors were represented without the soleus and the gastrocnemius in the lowest filaments, but in the upper filaments the soleus and gastrocnemius as well were present.

Again, excitation of the two lowest (most posterior) of eight filaments into which a 6th anterior root had been separated gave extension of the ankle; while excitation of each of the remaining six gave flexion of the ankle.

Again, the higher (more anterior) filaments of the 7th will sometimes give a better action of the short extensor of the second toe than do the most posterior filaments of the 7th. And the most posterior filaments of the 5th give a better extension of the hallux than the more anterior filaments of the 5th.

Again, on two occasions the motor outflow to the internal group of thigh muscles, supplied by the obturator nerve, has had its lower limit about one-third of the distance up the 5th lumbar rootlets, the root filaments below that point passing to the semimembranosus and the pretibial muscles, but not to the adductor group.

In one experiment the extensor muscles of the thigh were represented in the upper half of the rootlets of the 5th lumbar segment, but not in the rootlets of the lower half.

The deep inner hamstring is frequently represented in the lower but not the upper half of the 5th lumbar segment.

It is curious to note that *the region of outflow of the efferent fibres to a group of muscles or the representation of a particular movement at a joint often ends not conterminously with the spinal segment, but somewhere within the spinal segment, either as it were overstepping or falling short of the anatomical limits of a segment.* The representation then stops short not at the interval between two segments of the cord, but midway within a segment of the cord. This fact may modify considerably our conception of the spinal root as a guide in studying the segmental arrangement of the limb, and on the other hand our conception of the morphological construction of the limb itself.   The ankle and wrist, which seem at first sight natural boundaries marking the division between fundamentally distinct portions of the limb, are not regarded as such in the segments of the spinal cord.   On the sensory side much evidence of a similar kind is obtainable, and I will reserve the point for discussion in a paper dealing with the sensory evidence.

E. Remak[1] concluded that most muscles are represented in the cord by vertical tracts, so that as Gowers[2] remarks the whole anterior grey matter at any one nerve-segment contains cells that are concerned with different movements.   The length of the region of outflow of motor fibres for certain primary movements in the lower limb of the species Rhesus may be thus tabulated, the table being formed by combining the results from various individuals.

	XI	X	IX	VIII	VII	VI	V	IV	III	II	I
Hallux :											
Flexion			——	——	——	——	—				
Extension					——	——	—				
Digits :											
Flexion			——	——	——	——	—				
Extension					——	——	—				
Ankle :											
Flexion					——	——	—				
Extension				——	——	—					
Knee :											
Flexion				——	——	——	—				
Extension							——	——	—		
Hip :											
Extension			——	——	——	——	—				
Flexion							——	——	——	—	
Adduction						——	——	——	—		

It is clear that the region of outflow for movement at the hip is longer than that for movement of any other joint in the lower limb, especially

---

[1] *Arch. Psychiat. Nervenkr.*, 1879, **9**, 510.
[2] *Diseases of the Nervous System*, 2nd ed., London, 1892, **1**, 192.

than that of the ankle. It runs through at least seven segments of the cord instead of four. But if each of the main movements of the joints be considered individually it is seen that the region of representation in the spinal roots of Macacus is as long in the case of the small joints of the toes, such as the metatarso-phalangeal of the thumb, as it is for the hip, or knee, or ankle. It is noticeable that with all the joints mentioned the region of outflow for any individual main movement extends into at least three segments of the cord. The long region of outflow for movement at the hip is due to the *flexion* outflow being more separated from the *extension* outflow in the case of the hip than in the case of the other joints, especially than in the case of the joints of the digits. One might express the difference by saying that the spinal nuclei for flexion of the hip and for extension of the hip overlap each other very slightly, but that the nuclei for flexion and extension of the digits overlap each other very largely.

This fact is merely the physiological side of an anatomical disposition of the musculature of the limb which has considerable morphological significance. In the proximal portion of the limb (the thigh) the nerve-roots supplying the musculature are not common to muscle-groups both of the anterior and posterior aspects of the limb. But the nerve-roots entering the foot and leg each supply muscles both on the posterior and anterior aspects, more markedly so in the foot than in the leg. In the foot the dorsum is distinctly segmentally anterior to the sole; and there the rule is broken (and the same may be said of the hand) by the lowest root which enters the foot or hand frequently supplying the musculature on one aspect only, that aspect always being posterior—the plantar or palmar—unless by some straining of anatomical principle the dorsal interossei may be considered to belong not to the plantar but to the dorsal side.

THE MOTOR INNERVATION FROM THE BRACHIAL PLEXUS

Method:

For examining the distribution of the motor roots of the brachial nerves, one mode of procedure adopted was similar to one previously used in my examination of the lumbo-sacral plexus.

The vertebral canal was opened, and a short series of the spinal nerves immediately above and immediately below the one to be investigated were divided; a sufficient time, usually twenty-eight days, sometimes longer, was allowed for degeneration to have play; and finally, electrical excitation of the various nerve-branches in the limb itself was carried out. Strict asepsis and profound anæsthesia were maintained throughout the operative procedure.

In a certain number of experiments on motor distribution, the Wallerian degeneration was employed: the segmental nerve, the distribution of whose motor fibres it was desired to investigate, was cut completely through just after its exit from the spinal dura as far proximal to its spinal ganglion as possible. A sufficient number of weeks was then allowed for the progress of the degeneration: this time varied from eighteen to thirty days. The animal was then killed and dissected. The nerve twigs to the muscles were fixed and stained with osmic acid and then allowed to dissociate in methyl alcohol 40 per cent. in water. They were then exhaustively examined in teased preparations. Each nerve twig was completely examined—*i.e.*, the whole thickness of it teased up, mounted and preserved in a series of preparations. The accuracy, delicacy, and ease of this method surprised me not a little. It is greatly superior to the most perfect serial preparations of cross or longitudinal sections.

4th Cervical Motor Root[1]

Examined in four individuals.

The dorsal primary division supplied: Complexus, splenius, trachelo-mastoideus, cervicalis ascendens, transverso-spinales.

The ventral primary division supplied: Levator scapulæ, longus colli, levator claviculæ, scalenus medius, trapezius, subclavius. In three individuals the front, especially sternal, portion of the diaphragm. In one experiment this was examined by degeneration; the degeneration in the ventral division of the phrenic nerve on the diaphragm was much heavier than in the dorsal division.

5th Cervical Motor Root

The method of examination adopted for the motor root was section of the motor roots adjoining that to be examined, then, after a lapse of at least fourteen days, excitation with the faradic current of the remaining sound root in the vertebral canal, and of the various nerve-trunks composing the brachial plexus.

On the motor root of the 5th cervical nerve four such experiments were carried out, one on *M. sinicus*, the rest on *M. rhesus*.

The root was found to be distributed to the following muscles:

Dorsal primary division: *erector spinæ* and *transverso-spinales.*

Ventral primary division:
longus colli.
rhomboidei.
levator anguli scapulæ.
serratus magnus.
pectoralis major (clavicular portion only).
deltoideus (clavicular and acromial portions).
teres minor.
supraspinatus.
infraspinatus.
subscapularis.
scalenus medius.

biceps (both heads).
brachialis anticus.
coraco-brachialis (slightly only).
supinator longus (feebly) and *brevis* (very feebly).
extensor carpi radialis longior (feebly; in one experiment not at all).
extensor carpi radialis brevior (feebly; in two experiments not at all).
diaphragma : degeneration heavy in both sternal (ventral) and vertebral (dorsal) divisions of the phrenic on diaphragm.
subclavius.

6th Cervical Motor Root

Three experiments, all on *Macacus rhesus*, by the combined degeneration and excitation method.

---

[1] *Philos. Trans.*, 1898, **190B**, 73 *et seq.*

The distribution of the root was found to include the following muscles:

The dorsal primary division innervated the following, as tested by experimental excitation:

erector spinæ.   *transverso-spinales.*

The ventral primary division as given below:

scaleni (not always).   *coraco-brachialis.*
teres major.   *supinator longus.*
teres minor.   *supinator brevis.*
rhomboidei.   *extensor carpi radialis longior.*
serratus magnus.   *extensor carpi radialis brevior* (slightly).
pectoralis major.   *pronator radii teres* (slightly).
deltoideus (apparently the *whole* of the   *flexor carpi radialis* (slightly).
   muscle).   *latissimus dorsi.*
supraspinatus.   *diaphragma* (especially the portions
infraspinatus.   nearer the vertebral column and
subscapularis.   lateral part attached to lowest
biceps caput longum.   ribs).
biceps caput breve.   *longus colli.*
brachialis anticus.   *triceps.*

In one experiment a part of the outer head of *triceps* contracted feebly but distinctly.

In two experiments the distribution was further examined by tracing *microscopically* the Wallerian degeneration in the nerve-twigs of the limb twenty days subsequent to section of the motor root of the inside of the vertebral canal.

Degeneration was found in the nerve-twigs to the following muscles:[1]

subclavius.
extensor carpi radialis brevior.

In both experiments { *triceps*, in outer and inner heads (but slight degeneration only).
{ *supinator brevis.*

In one experiment, } *flexor carpi ulnaris* (slight degeneration).
not in both }

In both experiments: *extensor communis digitorum* (a few fibres only).

In one experiment,   { *extensor longus pollicis* (a few fibres only).
not in both   { *extensor ossis metacarpi pollicis* (six fibres only).
                     { *flexor longus pollicis* (a few fibres only).

It will be seen that the five last mentioned groups were not noticed by the previous method to respond to the excitation of the 6th cervical root; the teasing method was carried out only after the examination made by the excitation method above described, and it is possible that if its results had been known, and particularly minute attention paid to the above muscles, some trace of contraction might have been found; but it seems clear that, if detectable, it was so slight as to have escaped a careful search.

[1] In addition to a list including most of the muscles given above, given in original paper. The serratus magnus and pectoralis major were not included in the search by teasing, partly on account of their size, partly because the labour was believed to be superfluous.—ED.

I am, therefore, inclined to consider the amplification of the list obtained by the purely microscopical method of teasing to be explicable not by individual variation, but by a greater delicacy of the " teasing " than of the previous method.   Allowing twenty muscle fibres to each neurone, the six neurones contributed by the 6th cervical segment to the motor innervation of the extensor ossis metacarpi pollicis might—especially if, as is most probable,[1] scattered about the thickness of the muscle—under excitation evoke no *appreciable* contraction in the muscle.

My experiments on this nerve bear out the statement by Forgue and Lannegrace,[2] that the hinder part of the diaphragm is supplied by the 6th cervical nerve; so also my degeneration obtained of the 4th cervical bear them out that that root supplies the front of the diaphragm; but the degenerations show that there is much intermingling of the two nerves, both with each other and with the 5th in their distribution both to back and front.

My observations on this nerve bear out Thorburn's[3] statement, based on clinical observation, that the nerve supplies the teres major, latissimus dorsi, sternal portion of pectoralis major, and the triceps—a statement contrary to Forgue and Lannegrace's[4] experiments.

The Diaphragm.—The degeneration in the phrenic after section of 6th cervical in Macacus is heavy.   Of the two main divisions into which the phrenic divides on reaching the diaphragm, the degeneration is considerably greater in that (dorsal) which turns backward toward the vertebral column than in that which turns forward (ventral).

Degenerated fibres I found in considerable numbers in the phrenic twenty days after section of the motor root of the 4th cervical; but in this instance the amount of degeneration was greater in the division of the nerve which turned forward toward the sternal border of the muscle than in that turning backward.   The diaphragm in all my experiments proved to be a trimeric muscle—that is to say, drew its innervation from a series of three consecutive spinal nerves, resembling in this character the majority of the limb muscles.   The elements of the individual metameres are also, as in the limb muscles, much commingled and not strictly territorially arranged.

7th Cervical Motor Root

Three experiments, two on *Macacus rhesus*, one on *Macacus sinicus*; all by degeneration method with stimulation of the remaining root.

Dorsal primary division: *erector spinæ* and *transverso-spinales*.

Ventral primary division:

   scaleni.
   serratus magnus.

pectoralis major (the whole muscle apparently).

pectoralis minor (less vigorously than *pectoralis major*).

deltoideus (especially the portion from the scapular spine).

[1] Sherrington, *J. Physiol.*, 1892, **13**, 751.
[3] *Brain*, 1886-7, **9**, 510; 1888-9, **11**, 289.

[2] *C. R. Acad. Sci.*, Paris, 1884, **98**, 829.
[4] *Loc. cit.*

longus colli.

latissimus dorsi.

triceps (especially the long and outer heads) anconeus.

teres major.

subscapularis.

infraspinatus.

coraco-brachialis.

supinator longus.

extensor carpi radialis longior.

extensor carpi radialis brevior.

flexor sublimis digitorum.

flexor profundus digitorum.

flexor carpi radialis.

pronator radii teres.

extensor communis digitorum (feebly, but distinctly).

extensor carpi ulnaris (feebly, but distinctly).

extensor ossis metacarpi pollicis (feebly, but distinctly).

extensor longus pollicis (feebly, but distinctly).

flexor brevis pollicis (superficial head only; feebly, but distinctly).

biceps (feebly; in one experiment not at all).

brachialis anticus (feebly; in one experiment not at all).

flexor carpi ulnaris (feebly; in one experiment not at all).

flexor longus pollicis (feebly; in one experiment not at all).

supinator brevis (feebly; in one experiment not at all).

In one experiment further the degeneration method was completed by teasing nerve-twigs to muscles, and the following muscular branches revealed degenerate motor fibres, the right hand 7th cervical nerve having been severed in the vertebral canal twenty days previously:

Supraspinatus.*

palmaris longus.*

flexor carpi ulnaris.

extensor brevis pollicis.*

extensor indicis.*

superficial short muscles of thumb. Lumbricals (2) and interossei (2).

extensor minimi digiti.*

pronator quadratus* (two degenerated fibres).

supinator brevis (two degenerated fibres).[1]

The six muscles marked with an asterisk have, therefore, to be added to those given in the previous list in order to complete the motor distribution of the 7th cervical segment.

In this experiment not a single degenerate nerve-fibre was detected in the cervical sympathetic trunk.

The phrenic trunk contained no degeneration after section of this root.

8th Cervical Motor Root

Three experiments, all on *Macacus rhesus*, and by combined degeneration and excitation method as above.

The root is distributed to the following muscles:

scaleni.

pectoralis major.

pectoralis minor.

triceps (all three heads, especially, perhaps, to the long head).

latissimus dorsi (especially to a portion near the humeral attachment).

extensor carpi ulnaris.

extensor communis digitorum.

extensor ossis metacarpi pollicis.

[1] With many of the muscles listed above (see original article for complete list).—ED.

extensor longus pollicis.
extensor brevis pollicis.
extensor indicis.
extensor minimi digiti.
flexor carpi radialis.
flexor carpi ulnaris.
flexor sublimis digitorum.
flexor profundus digitorum.

flexor longus pollicis.
palmaris longus.
pronator quadratus.
the intrinsic muscles of the hand, including the interossei.
teres major—in one experiment only.
coraco-brachialis—in one experiment only.

In two further experiments the 8th cervical ventral (motor) root having been severed twenty days previously, degenerate fibres were found in nerves to the following muscles:

superficial short muscles of thumb.
1st, 2nd, 3rd lumbricales.
1st, 2nd, 3rd palmar interossei.
all the dorsal interossei.
extensor carpi radialis brevior ⎰ A few degenerate fibres were present in one of the
pronator radii teres ⎱ experiments, but were absent in the other.

4th palmar interosseus muscle; it was doubtful if any degenerate fibres existed in the nerve of this muscle in the experiment in which some were present in the nerve to *extensor carpi radialis brevior*, but in the other experiment there were some undoubtedly present.

In each of these experiments degenerate fibres existed in the cervical sympathetic—in the former case two fibres, in the latter five; the degenerate fibres were small myelinate (less than $3.5\ \mu$).

When the motor root of this nerve has been completely destroyed by degeneration a number of perfectly sound myelinate fibres are still to be found in the small *primary dorsal division* of it, although that division supplies no cutaneous branch. The sensory fibres in this division must be destined for muscles, ligaments, and connective tissue endings. The motor fibres in the division supply the *erector spinæ* and *transverso-spinales*.

1st *Thoracic Motor Root*

Two experiments, both by degeneration method: one performed on *Macacus rhesus*, one on *Macacus sinicus*. The muscular distribution was in this way found to include the following:

scaleni.
pectoralis major (lower body only).
pectoralis minor.
triceps (inner head, long head less).
latissimus dorsi (in part).
serratus posticus superior.
palmaris longus.
flexor carpi ulnaris.
flexor profundus digitorum.
flexor sublimis digitorum.
flexor longus pollicis.

pronator quadratus.
extensor ossis metacarpi pollicis.
extensor longus pollicis.
extensor brevis pollicis.
extensor communis digitorum.
extensor indicis.
extensor minimi digiti.
extensor carpi ulnaris.
intrinsic muscles of the hand, including the interossei.

A further examination of the distribution of this motor root was carried out as before by degeneration and teasing nerve-trunks. Degenerate nerve-fibres were traced to the following muscles:

flexor carpi radialis.
extensor indicis (not always).
extensor internodii (longus et brevis) pollicis (not always).
1st, 2nd and 3rd lumbricales.
all the palmar } interossei { The amount of degeneration was greater in the 4th
all the dorsal }   { palmar interosseus than in the 1st.

In this experiment seventy-three degenerate fibres were present in the cervical sympathetic—fine myelinated all of them.

After this motor root has been destroyed by degeneration, a considerable number of perfectly sound nerve-fibres still persist in the first intercostal nerve. This latter must therefore contain a number of afferent nerve-fibres, although in the monkey it does not give any lateral or other cutaneous branch—at least, I have found none. In the same way the small dorsal primary division of this nerve is found to contain a number of fibres from the spinal root-ganglion, although it gives off no cutaneous branch. The motor fibres in the small *posterior primary division* innervate the *erector-spinæ*, *levator costæ*, and *transverso-spinales*.

2nd Thoracic Motor Root

I have never, in Macacus, found wanting a distinct contribution from the 2nd thoracic to the brachial plexus. I ascertained by degeneration experiments that this, which is too short to stimulate without some risk of escape of current, contains both motor and sensory fibres. In full accord with the distribution of the degeneration, excitation of the 2nd thoracic motor root gives contraction of a number of hand muscles. W. Krause, although he noted the presence of this branch in the rabbit, did not discover its importance to the plexus. Forgue and Lannegrace overlooked it altogether in dog and monkey. Ferrier and Yeo (1884) were the first to demonstrate that it contributes to the hand: they describe it as supplying the *interossei* and evoking " interosseous flexion." In my own paper I noted instances in which it evoked flexion and pronation at wrist, as well as full flexion of the thumb and fingers, both in *M. rhesus* and in *sinicus*; also in Cercopithecus and in Cynocephalus. I have also seen slight flexion of the wrist as a willed movement in a Macaque in which the 6th, 7th, and 8th cervical and 1st thoracic roots had been cut through. In fact, it supplies *flexor profundus*, *flexor sublimis*, *palmaris longus*, *pronator quadratus*, as well as the muscles of the hand.

In all cases the *scaleni* (not *medius*) muscles contained degenerated nerve-fibres; as also, via the posterior primary division of the nerve, the *erector spinæ* and *transverso-spinales*.

Examined by the degeneration method and the teasing of muscle-nerves for detection of breaking down nerve-fibres, the following results were obtained in two Macaques:

Experiment 1.	*Experiment 2.*
palmaris longus.	flexor longus pollicis.
pronator quadratus.	flexor sublimis digitorum.
flexor longus pollicis.	flexor profundus digitorum.
flexor sublimis digitorum.	deep short muscles of thumb.
flexor profundus digitorum.	short muscles of little finger.
deep short muscles of thumb.	all the lumbricales.
all the lumbricales.	all the dorsal ⎱ interossei.
all the dorsal ⎱ interossei.	all the palmar ⎰
all the palmar ⎰	
short muscles of little finger.	

The fact that after degeneration of the lowest four cervical and of the 1st thoracic nerves, excitation of the 2nd thoracic or of the cords of brachial plexus still evokes a flexion of the wrist and of the digits, in which the terminal phalanges of the latter are flexed on the middle phalanges as well as these last on the proximal, might be taken to prove that the flexor profundus digitorum was in action, and therefore innervated by the 2nd thoracic. The flexor profundus is, it is true, usually innervated in part by the 2nd thoracic, but the above fact is not the proof of it. In man the flexor profundus (perforans) is the flexor of the terminal phalanges on the middle phalanges, and the sublimis does not flex the former. In the Macaque both profundus and sublimis flex similarly the terminal and middle and proximal phalanges; if the middle phalanges are prevented from flexion (as presumably under action of the interossei and lumbricales), the sublimis cannot flex the terminal phalanx, although the profundus can. This action can be easily examined by pulling on the respective tendons in the Macaque.

In all the Macaques I have examined in reference to the point, the 2nd thoracic innervates the hand not only via the ulnar nerve, but also via the median. Hepburn has described that in monkeys the ulnar gives a considerable branch to the median in the upper part of the forearm. It is through this that the above-described distribution takes place. Although present in the Macaque, I have never met with this forearm branch in Cercocebus nor in Cynocephalus. These latter forms do possess, however, the somewhat similar communication between external saphenous nerve and external plantar at the heel deep to the tendo Achillis, which I described and figured in my former paper in Macacus.[1] The contribution from ulnar to median contains cutaneous sensory fibres as well as motor efferent (see p. 70, and Fig. 19, p. 71). The communication between ulnar and median is normal in most mammals.[2] In man it occurs in 20 to 25 per cent. of individuals,[3] a fact which lends more interest to the physiological analysis of the communication as it exists in Macacus.

[1] *J. Physiol.*, 1892, **13**, 643, Plate 21, fig. 7.   [2] Bardeleben.
[3] Quain's *Anatomy*, vol. iii., part 2, p. 302. Thane, 1895.

It will be noted that although the 2nd thoracic nerve contributes to the innervation of the muscles of the hand and lower forearm, it does not contribute to the sensory innervation of any part of the skin of the hand, nor even to that of the lower part of the forearm. Also, although it supplies the muscles of the second intercostal space, the skin overlying the second intercostal space is not innervated by it. I have already pointed this out as a striking illustration of the want of real basis for the so-called " law " (Van der Kolk, Hilton), which states that muscles and their overlying integument are supplied by the *same* segmental nerves. The skin over the first and second intercostal spaces is in great part innervated from segments five and six, segments further headward than the source of innervation of the underlying muscles—*e.g.*, first intercostal space: muscles, 1st thoracic, skin, 4th cervical.

THE PATTERN OF SUPPLY OF THE BRACHIAL LIMB

[*The muscular structure of the brachial limb, similar to that of the lower limb, is also that of a number of fused parallel plates, or rays, of muscle substance extending from the base of the limb to its tip.*]

The mode of distribution of the motor roots to the skeletal muscles[1] of the brachial limb indicates that the limb is composed of a number of rays placed at right angles to the long axis of the body, and parallel with the long axis of the limb. The most posterior of these muscular rays are the longest ones, and the most anterior the shortest ones of the limb series. The prominence of the limb from the body is of such a form that the anterior edge of the prominence is thrust out less abruptly from the side of the trunk than is the posterior. Into the anterior edge enter a number of rays; taking six to be the number of muscular rays in the fore-limb of Macacus, into the segmental composition of its anterior edge there enter four out of the six.

If by a ray be meant a band of muscular tissue extending lengthwise through the musculature of the limb, it is not difficult by the degeneration method to trace in the limb the rays of the 5th, 6th, 7th, 8th, and 9th (D. 1) spinal segments, and to see that of these the last two extend out even to the extreme free end of the limb. The ray of the 10th segment is less easily traced throughout its extent continuously. The distal part of it is obvious enough in the intrinsic hand muscles; it is also clear in that part of it stretching between elbow and wrist, for there in Macacus it supplies the flexor muscles. But in Macacus it is unrepresented in the musculature of the upper arm, and in the cat and dog it is generally absent from the musculature of the forearm also. Indeed, in the cat it is often absent from the musculature of the hand itself. In man it appears, as in the cat, to be sometimes wanting altogether from the musculature of the limb,

---

[1] Extract from *Philos. Trans.*, 1898, **190B,** 119. A large detailed chart recording the muscular distribution and variation is here included in the original paper.

although not unfrequently it undoubtedly does contribute to it, then probably, as in the other types, occurring chiefly in the hand and flexors of the forearm.   It is clear that, broadly described, the musculature of the fore-limb is built up by successive contributions of segments, which reviewed in series passing from the segmentally anterior to the segmentally posterior, first extend stepwise down the deltoid scapular group, including in that the clavicular part of pectoralis major.   That the next step takes in the biceps and brachialis anticus and part of supinator longus, and the descent then follows down the radial side especially, until with the 8th cervical ray the whole length of the musculature of the limb is reached even to its extreme apex.   The length of the limb thus having been attained, and occupied by successively longer and longer out-thrusts of four segments (just as I have described for the hind-limb), a number of other segments, usually two (dog, Macacus), thrust out each a process, which extends along the back of the process of the segment immediately anterior to it, and throughout the whole length of the limb.   These segments are so intimately fused in the hand region that it is difficult to pick out from the rest any one muscle which shows more of this or that constituent.   But in the forearm and arm it is less difficult; thus, in the former, the extensor communis digitorum receives a root which does not contribute to either of the long flexores digitorum, and the latter often receive a root which never contributes to the long extensor digitorum; in the arm triceps receives supply from two roots which never supply the biceps, the latter from one root which never supplies the triceps.

OVERLAPPING OF MOTOR FUNCTION IN THE GREY MATTER OF THE CORD

From the foregoing it is seen that by collating the combined movements obtained from each of the brachial series of roots a *sketch* of the motor localisation of the limb movements is indicated; but the sketch is an *imperfect* one.   As to the topographical order of the groups of motor nerve-cells executing the simple movements of the limb-joints, the analysis of the muscular fields of the motor roots carried out in my degeneration experiments yields a fuller and more accurate view of spinal localisation, considered in its fore-and-aft arrangement.   The information from the combined movements evoked by nerve-roots is complicated by algebraic summation of component antagonistic factors, which, as I have shown elsewhere, is not of physiological value.   Taken in longitudinal direction, the order of spinal localisation of simple limb movements in the brachial enlargement of the ape is:

protraction of shoulder.
abduction of shoulder.
outward rotation of shoulder.
flexion of elbow.
supination of forearm.

adduction of shoulder.
radial abduction of wrist.
extension of wrist.
inward rotation of shoulder.
extension of and abduction of thumb.
extension of elbow.
extension of fingers.
flexion of wrist.
retraction of shoulder.
pronation of forearm.
flexion of fingers.
interosseous flexion of fingers.
adduction and abduction of fingers.
abduction of little finger.

So much mutual overlapping of the spinal representation of the simple limb-movements is present that the above list does not give a very intelligible picture of the real topographical relationships of these motor centres.   These are better represented in the scheme shown on p. 28.

Certain simple movements of the limb are not seen at all on the stimulation of individual motor roots—e.g., in many monkeys no *root* gives extension of the pollex, and in some monkeys no root gives extension of the wrist, and I have met with an individual in which no root evoked extension of the fingers.   In the dog often no motor root dorsiflexes ankle or flexes the knee.   In the monkey, again, no root gives abduction of the pollex or little finger.   If the muscles producing one movement at a certain joint predominate in one root, it does not follow those producing the opposite movement of the joint need predominate in another.   Nor is the supposition borne out that muscles whose action predominates in one root always predominate in that root; thus, in the cat, the 6th subthoracic root occasionally gives flexion of knee, though usually extension.   In the dog the 7th subthoracic root generally produces extension of the knee, and generally spreading of the toes, but occasionally flexion of knee, and occasionally flexion of the toes.   The 6th cervical root of Macacus usually produces extension of the wrist, but sometimes flexion; the 2nd thoracic of Macacus usually produces flexion of the wrist, but occasionally only flexion of the fingers and thumb.

The fibres in the motor roots of the brachial region are, as I have pointed out also for those of the lumbo-sacral region, from their very origin commingled in such a way that any one root-filament contains motor fibres for a variety of muscles, and often for muscles not concerned with the same simple movement of the limb.   Commingled in this way at their source, they, after entering the nerves of the plexus, become sorted out into proper groups destined for particular muscles; hence the possibility of carrying out such dissections as those of Herringham[1] in spite of the difficulties on which W. Krause[2] has so much insisted, and indeed stated to be insuperable.

[1] *Proc. roy. Soc.*, 1886, **41,** 423.
[2] *Beiträge zur Anatomie der oberen Extremität.* Leipzig u. Heidelberg, 1863.

The scheme represents, by horizontal lines, the longitudinal localisation in the ape's brachial spinal segments of the motor nerve-cell groups for the simpler functional muscle-groups of the limb.

	DII / X	DI / IX	VIII	VII	VI	V	IV
Protraction of shoulder						———	———
Abduction of shoulder				———	———	———	
Outward rotation of shoulder				———	———	———	
Flexion of elbow				———	———	———	
Supination of forearm				———	———	- - -	
Adduction of shoulder		———	———	———	———	———	
Radial abduction at wrist			———	———			
Extension of wrist			———	———			
Inward rotation of shoulder			———	———			
Extension of elbow			———	———			
Extension of fingers		———	———				
Flexion of wrist		———	———				
Retraction of shoulder	———	———	———	———			
Pronation of forearm	———	———	———	———			
Flexion of fingers	———	———	———				
Interosseous flexion of fingers	———	———	———	- - -			
Adduction of fingers	———	———	———	- - -			
Abduction of fingers	———	———	———				

But within the motor-roots themselves the fibres are so commingled that it is impossible, in one and the same root, to obtain, for instance, a bundle of fibres in one part of the root which represents flexion of the wrist, and a bundle in another part of the root which represents extension of the wrist.

CONCLUSION[1]

Regarding the efferent root-cells of the spinal cord, these, like the afferent, are divisible into three groups—those related to the skeletal musculature, to the skin, and to the viscera. The position of the nerve-cell bodies or perikarya of these efferent neurones, unlike that of the afferent, is intraspinal. There is good evidence that they lie embedded in the cord at the same segmental level as the point of emergence from the cord of the nerve-fibres they originate.[2] If into the cord a clean incision be made transversely to its length, there ensues degeneration of the motor root-fibres immediately at the site of the trauma and not in front of or behind that level; the root-fibres therefore do not take their origin any distance in front of or behind their point of exit or they would suffer degeneration. This is well seen in regions where each motor root consists of a series of rootlets. It proves each rootlet to be a collection of fibres which represents the nerve-cells lying in its own particular level of the grey matter—in fact, so to say, which drains only one particular cross-level of the cord. This fact can be combined with the further observation that each constituent natural rootlet of the motor root contains fibres which, broadly speaking, are distributed to all the structures which the entire root innervates. Each rootlet of the root can thus be described as representing in miniature the entire root. It follows that the position of the nerve-cells sending motor fibres to any one skeletal muscle is a scattered one, extending throughout the whole length of the spinal segments innervating that muscle; in the limb regions many muscles receive their motor fibres from as many as three consecutive spinal roots, and the bodies of the nerve-cells innervating those must therefore, inside the cord, extend through the length of three whole segments of the cord as a continuous columnar group, and in each transverse level of the cord these cells must lie commingled with nerve-cells innervating many other muscles. Hence no traumatic injury of the spinal cord can ever paralyse a single muscle alone and apart from others. Even the severance of any one whole motor nerve-root cannot paralyse a single limb muscle; the effect of such an injury is to partially impair a large number of the muscles.

Analysis of the spinal nerve-supply of the muscles of either limb demonstrates that the muscular tissue of the limb is arranged in a number of rays, there being one ray for each one metamere contributing to the limb. Of these rays the tailmost in the fore-and-aft series are the longest; they extend to the extreme free apex of the limb, whereas the foremost, the most rostral, pass only as far as the thigh, the next hindward as far as the knee, the next hindward as far as the ankle. In the fore-limb of *Macacus rhesus*, the common *rhesus* monkey, the four hindmost, most aboral rays all contribute to the musculature of the hand. When we inquire how these units of the segmental

---

[1] Extract from *Med.-chir. Trans.*, 1899, **82**, 455.

[2] Sherrington, *J. Physiol.*, 1892, **13**, 621; and A. S. F. Grünbaum, *ibid.*, 1894, **16**, 368.

architecture of the limbs, these muscular rays, are related to the physiological or functional units of the limb musculature, it is at once obvious
that the extent and boundaries of the two do not coincide.   The definitely
bounded, individual and circumscribed masses of muscular tissue which
are known as " the muscles " of the limb are functional elements of its
structure as a physiological machine.   But each of these functional elements
is compounded and pieced together out of several rays or myotomes.   Moreover, the boundaries between the myotomes do not correspond with the
intervals between muscles nor even with those between muscle-groups.

Another feature of the distribution of the motor fibres of the spinal root
to a muscle is the remarkable frequency with which it is subject to slight
individual variation.   In examining a series of individuals (cats, monkeys)
it is almost rare to meet two consecutive members of the series in which
the root-distribution is not by the degeneration or experimental method
demonstrably somewhat different.   Thus as instance I found in some
individuals supinator brevis innervated from the 6th and 5th cervical nerves,
in others, from the 6th and 7th.   In the former case the innervation of
the muscle may be termed " *prefixed* " type, in the latter " *postfixed*."   The
absolute segmental level of a muscle is variable over the range of nearly a
whole segment's length; the *relative* segmental position is, however, preserved
inviolably constant.

II

ON THE DISTRIBUTION OF THE SENSORY
NERVE-ROOTS

[The exact plan of segmental innervation of the skin was established in a series of experiments in the monkey, published chiefly in two papers, in 1893 and 1898. Full historical notes will be found in the original papers. Extracts from both are printed here. With the exception of the isolated observations of Krause (1865) in the rabbit, Türck (1856) in the dog, dissections of the brachial plexus by Herringham (1887), and certain clinical observations in man (Thorburn, Starr) the cutaneous segmental fields had not been charted. Previous investigators had described variability in area of supply by some particular sensory nerve-roots, but only Herringham[1] had noted that the plexus as a whole varied in relation to the vertebræ. Türck[2] had described bands of segmental innervation in the skin of the limbs of the dog, and the displacement of some segments away from the trunk. Independently of Sherrington's complete survey, Bolk[3] was investigating the cutaneous innervation of the brachial limb by morphological method, and the publication of both researches on this limb in 1898 showed substantial agreement in the respects in which they coincided. The amount of overlap is more accurately shown by the physiological method.

The difficulties attendant upon experiments designed to estimate sensation in animals are discussed. The method of root section in the cat, and the method of isolation of one sensory root by section of its neighbours (called later by Head[4] the method of "remaining æsthesia"), as used in the monkey, are described. The sensory root is found to serve an area of skin which derives its form from anatomical segmentation. Sample experiments from both lower and upper limb are quoted from the original series. The nature of overlapping of segmental skin areas is defined. The segmental supply of the skin was shown, in contradiction to Krause and others, to be in places widely divergent from that of the motor supply of the muscles underlying it. The effect of section of only one sensory nerve-root is later described.—ED.]

METHODS OF OBSERVATION[5]

By exciting in an anæsthetised animal the central end of a nerve-trunk containing afferent nerve-fibres, reflex actions of various quality and degree may be initiated. By severance of the afferent rootlets of the spinal nerve

---

[1] *Proc. roy. Soc.*, 1887, **41**, 440.

[2] Türck, L., *S. B. Akad. Wiss. Wien*, 1856, p. 586; and *Denkschrift der Wien. Akad.*, 1869. See Sherrington, *Philos. Trans.*, 1893, **184B**, 641.

[3] See Postscript note, *Philos. Trans.*, 1898, **190B**, 180. [4] *Brain*, 1894, **17**, 461 (see p. 469).

[4] Extract from *Philos. Trans.*, 1893, **184B**, 654.

or nerves by which a peripheral nerve-trunk is connected with the cord the reflexes originated through it can be diminished or set aside completely; diminished if the peripheral trunk communicate with the cord through the channel of several roots and one but not all of these be severed, set aside completely if the severance include all the lines of the connection. This plan of observation was adopted for the exploration of the spinal connections of the afferent nerve-trunks of the lower limb in the cat.

Choice of a Reflex.—It is evidently desirable for the purpose to choose as criterion of the existence of afferent nerve-fibres a reflex the quantitative amount of which is at least roughly estimable, a reflex not easily fatigued by repetition, not liable to be occasioned by extraneous occurrences during an experiment nor to be simulated by nervous actions arising intrinsically, and, above all, a reflex capable of being evoked to a clearly detectable extent by excitation even feeble in character. Some trial experiments convinced me that the reflex I had looked forward to as probably the most satisfactory was not so; I had thought that in the arterial blood-pressure, admitting as that does of continuous graphic record, and affected as it is by many afferent channels, a most suitable index could be obtained. However, as my friend Dr. Rose-Bradford early foretold me, it proved unsuitable, and for several reasons. In an afferent limb-nerve excitation sufficient to cause a marked reflex contraction in the musculature of the limb often leaves the blood-pressure trace completely without alteration; the difficulty of maintaining the anæsthesia at so constant a depth that the mean arterial pressure remains the same from half-hour to half-hour is very great; the experiment involves frequently cutting large nerve-roots, and this, with the usually somewhat severe operation and the prolonged employment of the anæsthetic, combines to induce a tendency to Traube-Hering undulations, destroying the regularity of mean pressure desirable in the detection of transient reflex elevations and depressions. Another reflex sign elicitable is alteration of size of the pupil (Schiff,[1] Ott[2]), but under anæsthesia the pupil soon becomes widely dilated and sluggish, and a short trial sufficed to show that as a sign it is neither reliable nor easily legible. Modification of the respiratory rhythm induced by excitation of an afferent limb-nerve was next tested as a guide. It was found more delicate in this respect than either arterial pressure or size of pupil, but it appeared less amenable to excitation of the great sacral roots than to that of the lumbar, especially of the upper lumbar. Indeed, it became evident, when experimenting on respiratory reflexes, that local muscular movement was the least variable and the most obvious evidence of the arrival of impulses in the cord by afferent fibres from the *limbs* and body wall, and that the *occurrence* of the local movement was a more reliable token than was the *absence* of it, considered as a negative.

The locality of the reflex movement varies with the locality of source of the afferent impulses and the intensity of them. With weak stimulation

[1] *La Pupille considéré comme Esthésiométre*, Paris, 1875. [2] *J. Physiol.*, 1879-80, **2,** 443.

the movement tends to be confined to the muscles innervated by the same spinal segment irritated,[1] but it also tends to appear with especial ease in the muscles antagonistic to those, even when of other segments. When the central end of the external saphenous nerve is excited by currents somewhat stronger than, if applied to the posterior tibial trunk, would produce contraction of the gastrocnemius, contraction of the gastrocnemius is evoked, and the contraction of the gastrocnemius may be apparently limited to one head of the muscle if the currents employed be of minimal efficiency. Somewhat stronger excitation produces a reply less locally restricted but still distinctly local in character. These limited reflex movements can be evoked from pure muscular nerves—e.g., the nerve-twigs entering muscles. From the central end of the nerve entering the outer head of the gastrocnemius a contraction of the inner head of the muscle can be obtained which is immediately cut out by severance of certain roots in the spinal canal. So quick appears the reply thus obtained that it was for some time disregarded, as I thought it but an example of the " paradoxical " contraction. On some occasions it may have been of of that nature, but more frequently it ceased directly the posterior roots were severed in the spinal canal. Attention has been called recently to such reflex movements by Chauveau;[2] in the present paper I refer to them merely as constituting the criterion which was employed as best for my purpose, because delicate, readily detectable, and practically unexhausted by the course of experiment.

My experiments were conducted as follows: The animal was wrapped in cotton-wool with the exception of the head and back. The back was shaved and one of the limbs in the region to be examined. The animal was then deeply anæsthetised, and placed on a warm water stage upon the operating table. The spinal cord was then in requisite length exposed in the vertebral canal by removal of a sufficient number of spinous processes and laminæ. The dura mater is usually covered in the lumbar region by a layer of fat, in which there lie embedded largish veins. When this layer is turned back by a blunt " seeker " the cord is seen through the transparent membrane, and the pulsation of the vessels on it is very obvious. A little further preparation suffices to bring into view the nerve-roots at their emergence from the dural sheath. The nerve-root can be divided outside the dural sheath or inside it. The former plan has the advantage of not letting out much of the cerebro-spinal fluid, a condition of prime importance for the prolonged preservation of the normal state of the cord. The latter plan has the advantage of presenting no difficulty to severance of the whole of the afferent root of the spinal nerve without injuring the efferent root, whereas if the severance be made outside the theca, it is, in order to be certain that the whole afferent root is divided, best to sever the entire spinal nerve trunk altogether, and this entails a reduction of the efferent field for motor play by a part. In my experiments, unless otherwise stated,

[1] Sherrington, *J. Physiol.*, 1892, **13**, 730.   [2] *Brain*, 1891, **14**, 145.

the root was cut inside the theca, and the afferent portion alone was severed. Before carrying out the section of a nerve-root it is important to pass a thread round the root in order to ensure the inclusion of all the root filaments in the section. The large nerve-roots of the lumbo-sacral region are accompanied by veins proportionately large, which may after section give sufficient hæmorrhage to obscure the position of the root; it is therefore necessary to perform the desired section at one closure of the scissors. After the section a pledget of wool with normal saline at 38° C. is laid over the cord, and the soft parts are brought together with accurate adjustment. The peripheral nerve, the root constitution of which is to be examined, is then rapidly exposed at a suitable point through a small incision. Beneath it two threads are carefully laid, the more distal is tied, and the trunk divided just distal to it. The other ligature is drawn tight, and the character of the resulting reflex movement noted. Then one of the nerve-roots already exposed in the vertebral canal is severed, and again the nerve-trunk excited by tying a thread ligature. If, as before, the local movement follow in a clear manner, the test is considered to have given an affirmative, and another root is proceeded with by section. If the local movement is not clearly obtained, the test is repeated with a second ligature applied to a point rather higher up the nerve than was the former one. If a local movement is again not clearly obtained, the trunk is well cleared from tissue with the scissors, and lifted up to sheathed electrodes, and weak induction shocks in series of a rate of 100 per second are applied. If this stimulation is followed by no movement even when strong enough to be distinctly unpleasant to the tongue, then it is considered that the afferent connections of the peripheral trunk with the cord had been broken completely through. On the other hand, directly a clear local movement has been observed to follow the excitation, the test is considered to have replied that the nerve has probably still afferent connections with the cord, and another of the spinal roots already exposed is severed. If this severance is immediately followed by inability to re-obtain the movement elicited before, or, indeed, any movement with the strength of stimulus previously employed, it is considered that the previous movement was truly reflex, and that at the last root-section the nerve-trunk under examination lost its last afferent connection with the cord. In each experiment the sections of the posterior roots were made successively in an ascending direction or successively in a descending direction, unless expressly stated otherwise. In most cases in each experiment the corresponding peripheral trunk of the right and left sides was examined at a corresponding point both right and left, and on the right hand the roots were severed in the ascending direction, on the left hand in the descending direction. The result on the right side gave for the individual the upper limit of root connection of the trunk examined, the result on the left side the lower limit for the connection. By observing the difference in the strength of excitation required to elicit the reflex before and after intermediate sections of roots, it was possible to judge roughly the share which the root took in the composition of the peripheral trunk. But the indication so obtained is apt to be fallacious because the degree of anæsthesia influences the amount of reflex obtained.

Two examples will make clear the above description.

March 3, 1890. *Cat.* 4 lb. 6 oz. Ether and chloroform.

Tracheotomy, carotid exposed. The 3rd, 4th, 5th, 6th and 7th lumbar, and the 1st, 2nd, and 3rd sacral, and 1st and 2nd caudal nerve-roots exposed and looped in the spinal canal right and left. The 4th dorsal digital nerve and the musculo-cutaneous exposed on the right foot.

11.16. Carotid connected with manometer. Mean pressure 118 mm. Hg. Both vagus nerves divided in the neck.

11.20. Secondary at 15 cm. Current just perceptible to tongue. Excitation of musculo-cutaneous for 30 seconds. Rise of blood-pressure.

11.23. Secondary at 15 cm. Excitation of 4th dorsal digit for 30 seconds. Rise of blood-pressure, not half the increase obtained from musculo-cutaneous.

11.28. Right 2nd caudal root cut in the spinal canal.

11.33-37. Excitation of each nerve as before gave results as before.

11.42. Right 1st caudal root cut.

11.46-51. Excitation of each nerve as before.

11.54. Right 3rd sacral root cut.

11.58-12.2. Excitation of each nerve gave rise as before.

12.5. Right 2nd sacral root cut.

12.8-15. Excitation of each nerve gave rise as before.

12.18. Right 1st sacral root cut.

12.23-30. Excitations of each nerve gave rise as before.

12.33. Right 7th lumbar root cut.

12.36. Excitation of musculo-cutaneous gave rise as before.

12.38. Excitation of 4th digital evoked no alteration in blood-pressure.

12.40. Repeated—no rise obtained.

12.42. Repeated—no rise obtained.

12.45. Right 6th lumbar root cut.

12.50. Excitation of musculo-cutaneous as before gave now no rise of blood-pressure.

12.55. No rise of blood-pressure from musculo-cutaneous.

12.58. Repeated, with same absence of effect.

1.3-12. Left 4th plantar digital and left musculo-cutaneous exposed as on right side.

1.15. Excitation of each gives rise of blood-pressure. The mean blood-pressure is now 97 mm. Hg.

1.18. Left 5th lumbar root cut in spinal canal.

1.20. Excitation of each nerve gives rise on blood-pressure tracing, but the rise is hardly perceptible from the 4th plantar digital.

1.22. Again, with same result.

1.25. Left 6th lumbar root cut in spinal canal. Blood-pressure falls somewhat. Mean pressure at 1.30 is 93 mm. Hg.

1.32. Excitation of musculo-cutaneous nerve gives no obvious indication of blood-pressure trace.

1.35. Traube-Hering undulations have set in. These are not broken by excitation of either musculo-cutaneous or 4th digital nerve. No indication of the excitation is legible on the trace.

1.45. Traube-Hering undulations and somewhat falling blood-pressure. Excitation of 3rd and 4th digitals (plantar) and of whole musculo-cutaneous above ankle are without effect.

This example illustrates the difficulty constantly presenting itself in the method. The plantar digitals gave way on the left side before their roots had been interfered with at all, and the result from the musculo-cutaneous was vitiated to an indeterminable extent by the same failure.

In contrast with this stands the first experiment in which a local muscular contraction was used as index instead of an alteration on the blood-pressure trace.

April 28, 1890. *Cat.* Small. Ether and chloroform.

Six roots exposed and looped in the spinal canal right and left, and found by *post-mortem* dissection to be the 2nd and 1st sacral and the lowest four lumbar. The 1st and 4th plantar digital nerves exposed on right side.

11.43-45. Thread round 4th digital drawn tight gives slight flexion at ankle. Thread round 1st digital drawn tight gives same movement.

11.48. Lowest root on right side (*i.e.*, 2nd sacral) divided.

11.52-54. Threads tightened on 4th and 1st digitals give slight flexion at ankle as before.

11.59. 1st sacral root on right side cut. A thread tightened on each nerve gives the flexion as before.

12.5. 7th lumbar on right side cut.

12.8. Thread tightened on 4th digital gives no movement at ankle or elsewhere.

12.10. Another thread—also without result.

12.12. Thread tightened on 1st digital gives movement at ankle, but feebler than before.

12.15-20. Currents with secondary at 14 cm. applied to 4th digital give no movement, applied to 1st digital give flexion at ankle stronger than with thread at 11.45.

12.23-30. 6th lumbar root on right side cut. Thread tightened on 1st plantar digital evokes no movement anywhere.

12.33. Currents applied as before give no movement.

12.40-50. 1st and 4th plantar digital nerves exposed on left side. When thread is tightened each evokes flexion at ankle.

12.54. 6th lumbar root on left side cut.

12.58-1.9. Thread tightened on 1st plantar digital evokes a dubious movement at ankle. Thread tightened on 4th plantar elicits flexion at ankle, perhaps, weaker than 10 minutes ago. Repeated with threads a centimetre higher up nerve—same effect as before.

1.12. Weak induced currents (perceptible to tongue) evoke a perceptible flexion at ankle from 1st plantar digital; a fairly good flexion at ankle from 4th digital.

1.20. 7th lumbar root cut.

1.24-35. No movement elicitable through either of the plantar nerves with secondary at 10 cm.

The experiment showed, therefore, clearly that in this individual the 1st plantar digital nerve was connected with the cord mainly by the 6th lumbar root but also by the 7th root; and that the 4th plantar digital was connected with the cord mainly by the 7th lumbar root but also by the 6th lumbar root.

By this method the root-constitution of most of the peripheral nerves of the lower limb was studied; usually in each experiment two small nerves and one large one were taken for analysis.

ROOT CONSTITUTION OF THE PERIPHERAL NERVES OF THE HIND LIMB (SAMPLE EXPERIMENTS AND TABLE)

I will give the experiments in the order in which they were made. From Experiment V. onwards the cord was severed at 6th thoracic segment prior to test of the reflexes.

Experimental Series I. A.

1. *Cat.* Male.

1st and 4th plantar digital explored, right and left. Movement obtained from each nerve was slight flexion at ankle. 2nd section did not obviously affect either 1st or 4th plantar. 3rd section destroyed 4th plantar, diminished 1st. 4th section destroyed 1st plantar. 5th section diminished 1st plantar very greatly, and 4th plantar dubiously. 6th section destroyed both. Therefore, 4th plantar digital constituted from the 7th and (?) 6th afferent roots; 1st plantar, from the 6th and 7th roots.

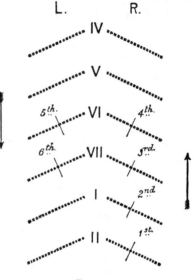

FIG. I

The above experiments[1] were made in uncertainty of the exact segmental numbers of the roots which had been divided. This was ascertained in each case by *post-mortem* dissection, in the following manner. The first rib on each side was exposed and the right and left ribs counted, and the number of the lumbar roots was taken from the last rib. In my notebook no attention was paid to the distinction between lumbar and sacral vertebræ, but all the roots below the last thoracic were termed post-thoracic. In quoting the experiments I have considered that the lumbar roots are seven and the sacral three, in the cat, because those numbers are in use by mammalian anatomists. In only one of twenty-two individuals examined was the number of ribs found to be twelve instead of thirteen, but in one there were fourteen ribs instead of thirteen. Among the individuals used in the above experiments one had a postfixed plexus in which root 6 gave no discovered contribution to the sciatic trunk, but root 7 gave a small branch to the obturator nerve, and a smaller twig to the anterior crural —and this was traced by experiment into the internal saphenous nerve. This degree of postfixture is not common; I have found and figured it in the monkey, and I have seen other instances in the cat. The anterior crural and especially the obturator were found by dissection to receive

[1] For the remaining twenty protocols see original paper, *loc. cit.*, p. 667.

each a branch from the nerve-root lower than the lowest usually entering them, and in one of these individuals I had found by experiment the gracilis muscle supplied with motor fibres from root 7, the last lumbar, although the lowest root usually supplying the gracilis in the cat is root 6, the lowest lumbar but one.   It is thus clear that individual variation occurs in the building of the peripheral trunks from the sensory roots just as it occurs in the building up from the motor roots.   Further, the degree of this varia-tion is often sufficiently great to be revealed by naked-eye dissection of the roots of the plexus.   When one finds by naked-eye dissection a plexus of obviously postfixed or prefixed type the character of its conformation may be impressed not only on its motor composition but on its sensory, and probably on both together, and in the same sense (*cf.* Experiment XX., and also experiment of January 19, 1891).[1]

A certain number of experiments were made on the monkey by exactly the same method as those above related in the cat.   The species of monkey employed was, without exception, *Macacus rhesus*, and, for the most part, immature individuals—*e.g.*, in the females menstruation had hardly com-menced.   In regard to *Macacus rhesus*, it will be remembered that the lumbar vertebræ are seven as in the cat, and that the sacral vertebræ are three, but that there are twelve pairs of ribs instead of thirteen as in the cat.   As stated in my paper on the efferent fibres of the lumbo-sacral plexus, the correspondence between the roots of that region in cat and monkey, respectively, seems as follows:

Cat.	Macacus rhesus.	Man.[2]
2nd lumbar root (? + 1st)	= 1st lumbar.	
3rd „ „	= 2nd „	= 1st lumbar.
4th „ „	= 3rd „	= 2nd „
5th „ „	= 4th „	= 3rd „
6th „ „	= 5th „	= 4th „
7th „ „	= 6th „	= 5th „
1st sacral root	= 7th „	= 1st sacral
2nd „ „	= 1st sacral	= 2nd „
3rd „ „	= 2nd „	= 3rd „

Further, it must be noted that the foot of Macacus has five well developed digits instead of the four of the hind-foot of the cat; I have, therefore, attempted the analysis of twenty instead of sixteen collateral digital nerves.

The segmental number of the individual root could only be positively ascertained by *post-mortem* dissection.   As with the cat, the numbering of the roots was always commenced from the first, not from the last rib, and the counting was carried out on both sides.

---

[1] Details of these experiments and a table summarising them will be found in the original account, from which only sample experiments are quoted here.—ED.

[2] The table is compounded from two tables in the original paper, *loc. cit.*, pp. 647, 669.—ED.

Experimental Series I. B.

1. *M. rhesus.* Young female.

1st, 2nd, and 3rd, and 8th, 9th, and 10th dorsal collateral digital nerves analysed for root-composition. The reply obtained from each was flexion with adduction of the hallux, occasionally accompanied by slight flexion of other digits as well.

1st section produced no obvious alteration in the reflex replies. 2nd section produced no obvious alteration in the replies. 3rd section cut down the replies from 10th and 9th digitals, the former almost to extinction, but did not affect the other replies at all. 4th section destroyed reply from 10th, 9th, and 8th, and reduced replies from 3rd, 2nd, and 1st, the last very slightly; the character of the reply when obtained was now a slight flexion at the ankle. 5th section destroyed the reply in all. 6th section (left) much reduced the reply in the 1st digital obviously, in the 2nd slightly, hardly at all in 3rd; the three degrees of reduction were a striking series; left the other replies unaffected. 7th section destroyed the replies form 1, 2, and 3, and reduced the replies from the external three, nearly, but not quite, abolishing reply from 8th. 8th section abolished all reply.[1]

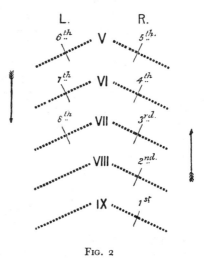

FIG. 2

The collective results of the foregoing series of experiments are for the sake of clearness of comparison placed in tabular form, as were the results obtained on the cat. Each large cross denotes that the spinal root it lies opposite contributed largely to the nerve. (See table on p. 41.)

SAMPLES OF SKIN-FIELDS SUPPLIED BY ROOTS ENTERING INTO THE LUMBO-SACRAL PLEXUS

The Method of Analysis of Sensation in the Skin[2]

From the above observations on the cat and *Macacus rhesus* it appeared clear that each branch of many of the sensory nerve-trunks in the limb consists of fibres which enter the cord by two or three distinct posterior roots, and that, therefore, just as there is a great interlapping of the limb territories of adjacent spinal nerve-roots judged by their distribution to the skeletal muscles, so also a great interlapping is evidenced in the distribution of the afferent fibres from the skin. It was also clear that as in the afferent roots of the frog,[3] so also in cat and monkey, some amount of individual variation is frequent. Points of interest especially requiring confirmation as unexpected and not in harmony with the observations on

---

[1] The remaining experiments, including some on the fore-limb, are omitted here for considerations of space.—ED.

[2] From *loc. cit.*, p. 685.   [3] Experiments on the frog described in the same paper.—ED.

the frog, or with the scheme of distribution of efferent fibres of the plexus, were the following. Among the conclusions arrived at from the experiments on the frog is this: the cutaneous field for each posterior root meets the middle line of the body both ventrally and dorsally. In the cat and monkey after the above analysis of the constitution of the peripheral branches of the plexus it was clear the skin field of post-thoracic root 6 could not possibly attain the dorsal or the ventral lines, it seemed roughly speaking to be distributed entirely to the apex of the limb—again, in the scheme of distribution to the musculature of the limb, the most segmentally posterior of the rays composing the limb penetrates to the very apex of the limb, both in the arm and leg. To judge from the above experiments this does not appear true for the segmental constitution of the *skin* of the limb. The posterior root of the 8th nerve does not appear to penetrate so far into the limb as does that of the 6th. That is to say, the limb being considered as a fin-like appendage, the musculature has a posterior border which is straight and abrupt and formed out of one ray, the overlying skin has a posterior border which is slanting and gradual and composed of more than one ray. Again as regards the musculature it was often the case (in the postfixed type of plexus) that root 9 contributed well to the innervation of the limb. This root does not (according to the above experiments) contribute to the skin of the limb proper; therefore the skin to which it supplies afferent fibres and the muscle to which it supplies motor fibres are separated by nearly the whole length of the limb, breaking the rule set down by Van der Kolk,[1] Peyer, Krause,[2] and others. In order to obtain a clearer answer on these points I attempted a direct delimitation of the spinal sensory root-fields in the mammal, in the same way as in the already cited experiments on delimitation of the root-fields in the frog. An essential feature in these experiments consisted in severance of a sufficient number of nerve-roots immediately above and below the root examined to make a field of anæsthesia, on which as on a blank surface the territory of the anæsthesia subserved by the isolated root could be mapped. The preparatory procedure of experiment was the same as for the observations on the root-composition of the various peripheral nerves, but of course no exposure of peripheral nerves was employed or necessary, mechanical excitation of the skin being substituted for mechanical and electrical excitation of the nerve-trunks. The same recording method was employed in the frog's experiments—that is, each point of the previously shaved skin that gave a reply was marked (with ink) at the time, and no other points were ever marked. After the whole area had been once explored in this way, a process which might occupy two or three hours, the extreme limit of the area was indicated by a white line carried on from reply spot to reply spot. After an interval of perhaps an hour this boundary-line was

---

[1] Froriep's *Notizen*, 3rd series, Oct., 1848.

[2] " That a muscle is supplied with nerve-fibres by the same spinal nerve that innervates the skin overlying it." Krause, *Beit. z. Neurol. d. oberen Extremitat*, Leipzig, 1865.

DISTRIBUTION of the Fibres of the Afferent Roots in some Nerve-trunks of the Lumbo-sacral Plexus of *Macacus rhesus* based on Experimental Series I. B.

		Lumbar					Sacral		
Number of the nerve-root		IIIrd	IVth	Vth	VIth	VIIth	Ist	IInd	Experiments
Collateral digital nerves. Dorsal.	1st	⋮	⋮	×	+	⋮	⋮		I, II, III, V, VIII.
	IInd	⋮	⋮	×	+	⋮	⋮		I, II, III, V, VIII.
	IIIrd	⋮	⋮	×	×	⋮	⋮		I, II, III, V, VIII.
	IVth	⋮	⋮	×	×	⋮	⋮		II, III, V, VIII.
	Vth	⋮	⋮	+	×	⋮	⋮		II, III, V, VIII.
	VIth	⋮	⋮	+	×	⋮	⋮		III, VI.
	VIIth	⋮	⋮	⋮	×	(+)	⋮		III, VI.
	VIIIth	⋮	⋮	⋮	×	+	⋮		I, II, III, VI.
	IXth	⋮	⋮	⋮	+	+	⋮		I, II, VI.
	Xth	⋮	⋮	⋮	+	+	⋮		I, II, III, VI.
Plantar.	1st	⋮	⋮	×	×	⋮	⋮		IV, V.
	IInd	⋮	⋮	×	×	(+)	⋮		IV, V.
	IIIrd	⋮	+	×	+	⋮	⋮		IV, V.
	IVth	⋮	+	×	+	⋮	⋮		IV, VII.
	Vth	⋮	+	×	×	⋮	⋮		IV, V, VII.
	VIth	⋮	⋮	×	×	⋮	⋮		IV, VI, VII.
	VIIth	⋮	⋮	+	×	⋮	⋮		IV, VI, VII.
	VIIIth	⋮	⋮	+	×	⋮	⋮		IV, VI, VII.
	IXth	⋮	⋮	+	×	⋮	⋮		IV, VI, VII.
	Xth	⋮	⋮	+	×	⋮	⋮		IV, VI, VII.
Int. plantar.		⋮	⋮	+	+	+	⋮		IX.
Ext. plantar.		⋮	⋮	(×?)	+	+	⋮		IX, X.
Anter. tibial.		⋮	⋮	+	+	⋮	⋮		XIII.
Musc. cutan.		⋮	⋮	+	+	+	⋮		IX, XIII.
obturator. Thigh		(+)	+	+	(+)	⋮	⋮		XII, XIII, XIV.
obturator. Pelvis		(+)(+)	+	+	(+)(+)	⋮	⋮		XII, XIII, XIV.
int. saph. Thigh		+	+	+	⋮	⋮	⋮		VIII, X, XII, XVII.
int. saph. Knee		×	×(+)	+	⋮	⋮	⋮		VIII, X, XII, XVII.
int. saph. Ankle		+							VIII, X, XII, XVII.
Post. tib.		⋮	⋮	+	+	+	+		IX.
Ext. saph.		⋮	⋮	+	+	+	+		V, VII, XVII.
Int. popl.		⋮	⋮	+	+	+	+		XI, XVI.
Ext. popl.		⋮	⋮	+	+	+	⋮		XI, XVI.
Hamstring N.		⋮	⋮	⋮	⋮	+	⋮		XV, XVI.
Ext. plantar (deep).		⋮	⋮	+	⋮	⋮	⋮		X.
Ext. br. of ant. tib. N. on the ankle.		⋮	⋮	+	⋮	⋮	⋮		XIII.
Cutan. br. from ext. popl. over head of fibula.		⋮	⋮	+	+	⋮	⋮		X, XVI, XVII.
Br. from ext. saph. to ext. plantar.		⋮	⋮	⋮	⋮	+	⋮		X.
ext. cuta-neous. Above patella		⋮	+	+	⋮	⋮	⋮		VIII, XI, XIII.
ext. cuta-neous. Below patella		⋮	+	+	⋮	⋮	⋮		VIII, XI, XIII.
genito-crural. Crural		+.							XV.
genito-crural. Genital		+							XV.
int. cuta-neous. Above knee		×	+						XII, XIV, XV.
int. cuta-neous. Below knee		+	×						XII, XIV, XV.

× Denotes that the root has a major share in the nerve-trunk.

(+) Denotes that slight but distinct evidence of the root was *sometimes* found.

(× ?) Denotes that evidence obtained was never better than dubious.

then very carefully and minutely explored at about 5-minute intervals, and the first white line was thus corrected as regards its detailed contour. After a few experiments on certain roots, especially root 6, it became evident that in this way a fairly constant figure was arrived at for the same root, subject to comparatively minor variations; it also became evident that the root-distribution was such that in order to isolate one root-territory, in some cases as many as seven consecutive posterior roots above or below had to be severed. Some time and labour were wasted by my not recognising this fact early enough, and its explanation will be dealt with after relating the experiments in which it occurred.

Regarding the form of stimulus used, the skin was pinched with a fine-pointed pair of dissecting forceps, and sometimes a mere touch sufficed to elicit a reflex; at other times, especially near the edge of the root-territory, a hard pinch had to be employed. At first I attempted to keep a record of the areas obtained by transferring them to " proportional paper " as in mapping from the microscope by means of the movable stage and squared eye-piece: difference of size and proportion between individual and individual frustrated this attempt, the maps becoming too confusing from necessary absence of perspective and inability to follow accurately the two superficial dimensions of a very irregular solid figure. I then proposed to content myself with accurate measurements from comparatively fixed points and written description, illustrated with pencil sketches; the difficulty of obtaining accuracy with the latter induced me to record with photography at the latter part of each experiment or immediately after it. As it was found that for photography in winter in London the ink marks often did not show up sufficiently on the pigmented skin, in the later experiments the boundary of the territories was usually indicated by a double line of white and black, the white border turned toward the side which yielded reflexes, the black toward that which did not yield reflexes. Finally, plaster casts of *Macacus rhesus* were made under my own direction by Messrs. Brucciani, and the position of the chief bony points accurately transferred from the individual whence the casts had been taken to the casts. Then the territory of the nerve-root desired to be transferred to the plaster model was delimited on an individual of approximately the same size as the cast, and in that way the model was gradually covered with the pattern of the various root-territories. It was only when that had been done that certain important points in the scheme of their arrangement became salient. Several reasons led me beyond the limits of the lower limb in this part of the research.

In the series of experiments in which analysis of peripheral nerves into their root-composition was attempted by electrical excitation of the nerve and successive sections of the contributing roots, it was usually found that when one of the roots that contributed largely to, for instance, a small digital collateral nerve had been severed, a very weak reply or no reply could be evoked from the proximal end of the digital nerve for a few minutes

immediately subsequent to the section of the root; but if tested about twenty
minutes later it gave a better reply, or even a smart reply, when previously
there had been none.   At first I imagined this the result of some adventitious
error in the excitation.   Later, one recognised the phenomenon as in some
degree or other of constant occurrence.   The same phenomenon has recurred
in the last quoted series of experiments in which instead of analysis of nerve-
twigs under electrical excitation, analysis of root-fields under mechanical
excitation has been the method.   If the isolated *field of response* was
delimited very soon after the posterior roots immediately above and below
that distributed to the root-field under examination had been severed, a field
was obtained of the approximate shape of the true root-field but smaller
than it, and curtailed especially in certain directions.   When examined later,
the field of response, determined by exactly the same method as before, was
found to have extended.   The following instances exemplify this phenomenon.

Experiment.—*M. rhesus.*   October 20, 1890.

The 5th, 6th, 7th, 9th, and 10th roots (posterior) of the post-thoracic region severed
on the right side, at 10.50.   At 11 o'clock the delimitation of the areas carried out first.
At 9.30 p.m. the delimitation of the areas carried out finally.   The lower limit of the

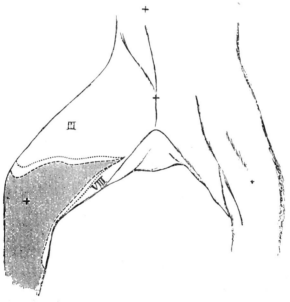

FIG. 3

8th root-field has travelled downward 3·5 cm., that of the 4th about 1·4 cm. at greatest.
The upper limit of the 6th and 8th root-fields combined had advanced about 0·8 cm.
toward the perineum at greatest.

Experiment.—*M. rhesus.*   May 4, 1891.

The posterior roots of the 4th, 5th, 6th, 7th, 9th, and 10th post-thoracic spinal nerves
of the right side severed in the spinal canal at 9.10 a.m.   At 9.20 the delimitation of the

field of the 8th post-thoracic root was carried on.   The result was that the lower margin was placed distinctly above the flexure of the knee.   (See Figs. 3 and 4, sketches made at the time.)   At 4 o'clock the field of the 8th root was delimited again, and without hesitation the lower margin of the area was placed distinctly in the flexure of the knee and in part for a certain distance below it.   (Figs. 3 and 4, the same sketch as before.)   The upper margin had also extended, but not so far, in the direction of the perineum and along the labium of the vulva.   It was especially noticeable that there had been no obvious extension along the border turned toward the field of the 3rd lumbar.   That is to say, the advance had been confined to the anterior and posterior borders of the root-field and had occurred but little at the dorsal and ventral borders.

The second of the two experiments quoted was performed to determine the nature of the " extension of the field " in regard to the two borders, and the rate of extension at different periods; regarding the latter point it was

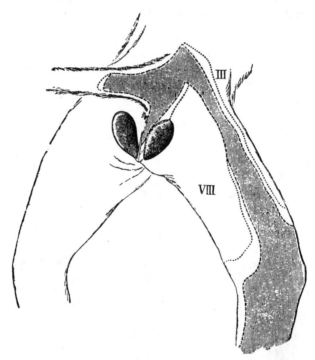

FIG. 4

found that the rate of " extension " was greatest in the first half-hour, and that in the third hour and afterwards there was little if any further progress of the field.   I have been used to call the initial lowering of response, the " local spinal depression," and the subsequent increase of response and the accompanying increase of the area of reply, the " local spinal exaltation," and the " extension of the field."   During the period of " local spinal depression " the responses besides being enfeebled are often of curiously long latency.   The period of " local spinal depression " has often seemed to me to be shortened in duration by repetition of excitations, even when these are at first inefficient to evoke obvious responses.[1]   The whole phenomenon appears quite comparable to the transient depression and subsequent exaltation of the " knee jerk " produced in, for instance, the cat by section of the spinal cord above the lumbar region.   And the briskness of the " jerk " may in like manner be increased by section in the spinal canal of the spinal roots, either sensory or motor, adjacent to that one most intimately concerned with the jerk, and especially of the muscular nerves to the antagonists of the " jerk " muscles.   In the field of a root immediately above severed roots, or immediately below severed roots, a marginal area of unmistakably exalted reflex reply is sometimes found.   This is due, I imagine, to the " local spinal exaltation " and is an evidence of the local character of the exaltation.   It may be essentially the same phenomenon as the hyperæsthetic zone bordering a paralysed area (Fodéra, 1823[2]) after lesions of the spinal cord itself.   The " local spinal exaltation " is of great assistance to the above method of delimiting the cutaneous spinal root-fields; the whole field of the root isolated by sections of adjacent roots is more or less affected by the exaltation.   In one of the experiments in which one-half the rootlets of the posterior division of the 6th lumbar spinal root were cut through after previous section of the adjacent roots, it seemed clear that in the plantar region the reflex response was *increased further* after the section of half the rootlets of the spinal root.   As to the length of time which the phenomenon lasts I can say little, but the exaltation of the knee jerk after section of adjacent roots I have seen persist for more than three months. Of course it must be remembered that in that case the loss of the tone of the muscles antagonistic to those on which the jerk depends may play a main part in the production of the exaggeration of the jerk.   The influence of a sensory root on the activity of the motor, or of blocking one motor root on the activity of another, is too far from the present experiments to be entered upon here, but I have attempted to see whether the " local spinal depression " could be demonstrated to affect the reaction of the anterior root to cortical excitation, and I have not been able to show that it does.

Further Samples of Lumbar and Sacral Segments

4th Post-thoracic.[3]

   Experiment.—M. *rhesus.*   Female; small.   November 17, 1890.   Figs. 5 and 10.
Measurement 8·5 cms. umbilicus to crest of pubes.
   The 10th and 11th thoracic and the highest three lumbar roots of the right side severed at 10.50.   Final determination of the anterior border of the 4th lumbar root at 7.10.
   " The anterior edge of the lower field of reply starts from the mid-dorsal line 0·2 cm. above the level of the crest of the ilium, descends to that crest, meeting it 1·2 cm. dorsal to the anterior superior spinous process; it crosses to 1 cm. below the anterior superior spine, running close below Poupart's ligament in its outer half, and turns down the limb

---

[1] An example of the physiological process called by Exner " Bahnung " (facilitation), *Pflüg. Arch. ges. Physiol.*, 1882, **28**, 487.
   [2] Magendie's " Journal de Physiologie," 1823, vol. 3, p. 191.   [3] From *loc. cit.*, p. 711.

just on the crest of the prominence of the rectus femoris; it follows that direction to as far as a point rather more than 3 cm. below the inguinal flexure, and then turning inwards soon doubles back across Scarpa's triangle to 1·4 cm. below Poupart's ligament. Then again it sweeps inward, and running for a short distance almost horizontally, approaches

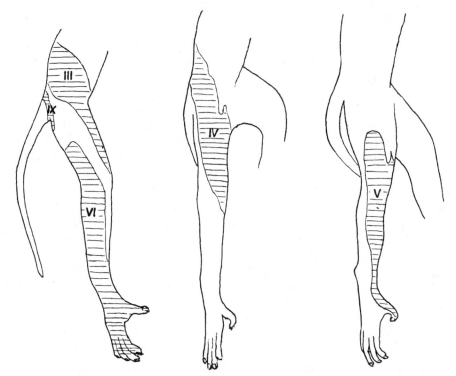

FIG. 5.—MACACUS

To show the extent of the 3rd, 4th, 5th, and 6th post-thoracic skin-fields (corresponding to 2nd, 3rd, 4th, and 5th L of man). Traced from photographs figured in the original plates (Figs. 7, 8, 16, Pl. 44, 47, *Philos. Trans.*, 1893, **184B**)

the mid-ventral line, not, however, to reach it, for turning downward about 1 cm. away from the mid-ventral line it strikes the genital fold 1·5 cm. from the angle of the notch."

Ribs twelve in number each side.

5th Post-thoracic.

Experiment.—*M. rhesus.* Male; young. November 24, 1890. Figs. 5, 8, and 10.

The two lowest thoracic nerve-roots and the 2nd, 3rd, 4th, 6th, 7th, 8th, 9th, and 10th post-thoracic roots of the right side severed at 9.10.

The isolated area of the 5th lumbar delimited at 5.20.

" The edge of the isolated field of reply passes from a point 1 cm. from the mid-ventral line, halfway between the top of the symphysis pubis and the root of the penis downward and outward, sloping across the inner aspect of the thigh to the mid-quadriceps line, which it crosses above the top of the patella about 1 cm. above the patella, and then retires up the thigh again for about 2 cm. to gain the outer aspect of the thigh and descend along the middle of it and the middle of the outer aspect of the knee over the peroneal group of muscles to the groove in front of the external malleolus; it enters the dorsum of the foot close to the outer side of the head of the astragalus, and somewhat distal to the tarso-metatarsal joint sweeps inwards, bisecting the first interdigital web. It curves round the hallux along the extreme limits of the aspect of the phalanges of the hallux, encroaching somewhat on the plantar surface along the inner edge, and passing distinctly on the plantar face of the foot about 1 cm. from the inner edge. It leaves the sole of the foot midway between calcaneum and internal malleolus to ascend on the inner edge of the tendo Achillis for 3 cm. before turning backward, always ascending, over the inner belly of the gastrocnemius to reach the fold of the inner hamstrings. The crest of that fold it gradually crosses, appearing on the prominence of the inner hamstring group at the postero-external aspect, about 2 cm. behind the scrotal flexure. It turns backward and inward so as to cross that fold again, and just in front of it, or on it, meets the point whence it started about 1 cm. from the ventral median line."

At the autopsy the ribs were found to be twelve in number.

9th Post-thoracic.

Experiment.—*M. rhesus.* Male. January 27, 1891. Figs. 5, 6, 7, and 10.

The posterior divisions (roots) of the 3rd, 4th, 5th, 7th, and 8th post-thoracic spinal nerves divided in the vertebral canal at 12.25 p.m. The anterior border of the 9th post-thoracic field delimited at 6.30.

"The upper edge of the lower field of reply starts from the mid-dorsal line about 5 cm. below the level of the anterior superior spine of the ileum; the lower edge of the

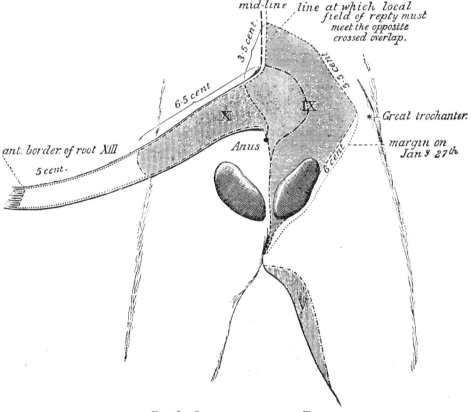

FIG. 6.—SKETCH MADE AT THE TIME

upper field of reply starts from the mid-dorsal line about on a level with the anterior superior spine, and the level at which the upper edge of the lower field lies at the mid-dorsum is about midway between the anterior superior spine and the ischial tuberosity.

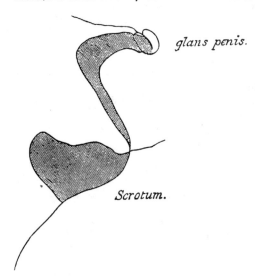

glans penis.

Scrotum.

FIG. 7.—SKETCH MADE AT THE TIME

From that point the margin runs outwards, at first sloping downwards, then sloping more abruptly, and then turning inwards and downwards, so as to sweep about 0·5 cm. outside the lower and lateral edge of the callosity and then runs forward under the inner edge of thigh up on to the front of the trunk along the lateral edge of the scrotum nearly as high as the root of the penis; at the root of the penis it meets the field of the upper roots."

At 7.30 the 1st lumbar root was severed on right side.

" The lower field of reply on scrotum extends to same points as before, and it is now clear that replies from the side of the penis and from the glans penis which were taken to be part of the field of the upper roots belong to the lower roots. It is not clear that the little area of reply which extends along the side of the penis and one-half the glans composes a field quite continuous with the scrotal field, because the replies are not obtained from absolutely the root of the organ; the penile field and the scrotal field are nearly continuous, but not quite, in this individual." (Fig. 7.)

The penile and scrotal fields disappeared on section of the 9th post-thoracic root.

CONCLUSIONS AS TO THE SEGMENTAL ARCHITECTURE

Conclusions

When the facts of the above arrangement are compared with those found to exist in the frog,[1] it will be seen that considerable differences between the two schemes of distribution become apparent. It seems well to return to the conclusions arrived at for Rana, and examine the extent of their applicability to Macacus.

1. Although in a plexus each spinal nerve-root affords separate contributions to many several nerve-trunks in the plexus, the cutaneous distribution of the root is composed, not of patches which are disjoined, but of patches which are so joined that the distribution of the entire root forms one continuous field.

Looking over the areas determined for Macacus in the foregoing experiments, it is seen that, just as in the leg of the frog, so with the nerve-roots of

[1] The segmental innervation of the skin of the frog is described earlier in the same paper. *Philos. Trans.*, 1893, **184B**, 652.—ED.

the trunk and lower limb of *M. rhesus*, each root possesses a single undivided field of cutaneous distribution, not a field composed of separated patches. This is a point to which attention was always paid in the experiments, because it was remembered that Türck found evidence of such " divided " fields in the case of certain nerve-roots—viz., the 2nd and 3rd thoracic roots of the dog; also because such an arrangement might exist with the more completely branched plexus of Macacus, although absent from the simpler type of the frog. In Maca-

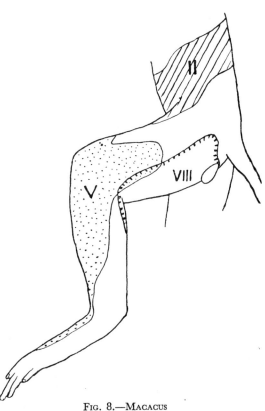

cus no evidence of this division of the skin-field of the root was found. There was once noticed, it is true, in an experiment upon the 2nd thoracic root, a small area, about an inch long, which *appeared* to be not perfectly continuous with the otherwise perfectly continuous field of reply referable to that root; but this outlying islet did not appear in other delimitations of the 2nd thoracic field, and it was well within the limits of error which must be acknowledged for the experiments. My experimental fields probably understate, perhaps in certain directions considerably, the real area of skin-field of the root. The above apparent exception to the general statement is therefore mentioned, but is not believed to really modify the statement. Another instance of an outlying islet

FIG. 8.—MACACUS

To show lateral view of 2nd and 5th lumbar (1 and 4L of man) skin segments and the overlapping between 5th and 8th post-thoracic (4L and 2S, man) along the dorsal axial line (*Philos. Trans.*, 1893, **184B,** tracing of Fig. 18)

of æsthesia, apparently detached from the general field at the rest of the root, occurred in an experiment on the 9th post-thoracic. One-half of the scrotum is included in the field of the 9th post-thoracic, and also the corresponding half of the penis, but I could not demonstrate the conjunction of the scrotal and penile fields at the root of the penis. I think this probably due to my experimental field being a minimal representation of the true root-field, and that probably the skin at the root of the penis is included in the root-field, and through it the penile and scrotal fields are conjoined.

Similarity of the root-compositions of neighbouring nerve-twigs that are near their destination is a necessity of the above arrangement. Thus, the dorsal collateral digital nerve on the tibial side of a digit will resemble in composition the plantar collateral digital on the tibial side of the same digit, and this is exemplified in the table of analysis of peripheral nerves given above. This is comparable to the similarity of root composition exhibited by the several motor twigs entering a skeletal muscle in the limb. Thus, the tibialis anticus receives fibres from the anterior roots of at least two spinal nerves entering the plexus, and receives those fibres by several separate nerve-branches entering the muscle; in each of the nerve-branches will be found a proportion of fibres from each of the roots supplying the muscle, and in fairly similar proportions in all. But there are exceptions, thus the upper and lower nerves to the sartorius, the upper nerves containing the fibres from the 3rd and 4th lumbar roots, the lower from the 4th and 5th lumbar roots. So also adductor magnus.

On the dorsum of the foot a somewhat curious anatomical arrangement of the peripheral nerves to the skin of the toes is the interposition between the digitales communes from the musculo-cutaneous trunk of a similar trunk for the cleft between hallux and 2nd digit supplied from the anterior tibial nerve. I looked with some interest to see whether the root-composition of the branch from the anterior tibial would fall into series with the arrangement of the root-composition of the digitals from the musculo-cutaneous. In the latter, as traced from the tibial toward the fibular edge of the foot—*i.e.*, from the preaxial toward the postaxial border—the proportion of fibres from the 5th lumbar root rapidly diminishes to disappearance, a proportion of fibres from the 7th lumbar root appears and gradually increases. In Rhesus (and also in cat) experiments disclose that the branch from the anterior tibial falls into perfect series with the rest as far as its root-composition is concerned, and can be analysed by the experiments above. The case is comparable with that of the external saphenous nerve in Macacus and the plantar muscles.[1] Despite the existence of some latitude of individual variation (*vide infra*), the connection between the position of the central end of a sensory nerve-fibre and that of the peripheral end is, in one and the same individual, definite and fixed enough. In other words, the mutual relationship between the position of points composing a region of the body is specific, the absolute position of the whole region is largely individual.

2. The field of skin belonging to each sensory spinal nerve-root overlaps the skin-fields of the neighbouring spinal nerve-roots to a remarkable extent. The disposition is such that the field laps to a certain extent over the field of the root or roots immediately in front of it, and to a certain extent over the field of the sensory roots immediately behind it. These two overlaps may be termed respectively the anterior overlap and the posterior overlap of the sensory root-field.

The above conclusion is applicable without modification to the arrange-

[1] Sherrington, *J. Physiol.*, 1892, **13**, 739.

ment existing in Macacus. The overlap is very great, so great indeed that each point of skin is supplied by two spinal nerve-roots, and some, it would appear, by three. And this overlap is true for the nerves of the trunk as well as for those of the limb. Thus the nipple is a point of skin which lies in the field of the 4th thoracic root, often a little nearer the posterior than the anterior border of that field. Now the nipple is included also in the experimental field of the 5th thoracic root, the anterior border of which passes above it; and the nipple was found on two of three occasions on which the posterior border of the field of the 3rd thoracic root was examined to lie demonstrably in the experimental field of that root, although on one occasion the border passed just above the nipple itself, including only the areola above the nipple. In the foot the mid-point of the border of the web between hallux and 2nd digit is included in the experimentally demonstrable field of the 5th lumbar root; it is also generally included in the experimentally demonstrable fields of the 5th lumbar and 7th lumbar roots, but it lies at

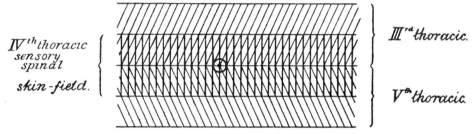

FIG. 9.—DIAGRAM OF THE POSITION OF THE NIPPLE IN THE SENSORY SKIN-FIELDS OF THE FOURTH, THIRD AND FIFTH THORACIC SPINAL ROOTS

the very confines of those fields. The skin of the upper part of the ham is included in the fields of the 7th and 8th post-thoracic roots.

Acknowledging that the size of the experimental skin-fields is somewhat smaller than the size of the skin-fields in reality, I conclude that the anterior and posterior overlaps are extensive enough in the monkey to provide that the skin, taken along any line parallel with the plane of segmentation of the body in the region in which the line is taken, is supplied by two adjacent posterior roots. It further seems certain that in several places the skin is supplied by three adjacent posterior roots, more by the middle of the three roots, less by the foremost and by the hindmost of the three roots individually taken. Possibly skin in which the interlap is thus triple instead of double exists along the centre of the cutaneous segments of the body. In the sole (cat) the anterior border of the skin-field of the lowest of three[1] roots overlaps the posterior border of the skin-field of the highest root of the three. The amount of supply given to its skin-field by any one root appears to vary in different parts of the field, and it is usual for the border of the field to be less richly supplied than the rest of the field. Thus

[1] These are 6th, 7th, and 8th post-thoracic.

the nipple lies about midway in the field of the 4th cutaneous segment of the thorax, and it is in each normal individual probably supplied by the 5th thoracic and the 3rd thoracic afferent roots, as well as by the 4th. It would therefore lie in one of the narrow zones of triple interlap above mentioned. I have met with an instance in which it was included in the anterior edge of the 6th thoracic skin-field.[1] In the trunk the degree of overlap of the skin-fields often seems to be less near the mid-dorsal and mid-ventral lines than on the lateral aspect at some distance from those lines. It must be remembered that the nipple lies in this lateral region, and so also, as I shall point out later, does the foot with its digits, again a region of remarkable overlapping.

Beside the anterior and posterior overlaps, the cutaneous field of each posterior root oversteps the median line of the body both ventrally and dorsally. This crosslap of right- and left-hand nerves is not so extensive as the overlap fore and aft. It is comparable with the lapping across the dorsal median line of the distribution of the pilomotor nerves in the monkey and cat described by Langley and myself.[2] It seems to vary in Macacus in different regions. It seems more marked along the mid-ventral line than along the mid-dorsal line, and I have seen it remarkably extensive on the penis and close below the xiphoid. I do not think I have ever seen it amount to more than a full centimetre in Macacus, but all the specimens have been small and the crosslap might be larger in larger individuals. The amount of supply by the root to the cross-lapping border of the field appears relatively small compared to elsewhere in the field, in fact it resembles in this way the extreme border of the forelapping and after-lapping portions of the skin-field.

[3]On comparing the segmental arrangement of the skin of the limb with that of the musculature of the limb, a difference becomes evident between them that is true of the fore limb as well as of the hind. I have in a previous paper shown that the limb, as regards its musculature, is composed of rays extending at right angles to the long axis of the trunk, and arranged in fore-and-aft series in such a way that the pelvic limb has a sloping anterior edge, into the composition of which enter four rays, each extending further into the limb than the ray preceding it. The posterior edge of the limb is abrupt and composed in its whole length by one ray only, the 6th, or most posterior of those which contribute to the limb musculature at all. The 5th ray, like the 6th, extends from the base to the free apex of the limb. A similar scheme of structure for the anterior limb is evidenced by the root-supply to the musculature of it; there also the posterior border of the limb is not formed by segments extending stepwise down into it, but is abrupt and formed by the ray of the 2nd thoracic segment. With this arrangement of the musculature the segmentation of the skin of the limb does not correspond. In the skin of the limb the posterior border, like the anterior

[1] The difficulty is to estimate coincidently the overlapping and the individual variation.
[2] *J. Physiol.*, 1891, **12**, 278.   [3] From *loc. cit.*, p. 749.

border, is constituted by a series of overlapping segments and not by a single segment; and this is true of both anterior and posterior limbs alike (Figs. 10 and 11.) The segmental arrangement of skin and musculature is also different in another respect.

The motor spinal roots supplying the muscles of the limb, even those

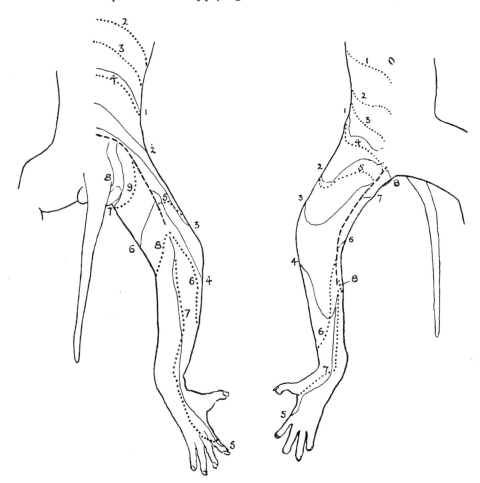

FIG. 10.—MACACUS: THE LUMBO-SACRAL SKIN-FIELDS

The headward border of each field is shown as a dotted line marked with corresponding number. The hinder border is shown as a continuous line. The numbers are in consecutive post-thoracic segments (6L monkey—5L in man, 7L monkey—1S in man). The mid-dorsal and mid-ventral lines are shown as heavy broken lines. Traced from the original photographic figures (Figs. 20, 21 with details 22, 23, *Philos. Trans.*, 1893, **184B**, Pl. 49-51)

roots which penetrate farthest into the limb, all of them contribute still to the supply of the muscles of the trunk. That is to say, the segments of the limb musculature are not detached from the mid-axis of the trunk. The 5th muscular ray of the pelvic limb which contributes to the musculature of the limb in even the free apex of the limb never loses its base in the axial muscles of the trunk, and gives a share to such axial trunk muscles as the sacro-coccygeus. So also does the 6th ray.

On the other hand, at the surface of the limb the segments of the skin seem to be actually dislocated from their attachment to the dorsal and ventral axes of the trunk; they appear to be detached from the mid-dorsal and mid-ventral lines of the body. Into the base of the limb the mid-dorsal line of the body thrusts sidewise a branch, a secondary lateral axis, almost at right angles to its own direction. The mid-ventral line behaves in a like manner. These are the *mid-dorsal* and *mid-ventral lines of the limb* (see Fig. 10). Upon these secondary dorsal and ventral axes the cutaneous segments of the limb are ranged, as though upon folded portions of the axial lines of the trunk itself. It must be remembered the distribution revealed in the cutaneous fields is probably an arrangement literally *only skin deep*. The difference between the arrangement shown for the motor root and that for the sensory root may be really *less* due to the comparison being of *efferent* with *afferent* distribution, than to the comparison being of *muscle* with *skin*. From such glimpses as I have occasionally obtained of afferent fibres from muscles (*e.g.*, afferents for knee jerk, afferents of antagonistics of "jerk" muscles), these afferent fibres seem to belong strictly to the same segments as supply motor fibres to their muscles.

It is interesting to note that no cutaneous branches can be found by dissection to be given from the posterior primary divisions of the 5th and 6th post-thoracic nerves of *Macacus rhesus*—at least, I have failed to find any. The muscles of the back do receive branches from the posterior primary divisions of these nerves, and in the musculature of the back the nerves end. Swan[1] says of the 4th and 5th lumbar nerves of man that the posterior primary divisions of them give off no cutaneous branches. The same is true of the 7th, 8th, and sometimes 6th cervical nerves. Türck[2] says that in the dog the 4th, 5th, 6th, and 7th lumbar nerves yield no supply to skin by their posterior divisions. This apparent absence of cutaneous distribution by the posterior primary divisions of these nerves is, I would suggest, a sign that they are at the very centre of the limb region—the region in which the skin segments have slipped outward down the limb. It is a point which apparently escaped Ross,[3] and is unrecognised in his suggestive essay.

In *Macacus rhesus* to the cutaneous surface of the anterior aspect of the hind-limb six segments contribute, the 1st, 2nd, 3rd, 4th, 5th, and 6th post-thoracic; to that of the posterior aspect four segments, the 6th, 7th, 8th, and 9th post-thoracic; to the cutaneous surface of the posterior aspect of the fore-limb five segments contribute, the 5th, 4th, 3rd, 2nd, and 1st thoracic; to that of the anterior aspect of the limb six segments contribute, the 3rd, 4th, 5th, 6th, 7th, and 8th cervical. There is thus a curious agree-

[1] Joseph Swan, *Demonstration of the Nerves*, London, 1834.
[2] *Denkschrift der Wien. Akad.*, 1869, **29.**   [3] *Brain*, 1888, **10,** 333.

ment in the number of segments contributing to the surfaces of the fore- and hind-limbs. And in each the anterior aspect is seen to be segmentally more extensive than the posterior, just as was found to be the case with the musculature of it.

The number of segments contributing to the skin of the limb is seen to be greater than the number of segments contributing to its musculature. From the examination of the motor fibres of the lumbo-sacral plexus, it was concluded that the limb, " plastic, like the rest of the body, has been moulded by variation and by function, but not so rudely as seriously to obscure its segmental plan." The segmentation at the surface of the limb

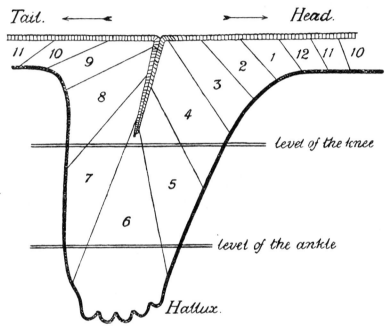

FIG. 11.—SCHEME OF THE SENSORY SPINAL SKIN-FIELDS OF THE HIND-LIMB OF *Macacus rhesus*
The overlapping is not indicated

presents, as has just been shown, certain characters different from the segmentation of the deeper parts. From examination of the segmentation of the skeletal muscle of the limb, it was concluded that " the quadrifid or quinquifid digital partition of the free end of the limb does not imply that respectively four or five segments are prolonged into the apex of the limb."[1]

In like manner, with the cutaneous segmentation of the limb, the quadrifid or quinquifid digital partition at the end of the limb has nothing to do. The skin of the four pedal digits of the cat belong to three of the cutaneous segments in common (6th, 7th, 8th post-thoracic). The skin of the five pedal digits of Macacus belong to three of the cutaneous segments

[1] Sherrington, *J. Physiol.*, 1892, **13**, 767.

in common (the 5th, 6th, 7th lumbar). I have shown elsewhere and in the present paper that the 5th segment of Macacus is the 6th of cat. The skin of the hallux, therefore, of Macacus is produced by an extension of the skin of the segment, which is the 6th in the cat, and is formed by the excrescence of another digit from a segment already bearing digits, and not by the introduction of another segment into the foot.

In describing experiments on the motor fibres to the muscles of the foot and hand, I have mentioned that it is extremely difficult to get any evidence that the intrinsic musculature of the 1st digit is segmentally anterior to the intrinsic musculature of the 5th digit. But the evidence that the skin of the 1st digit is segmentally anterior to the skin of the 5th digit is from the above experiments definite enough; the skin of hallux is shown to be segmentally anterior to skin of secundus, that of secundus to that of tertius, and so on; the skin of the dorsum of the foot is shown to be segmentally anterior to the skin of the plantar aspect.

SAMPLES OF SKIN-FIELDS SUPPLIED BY ROOTS ENTERING INTO THE BRACHIAL PLEXUS

6th Cervical Dorsal Root[1] (*Figs.* 12 *and* 13)

This skin-field has been delimited completely in four individuals, and incompletely in two more.

Example.—*M. rhesus.* ♀, young. At 9 a.m. the posterior roots of the 3rd, 4th, 5th, 7th, and 8th cervical, and of the 1st, 2nd, and 3rd thoracic nerves were severed in the vertebral canal. The isolated field of response, due to the intact 6th cervical root, was finally delimited about 5 p.m. See Figs. 12 and 13.

" The field of response is limited by a line which starts from a point on the infraspinous fossa of the scapula near the edge of the deltoid muscle. The line crosses the lateral part of the infraspinous fossa obliquely and turns down the arm behind the posterior border of the deltoid muscle. It descends the arm lengthwise, well on the triceps side of the furrow, between the masses of the extensors and flexors of the elbow. It enters the forearm close behind the outer condyle, and thence passes in an almost straight line to reach the radial side of the index finger, where on the proximal phalanx it recurves. The line returns across the palm to the forearm over about the middle of the thenar eminence; it crosses the wrist on the radial side of the lower radio-ulnar joint. On the flexor aspect of the forearm it ascends close to the ulnar side of the prominence made by the supinators of the wrist and long extensors of the fingers. It crosses the flexure of the elbow about the middle of it, and climbs the prominence over the flexors of the elbow somewhat to the ulnar side of the middle line of the biceps. Close above the junction of the limb with the trunk the line turns outward and downward, and sweeping below and round the deltoid muscle reaches the spot on the infraspinous fossa whence it was traced."

Variation

In the first experiment the field traced was closely similar to the above; in a third experiment it did not appear to extend lower than the styloid

[1] From *Philos. Trans.*, 1898, **190B**, 82, where the skin segments of all the cervical nerves are described and illustrated.—ED.

process of the radius, and I convinced myself it did not include the thumb, for the observation was repeated many times in the course of twenty-four days. When the animal was finally examined, electrical excitation of the central end of the musculo-cutaneous nerve, about 3 inches below the elbow, elicited smart reflexes. In a fourth individual nearly the whole length of the radial side of the index finger was included in the field.

There must, therefore, be a considerable degree of variation in the extent to which this nerve contributes to the sensation of the skin of the hand. The thumb, and even one-half of the index finger, in some individuals, enter into the composition of the field, but in some they do not.

7th Cervical Dorsal Root

This skin-field has been delimited completely in four individuals and incompletely in a fifth.

Example.—*M. rhesus.* ♀, young. At 11.15 a.m. the posterior roots of the 3rd, 4th, 5th, 6th, and 8th cervical, and of the 1st, 2nd, 3rd, 4th, 5th, and 6th thoracic nerves of the right side divided. The isolated field of response due to the 7th cervical being intact was finally delimited at 4.30 p.m.

"The field of response is limited by a line which is traceable from the radial side of the cleft between the 3rd and 4th digits, and runs along the palm on the radial edge of the main longitudinal furrow. From the palm it takes an almost rectilinear course ascending the flexor aspect of the forearm along the hollow between the flexor and the supinator groups of muscles. It attains the radial side of the biceps tendon and then mounts the swelling prominence of the biceps muscle; at first it fairly bisects the surface of this prominence longitudinally, but higher up the line tends outward and ascends over the insertion of the deltoid muscle, and then recurves abruptly downward below the insertion of the deltoid and again bends upward behind the deltoid: once more abruptly recurving it descends and follows the groove between extensors and flexors of elbow-joint. The line enters the extensor surface of the forearm closely behind the head of the radius and well in front of the olecranon process of the ulna. It runs down the back of the forearm nearer the ulnar than the radial edge, especially in the distal half of the region. The line enters the dorsal surface of the hand by passing over the joint between ulna and radius, and runs to the mid-point of the knuckle of the ring finger and down the back of the proximal phalanx of that finger for a short distance. Finally, the line turns abruptly outward to reach the cleft between the middle and the ring fingers, and attains there the point from which it was traced."

The individual variation met with in examining this field has been slight, but in two cases the field included all but the ulnar face of the ring-finger. In another (Fig. 16, p. 68) it included part of ring-finger.

8th Cervical Dorsal Root

This skin-field has been delimited completely in three individuals, incompletely in a fourth and fifth.

Example.—*M. rhesus.* ♂ strong, young. At 10 a.m. the 5th, 6th, and 7th cervical, and the 1st, 2nd, 3rd, 4th, and 5th thoracic roots of the right side severed in the vertebral canal.

" An isolated *field of response*, that supplied by 8th cervical root, was finally delimited at 4.30 p.m.   This field was contained within the following boundary.   From a point about one-quarter the way up the outer edge of the upper arm in the furrow between the biceps and triceps muscles the boundary slopes abruptly back across the triceps for

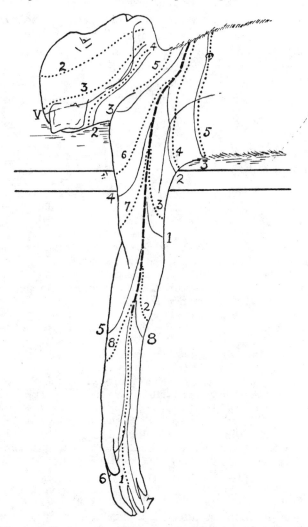

FIG. 12.—MACACUS: TO SHOW THE EXTENT OF THE CERVICAL AND UPPER THORACIC
SKIN-FIELDS

The headward border of each field is shown in dotted line marked with corresponding number, the hinder border is shown as a continuous line numbered at the periphery.   The mid-ventral axial line is shown as a heavy broken line (*Philos. Trans.*, 1898, **190B,** Figs. 4 and 5, redrawn)

about 2 centimetres, and then recurves at less than a right angle to pass downward between the olecranon and the outer condyle of the humerus and gain the forearm.   It descends the outer side of the extensor surface of the forearm for about one-third the way to the wrist, and then slants toward the ulnar side and attains the ulnar edge about one-third up the forearm.   It slopes round as far as the flexor aspect of the ulnar edge and then sharply recurves on itself, tending upward and outward across the face of the flexor aspect of the forearm to a point about two-fifths up the flexor aspect of the forearm and midway between its radial and ulnar borders. Thence the line of boundary returns and descends just to the ulnar side of the pronator longus tendon. Close above the wrist it slopes outward and attains a point 1 centimetre above the styloid process of the radius; from that

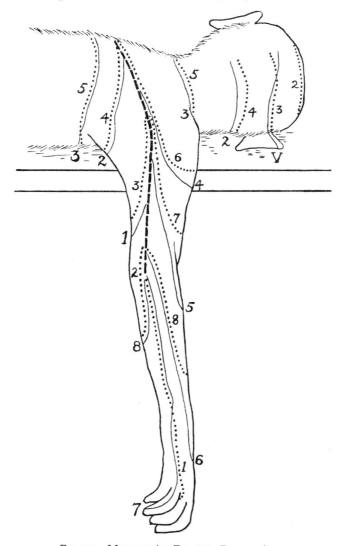

Fig. 13.—Macacus (as Fig. 12): Dorsal Aspect

the line runs up the forearm on the outer face of the prominence caused by the prominence of the group of supinator muscles, and it ascends finally the furrow between biceps and triceps to the point whence it was originally traced."

The agreement between the limits of this field in the individuals observed has been singularly close; the discrepancies have been too small to be clearly outside the limits of errors inherent in the experimental testing of the skin. The analogy between the cutaneous distribution of the 8th cervical in the fore-limb, and of the 6th lumbar (5th lumbar of man) in the hind-limb, is curiously great. Each supplies the skin covering the whole free apex of the limb to which it belongs, and each has anterior to it a nerve-root which supplies the skin of only the anterior side of the free apex of the limb, and each has next behind it a nerve-root that supplies the skin of only the posterior portion of the free apex of the limb.

Although this (8th cervical) skin-field extends further along the radial edge of the forearm than along the ulnar edge, it was noted in each of the experiments made that when the " contracted field " was examined, the reply from the pollex was much less brisk than from the fifth digit; also, the reply from the radial side of the forearm was gradually developed under " extension of the field." The centre of the field in the hand lies, therefore, in all probability nearer to the ulnar than to the radial border.

1st Thoracic Dorsal Root (Figs. 12 *and* 13)

Example.—M. rhesus. At 9.30 a.m. the posterior roots of the 5th, 6th, 7th, and 8th cervical and of the 2nd, 3rd, and 4th thoracic nerves of right side cut in the spinal canal. At 6 p.m. the skin-field of the 1st thoracic was finally determined.

" The field of response isolated is limited by a line traceable as follows: From a point in the flexure of the elbow superficial to the biceps tendon and thence down the front of the forearm and across the wrist a little to the radial side of the inferior radio-ulnar articulation along the palm in a straight line to the cleft between middle and ring fingers, thence along the radial side of the ring-finger as far as the last phalanx, on the radial face of which it recurves and runs back along the dorsal face of the middle and proximal phalanges to the hand. On the dorsum of the hand it takes a fairly straight course, passes over the back of the inferior radio-ulnar joint, and climbs the forearm along the extensor aspect to the external condyle of the humerus, and passes a centimetre or more above that. The line then makes a curious and characteristic rectangular bend, winding round the olecranon to the inner condyle of the humerus, and then tending up the arm along the axillary face of the coraco-brachialis, and making for a point just below the insertion of the deltoid. The line, when it has nearly reached the deltoid insertion, recurves and then passes down the skin over the biceps to the point whence it was traced; it thus includes a tongue-shaped area pointed upwards on the lower part of the flexor and axillary surface of the upper arm."

Varieties.—In one individual a little of the ulnar side of the middle finger and the whole of the ring finger, and in another individual (Figs. 16 and 17, pp. 68 and 69) the whole of the ring and middle fingers and a piece of the ulnar side of the root of the index, were included in the field of the 1st thoracic. This is not usual.

This skin-field has been delimited in eight individuals—in five for the present paper, in three for my previous communication.

I am inclined to think that on this skin-field, which seems a little post-fixed as compared with the human, rests some of the best evidence that the human brachial plexus, and therefore the skin and musculature of the arm of man, are somewhat prefixed as compared with Macacus. In man the 1st thoracic sends a branch back to join the 2nd thoracic (cutaneous), but it does not do so in the Macaques I have dissected.

COMPARISON OF SEGMENTAL ANATOMY OF MACACUS AND MAN[1]

A few words are desirable regarding the comparison between the segmental anatomy of man and of Macacus in this region. Beyond question the similarity between the two is almost minutely exact. The most salient point of difference appears in the motor distribution of the 2nd thoracic root, which is not generally considered to contribute to the brachial plexus in man. Its contribution is of almost universal occurrence in the animals used in the laboratory. I have tested the point by dissection and stimulation in the dog, cat,[2] horse, rabbit, and rat, as well as in monkeys, and find it among the types examined of inconstant presence in the cat and dog only: it is more frequently absent in cat than in dog, and sometimes on one side only. That a communicating branch often passes in man from 2nd thoracic to 1st thoracic has been seen by Cunningham,[3] who found it in 70 per cent. of the individuals examined. If the 2nd thoracic does not really contribute to the human brachial plexus, the plexus of man is prefixed as compared with that of the other types. Now in the Macaque the rectus capitis anticus major is supplied not from the 1st cervical root as in man. The *scaleni*, all three, are present in Macaque as in man, but they receive a more posterior root supply than in man, the upper two thoracic roots contributing to their innervation, whereas the 2nd and 3rd cervical roots do not contribute to them in Macacus, though they do so in man. In the Macaque I have in one individual found the 3rd cervical motor root innervating the diaphragm (ventral part), but in one instance only. Concordantly with this the 6th cervical in Macacus I have found to supply the diaphragm regularly (examination by degeneration and " teasing," as well as by excitation method). In a Macaque in which the 7th right cervical nerve had been severed twelve days, I failed to discover degenerate fibres in the phrenic trunk. In man the phrenic " arises mainly from the 4th nerve, also receiving in the majority of instances an additional root from either the 3rd or the 5th nerve " (Thane).[4] On the other hand, in his *Anatomy of Domesticated Animals*, Chauveau describes the phrenic as arising mainly from the 6th and 7th nerves, with a subsidiary branch from the 5th. As judged by the root-constitution of the phrenic nerve, therefore,

---

[1] Extract from *Philos. Trans.*, 1898, **190B**, 89 *et seq.*

[2] My results on this point were demonstrated to the Physiological Society, February 13, 1892. At that date Dr. Langley had already (January 20) sent in a paper to the Royal Society (" Origin of the Cervical and Upper Thoracic Fibres of the Sympathetic." Read February 18. *Philos. Trans.*, B, 1892) in which, as regards the cat and rabbit, results similar to my own had been arrived at. July 10, 1897, C. S. S.

[3] *J. Anat. and Physiol.*, 1877, **11**, iii., 539.   [4] Quain's *Anatomy*, 1895, **3**, pt. 2, 288.

the muscles innervated by the brachial region of the cord are more prefixed in man than in the other mammalian types coming under observation, including monkey. It may be, therefore, that in a certain number of human brachial plexuses the 2nd thoracic does not contribute to the innervation of the hand muscles; and certainly in Macacus the amount of contribution by it varies, for I have in some individuals failed to evoke contraction of the deep flexor of the forearm through it, though this is often readily done. On the other hand again, it is possible that the segmental position of diaphragm (or rather of phrenic nerve) may vary independently of that of the musculature (or nerve-trunks) of the limb; but this supposition is not in harmony with the rule I found deducible from the lumbo-sacral plexus —viz., " the shifting up or down of the region of outflow along the cord applies to all the efferent fibres of that length "; in other words, although each muscle (nerve-trunk) is displaced absolutely, it is not displaced relatively to its neighbours. Langley's researches on the sympathetic show that, to use my own nomenclature, the cervical sympathetic is more prefixed in the cat and dog than in the rabbit, a fact in accord with the not infrequent absence of the contribution from 2nd thoracic noted above in the cat (and dog). Klumpke's conclusion from clinical data, that in man the dilatators of the pupil emerge from cord *entirely* in the 1st thoracic root, is almost certainly not correct. We know of no type, including monkey, in which the outflow of dilatators is limited to one root, and Brun's case[1] shows that in man some leave by a root lower than 1st thoracic. Yet Klumpke's evidence makes it probable that they leave in man *chiefly* by 1st thoracic. If so, then the evidence from the sympathetic, and also from the phrenic, points to the nerves and muscles of this region in man being prefixed as compared with Macacus and the laboratory types. This fact may be remembered in connection with the reduction of sensory roots which seems to be in progress at the top of the neck; the ganglion of the hypoglossal and that of the 1st cervical roots, both present in Ruminants, the latter present in the cat and rabbit, have both disappeared in Macacus and in man.

As to the spinal skin-fields of Macacus and of man, clinical opportunities arise for observing some of the latter sufficiently to give ground for brief examination of the correspondence between the two. The opportunities of the bedside have afforded the basis for the admirable papers of Thorburn, Head, James Mackenzie, Starr, and Kocher. In regard to the 4th cervical, Starr's[2] determination of the posterior edge tallies closest in general level with that of Macacus; Head's[3] determination in shape of contour, the curious double shoulder peak of Macacus appearing with fidelity in man. In regard to the 5th cervical, there is close agreement between all the clinical observers and the experiments on Macacus; in the photograph of one of my experiments the posterior border of Macaque's skin-field must have agreed point for point with Thorburn's figure of that border;

[1] *Arch. Psychiat. Nervenkr.*, 1893, **25**, 759.   [2] *Brain*, 1894, **17**, 481.   [3] *Ibid.*, 1894, **17**, 339.

Mackenzie's[1] figure also gives almost exactly the same situation for it. In the clinical determination of the posterior border of 6th cervical the limit given it on the hand in Brun's case agrees absolutely with that part of one of my photographs of Macacus. But, as stated above, I found frequent slight variation of this border in Macacus, and the more usual position of the border in Macacus is one agreeing accurately with Williamson's case, and with the right hand in Herter's case.[2] These cases go far to show that the agreement in this region between Macacus and man is very close, extending even to details of individual variation. Head's upper patch—a deltoid patch—of the 6th cervical field is included quite identically by Macacus. As to the 7th cervical, Thorburn's Fig. 5, which he suggests[3] is the 7th cervical (of course, its posterior border only), closely follows the lines of Macacus, except that it takes in the ulnar edge of ring finger, which I have never seen quite reached by it in Macaque. The 7th cervical area of Head in the hand represents with remarkable accuracy the central strip of the same field in Macacus, for it is a strip equidistant from the anterior and posterior borders of that field. Also the 8th field of Macacus has extensor and flexor peaks resembling those of Head's field. Between the fields of the 1st thoracic in man as determined by Head and that experimentally delimited in Macacus the correspondence is again strikingly close, the latter being, as is inseparable from the difference of the two methods of determination, rather the more extensive; the determinations of the other clinicians for this root are not in good agreement with Macacus. In view of the above discussion as to whether the 2nd thoracic nerve contributes to the muscles of the arm in man as in Macacus, the degree of correspondence between the skin-field of the root in the two cases is of special interest. Now, Mackenzie's figure (a case of herpetic eruption) displays a distribution of the root closely similar to that in Macacus, and Head's area, determined both by herpetic eruption and by reference in visceral disease, gives a still completer correspondence. Other clinical observers do not describe the 2nd thoracic field. The correspondence between this field in man, as described by Head and Mackenzie, is so close as not to indicate that man's plexus is more prefixed than Macaque's. It is true that one occasionally meets with sensory roots and motor roots varying independently as regards pre- and postfixture; but that is not the rule. I cannot, therefore, help suspecting that our textbooks on human anatomy may err in omitting the 2nd thoracic nerve from the human brachial plexus, although I think the above observations prove a certain degree of prefixture in the prevailing type of human brachial plexus as compared with Macaque's—in this point resembling the cat's plexus—as compared with Macacus, rabbit, dog, and rat. The fact that in Macacus the 1st thoracic does not, as it does in man, send usually a branch to join the 2nd thoracic, points in the direction of slight prefixture in man, as does the muscular analysis. But Head's and

[1] *J. Path. Bact.*, 1893, **1**, 332.   [2] *Brain*, 1886-7, **9**, 510, and 1888-9, **11**, 289.
[3] See Starr, *loc cit.*, for summary and diagram.

Mackenzie's observations of the area of the 2nd thoracic in man seem to prove that the amount of his prefixture is after all small. It is certainly smaller in this region than in the lumbo-sacral, where, as I have shown in my previous papers, both in regard to muscle and skin the human lies one whole segment in front of (*i.e.*, prefixed in comparison with) the Macaque type.

VARIATION IN THE EXTENT OF OVERLAPPING OF THE SEGMENTAL SKIN-FIELDS IN DIFFERENT REGIONS[1]

In my previous paper[2] I stated that " I conclude that the anterior and posterior overlaps are extensive enough in the monkey to provide that the skin taken along any line parallel with the plane of the segmentation is supplied by two adjacent posterior roots. It further seems certain that in some places the skin is supplied by three adjacent posterior roots." In instance of skin receiving a triple root supply, I mentioned a part of the planta of the cat and the nipple of the monkey. To these I will add portions of the skin of the hand, where a triple overlap is clearly demonstrable by the following experiment: The 8th cervical dorsal (sensory) root of Macacus having been severed both on left and right sides in the vertebral canal, there are further severed on one side (*e.g.*, right) the dorsal (sensory) roots of the 7th, 6th, and 5th cervical nerves, on the opposite side (*e.g.*, left) the dorsal roots of the 1st, 2nd, and 3rd thoracic nerves. The field of remaining æsthesia is then delimited in each hand. The lines of boundary will on the one hand be those of the posterior border of the 7th cervical field, on the other hand, those of the anterior border of the 1st thoracic field. Now, as shown above, the field of the 8th cervical nerve includes every portion of the surface of the whole hand. Further, although a certain amount of asymmetry can be detected in some individuals in the root-distribution of right and left sides, it is of great rarity in the lower extremity, and even more uncommon in the upper extremity, and is always quite small in extent. If, therefore, in a series of experiments of the kind under description the field of the 7th cervical root is found to include in the left hand portions of skin included by the field of the 1st thoracic in the right hand, a triple overlap of the fields of the 8th cervical, 7th cervical, and 1st thoracic may be taken to be proven to exist there. And such is actually the case. The triangular area of skin on the dorsum and palm of the hand shown in Figs. 12 and 13 between the two border lines marked 7 and 1, is an area of triple root supply. It is notable that the area increases in width as followed from the wrist to the fingers, including in the latter position the whole of the medius and the adjacent sides of index and annulus (Figs. 16 and 17). The area lies along the dorsum and palm somewhat, but not much, towards the ulnar side of the mid-line of the hand.

Again, the pinna of the ear is in part a region of triple overlap—namely,

[1] From *loc. cit.*, p. 100.   [2] On the lumbo-sacral plexus, here p. 51.

in the fossa triangularis, tragus, opening of the meatus and part of the fossa of the anti-helix. In this latter portion it is probably a region of quadruple overlap, the curious little skin-field of the vagus coming into combination with the fields of the cranial 5th, and of the 2nd and 3rd cervical nerves.

On the other hand, in certain regions—e.g., along the back of the trunk about midway between the mid-dorsal and mid-lateral lines of the body— I think the amount of overlap of the root-fields in the skin of the monkey is not so great as to amount to a full half of the contiguous field of each of the two consecutive nerve-roots. This point is, however, a difficult one to feel satisfied upon; experiments upon animals are really hardly suitable for deciding it, chiefly because in this region the degree of sensitiveness of the skin is comparatively low, and to obtain clear evidence of sensation, and therefore to have distinct knowledge of the extreme boundary of the field of remaining æsthesia, is often by no means easy. The observations on which I rely do, nevertheless, distinctly indicate that in the dorsal region above mentioned the amount of overlap of the consecutive skin-fields is less than, for instance, in the hand. It is, therefore, safe to say that the amount of overlapping of the fields of distribution of adjacent sensory spinal roots is not equally great in all regions of the body.

Comparison of the Overlapping of the Fields of the Spinal Nerve-roots with that of the Territories of Peripheral Nerve-trunks.—That the skin-fields of neighbouring peripheral nerve-trunks do overlap is generally recognised, but very little experimental evidence exists on the subject. I have, therefore, made some observations on the foot and hand of *Macacus rhesus* and *sinicus*. I find the results much less open to individual variation than in the experiments upon the spinal nerve-roots innervating the same region. Figs. 14 and 15 illustrate the areas of anæsthesia obtained by section of the musculo-cutaneous and anterior tibial nerves, combined on the one side with section of both the plantar nerves, on the other with section of the external plantar only. It will be noted that the field of the internal saphenous nerve in the monkey reaches along the tibial and dorsal aspect of the hallux very nearly to the tip of that digit. This is in agreement with the fact that, as shown in my previous paper, the 5th lumbar of *Macacus rhesus* has a skin-field which runs down upon that aspect of the hallux.

In Macacus the nerve seems to descend further along the hallux than it does in man, where the skin-field of the internal saphenous nerve[1] does not descend (in some individuals at least) much further upon the foot than to include the inner aspect of the ankle; also that on the front of the leg it includes more of the peroneal aspect than is supposed. It makes probable the greater wrapping round the thigh and knee of the cutaneous branches of the femoral and obturator nerves, so that the internal cutaneous

[1] In the original description a full account of the distribution of the internal saphenous nerve in the foot in man, in a case where a portion of the sciatic nerve had been excised, is given here. This is apparently the first recorded description.—ED.

and obturator sweep from the inside back as far as the middle line of the ham, calf, and thigh, while on the outer side the external cutaneous innervates skin over the outer hamstring head of the fibula, and a portion of the outer head of the gastrocnemius and extends, perhaps, a fourth of the way from knee to ankle, instead of being confined to the thigh. This

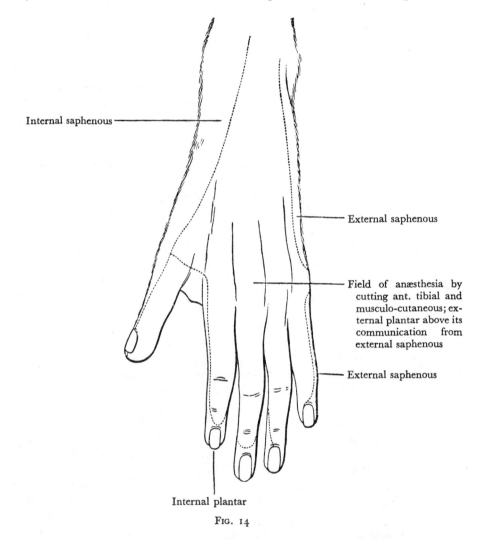

Internal saphenous

External saphenous

Field of anæsthesia by cutting ant. tibial and musculo-cutaneous; external plantar above its communication from external saphenous

External saphenous

Internal plantar

Fig. 14

distribution in these directions, more extended than is usually supposed, favours the supposition that the overlapping of the skin-fields of the peripheral nerve-trunks is greater than is generally thought.

Returning to the skin-fields of the peripheral nerve-trunks supplying the monkey's foot, the remaining sensation indicates that the field of the internal saphenous is larger in the foot of the monkey than in that of man.

Section of the musculo-cutaneous and anterior tibial nerves leaves the whole of the thumb, the plantar face, the sides, the nails and chief parts of the dorsal aspect of the end phalanx of each of 2nd, 3rd, 4th, and 5th digits, and the outer third as well of the dorsum of the 5th digit still sensitive. Section of the external plantar being then performed adds to the existing area of anæsthesia (1) the contiguous sides of the 4th and 5th digits, (2) the corresponding lateral halves of their plantar aspects (3) and of their terminal phalanges, dorsally as well, together with (4) an oblong strip

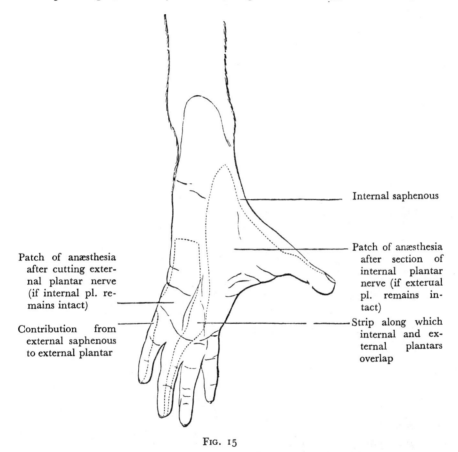

Internal saphenous

Patch of anæsthesia after section of internal plantar nerve (if external pl. remains intact)

Strip along which internal and external plantars overlap

Patch of anæsthesia after cutting external plantar nerve (if internal pl. remains intact)

Contribution from external saphenous to external plantar

Fig. 15

of the outer part of the sole extending half-way to the heel. If, instead of section of the external plantar, the section be of the internal plantar, then the additional area of anæsthesia includes (1) the tip and all but a small dorsal strip of the rest of the hallux, (2) the tips, sides, and plantar surfaces of the 2nd and 3rd digits, (3) the tibial side of the whole length of the 4th digit, and (4) a triangular patch of the planta, including almost all the hairless part of the thenar eminence and inwards up to the middle line of the planta, except that the outer edge of the patch is, in its more proximal part, directed toward the median line of the 3rd digit, and only over the distal end of the 3rd metatarsal bone curves outward to the outer side of the cleft between 3rd and 4th toes, to run along the plantar aspect of the 4th, distinctly on the tibial side of the middle line of that digit.[1]

In my experiments, the field of æsthesia persisting upon the fibular edge of the foot, and extending to the end of the 5th digit, has each time

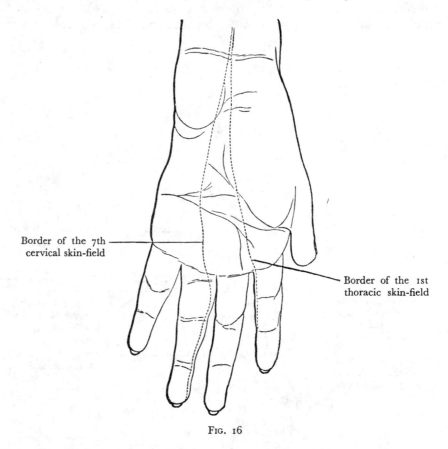

Border of the 7th cervical skin-field

Border of the 1st thoracic skin-field

FIG. 16

been distinctly separable into a smaller part on the digit, and a larger on the lateral edge of the metatarsus.

The distribution is more clearly understood by reference to Figs. 14 and 15 than by verbal description. It must be remembered, in comparing them with man, that, as I have pointed out, there is a communication between external plantar and external saphenous of regular occurrence in Macacus, of which I find no record, even as an exceptional variety, in man.

[1] After section of the anterior tibial and musculo-cutaneous the remaining area is supplied by the two plantar nerves. The description illustrates the smallness of area of additional anæsthesia by further section of either of the plantar nerves. The discrepancy is due to the overlap in their distribution.—ED.

The strip of overlap of the skin-fields of the external and internal plantar nerves is seen to be distinctly smaller than the overlap of skin between the 6th post-thoracic and the 7th and 5th post-thoracic nerve-roots, indeed trifling as compared with that. In position it does not lie in such a way as to suggest any commensuration at all between the two systems of overlap.

In the hand of Macacus the mutual overlap of the ulnar and median were examined after section of the musculo-cutaneous and musculo-spiral and internal cutaneous trunks in the upper arm. After the section of

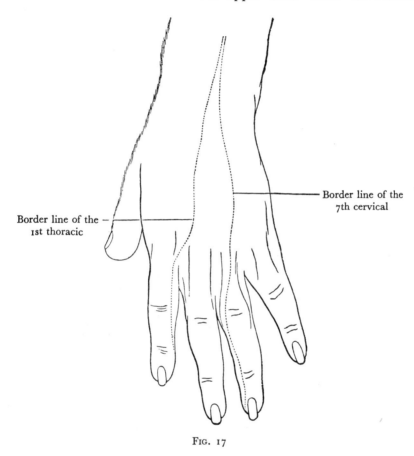

Border line of the 7th cervical

Border line of the 1st thoracic

FIG. 17

these nerves, the field of remaining æsthesia on the dorsum of the hand is that shown in Fig. 18 by the dotted line along the middle of back of the hand and the dotted lines on the pollex and 2nd and 3rd digits. If the dorsal branch of the ulnar be then severed, the field of æsthesia is further reduced, and confined by the dotted lines on the annulus and minimus as on the three radial digits. On the palm, section of the median nerve in the forearm produces a patch of anæsthesia, the limits of which are shown on Fig. 19 by the line " ulnar." Section of the ulnar trunk half-way down the forearm produces a patch of anæsthesia with the limit marked by the line " median " in the figure.

It is then clear that in the hand, as in the foot of Macacus, the extent of overlap of the skin-fields of the peripheral nerve-trunks, even on the exquisitely sensitive plantar and palmar surfaces, is much less than that of the cutaneous areas of the nerve-roots; it is, in fact, not so great as may be the overlap of the fields of nerve-roots three segments distant one from

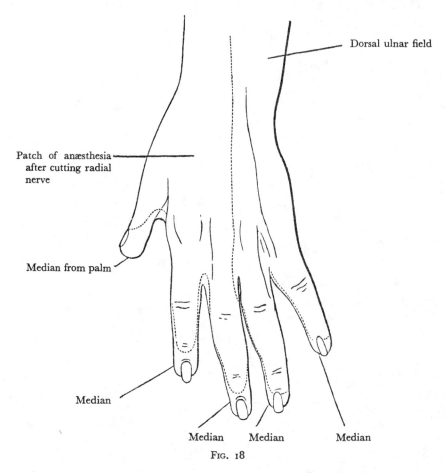

FIG. 18

another. If (as in Fig. 20) Fig. 16, p. 68, be compared with Fig. 19, p. 71, it will be seen that in the palm the region of triple overlap marked in the latter is greater than the medio-ulnar overlap in the former; and similarly in the fingers, if we set aside the communication between ulnar and median in the forearm, which is of only exceptional occurrence in man. It is also notable that the region of triple overlap, which is the central region of double overlap, strikes a line on the palm which leads to and includes the medius digit, whereas the peripheral nerve-trunk overlap strikes a line leading to and taking in part of a different digit—namely, the annulus.   This, again, points to there being no real correspondence between the two systems of overlap.

Where examined an overlap of the skin-fields of adjacent peripheral nerve-trunks has been found, but it is very small as compared with the overlapping of the skin-fields of adjacent nerve-roots and bears no

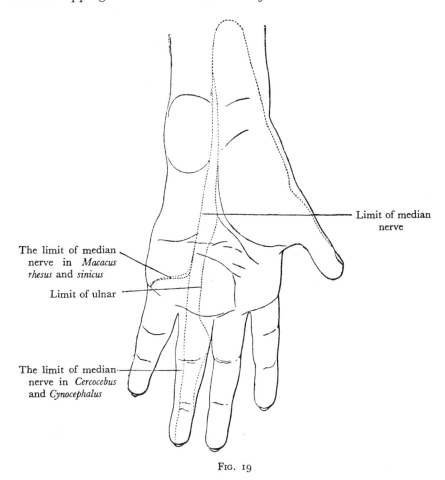

FIG. 19

significant topographical relation to the overlapping of the root-fields.   On the other hand, I have shown previously[1] that the overlap of distribution of the constituent fibres of each nerve-root itself is even greater than that of the overlapping of contiguous nerve-roots.

Comparison between the Overlapping of Segmental Skin-fields and the Overlapping of Segmental Supply of the Musculature by the Motor Nerve-roots.—In the hind-limb of Macacus I was able to confirm Eckhardt's conclusions as

[1] *Philos. Trans.*, 1893, **184B**, 717, 744.

to the pluri-segmental innervation of the limb-muscles, although Eckhardt's observations had been confined to the hind-limb of the frog.   In the pelvic limb of Macacus I found but one muscle (tensor fasciæ femoris) with a nerve-supply from a single spinal nerve-pair.   The other muscles I found to possess a bi-segmental or tri-segmental nerve-supply, a fact since con-

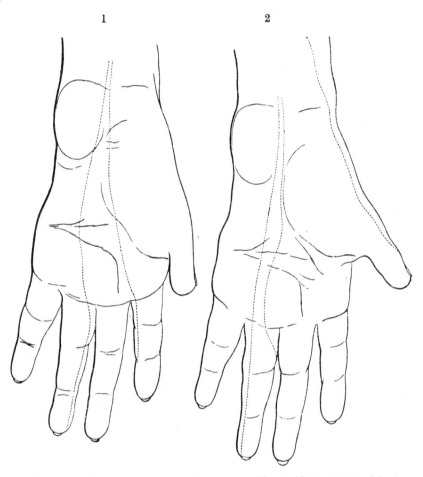

FIG. 20.—OVERLAP OF THE SKIN-FIELDS OF MEDIAN AND ULNAR NERVE-TRUNKS (2) COMPARED WITH OVERLAP OF THE SKIN-FIELDS OF THE SEVENTH CERVICAL AND FIRST THORACIC SEGMENTAL NERVES (1)

firmed for the same limb in the case of man by an anatomical research by Paterson.[1]   In the upper limb I find similarly that the muscles are pluri-segmental, a greater number being tri-segmental in the upper limb of Macacus than in the lower limb of that animal.   The *subclavius* muscle seems in some individuals, as I found also *tensor fasciæ femoris* and *rectus capitis postici*, to be uni-segmental, receiving its motor supply sometimes

[1] *J. Anat. and Physiol.*, 1894, 1895.

from the 6th cervical nerve alone: it is in so far the only muscle I find uni-segmental in the upper limb. As examples of bi-segmental muscles, I find the teres major and anconeus. The palmaris longus, the supinator brevis, the supinator longus, anconeus, and the extensor carpi ulnaris may serve as types of tri-segmental muscles, and of quadri-segmental muscles the pronator quadratus, and flexor profundus digitorum (in some individuals). Muscles innervated from longer series still are the pectorales and latissimus dorsi. On the other hand, in the intercostal spaces the intercostales externi and interni muscles appear, as far as I have yet examined them, to possess a strictly uni-segmental innervation, and somewhat similarly in the rectus abdominis, and in the sternalis these muscles have special zones for separate distribution of their motor roots. The multi-segmental nature of the nerve-supply, in the case of the large muscles at the attached base of the limb (pelvic and shoulder muscles), does not necessarily imply much actual overlapping or commingling of the muscular territories of the motor roots. I pointed out that in the case of the lower limb there is much " greater overlapping and intermingling of the root districts in the muscles of the foot than in those of the thigh." The same is the case in the arm: the intricacy of the commingling in the muscles of the hand is much greater than in those of the shoulder. In the muscles of the forearm and hand the manner in which the nerve-fibres of a spinal root are scattered through the small muscle-nerves, when examined by the degeneration method, gives a striking clue to the great commingling of the root territories in those organs.

It may therefore be replied that there is in the musculature of the limbs, and of certain, though not all of the trunk-musculature, an overlapping of motor-root territories quite comparable with that of the cutaneous sensory root-fields; and the former, like the latter, attains at least as great a development as it attains anywhere in the distal ends of the limbs.

What functional significance may be assigned to the overlapping ?—Mindful that the overlap is maximal in the hand, and that of the structures under consideration here the hand may be considered supreme in sentiency of skin and nicety of action, it might be imagined that the pre-eminence of functional delicacy and of polymeric character of nerve-supply were determinate one of the other. That the two features may be correlated I should be the last to deny, but I fail to find proof of a causal nexus between them in the sense that one is the result of the other. The overlap is as great in the skin of the back of the hand as it is in the palm, yet touch, as tested by localising power, is far the greater in the latter. It is medius not index which possesses the triple nerve-root supply, though medius is less sentient than index. The skin of the concha is not in Macacus apparently at all specially sentient, yet its sensory innervation is in part as regards nerve pairs a quadruple one. I am more inclined to connect the greater overlap in the hand and foot with degree of Lotze's " local sign " and with the fact, indicated by the arrangement of the nerve-fields, that they lie approximately in the region of the lateral line of the animal, as do the nipple and external auditory meatus, a line along which the amount of overlap seems to be great, perhaps as a heritage from old ancestral structure.

Examined by the degeneration method a somewhat greater degree of overlapping of root-distribution to the muscles of the limb is evidenced than examination by stimulation reveals. The degeneration method by its results explains the cause of the discrepancy between the observations by the two methods. The degeneration experiments show that in some muscles the number of motor nerve-fibres given by a spinal root to a muscle is too small to evoke from the muscle any contraction at all obvious to inspection. Cases occur where a limb muscle receives one, two, three, four, or five motor fibres from a particular root; allow to each of these motor nerve-fibres a dozen muscle-fibres, it is easy to understand that sixty muscle-fibres scattered in a muscle consisting of many thousands may cause no perceptible tightening of the tendon; they may simply stretch or compress adjoining inactive and elastic fibres. The degeneration of these few fibres I regard as strong evidence of the *morphological* character of the overlap; the fewness of the fibres is one of the many facts which indicate that the distribution of the motor roots is arranged on a segmental plan in accordance with the terms of a bequest dating back to a time when the present environment of the limb, especially in its mammalian form, had no preponderant weight in the shaping thereof. As regards functional value this character of the mammalian limb is on a par with details of structure which are not specific, and, therefore, with other details of structure outside those immediately acquired by the species, not to be considered as of necessity of present functional importance. The functional use of the contribution of one or two nerve-fibres to a muscle requiring hundreds is difficult to see; the probability of the occurrence of such poverty-stricken contributions is, on the view of the morphological necessity of the ray-arrangement of the limb-musculature, so high as to be only what might have been expected from theoretical considerations. The fact that certain of the motor roots of the limb contribute fibres to the innervation of certain muscles in such scanty number as to be ineffective for movement is a further argument for the morphological rather than functional character of the motor-root distribution in the mammalian limb. A number of motor fibres, too small to evoke appreciable movement in a muscle, when excited electrically, will hardly be effective for movement under the action of the will.

As to the relation between delicacy of co-ordination and number of nerve-roots contributing to motor innervation, one remembers that no muscles are more delicately adjustable than the ocular, although their individual innervation must be considered uni-segmental.

INDIVIDUAL VARIATION

A point that is very necessary to bear in mind in the discussion of generalisations obtainable from the above data remains to be insisted on before entering on that discussion. In the innervation of muscles and of skin-surface in regard to the nerve-root which supplies the innervation, a certain degree of latitude of individual variation occurs with quite remarkable frequency. In the fore-limb as in the hind-limb this is the case, and examples have been mentioned above. In the experimental basis of this paper instances have been particularly numerous with the 7th and 6th cervical roots; that may, however, be a fortuitous result. It would require a very large number of experiments to ascertain conclusively whether the peripheral distribution of these roots is more variable than that of the other brachial nerve-roots. I have already given evidence that individual variation affects not one root alone but a series of consecutive roots; but it may, perhaps, reach its maximum at some one root of the series.

Since writing my previous paper I have met in the skin-fields of the lower limb a particularly pronounced example of individual variation in the distribution of the 2nd lumbar nerve of *Macacus rhesus*. In two Rhesus monkeys I severed the dorsal (sensory) roots of the 3rd, 4th, 5th, 6th, 7th, 8th, and 9th post-thoracic nerves of the left side inside the vertebral canal. It is difficult in the region of the cauda equina to judge at the time of operation as to the exact segmental level of the nerve-roots exposed, and that has to remain, for the time being, a matter of doubt. When the operation wounds had well healed the field of remaining æsthesia was in each of the two monkeys determined, not on one occasion only, but on many, indeed, almost daily for some weeks. In the one animal (A) the anæsthetic area did not extend up the front of the leg quite so high as to the patella—that is, the skin of the front of the thigh and over the patella (covering the patella) still retained sensation, distinct though impaired. In the other animal (B) the field of the anæsthesia extended fully two-thirds up the front of the thigh; sensation was retained in a tongue-shaped field of skin covering Scarpa's triangle, and lower down sensation was completely wanting. In (A) the skin between the anus and the tuberosity of the left ischium was anæsthetic, although between the anus and root of the tail cutaneous sensation was distinctly present, though blunt. In (B) the skin lying between anus and left ischial tuber was for its half nearer to the anus distinctly sentient, as also above the anus between it and the root of the tail. From this, I did not hesitate to conclude that in animal (A) the 4th post-thoracic root, but not the 3rd, had been included in the series severed, and that in (B) the 3rd post-thoracic had been severed as well as the 4th, and I thought (B) in all probability an individual with a pelvic plexus of markedly postfixed type. I knew I had divided the same number of roots in the two individuals. The animals were kept after the operation wound was fully healed (ten days) for six weeks, and frequently compared;

no obvious alteration in the extent of the anæsthesia was found to take place, although there were the usual small oscillations of briskness of reaction from day to day. The boundary remained stationary. On terminating the experiments and dissecting the two animals, it was found that in reality in both individuals the roots cut had been exactly the same. No spinal complication was detected to explain the difference, but in (A) the plexus was extremely prefixed, in (B), as I had expected, it was markedly post-fixed.

In monkey (A)—   *Post-thoracic Roots.*

    External cutaneous nerve was formed from . . . 2nd, 3rd, 4th.
    Anterior crural nerve was formed from . . . . 3rd, 4th, 5th.
    Obturator nerve was formed from . . . . . . 3rd, 4th, 5th.

In monkey (B)—

    External cutaneous nerve was from . . . . . . 3rd, 4th.
    Anterior crural nerve was from . . . . 4th, 5th.
    Obturator nerve was from 4th, 5th, 6th,

the contribution from 6th being a very small slip.

I have not met in the brachial limb with any instance of individual variation so extreme in degree as the just-mentioned example from the lower limb. Slight degrees of variation appear to me about as common in the brachial as in the lumbo-sacral region. I also find them in the upper neck muscles. Does the individual variation affect the spinal root supply of muscles as much as it influences that of skin? In the case of the lower limb of monkey and cat I have already pointed out that it does do so; and the observations on the upper limb confirm the information obtained from the lower to the same effect. One and the same muscle, just as one and the same skin-point, is in many individuals distinctly differently innervated, as regards relation to spinal segments, from its segmental innervation in other individuals. For example, the extensor carpi radialis brevior receives in some specimens of *Macacus rhesus* motor nerve-fibres from the 5th cervical root; in many specimens, on the contrary, it does not. The extensor longus pollicis in some individuals receives motor fibres from the 6th cervical root, in many it does not. The extensor carpi radialis brevior in some individuals receives fibres from the 8th cervical root, in many it does not. And so on.

Before leaving this subject I will add that one meets certain instances of bilateral asymmetry of segmental innervation. Occasionally I have seen the extreme form of postfixed lumbo-sacral plexus of Macacus, in which the 9th post-thoracic root innervates the muscles of the foot, occur on one side of an individual and not upon the other, although usually, of course, bilateral. In the cat I have altogether met with five individuals in which the 2nd thoracic root contributed to the innervation of the palmar muscles upon one side and not upon the other; and it is noteworthy that the post-fixed side was in some left, in some right.

THE AXIAL LINES AND TORSION OF THE LIMBS

In the light of the observations recorded here it is instructive to compare the general scheme of root-distribution in the arm with that in the leg. As in the latter, so in the former, the cutaneous spinal fields become distorted from the simple zonal figure obtaining in neck and trunk. In the limbs they are displaced, and in the fore-limb in a manner similar to that obtaining in the pelvic limb. In each limb the cutaneous spinal segments are dislocated. Instead of each being by one of its borders attached to the mid-dorsal line of the body, and by one of its borders to the mid-ventral line of the body, the fields are ranged along certain dorsal and ventral lines in the limb surface. It is as though into the base of the dorsal surface of the limb the mid-dorsal line of the body thrust a spike sidewise, a lateral branch, set in a direction almost at right angles to the long axis of the body itself, but corresponding with the long axis of the limb. On the ventral surface similarly the mid-ventral line of the body thrusts out a lateral branch. These lateral branches are what I have termed the *mid-dorsal* and *mid-ventral lines of the limb*. I have brought forward evidence to prove that they are not merely hypothetical, nor even merely theoretical, but are existent, and govern skin-markings[1] in certain animals to a certain extent. On these secondary dorsal and ventral lines the skin segments of the limb are ranged as though on folded pieces of the axial line of the trunk itself.

These great ventral and dorsal lines lie presumably along the centres of the primitive or true ventral and dorsal surfaces of the limb. As regards the primitive position of the forearm and hand, it is shown by the skin-fields of the spinal nerves to be that of supination. The skin of the pollex is shown to be segmentally anterior to that of the middle finger, that of the middle finger to that of the minimus. In the skin of the chest, just above the nipple, it is evident there is a meeting place of spinal nerve-fields, which, segmentally considered, lie wide apart; the 3rd thoracic there meets the 4th cervical, or, in some individuals, the 4th thoracic there meets the 5th cervical. Where are the intervening nerve-fields to be sought? In part in the muscular tissue lying beneath the skin in this region; but, as regards skin, they are to be found in the limb proper, and the midmost of the fields—*i.e.*, the 7th cervical—is placed almost entirely in the hand and forearm—that is, lies widely separated from the trunk, being confined to the apex of the limb. These lines of shed between anterior and posterior groups of skin-fields descend behind and in front of the shoulder along approximately the middle of the extensor and flexor aspects of the upper arm, and to a certain distance down the similar aspects of the forearm. In fore-limb, as in hind-limb, the skin of the anterior side of the limb is found to be segmentally rather more extensive than that of the posterior side—that is to say, more segments participate in it. In the musculature

[1] *Philos. Trans.*, 1893, **184B**, 756.

the preponderance of the segmental length of the anterior aspect over that of the posterior is still further marked.

I must here, however, to avoid misapprehension, repeat my previously expressed conviction, that it is altogether idle to look for exact homologies between the component parts of the brachial and pelvic limbs. " The ontogeny of the brachial limb is distinct from that of the pelvic limb. The correspondence between the two is similarity, not identity. A general, but not a particular, resemblance is to be expected between the segmental components of the two,"[1] and that is all that has been found. More instructive than to attempt to construe identity out of approximate resemblance is to note the fact that broad similarity of requirement and use has from broadly similar segmental material evolved, at two places of the ventro-lateral aspect of the quadruped, two separate structures so curiously alike as are the brachial and the pelvic limbs. The details of this resemblance between the two appear to me absolutely insufficient criteria for establishing detailed homologies between their parts.

A *torsion* of the fore-limb about its own axis is traced by anatomists as having brought the distal end of the pre-axial border of that limb, during the pronate position of the fore-limb, into a position facing inwards. This view is borne out by the observations in my work. But the nerve-analysis in the monkey indicates a slight torsion in the more proximal part of both limbs, for the distal end of the mid-dorsal line of the fore-limb is turned a little backwards as well as dorsally when, in a fore-limb capable like the monkey's of supination at the wrist and elbow, the pollex is placed so as to correct the pronating torsion of the limb; and correspondingly the mid-ventral line passes on the flexor side of the inner condyle—that is, looks a little forwards as well as ventral. In the hind-limb the proximal part of the limb also exhibits a little torsion, and in the opposite direction to that evidenced in the fore-limb. The distal end of the mid-ventral line is set a little backward, that of the mid-dorsal line a little forwards. But in both the limbs the amount of torsion thus indicated is quite small, and the indication is of slight twisting, not of any rotation of the limb as a whole. The torsion accounts for the tongue-shaped extension from the posterior border of the successive spinal skin-fields in the brachial segments shifting its position from—as followed along the limb—the point of the shoulder and the deltoid eminence to flexor aspect of the forearm, although assuredly the radial part of that. Conversely, in the lower limb the tongue from the hinder edge of the spinal skin-field in the upper crural segments occupies the middle of the groin, and in lower segments gradually comes to lie over the subcutaneous surface of the tibia, and finally includes the hallux. But this torsion altogether is very slight.

[1] *J. Physiol.*, 1892, **13**, 621.

THE SKIN-FIELD OF THE FIFTH CRANIAL (TRIGEMINAL) NERVE

[*The skin-field of the 5th cranial nerve is that of a segmental nerve. The fields of the separate ophthalmic maxillary and mandibular divisions resemble those of peripheral nerve-trunks rather than those of nerve-roots.*]

[1] Of the whole 5th nerve only the *ramus mandibularis* includes in its sensory field the pinna, and it includes, as above mentioned, only a portion of the pinna. The boundary of the skin-field of the 5th at first sight seems, where it crosses the pinna, curiously irregular and arbitrarily placed. I find its course is, however, such as to include all those parts which are traceable to the tissue of the mandibular arch and none of those traceable to the hyoidean. This can be well appreciated by tracing the boundary of the skin-field of the 5th on the figures of the development of the human pinna by W. His, jun.[2] On the pinna, therefore, the field of the 5th cranial nerve extends to, but does not trespass across the first visceral cleft, and the skin-field of the third division of the nerve (*ramus mandibularis*) in so far accurately justifies the name mandibular.

The field of cutaneous distribution of the *trigeminus* possesses particular interest from Gaskell's suggestion that the huge sensory root of the nerve is compounded of a series of originally separate cranial sensory nerves secondarily massed together. The large area of the cutaneous field would then be really compounded of several segmental fields; each of these it might be possible to separately determine by appropriate section of the other divisions of the nerve. The intra-medullary course of the nerve-fibres arising from the Gasserian ganglion has for some of them been traced down to the level of the 2nd cervical segment of the spinal cord. As regards juxtaposition and overlap, it will be shown that the skin-fields of the 5th cranial and of 2nd cervical mutually behave as if the two nerves were immediately juxtaposed members of a spinal series, without intercalation of any intermediate segment.[3] All that part of the skin-field of the 5th cranial which is overlapped by the field of the 2nd cervical is, of course, segmentally posterior to the rest of the field. Of the large area not so over-lapped it was interesting to inquire from the sensory cutaneous supply which part might be segmentally anterior, which posterior. The sensory fibres for even the conjunctiva and cornea are traceable to quite low in the floor of the fourth ventricle, and even to the top of the spinal cord itself. I have seen anæsthesia of the conjunctiva and cornea ensue upon section of the so-called ascending, really descending, root of the 5th at the level

[1] From *Philos. Trans.*, 1898, **190B**, 57-63. The innervation of the tongue, palate, and cheek, and the distribution of the 12th cranial nerve are also discussed in this paper, which then goes on to describe the distribution of the 1st, 2nd, and lower cervical nerves and brachial plexus.—ED.

[2] W. His, jun., " Zur Entwickelungsgeschichte des Acustico-facialis Gebietes beim Menschen," *Archiv f. Anat. u. Physiol.*, Anat. Abth., 1889, Supplement-Band.

[3] In this statement the tiny and segmentally incomplete field of the vagus, described on p. 84, is intentionally left out of account.

of the *calamus scriptorius*.[1]   It is worth inquiring whether the three great divisions of the trigeminus springing from the Gasserian ganglion may not themselves be segmentally collected portions of the nerve, each representing one or more complete cranial sensory roots.   If so, the three great peripheral divisions will each possess a zonal skin-field extending from mid-dorsal line to mid-ventral line.   To examine this point, the delimitation of the skin-field belonging to each of the three divisions of the 5th was undertaken.

The Boundaries of the Three Divisions

I. The skin-field belonging to the first division (*Ramus ophthalmicus*) of the 5th cranial nerve (see Fig. 21) has been separately isolated[2] in two individuals.   The results of the two experiments agree very closely indeed.

Experiment.—*M. rhesus.*   Male, young.   September 15, 1893.   Measurements: Supra-sternal notch to pubic crest, 25 cm.   Acromion process to tip of middle digit, 31 cm. At 9.20 a.m., the posterior roots of the 2nd, 3rd, and 4th cervical nerves of the right side, and the inferior and middle divisions of the right 5th cranial nerve, severed after the dura mater had been opened.   At 5.30, the isolated field supplied by the *ramus ophthalmicus* finally delimited.

" The isolated field of response lies above and lateral to the palpebral fissure.   It is bounded by a line which, starting from the mid-dorsal line of the head at a level about 1 cm. behind the bregma and just in front of a transverse line joining the highest points of the roots of the right and left pinnæ, sweeps laterally in a rectilinear manner.   Having reached a point about 0·5 cm. above the level of a line drawn from the outer canthus of the palpebral fissure to the external auditory meatus, and in a vertical about 13 mm. in front of the front edge of the root of the pinna, the boundary of the field slopes down-ward and forward to a point at which the following two lines cross: (*a*) line from angle of mouth to top of root of pinna; (*b*) line from outer canthus to the angle of the lower jaw.   From this point it runs horizontally forward for a centimetre or more, and finally it ascends, sloping forward, to the free edge of the lower lid, attaining it a little to the lateral side of the middle point.   Winding over the free edge of the lid, it continues to slope inwards on the conjunctival surface, and finally emerges at the inner canthus, without the border having invaded at all the ocular conjunctiva; that is, the whole ocular conjunctiva is included in the field of the first division of the 5th.   On the bridge of the nose the boundary slopes downward and inward, so that it reaches the crossed overlap from the field of the nerve of the opposite side.   It was not found that the tip or any part of the lower 3 cm. of the nose was supplied by the ophthalmic division of the trigeminus.   About 1·5 cm. above the opening of the nostril, the internal surface of the nose, both on the septal and on the lateral walls, responded to touch; these must, therefore, be supplied by the *ramus ophthalmicus*.   The hard palate and the greater part of the soft palate gave no response; the extreme posterior edge of the soft palate certainly responded to touch; this response persisted after final section of the whole trigeminus.   There was distinct photophobia of the right eye, but no vascular injection and no abnormal degree of lacrymation.   There was no obvious difference in size between right and left pupils."

Another experiment yielded almost absolutely identical results.

II. To ascertain the field of the 2nd division (*ramus maxillaris*), the 2nd cervical nerve was divided, and the 1st and 3rd divisions of the 5th.   The area of response upon the face obtained in this way was bounded by a line which commenced at the crossed overlap

---

[1] *J. Physiol.*, 1893, **14**, 293.

[2] Technical details of operation described in original paper, p. 52.—ED.

on the middle line at the top of the root of the nose—*i.e.*, on the frontal bone about the level of the superior edge of the orbits, or about the region of the human glabella. From this point the boundary sloped rapidly down to the inner canthus of the eye, crossing the most median portion of the upper lid to attain the canthus: it then ran along the conjunctiva of the inner face of the lower lid, and at the outer canthus crossed upward over the upper lid, so as to include in the field the most lateral sixth of that lid. It then turned horizontally outward over the malar prominence, and, after extending along a good third of the line from the outermost point of the orbital opening to the external auditory meatus, bent downward and then swept toward the angle of the mouth; this it reached from below, so as to include the extreme lateral edge of the lower lip; it runs almost horizontally along

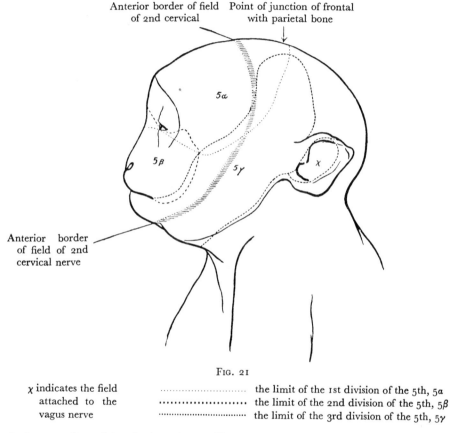

Fig. 21

χ indicates the field attached to the vagus nerve

.... the limit of the 1st division of the 5th, 5α
.... the limit of the 2nd division of the 5th, 5β
.... the limit of the 3rd division of the 5th, 5γ

the inner surface of the cheek to the maxillary gums. Along the middle line, both at lip and nose, the crossed overlap is very small indeed.

III. To delimit the 3rd division (*ramus mandibularis*), the following experiments were made: The 2nd and 3rd cervical roots were cut in the vertebral canal, and the 1st and 2nd divisions of the 5th just distal to the Gasserian ganglion. The anterior boundary of the field of response then ran from the angle of the mouth to the anterior end of the lower border of the zygomatic arch; between these points the lower part of the curve is slightly concave forward, the upper part slightly convex forward. Ascending then upon the temporal muscle, the course taken is again that of a line with a slight concavity forwards. The vertex is approached most nearly opposite the junction of the coronal and sagittal sutures (bregma); the middle line is, however, not actually reached.   I have paid particular attention to this point in three experiments, and am convinced that the field of the mandibular division of the 5th, although it approaches near to the middle line of the scalp, does not actually attain to it.   It, however, extends higher than as given for man in Flower's atlas of nerve-fields.   The boundary becomes identical with the posterior boundary of the skin-field of the entire 5th about 3 cm. from the mid-dorsal line; after that junction the boundary is that described earlier under the posterior boundary of the skin-field of the entire 5th.   The control experiment of estimating the field of the 3rd division, and then severing the nerve, I have carried out once.   On severing the 3rd division, the anterior boundary of the field which had previously lain between the angle of the mouth and the zygoma retreated to the pinna of the ear, ramus of jaw, and thyroid cartilage.

From these experiments it becomes obvious that if to the three divisions of the 5th cranial we apply as a test for complete segmental character the fact found to hold good for all complete spinal sensory nerves—i.e., that the skin-field of a complete segmental nerve extends continuously from the mid-dorsal line of the animal to the mid-ventral line—the test gives, as regards the three divisions of the 5th cranial, a distinct reply.   It is impossible to mark exactly the anterior polar point of the body—i.e., that point in the anterior end of the animal which occupies a position there similar to that held by the tip of the tail in the posterior end of the animal; that being so, it is impossible to say whether the skin-field of the *ramus ophthalmicus* does really reach the mid-ventral line of the body; it certainly occupies some of the mid-dorsal line, but the anterior pole of the body being the place of junction of the mid-dorsal with the mid-ventral line of the body, to admit ignorance of the position of the anterior polar point is tantamount to admitting that we do not know where the mid-dorsal line ends and the mid-ventral line begins.   Not being able to say, therefore, whether the field of the *ramus ophthalmicus* does extend to the mid-ventral line, we cannot apply the test confidently to it.   In the same way we cannot say whether the *ramus maxillaris* of the 5th extends to the mid-dorsal line, although we can be certain that it does extend to the mid-ventral line. The only conclusion that results from the application of the test to the skin-fields of these two nerves is, therefore, that if one of them is a complete segmental field, then the other cannot be, because there are not *two* anterior polar points to the body.

But if either of these two fields is a complete segmental one, and is at the same time overlapped by the field of the 2nd cervical nerve, then the remaining one of the two fields cannot be overlapped by the field of the 2nd cervical; at least, no such extent of overlapping is evidenced in other parts of the body.   On the other hand, if the two fields be neither of them, when considered separately, complete segmental fields, but be both merely portions of one segmental field, each of them might be well overlapped by the complete segmental field behind—namely, that of the 2nd cervical nerve.

Examination of the fields shows that each is overlapped by the field of the 2nd cervical nerve, though that of the *ramus ophthalmicus* constantly and to a greater extent than that of the *ramus maxillaris*, rarely and minutely overlapped. This part of the test indicates, therefore, that the combined skin-fields of the first and second divisions of the trigeminus may be together equivalent to the field of a complete posterior root of a segmental (spinal) nerve, but that neither of the fields is so when taken singly.

But the skin-field supplied by the third division of the nerve is, like those supplied by the first and second divisions, overlapped from behind by that of the 2nd cervical nerve, and to a far greater amount than they. This argues for the skin-fields of the first and third divisions of the trigeminus belonging to the same segmental level, and for no one of them by itself constituting a complete segmental area. Further, to the skin-field of the *ramus mandibularis*, the test for a complete segmental skin-field—namely, that it extends from mid-dorsal line without a break to the mid-ventral line—can be applied with certainty, since its position in regard to those lines is not dubious. The field, as a fact, occupies the mid-ventral line along a considerable length; but it does not actually attain the mid-dorsal line anywhere, although it approaches on the scalp at one point somewhat closely (see Fig. 21). It is, therefore, very unlikely that this field is of complete segmental character.

A third feature in which the separate skin-fields of the three divisions of the trigeminus differ from the fields of complete segmental (spinal) nerves is the following: The overlapping of fields of contiguous spinal nerves is regular and very considerable; the contiguous skin-fields may have half of their respective areas in common. With the fields of the three divisions of the trigeminus the extent of mutual overlap is irregular and not nearly so great. Thus, on the conjunctiva the fields of the first and second divisions meet, but *hardly overlap at all*; similarly those of the second and third divisions at the angle of the mouth. I do not know of detailed observations on the mutual overlap of the skin-fields of peripheral nerves, but in respect of their mutual overlap the skin-fields of the cranial 5th are very different from the skin-fields of complete segmental (spinal) nerves, and the skin-fields of peripheral nerve-trunks, as far as I have myself investigated them, resemble in this feature the divisions of the trigeminus.

Analysis of the sensory portion of the cranial 5th nerve, therefore, by this method fails to resolve it from a single segmental nerve into a series.

Taste[1]

After section of the 5th cranial nerve I have always failed to obtain evidence from the monkey of any persistence of any sense of taste. Monkeys normally react briskly to quinine or cayenne placed upon the tongue. After the intracranial section of the trigeminus the sensitiveness of the front two-thirds of the organ seems lost to these substances as well as to mechanical and thermal stimuli. Either the chorda tympani contains no gustatory fibres, or the gustatory fibres existing in it are in some way

[1] From *Philos. Trans.*, 1898, **190B**, 56.

derived from the trigeminus.   This latter supposition appears on anatomical and morphological grounds hardly possible.   It is difficult to obtain from experiment upon laboratory animals any minute evidence about the sense of taste, but my experiments point clearly to abolition—complete removal— of the sense of taste in the anterior two-thirds of the tongue—*i.e.*, in front of a line a few millimetres anterior to the circumvallate papillæ.   After intracranial section of the 5th the sense of taste *behind* that line still remains intact.   This indicates that the gustatory fibres in the glosso-pharyngeal are not traceable to the trigeminal root, and that the gustatory and tactile fields of the two nerves are, on the dorsum linguæ, coterminous.

The External Auditory Meatus

[1] After-cranial 5th and all the upper cervical posterior roots have been severed there still persists a small field of sentient skin, which includes the external auditory meatus and a part of the pinna (Fig. 21).   I think there is little doubt that this must be due to the still unsevered vagus nerve with the auricular branch from its " ganglion of the root."[2]   I have not, however, succeeded in obtaining an animal in sufficiently good condition after the operation of intercranial section of the vagus, in addition to intracranial section of trigeminus and section of the three highest cervical nerves, to ascertain with certainty the disappearance of the field after section of all those nerves.

This tiny area, confined to the lateral region and widely distant from both the mid-dorsal and the mid-ventral lines, differs curiously in these respects from the skin-fields delimited for all the other cranio-spinal nerves. The area lies on the opening of the first visceral cleft.   It is overlapped by the fields of the 5th cranial and of the 2nd and 3rd cervical nerves. The auricular branch of the vagus is, by some authorities, considered the *ramus lateralis* of the vagus of lower vertebrates; its skin-field points, however, rather to its being a branchial branch, just as the distribution of the glosso-pharyngeal nerve to the tongue and fauces shows it supplying the depth of the first visceral cleft.

THE LOSS OF SENSATION FOLLOWING SECTION OF ONE DORSAL NERVE-ROOT [3]

[*The loss of sensation when one root only is sectioned is of small area owing to the overlapping of neighbouring nerve-roots.   The area is largest for heat and pain sensation. The skin-field for each nerve-root therefore differs in size for different sensations.*]

For information regarding disturbances of sensation the evidence obtainable from animals is gathered under obvious disadvantages.   The

---

[1] From *Proc. roy. Soc.*, 1896-7, **60**, 409.
[2] Extract from *Philos. Trans.*, 1898, **190B**, 64.   Later experiments in the cat proved its origin from the vagus (*J. Physiol.*, 1917, **51**, 404, and on p. 190 of this volume).
[3] " The Spinal Roots and Dissociative Anæsthesia," *J. Physiol.*, 1901-2, **27**, 360-371.

first attempt at experimental discrimination of disturbance of the qualities of skin sensation in animals seems to have been Schiff's[1] notable description of a dissociative anæsthesia consequent on transection (i) of the dorsal columns of the spinal cord, (ii) of the whole cross-area of the cord except the dorsal columns. The dissociation noted was that of " pain " from " touch." There seems to ensue in limited areas a similar kind of dissociation after severance of dorsal spinal nerve-roots in monkeys.

In examining, in the Macaque, the skin distribution of the sensory spinal roots I employed[2] for the most part mechanical stimuli. A point of skin was touched or pinched lightly or more severely with fine forceps. In determining the delimitation of a root-field by the method of " remaining æsthesia " I confined myself to the simple issue of absence or presence of sensory response. Every response that seemed obviously sensory, no matter what the nature of the skin stimulus, was included; the field delimited was termed simply the field of æsthesia or of response.

In the course of the observations I received the impression that some dissociation of skin sensations does occur in the isolation of the skin-fields of the roots. " In a skin-field where one root only remains, punctiform stimulation at the edge is less bound up with pain than that nearer the centre of the field."[3] " Mechanical stimuli are felt by the skin with normal delicacy as ' touches,' while stimuli normally painful are felt merely as touches. This occurs at the edge of an isolated spinal root skin-field."[4] " The overlapping is greater for touch nerves than for pain nerves."[5] But the evidence I met in some individuals obtained little support from evidence in others. It became evident that only on particularly tame individuals could one hope for any reliable discrimination between qualities of their skin sensation. If an animal were in an excited state it often happened that no degree of intensity of the stimuli evoked any outward sign whatsoever of sensation. On the other hand, sometimes an animal seemed to be in a fretful condition, and then to show signs of complaint and resentment easily interpretable as pain in response to any stimulus whether or not painful. The risk of confusion from these sources of error, though never absent, is much reduced by employing absolutely tame animals in good nutritive condition. Only individuals answering to this description have been employed in the following observations, which have taken some time to accumulate, mainly from the difficulty of finding such suitable material.

Method of Observation.—The defect in sensation produced by section of a single root was the condition set up most usually for examination. In detecting the defect it would be necessary to make such an examination as might reveal dissociative anæsthesia if that existed to any considerable degree. In a few instances only was the method of " remaining æsthesia "

[1] *Physiologie*, Lahr, 1858; confirmed by Herzen, *Pflüg. Arch. ges. Physiol.*, Bonn, 1886, **38**, 93.
[2] *Philos. Trans.*, 1893, 1898 (extracts here pp. 39-78).
[3] Article " Common Sensation," in *Textbook of Physiology*, edited by Schäfer, 1900, **2**, 997.
[4] *Ibid.*, p. 979.   [5] Physiol. Introduction to Allchin's *Manual of Medicine*, 1901, **3**, 14.

adopted, as in the preceding delimitation of the root-fields of æsthesia or response.

General Precautions Adopted.—The examination was conducted in a perfectly quiet room distant from other occupied rooms. The room was always heated, generally to over 80° F.; the monkey was then more comfortable and quiet, inclined to repose rather than activity. The examination was made before feeding time, it being found that the animals seemed then more mentally alert. The animal was nursed all through the examination in the arms of the attendant by whom he was daily fed and his cage cleansed. From time to time during the examination he received morsels of food—*e.g.*, sugar or soft fruit. These he put in his cheek pouches and with them occupied himself. The animal was never allowed to see the application of a stimulus. The skin to be examined was always shaved completely. Each point of skin that replied to the kind of stimulus in question was marked with aniline colour at once without the eye being taken from it. It was usually necessary, unless the sitting was to be a very brief one, to break the monotony of the repetition of one kind of stimulus by variously introducing others. If monotonously applied a single kind of stimulus, of non-affective character, was found to cease to provoke obvious response; sometimes the failure was very rapid. A very favourable condition of the animal was light dozing, with the eyelids nearly closed, basking in the arms of the attendant. An unexpected touch, however light, then would cause the eyes to be opened without other movement. The touch over, the eyes would be closed again, and a renewed stimulus after a pause caused them to be reopened. Noises such as the closing of a distant door, a new footfall in the corridor, a street call, or a dog barking would render the examination difficult and untrustworthy for many minutes at a time.

Tests for Touch.—The following was found an excellent method for touch. The skin at some point known to be fully sentient was touched with a thermo-electric wire point sufficiently heated to be clearly unpleasant. The response was of course sharp; the part or the point was in a moment snatched away. The lightest touch then applied when the animal has settled down again evoked obvious attentive response. It was evidently expected that the new touch might, like the preceding, be dolorific. That expectation usually produced a condition of obvious response to each of a short series of even the lightest succeeding touches.

It was also useful to vary the touches, making some by a dry wire, and others with a wet camel's hair brush.

For *analgesia* a method of examination found to be good was as follows: A fine wire (platinum) bent sharply to a **V**-shape was mounted on an electro-cautery handle and connected with a couple of accumulator cells. The wire could be heated in 5 seconds at any desired moment by closing a silent screw-key within reach. With this instrument tactual sensitivity was examined by lightly resting the minute but not sharp point of the **V** on the skin. The animal would notice the touch. The wire was not then removed; it was, on the contrary, allowed to remain resting on the skin and the animal would generally soon cease to take further notice of it, its attention wandering elsewhere. At a suitable moment the concealed key was noiselessly closed. The thermo-electric wire then became warm and hot. If the skin thus stimulated were of some normal part the animal then snatched the limb away or snatched at the wire. In some areas of the skin examined in the experiments, although the first contact of the wire—the touch—evoked a response and drew the creature's attention, the application of the heat either provoked a second response merely inexpressive of any affective tone and as neutral as the former response, or it provoked no response whatever. This was considered evidence of defect of algesia. This was the test most frequently employed for detecting hypalgesia and analgesia.

Another test for algesia, also for thermo-æsthesia, was a dark-heat test. It was designed to discriminate between tactual sensation and algesia, by applying a stimulus suitable for the latter yet without any mechanical excitation. It was, however, difficult to localise minutely in its action, and was therefore only suitable where the area to be tested was at least a centimetre or more in width. Radiation from a strong source—e.g., arc lamp—was collected through a thin-walled hollow glass lens filled with carbon bisulphide containing iodine sufficient to render it opaque to light. The spot of skin to be examined was brought to the place of focus of the heat rays invisibly collected by the lens. A movable wooden shutter intervened between lens and skin, protecting the latter from the invisible beam for as long as desired. When the heat-beam fell upon normal skin the animal's attention was called to the spot usually in less than a couple of seconds. In the case of some of the skin areas examined the action of the beam attracted the attention of the animal not at all, although the injury done to the skin was subsequently found to have been great, causing immediate discoloration and severe after-effects locally. An outcome of this test was further that in some of the experimental areas where tactual stimuli provoked indubitable sensory response the heat-beam not only failed to evoke any sign of algesia, but also failed to evoke any sign whatsoever of sensation, thus indicating that heat sensation was also defective or wanting. The advantage of the invisibility of the beam was that there was no other sign than the sensation evoked by the heat which could attract the animal's attention to the part excited.

Another mode of testing algesia was to pinch a point of skin with fine-pointed forceps. This can be done with more minute localisation in most regions than can pricking, the latter causing a more widely spread deformation of the surface. Faradism by the unipolar method was also employed, but not found so useful as the above-mentioned tests.

For *cold* stimuli the ends of small test-tubes containing ice or of copper rods cooled with ice were used: a fine camel's hair brush with ice-cold water was also used.

EXPERIMENTS. The operative procedure was in every case entirely conducted under deep anæsthesia, obtained by ether and chloroform mixture.

I. TRUNK

1. *Macacus rhesus.* July 2, 1897. In the lower thoracic region one right and one left spinal root divided: these found by autopsy September 30, 1897, to be 8th and 9th thoracic respectively. Skin examinations commenced July 12.

In the post-axillary vertical line of the left side above the last rib a narrow area about 5 mm. wide gave very poor evidence of algesia: the wire point when warmed seemed felt as a second touch. The band of skin seemed analgesic to pinching. The band sloped downward ventrally. The area was not demonstrably a band of analgesia, for it was interrupted by places which were algesic. On the right side somewhat further headward a narrower less well-defined patch was demonstrable. These patches were examined in many repeated examinations. The existence of touch was proved throughout them, although dull in places; the defect of reactions indicating pain amounted to analgesia in many places, and in others to deep hypalgesia. The limits of the patches seemed to fluctuate somewhat from day to day, but there was no substantial constant difference in either of them from the end of the first fortnight to the end of the fourth month, when the animal was sacrificed.

2. *Calothrix.* October 9, 1897. Two thoracic roots cut: found at autopsy (January 29, 1898) to be 7th right and 10th left. Skin examinations begun October 17, 1897. On the right side no defect of sensation anywhere discovered. On the left equivocal signs of hypalgesia on several occasions observed near the tip of the last rib—but no absolute analgesia ever ascertained with certainty. Touch blunted slightly perhaps in same area. Autopsy proved both roots to have been completely severed.

3. *Macacus cynocephalus.* August 27, 1899. In lower thoracic region one right and one left root severed: found by autopsy October 23, 1900, to be 10th right and 11th left. Skin examinations commenced September 3, 1900. On right side no abnormality was ever clearly detected anywhere. On left side a band-like patch of distinct hypalgesia was discoverable below the last rib.[1] In the patch touches were everywhere felt—though it was not clear that they were felt in normal degree. In places the patch was absolutely analgesic, and it was everywhere hypalgesic. The patch extended—but in a broken manner—toward the mid-ventral line, which it could never be shown to reach. It seemed on many occasions clear that it did not reach to the mid-line of the dorsum. When the animal was killed thirteen months later the patch was still existent and of about the same size as a year previously. The root had been cut—as was also seen at autopsy—proximal to the root ganglion.

4. *Calothrix.* May 10, 1900. One thoracic root, right side, cut: found by autopsy February 2, 1901, to be 10th thoracic. Skin examinations commenced May 16, 1900. Below the tip of the last rib of right side was found an area—almost transverse but sloping downward and forward—about 7 mm. wide, in which contact sensation (touch), though distinctly blunted at middle of band, was present but algesia was deficient throughout. In this area painful pinching with forceps caused no sign of algesia, neither did the thermo-electric wire. When lightly touched with the thermal wire elsewhere the animal at once struggled and fought; but the wire applied to the band-like patch caused no more reaction than an ordinary contact. When the point of the wire at room temperature was laid on the patch the animal, usually drowsy from the monotony of the examination, would open his eyelids for a moment and close them again while the wire still rested on the skin; the wire being a few seconds later heated with the current the animal would at some moment as the wire grew hot open its eyes again for a moment as before and close them again, but would express no further interest in the matter although the wire continued to grow hotter even to the obvious injury of the point of skin to which it was applied and

_____
[1] Illustrated by photograph in the original.—ED.

of a continuously enlarging little skin area round about. Sometimes the heating of the wire-point did not appear to evoke a trace of any sensation whatsoever.

5. *Macacus rhesus.* October 6, 1895. Two roots divided in sacral region—found by autopsy December 20, 1895, to be 8th post-thoracic on right side, 9th post-thoracic on left. Skin examination October 7 revealed on right side a triangular area close below ischial callosity in which hypalgesia was marked. The base of the triangle lay close to the callosity, the apex extended about one-quarter down the back of the thigh. Within this area the hypalgesia amounted in places to analgesia, especially in the parts not far from the callosity. On the left side close to and partly occupying the root of the tail a small rectangular patch of hypalgesia was found amounting to analgesia near its posterior edge. The edge was nowhere quite abrupt in these patches, and over the whole of the patches evidence was forthcoming that touches were perceptible, although in the middle of the patches the touches seemed to evoke only feeble reactions, as if blunted. At the end of one week both patches seemed smaller than when first delimited, but from that time onward until the animal was sacrificed there seemed little change in the patches; both persisted as areas of hypalgesia amounting in parts to analgesia, but yet reacting to touch.

6. *Macacus cynocephalus.* September, 1899. In the upper thoracic region a root severed on the right side. Autopsy May, 1900, showed this to be the 4th thoracic. Skin in vertical line of the nipple was repeatedly examined at various levels, including the mammillary. No clear evidence of defect of sentience was found. The reactions from the right and left sides were compared, and on some occasions those of the right side were thought the more acute. No analgesia was ever proved, nor was there any unequivocal evidence of hypalgesia. The nipple itself and the skin all round it remained sentient to touch.

II. Limbs

7. *Calothrix.* September, 1899. In the brachial region one dorsal root of right side severed: found by autopsy February, 1900, to be root of 1st thoracic nerve. In repeated examinations of the skin of the right and left arms no defect of sentiency was discovered for right fingers, hand, or wrist, nor upper arm. On the right forearm there was found an oblong patch (Fig. 22) of deep hypalgesia amounting in places to absolute analgesia. The size and position of the patch are shown in the photogram, and there the extent is seen at its maximum. The extent seemed to fluctuate somewhat from day to day. When smaller than usual the curtailment was chiefly at expense of the upper ulnar peak of the forked border lying toward the elbow. A few millimetres within the edge of the patch the dark heat-test gave no sign of sensation, even when pushed to extreme. It seems therefore that the patch was thermanæsthetic as well as analgesic, for it often gave *no reaction whatever* to the thermal stimulus. Evidence of touch was easily obtained from it except near its central part, where touch reaction was evidently imperfect. The heating of the wire already applied (as described above) often gave a reaction as if from a second " touch."

8. *Macacus rhesus.* September, 1900. Two dorsal roots severed in the brachial region; autopsy, January 19, 1901, revealed roots to be left 8th cervical and right 1st thoracic. Skin examinations commenced day after operation. No loss of any kind of sensation detected in either hand. Fingers of each hand clearly sensitive all over to tangible, to thermal, and to algesiometric stimuli. On the left limb no unequivocal signs of impairment of sensation anywhere discovered. On the right limb no unequivocal evidence of impairment in wrist or upper arm, but on the forearm a restricted area sentient for touch but markedly hypalgesic and in many places absolutely analgesic (Fig. 22). Examinations repeatedly undertaken confirmed always the coexistence of tactual sensitivity with analgesia in many parts of this patch: it was sentient to touch everywhere, although the touch reactions were poor in parts of the patch, especially towards its centre. The extent of the patch varied very little from sitting to sitting, except in regard to the upper spur-like

extension on the ulnar side. Thus on November 14 this could not be demonstrated to be hypalgesic, but on November 28 it was deeply hypalgesic: again on December 4 the spur was hardly demonstrable. The photogram shows the patch when the spur was demonstrable. The similarity between this patch and that found previously in a Calothrix (Exp. 7) was strikingly close. It confused me, however, at the time because I had not supposed the root cut on the right side to be the 1st thoracic, as it proved to be at the autopsy. As with the Calothrix the dark heat-test elicited no evidence of sensory reaction. Also as with the Calothrix the thermo-electric wire-point usually elicited a response when first applied (at room temperature), and then when heated a second response seemingly as unfraught with affective tone as the first—a second " touch "—or elicited no evidence whatever of algesia even when its stimulation was extreme. From the left arm no unequivocal evidence of loss of sensitivity was at any time obtained.

9. *Macacus cynocephalus.* February, 1901. In the brachial region one right and one left dorsal root severed: these believed at time of operation to be 6th and 8th cervical, but found at autopsy (October 4, 1901) to be 5th left and 7th right cervical roots respectively. Whole of both hands examined exhaustively on many occasions failed to allow detection of any loss of sensitivity of any kind. The upper arms, more difficult to examine, also yielded no clear evidence of loss of sensation. It was especially noted that round each upper arm close below the shoulder and again close above the elbow a ring of closely set skin points could be demonstrated as being to all appearance fully sentient.

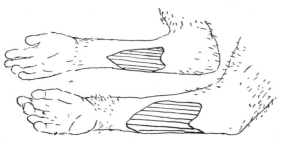

FIG. 22.—PATCH OF ANALGESIA AND LOSS OF HEAT SENSATION OBTAINED IN A CALOTHRIX (EXP. 7) AND A RHESUS (EXP. 8) RESPECTIVELY

The analgesia was perhaps not absolute at the extreme margin of this patch as marked, but amounted only to deep hypalgesia. Except near the margin the analgesia seemed absolute. A similar patch differing only in being a little lower down the forearm was found in a second Calothrix (Exp. 10). In all three instances the patch ensued on severance of the 1st thoracic root. (Traced from photograph, Fig. 2, Pl. X., *J. Physiol.*, 1901-2, **27**.)

10. *Calothrix.* December, 1899. Six dorsal roots cut on the left side, three above and three below a root (proved at autopsy March, 1901, to be the 1st thoracic) the fellow to which on the right side was cut. On right side the analgesic patch on forearm described in Experiments 7 and 8 was observed and delimited. It extended somewhat further down the forearm than in the other two instances, but was hardly larger than in them because it fell further short of the elbow-joint. Its shape resembled that found in the other experiments. In the left limb numerous examinations indicated that the thumb was sentient of touch but not of pain, and that its sentiency to touch was blunted. The index finger on its radial aspect was analgesic in the proximal phalanx and beyond that down to the tip was hypalgesic. The middle finger on its radial side was slightly hypalgesic. Index and medius were both sentient to touch. The little and ring fingers and the ulnar side of the medius did not appear in the least hypalgesic. The skin over the radial side of the wrist and forearm was anæsthetic completely, as also was the axillary aspect of the upper arm. The left nipple was sentient to touch: it was further certainly not analgesic, perhaps not hypalgesic. Above the nipple a strip of anæsthesia passed horizontally across the pectoral muscle. Both in the forearm, arm, and chest the field of anæsthesia was edged by a zone in which the skin though sentient to touch was deeply hypalgesic.

11. *Calothrix.* February, 1899. In the lower lumbar region two dorsal roots, one right and one left, cut: these found by autopsy (July, 1899) to be the 5th left and 6th right

post-thoracic. Both knee jerks remained good. No loss of skin sensation was anywhere detected despite repeated examinations. Brisk reactions were evoked by tactual and algesic stimuli when applied to tips of the digits, outer or inner edges of plantæ, heels, back of either calf and back of thighs. The whole of the feet and digits were repeatedly examined with punctiform stimuli and no loss of sensitivity detected. The skin of the left shin was several times suspected to be hypalgesic as compared with right, but the evidence was often dubious.

12. *Calothrix.* April, 1898. In the sacral region one dorsal root severed: this found by autopsy (December, 1898) to be the left 7th post-thoracic (= 1st sacral of man). The skin of the foot was repeatedly examined. The digits everywhere and the planta everywhere seemed well sentient to touch and temperature and dolorific stimuli. The examination of the skin elsewhere was not so thorough, but no loss of sensitivity was anywhere demonstrated, though there was often a question as to hypalgesia in the popliteal space.

In certain of the above experiments analgesia or marked hypalgesia (with loss of heat-sensation) ensued in a limited area of skin upon severance of a single root. The roots for which this was demonstrated (Group A) were in the trunk the 8th, 9th, 10th (in two individuals), and 11th thoracic respectively and the 9th post-thoracic (3rd sacral of man); in the limbs the 1st thoracic (in three individuals) and the 8th post-thoracic (2nd sacral of man). On the other hand, in the case of certain roots the experiments failed (Group B) to demonstrate any such patch after section of the single root; these roots were in the trunk the 4th, 7th, and (in one individual) 10th thoracic; in the limbs the 8th cervical, 7th cervical, and the 5th and 6th post-thoracic. In two experiments (on 5th cervical and 7th post-thoracic) the results left me altogether dubious. Experimental Group B may from the present point of view be considered negative in result. It has seemed right to include them in the record given. But such negative evidence has not the value of positive, nor is it of equal value from all skin regions. Certain regions are much more satisfactorily investigated in these animals than are others. Among the least unsatisfactory regions are the fingers, toes, palmar aspect of hand, plantar of foot, and the nipple; among the most unsatisfactory are the axillary aspect of chest and arm, the fold of the groin, and the popliteal fold. In unsatisfactory regions a defect of sensation might have existed and yet have in my belief possibly escaped detection in the examinations. The noteworthy part, therefore, of the negative evidence is this, that although severance of a single nerve-root does in certain regions produce a patch of analgesia, the severance singly of any one of the three sensory roots which together innervate the skin of the hand failed to render any part of the hand analgesic; and similarly that the single severance of any one of the three roots innervating the skin of the foot failed to render analgesic any part of that skin.

With regard to the experiments Group A they may from the present point of view be regarded as positive in result. They indicate that severance of certain single roots renders certain patches of skin analgesic, though not tactually anæsthetic. It is instructive to compare the extent and situation of the patch of analgesia consequent in *Macacus rhesus* on severance of the 1st thoracic root with the skin-field delimited for that root in the same species. The patch is seen to be equal in area to somewhat less than a sixth of the whole root-field and to lie about the middle of it—*i.e.*, to lie about midway between the borders which were argued in my paper to be the anterior and posterior borders of the 1st thoracic field in Macacus. Its place is that which would be left insentient were what was argued in my scheme to be the anterior border of the 2nd thoracic field not to reach what was argued to be the posterior border of the 8th cervical (see Fig. 12, p. 58). The radial edge of the analgesic patch comes just to where the " ventral axial line of the limb " was traced. On the extensor aspect of the limb the other lateral edge of the analgesic patch roughly though less well agrees with the position I accorded to the " dorsal axial line of the limb " in that region. The patch therefore, according to my scheme, forms a semi-zonal band half encircling the limb as it should if due to a want of complete approximation of the anterior border of the pain-field of the 2nd thoracic to the posterior of the 8th cervical. But the patch though analgesic was not tactually anæsthetic—though with in part blunted tactual sense. Therefore, if skin-pain and touch be in the nerve-roots subserved each by a separate set of nerve-fibres, we must conclude that in this region the area of terminal distribution of the former set of fibres is less wide than is that of the latter. In other words, in this skin-region of Macacus the overlap of the 2nd and 1st thoracic root-fields and of the 1st thoracic and 8th cervical root-fields is less for pain than for touch.

> To those unwilling to assume separate sets of nerve-fibres for " skin-pain " and for touch the analgesic fringe of a tactual root-field is perhaps explicable by the simple reduction of the number of sensifacient channels. That reduction might conceivably be so great in the fringe as to make it impossible there to evoke that full intensity of sensation perhaps necessary for development of marked affective tone. In my own view the evidence is in favour of the existence of a separate set of nerve-fibres that may be termed " pain-fibres," because particularly prone to evoke sensations fraught with disagreeable affective tone. But discussion of that question is not necessary to the point now raised.

If different skin-regions are compared the extent of overlap of the pain-fields of the roots seems to be unequal. This seems shown by comparison one with another of the results of experiments Group A and B respectively. In Macacus, just as with its " fields of æsthesia," so with its pain-fields their overlapping seems greater in the hand and foot than in some other regions—*e.g.*, in the lower part of the trunk, the upper forearm, the thigh.

It would be interesting to inquire—though of course to inquire it from animals is futile—what is the character of the sensation evoked when the electric wire already in contact with the paræsthetic skin is heated and then, as several times mentioned above, evokes a second response, apparently void of affective tone. Does this application of heat evoke a second " touch " from the nerve-fibres specific for so-called " touch proper " ? I have used the term " touch " in recording the phenomenon in my note-book, and that term reappears in the text here. I would, however, expressly disclaim all intention to urge in that way that the quality of the sensation was truly tactual. All I could infer regarding its character was its negativity in respect to affective tone. To know more of its character is urgently desirable. But the information is only obtainable from examination of the human subject.

Conclusions drawn are, then, the following:

(i) The disturbance of skin sensation produced in Macacus by severance of spinal roots is to some extent a dissociative one.

(ii) In Macacus the distinction of a single sensory spinal root, at least in the case of certain spinal nerves, entails in a limited skin-area, much smaller than the total skin-field of the root, an abolition of heat-sensitivity and of pain-sensitivity without abolition but with some concomitant impairment of tactual sensitivity.

(iii) In the skin of Macacus the " pain-" field and the " heat-" field of a single sensory spinal root, at least in the case of certain spinal nerves, are each less extensive than is the " touch-" field of the same root.

(iv) With the " heat-" fields and " pain-" fields of the roots the extent of overlap is greater in some skin regions than in others—e.g., in the hand and foot than in parts of the forearm, thigh, and trunk.

I recognise that the problem here attempted has been one imperfectly accessible by inquiry upon animals. It awaits fuller solution in the opportunities afforded by human disease where the attention of an instructed human subject can be enlisted and interrogated verbally.

III

ON THE SENSORY NERVES TO MUSCLES

[" *Charles Bell* [1] *was the first definitely to postulate the existence of a muscular sense on a physiological parity with the other senses. After his writings it began to be referred to as the sixth sense. He was not, of course, the first to suppose that consciousness of the position and movements of the body and of its parts is based on sensations. Neither did he, in speaking of ' muscular sense,' suggest that the muscles are the exclusive site of origin of the sensations ; but he was the first to postulate the existence of special afferent peripheral nerves for impulses evoked by the movements and postures of the body.*" [2] *Sachs* (1874) *had by degeneration in the frog shown the passage of some dorsal root (afferent) fibres to muscle, and Kölliker, Kuhne, Tschiriew and others had speculated on the nature of nerve-endings in muscle other than those of clearly motor type. In papers published in* 1893-94, *Sherrington demonstrated the dorsal root (afferent) origin of large numbers of nerve fibres in the muscular nerves, showed their root origin to correspond with that of the motor supply to the muscle and not that to the overlying skin, and proved the sensory nature of the muscle spindle by degeneration of its nerve-fibres. The muscles of the eyes, having no spindles in most animals, were the subject of a series of investigations and an interesting proof of muscle sense. Experimental sensory ataxia is described.—*ED.]

THE AFFERENT NERVE FIBRES FROM LIMB MUSCLES [3]

When previously pointing out the discrepancy between the arrangement of the fields of distribution of the motor and sensory roots, I added,[4] " It must be remembered that the fields of the sensory roots as delimited in the present research are cutaneous and literally only skin-deep. In such glimpses as we obtain of the distribution of sensory nerve-fibres to muscles they seem to correspond segmentally with the motor supply." " The difference between the arrangement found for the motor roots and that for the sensory may really be due less to the comparison being of efferent with afferent distribution than to the comparison being of muscle with skin." I have now observations which, I think, prove the above suggestion to be correct. The observations are as follows:

I. The phrenic, which may be taken as a muscular nerve, contains fibres from the 4th, 5th and 6th cervical spinal ganglia—*i.e.*, from the

---

[1] *Philos. Trans.*, 1826, **116**, 163.

[2] Sherrington, in Schäfer's *Textbook of Physiology*, 1900, **2**, 1006.

[3] Extract from *Philos. Trans.*, 1898, **190B**, 95.

[4] *Philos. Trans.*, 1893, **184B**, 641. I have since examined the sensory nerve-fibres in muscles, *J. Physiol.*, 1894, **17**, 211. (See p. 99 of this volume.—ED.)

sensory roots of exactly the same spinal segments as those whence motor fibres are furnished to it.

II. Afferent fibres in the nerve to vastus medialis and femoralis muscles are traceable to the spinal ganglia of the 5th and 4th lumbar nerves of Macacus—that is, to exactly the nerves which furnish the motor innervation of those muscles. I showed previously that the afferent nerve-fibres of these muscles pass through the 5th lumbar root, but I failed to demonstrate them with certainty in the root of the 4th lumbar, although in this latter root the corresponding motor fibres are easily detected. Returning to the experiments again, I have since found that by employing strychnia it is possible to distinctly detect the existence of afferent fibres from vastus medialis and femoralis in the root of the 4th lumbar, in addition to those in the 5th. The proof is furnished by the persistence of the knee jerk under strychnia poisoning, after severance of the obturator and sciatic trunks and of all branches of the femoral nerve, except that to vastus medialis and femoralis, *together with section of the sensory root of the 5th lumbar nerve*. The jerk persists, although in a crippled manner; it is completely (with the reservation explained in next paragraph) abolished by subsequent section of the sensory root of the 4th lumbar nerve.

The same appears true for the cat, if for 5th and 4th lumbar nerves 6th and 5th be substituted. But in the cat I have twice observed a phenomenon, recorded by Westphal, which might appear to invalidate the above evidence. Westphal states, on the strength of two observations on the dog, that after exhibition of strychnia the knee jerk is obtainable after section of *all* the afferent roots of the plexus; these observations form a part of his evidence that the jerk is not a reflex. In spite of their importance I cannot find the observations to have been ever repeated by Westphal or by others. Certainly, in the cat, after section of all the afferent roots of the plexus, if strychnia be exhibited, a tap upon the patellar tendon occasionally evokes an extension of the knee, indistinguishable, as far as inspection can judge, from a true knee jerk. But the phenomenon is exceptional, not the rule; thus it occurred in two out of six experiments.[1] The exceptional production of this condition by strychnia need not really confuse its regular effect of rendering sufficient for production of the jerk the comparatively slender afferent path in the 4th lumbar (Macacus) root, after section of which the jerk, even under strychnia, is as a rule absolutely lost.

III. In the case of the 6th post-thoracic nerve of Macacus and of the 7th of the cat, the discrepancy between sensory distribution, as examined in skin, and motor distribution, as examined in skeletal muscle, reaches its extremest degree; yet even there the sensory root supplies nerve-fibres to the same muscles which the motor root supplies.

Example.—M. sinicus : the motor and sensory roots, including the whole spinal ganglion of the right 3rd, 4th, 5th, 7th and 8th post-thoracic nerves excised; the motor and sensory roots of the 6th post-thoracic simply severed well proximal to the ganglion. Thirty-five days' interval allowed for degeneration; the animal then finally examined, and its nerves prepared.

[1] The " jerk " in these circumstances is part of a sudden " start " of the whole animal following percussion, and is now known to have a mechanism in the higher centres and a wider afferent path than the knee jerk.—Ed.

The lumbo-sacral plexus proved, on dissection, to be of prefixed type.

On excitation of the motor root of the 6th nerve of the intact side, contraction was noted in the following muscles: tibialis anticus, extensor longus digitorum, peronei, tibialis posticus, flexor longus digitorum, gastrocnemius, extensor brevis digitorum, flexor brevis digitorum, semimembranosus, semitendinosus, biceps, pyriformis, muscles of the back abducting the root of the tail.

The following nerves of muscles were microtomed for detection of some fibres; in most cases they were examined by teasing also:

Nerve-trunk.	*Number of Sound Myelinate Fibres.*
n. to *tibialis anticus* and *extensor longus*	hardly any.
n. to *peroneus longus*	hardly any.
n. to *extensor brevis digitorum*	a few sound fibres.
n. to *tibialis posticus*	few, but more than to tibialis anticus.
n. to *flexor brevis min. digiti*	a fair number.
n. to *gastrocnemius*, mesial head	a large number of sound fibres.
,, ,, lateral ,,	a large number of sound fibres.
n. to *semimembranosus*	a few sound fibres.
n. to *semitendinosus*	a larger number of sound fibres.
n. to *biceps*	a great number.
n. *to all the hamstring group*—14 *bundles*	no bundle without sound fibres.
6th post-thoracic nerve, including spinal ganglion and ventral and dorsal primary divisions of the nerve	the number of fibres in the ventral division must be more than half, and in the dorsal very nearly a half.

collateral cutaneous nerves of the toes—

2nd toe, mesial side, dorsal twig	five fibres.
,, lateral side, dorsal twig	seventeen fibres.
,, ,, ,, ventral twig	about sixty fibres.
cleft between 3rd and 4th toes, dorsal twig	plenty.
,, ,, 4th and 5th toes, dorsal twig	at least a half are sound.
5th toe, lateral edge, dorsal twig	more than half are sound.
,, ,, ,, ventral twig	more than half are sound.

Example.—Cat : the motor and sensory roots of the 5th, 6th, and 8th post-thoracic nerves excised, including the whole ganglion of each sensory root. The 7th post-thoracic severed well on the spinal side of the ganglion. Time allowed for degeneration, forty-three days. The animal then finally examined, and the various nerves prepared. The lumbo-sacral plexus was found by dissection to be a moderate example of the prefixed class. The 7th post-thoracic nerve contributed no twig to the obturator trunk. Excitation of the 9th post-thoracic root gave no contraction of the limb muscles.

The cutaneous distribution of the 7th post-thoracic nerve in the cat includes the foot (both dorsal and plantar aspects), and the lateral aspect of the leg below the knee, reaching above the knee for a short distance only on the postero-lateral surface of the limb. On excitation of the motor root of this nerve on the side of the body in which it was intact, contractions were noted in the following muscles: tibialis anticus, peroneus, tibialis posticus, flexor longus digitorum, gastrocnemius, semimembranosus, semitendinosus, biceps, and in muscles of the back moving the root of the tail. Of the muscular ray thus innervated by the motor root of this nerve the distal part only is, therefore, covered by the skin innervated by the sensory root of the nerve. But, on examining the following muscular nerves for undegenerate fibres, the sensory distribution of the nerve was found to include the following muscles: *gastrocnemius*, both heads; *semimembranosus, semitendinosus, biceps, tibialis anticus, tibialis posticus*, and muscles of the back. Examination of nerve-bundles:

Nerve Trunk.	Condition of Nerve-fibres.
n. to *sartorius*	no sound myelinate fibres.
obturator in pelvis	? a few minute myelinate fibres in the perineum: none sound elsewhere.
obturator in thigh, deep division . .	no sound myelinate fibres.
,, ,, superficial division .	no sound myelinate fibres.
n. to *tibialis anticus*	plenty of sound myelinate fibres.
n. to *extensor digitorum*	plenty of sound myelinate fibres.
n. to *tibialis posticus*	a number of sound myelinate fibres.
n. to *gastrocnemius*, lateral head, 5 bundles .	87 sound fibres, 17 μ—2 μ.
,, ,, median head, 4 bundles .	7 sound fibres, 12 μ—2 μ.
n. to *semimembranosus*, 3 bundles . .	94 sound fibres, 19 μ—2 μ.
n. to *semitendinosus*, 2 bundles . .	52 sound fibres, 19 μ—2 μ.
n. to *biceps*, 4 bundles . . .	37 sound fibres.
the most lateral plantar digital . .	many sound myelinate fibres.
the most lateral dorsal digital . .	very few sound myelinate fibres.
the most medial dorsal digital . .	a fair number of sound myelinate fibres.
the 5th post-thoracic nerve-trunk from the scar outward for a centimetre	no ganglion cells or sound myelinate fibres, except a few minute ones in or near the sheath.
the 6th post-thoracic	condition same as that of 5th.
the 7th post-thoracic nerve, with ganglion and ventral and dorsal roots and ventral and dorsal primary divisions of the nerve. The motor root	3 sound myelinate fibres, ? recurrent.
ganglion and adjoining piece of dorsal root .	no degeneration, except where the scar is approached; there plenty, traumatic.
ventral primary division . . .	great numbers of sound fibres.
dorsal primary division . . .	about a half of the nerve consists of sound myelinate fibres.
the 8th post-thoracic nerve . . .	condition as in 5th and 6th.

In the above evidence for the existence in the limb of complete sensory as well as complete motor rays, the most convincing item is perhaps that furnished by the primary dorsal divisions of the 5th, 6th, and 7th post-thoracic, and of the 8th cervical and 1st thoracic nerves of Macacus. I have previously pointed out that these divisions differ from the similar divisions of all the other spinal nerves in not entering the skin; they are devoid of cutaneous branches. Their anomalous behaviour is confirmed by the examination of the cutaneous distribution of the nerve, which shows that these particular nerves have skin-fields confined to the limb proper (to the leg almost exclusively below the knee). They have, therefore, no cutaneous territory at all along the middle line of the body. But by the experimental method it is seen that after section of the motor roots of these particular nerves more than a half of the nerve-fibres in their primary dorsal divisions still remain intact; the intact fibres are sensory; the primary dorsal division, although not cutaneous, is therefore nevertheless largely sensory. When in the same way the contribution given by the sensory roots of these nerves to the muscular parts of the limb is taken into account, a ray of muscular and other tissue is found to extend between the sensory skin-cap supplied by the nerves of the apex of the limb only and the median plane of the body. The proximal portion of the sensory ray exists, but buried beneath the surface; this proximal part is therefore nowhere cutaneous, but is mainly muscular; the sensory ray in the muscular and noncutaneous tissue stretches from its base in the muscles and ligaments of the vertebral column to an apex in the muscles and ligaments, etc., of the foot.

By the experiments cited this has been shown for the lower limb; it is also true for the upper limb and the 7th and 8th cervical and 1st thoracic nerves. The dorsal primary divisions of these nerves, like those of the 5th, 6th, and 7th post-thoracic, do not possess cutaneous branches, thus differing from the primary dorsal divisions of all the other cervical and thoracic nerves.

Experiment.—M. rhesus. The 5th, 7th, 8th cervical, and the 1st, 2nd, and 3rd thoracic nerves cut in the vertebral canal proximal to the root ganglia. Time allowed for degeneration twenty-eight days. The primary dorsal divisions of the 1st thoracic and 8th and 7th cervical nerves on excitation evoked no muscular contraction, but when teased and when examined in serial sections a number of sound myelinate nerve-fibres were found in them; these must have arisen in the spinal ganglia. The muscular branches of the ulnar nerve contained a certain number of sound myelinate fibres (not so many as in instance quoted from the lower limb); so also the inner head of the median nerve, but neither of these trunks on faradic excitation evoked muscular contractions.

It has been shown above that the distribution of the sensory root-fibres in the last two cervical, and in the highest thoracic nerve, is, as regards skin, confined to the hand, forearm, and lowest part of the upper arm, nowhere approaching to the median line of the body. If we include the sensory fibres distributed to the deep parts, the distribution of these nerves does, however, come right up to the median plane, including the muscles and ligaments of the vertebral column. Thus in the upper limb, as in the lower, the sensory ray when its nerves are examined by experimental degeneration is proved to extend from the apex of the limb to the median plane of the body—in fact, to be a complete ray. The proximal part of the ray, however, just as in the pelvic limb, nowhere reaches the body surface, but lies beneath the surface, and is composed of muscles and deep tissues. If judged by skin alone it is wanting.

It becomes clear that absence of cutaneous branches from the dorsal primary divisions of the 7th, 8th cervical, and 1st thoracic, and from the 5th, 6th, and 7th post-thoracic nerves proves to be simply a natural concomitant of their segmental position in the spinal series, and is a criterion indicating that they lie at the very centre of the limb regions, respectively brachial and pelvic.

IV. The spinal roots which are the source of the afferent nerve-fibres of the hamstring *muscles* can be determined by use of vasomotor and of respiratory reflexes. The individual dorsal (posterior) roots through which the afferent nerve-fibres from a muscle pass can be found by noting which are the roots whose section lessens or abolishes the reflex. In the case of the hamstring muscles of the cat, I find these roots, subject to individual variation, are the 7th, 8th, and 6th post-thoracic; now the 7th, 8th, and 6th nerves are exactly those the ventral (anterior) roots of which supply the innervation of the muscles in question. Further, the 7th is the chief root of the muscles, both as regards sensory fibres and motor. It is noteworthy that the effects of excitation of these afferent nerve-fibres from muscle, both on blood pressure and respiration, were not the converse of, but similar in character to, those from internal saphenous nerve, though not so extreme.

The conclusion arrived at by each of the four lines of observation is, therefore, that the *afferent* nerve-fibres distributed in a given muscle arise in the *root ganglia of exactly those spinal segments whence emerge the motor fibres for the same muscle.* In other words, the sensory nerve-cells directly connected with a given skeletal muscle are in any one individual always of the same segmental level as the motor nerve-cells connected with the same given muscle. The simplest reflex path connected with a muscle may, therefore, be expected to lie exactly in the particular segments whence issue the motor fibres to the muscle. In the " knee jerk " we have evidence of a muscular reflex arc, traceable usually principally *from* and *into vastus medialis* and adjacent part of *crureus*, and this affords, as it were, a test case for the above conclusions; it confirms them perfectly; it exemplifies them by its narrow local extent, and by the segmentally horizontal, correlative position of its motor and sensory components.

SENSORY FIBRES IN THE NERVES OF MUSCLES[1]

[*Conclusions as to the numbers and general distribution of sensory nerve-fibres in the nerves to muscle, their end-organs, and the question of efferent fibres in the dorsal nerve-roots, reached from a large series of degeneration experiments in cat and monkey.*]

1. In a muscular nerve-trunk from one-third to one-half of the myelinate fibres are from cells of the spinal root ganglion.

2. These fibres range in size (in fresh preparations) from 1·5 μ to 20 μ diameter.

3. The largest of them are not the largest fibres in the muscular nerve-trunk; the largest in the nerve-trunk come from the ventral (motor) spinal root.

---

[1] The conclusions from the paper in *J. Physiol.*, 1894-5, **17,** 211-258. This important paper is too long to be reprinted here entire, and the conclusions are alone presented. It established the sensory content of the nerves to muscles, enlarged the description of the muscle-spindle, and proved the afferent nature of the nerve to the end-organ. There is also described the " Sherrington Phenomenon " of contracture of a de-efferented muscle by stimulation of the sensory fibres supplying it, and the late re-appearance of nerve-fibres in the central stump of the dorsal root after excision of the root ganglion.—ED.

4. The largest root-ganglion fibres in the muscular nerve are larger than any fibres in the cutaneous nerves of the limb and than any in the articular nerves examined.

5. The smallest myelinate fibres in the muscular nerve are for the most part, perhaps entirely, root-ganglion fibres.

6. Macroscopic nerve-trunks are, as regards their myelinate fibres, in no case purely motor, all are sensori-motor or purely sensory. Such nerves as phrenic, hypoglossal, recurrent laryngeal, posterior interosseus contain abundance of fibres from sensory ganglia.

7. For the root-ganglion fibres in the muscles a special end-organ exists;[1] this is the so-called " muscle-spindle " (Kühne).

8. The muscle-spindles lie numerously imbedded in the muscular tissue, and are especially frequent in the neighbourhood of aponeuroses, tendinous intersections, and tendons.

9. The majority, perhaps all, of the larger root-ganglion fibres in the muscular nerves terminate in " muscle-spindles "; the small nerve-fibres do not appear to end in spindle-organs; some seem to terminate after branching in free fibrils.

10. After section of the nerve supplying the muscle the muscle-fibres inside the spindles do not degenerate like the fibres composing the rest of the muscle.

11. The skeletal muscles and their primitive fibres can attain a very complete structural development in absence of the spinal cord and its roots.

12. The peripheral limb-nerves contain no myelinate fibres derived from the sympathetic system; but they contain large numbers of pale fibres; all their sympathetic fibres must therefore be among these.

13. In the lumbo-sacral region there exist recurrent fibres in the ventral spinal root as shown in other regions by Waller, Schiff, etc.

14. Schäfer's ganglion cells in the ventral spinal root, although many of them lie in proximity to the recurrent sensory bundle in the root, do not for the most part appear to be connected with those fibres.

15. In the lumbo-sacral nerves near their commencement exist a few minute and scattered myelinate fibres which do not degenerate after section of the nerves at their origin; the fibres appear related to the sheaths of the nerve-trunk, and may be " sympathetic."

16. All the fibres of the dorsal (posterior) spinal roots of the sacro-lumbar nerves remain sound (apart from traumatic degeneration for a few millimetres) on the dorsal (ganglionic) side of a section carried out between the ganglion and the cord; all on the spinal side degenerate.

[1] " It was shown above that about two-thirds of all the afferent fibres measure above 7 μ diameter. Of these I imagine that considerably more than a half may be apportioned to the muscle-spindles, the majority of the rest belonging probably to Golgi's tendon-organs " (*Ibid.*, p. 247).

17. Four to seven weeks after excision of the spinal root ganglia large numbers of minute myelinate nerve-fibres (less than 4 μ) exist in the proximal (spinal) end of the dorsal (posterior) spinal root; these fibres resemble regenerate fibres.

A Further Note on the Question of Possible Efferent Fibres in the Dorsal Nerve-roots[1]

The present position of the question seems to be as follows:

In *Amphioxus* the dorsal (afferent) spinal root does not possess any extra-spinal ganglion. Retzius shows, however, that its root-fibres, which are all of intraspinal origin, are some of them processes of bipolar neurones imbedded in the spinal cord, and some of them processes from multipolar neurones imbedded in the cord.

In *Petromyzon* the dorsal (afferent) root possesses an extraspinal ganglion, this containing both bipolar and unipolar (T-processed) neurones. Some, however, of the dorsal root-fibres spring, not from cells of the ganglion, but from neurones imbedded in the spinal cord (Freud, Nansen, Retzius).

In *Pristiurus* some fibres of the dorsal root are not connected with any cells in the extraspinal ganglion and are believed to be of intraspinal origin (v. Lenhossek).

In *Myxine* all the dorsal root-fibres are derived from cells of the extraspinal root ganglion, none belonging to intraspinal neurones (Nansen).

In *Rana* distinct peripheral effects are said to be elicited by excitation of the peripheral ends of the dorsal (afferent) spinal roots (Steinach); all these effects appear to be visceral.[2]

In the *chick* an intraspinal origin for a few of the fibres of the dorsal root has been placed beyond all doubt, and the appearance of the cells of origin of these fibres does not differ from those of the multipolar motor neurones belonging to the motor root (Cajal, v. Lenhossek, Retzius, v. Gehuchten).

In the *mammal* (cat, dog, monkey) my own observations agree entirely with those of Singer and Münzer in upholding the original statement of Waller to the effect that none of the fibres of the dorsal (afferent) spinal root have their origin in intraspinal nerve-cells. That is to say, all are processes belonging to extraspinal cells. And the present communication extends that result to the roots of origin of the sympathetic system.

---

[1] Conclusions from *J. Physiol.*, 1897, **21**, 209, following an investigation by careful teasing of the osmic-stained mammalian dorsal root, searching for degenerate fibres peripheral to the section after about two weeks.—ED.

[2] An addendum to the original paper indicates some occasional motor fibres to skeletal muscle occasionally found in the frog by Horton-Smith, *J. Physiol.*, 1897, **21**, 101. See also Wana, *Pflüg. Arch. ges Physiol.*, 1898, **71**, 555; Dale, *J. Physiol.*, 1902, **27**, 350.—ED.

THE SENSORY INNERVATION OF THE EYE-MUSCLES[1]

In a former number of these *Proceedings*[2] I drew attention to the occurrence of reflex reactions evoked by mechanical and electrical excitation of individual eye-muscles and of their nerve-trunks. I was later somewhat surprised when, after the sensory nature of the structures originally termed muscle-spindles (Kühne) had been proved, I was unable to find in the eye-muscles any examples of these structures.[3] I had expected to find in those muscles, on account of the great delicacy of their control and coordination, and in view of the well-known richness of their innervation, a field peculiarly favourable for the examination and study of " spindles." It appeared to me possible, however, that spindles if of a *very* simple type— *e.g.*, containing a single muscle-fibre not enveloped in a distinct capsule, but with simply an unthickened perimysial sheath and without any circumfusal lymph space, in short, if reduced to a far simpler type than I have ever met actually existent—might, although present, yet escape recognition. I turned, therefore, to the production of degeneration for further information.

I had noted that the intra-fusal muscle-fibres, of the " red " variety as they are, undergo when the nerve-trunk of a muscle has been severed a much slower course of alteration than do extra-fusal muscle-fibres[3]—*i.e.*, I found no pronounced degeneration for even two years following section. I therefore cut through *n. oculomotorius* at its origin, and examined the resultant degenerations in the eye-muscles which it innervates and in their individual nerve-trunks. The degenerative process was allowed scope for various periods. This method of test failed, however, to give me distinct results because (1) the muscle-fibres of the eye-muscles (in monkey) exhibit normally a certain variable amount of fatty granulation, simulating degenerative change; and because (2) the resultant changes in the muscle-fibres, although the fatty granulation distinctly increased, did not even after a period of sixty days show the clearly distinctive characters I had hoped.

On the other hand, in the nerve-trunks, extra-muscular and intra-muscular, the Wallerian degeneration did clearly demonstrate a result of importance. With the exception of a few minute fibres, of variable number, derived perhaps from the ciliary ganglion, *all* myelinate nerve-fibres in all these eye-muscles were degenerated. Therefore these eye-muscles derive the vast majority of their myelinate nerve-fibres from *n. oculomotorius*. The sensory innervation of these muscles does not therefore seem derivable from the 5th cranial pair. In accord with this I found (*a*) that severance of both trigemini caused no obvious impairment of the movement of the eyeballs, (*b*) that the combined severance of both *nn. trigemini* and of both optic nerves even after section of the encephalic bulb did not severely

---

[1] From *Proc. roy. Soc.*, 1897, **61**, 247-249.
[2] *Proc. roy. Soc.*, 1893, **53**, 407-420. Reprinted here in Chap. VII, p. 244.
[3] *J. Physiol.*, 1894, **17**, 211.

depress the tonus of the eye-muscles. Now we know that section of the sensory spinal roots belonging to muscles does very severely depress the tonus of them.

At the same time I was struck with the long distance to which many of the nerve-fibres in these muscles travel forward toward the ocular tendons of the muscles. I was the more impressed with this fact because direct examination proved that the region of the distribution of motor end-plates in these muscles is almost confined to the middle portion of the fleshy mass of the muscle. Further investigation of the course and destination of the nerve-fibres at the tendon end of the muscle revealed them (both in cat and monkey) undergoing terminal subdivision, and in very numerous instances passing beyond into the bundles of the tendon itself. The terminations of many of these nerve-fibres lie within the tendons; many recurve again toward the muscular fibres, and end just at junction of muscle-fibre with tendon bundle. The nerve-fibres in so terminating frequently become thick— as I have described in the case of muscle-spindles—with shortened internodes.

The terminal arborisation which the nerve-fibres finally make is as a rule small as compared with the end-arborisation of ordinary Kühne-Ruffini " spindles " or the Golgi " tendon-organs," but closely resembles in numerous instances the form of arborisation of the latter.

In my former communication I wrote: " The question therefore arises whether the above cranial nerves (3rd and 4th) are not in reality sensori-motor."[1] In view of the additional observations now recorded I think it must be conceded that *nervus oculomotorius* is perhaps not a merely motor nerve, but although purely " muscular " may be sensori-motor.

My observations have included also the 4th cranial pair, and with like result. Investigation of the 6th cranial pair is also in progress.

It also appears clear from the above that the absence of the distinct Kühne-Ruffini " spindles " from a muscle does not exclude the possession by it of sensorial end-organs and of afferent nerve-fibres. This point is not without importance, because examination of various muscles has led me to the conclusion that the " spindle-organs " are absent from the following muscles: From all the orbital eye-muscles, from the intrinsic muscles of the larynx (though Pacinian corpuscles occur in these as in various other muscles), from the intrinsic muscles of the tongue, and from the diaphragm. It is notable that all these muscles belong to that set which are innervated by nerve-fibres of rather smaller calibre (Gaskell) than those supplying the skeletal muscles generally—that is to say, are innervated by the non-ganglionated splanchnic efferent nerves of Gaskell.

In a communication on the sensory nerves of muscles laid before the Society last year,[2] the question previously raised[3] as to the existence of

---

[1] *Proc. Physiol. Soc., J. Physiol.*, 1894, **17**, xix.

[2] Sherrington, *Proc. roy. Soc.*, 1897, **61**, 247 (reprinted above).

[3] Sherrington, *Proc. Physiol. Soc., J. Physiol.*, 1894, **17**, xix.

afferent nerve-fibres in the so-called " motor " cranial nerves for the muscles of the eye was advanced to the following position. Myelinated nerve-fibres from the 3rd cranial and 4th cranial nerve-roots were traced into the tendons of the recti and oblique muscles. Since then control observations have been made.[1] The ophthalmic division of the 5th cranial has been severed at its origin, and with it the 6th cranial trunk. This has been done in the monkey. The condition of the nerve branches going to and lying within the muscles and tendons has been examined after an interval of twelve to fourteen days. Those of the external rectus contained nothing but degenerate nerve-fibres, save for a few fine myelinate fibres, probably from the ciliary ganglion. Those of all of the other eye-muscles contained exclusively healthy nerve-fibres. The sensorial musculo-tendinous organs of the eye-muscles are, therefore, not innervated by the ophthalmic division of the trigeminus. On the other hand, the nerve-fibres of the external rectus muscle behave, after severance of the 6th cranial nerve, in the same way as my previous papers showed those of the other eye-muscles do after section of the 3rd and 4th nerves.

A contribution towards the physiological inquiry into the matter has been made as follows, and has given a clear reply.[2] The conjunctivæ, both palpebral and ocular, and the corneæ of both eyes have been rendered deeply anæsthetic to cold, warmth, touch, and pain by liberal applications of cocaine. Then in a completely dark room the power to direct the gaze with accuracy in any required direction has been tested. The person under examination is seated, with the head securely fixed, in front of a screen. One of his hands carries a marker. The hand is moved by an assistant, and is made to mark the screen at some one point; it is then passively replaced. The person under observation during this time keeps the eyes open in the primary position or sits with them closed. He is then required to direct his gaze to the spot marked on the screen. The light is then switched on, and the point to which the gaze is turned is noted. The power to direct the gaze under these circumstances has been found to remain good. If for co-ordinate execution and ability to perform the delicate adjustments for training the eyeballs correctly in any desired position the exercise of peripheral apparatus of muscular sense is required, the only possible channels under the above conditions would seem to be deep branches of the 5th nerve or the 3rd, 4th, and 6th so-called " motor " nerves themselves. As previously stated, the former are by both my earlier and later degeneration experiments excluded. The latter,

---

[1] Reprinted from *Proc. roy. Soc.*, 1898, **64**, 120-121.

[2] A review of the theories of muscular sense will be found in Schäfer's *Textbook of Physiology*, 1900, **2**, pp. 1001-1025. The physiological proof owes much to the demonstration of the reflex effects of muscular stimulation—the stretch-reflex and other proprioceptive reflexes—by Sherrington. The sense of relaxation of a muscle, as during inhibition, was also indicated by Hering and Sherrington, *Pflüg. Arch. ges. Physiol.*, 1897, **68**, 221-228.—ED.

therefore, are the only ones remaining, for the superficial branches of the 5th and the retinæ are put out of action by the conditions of experiment.[1]

THE PROPRIOCEPTIVE FUNCTION OF THE EXTRINSIC OCULAR MUSCLES[2]

The rich supply of afferent nerve-fibres existent in the muscles which move the eyeball invites inquiry as to what may be the contribution which these nerves make to visual reactions. Their reflex function should, like that of other proprioceptives, relate to the adjustment and maintenance of postures. Ocular posturing, such as the adjustment and maintenance of the gaze, is delicate and almost continual throughout the waking day. And the afferent nerves from muscles, as is known of them from other muscular fields, yield, besides their purely reflex taxis of local posture and movement, sensory impressions which are the basis of perceptions of postures and movements—in short, subserve muscular sense. Muscular sense being, along with vision, touch, and the " labyrinthine " sense, a chief source whence the mind manufactures sensual " space," the above is tantamount to saying that the proprioceptive nerves of the eyeball-muscles may be expected to contribute to space as perceived with the eye. In the literatures of muscular sense and of visual perception one does not, however, find, at least so far as my acquaintance with those literatures reaches, much advertence to a spatial rôle for the eye-muscle afferents, and if adverted to, such a rôle for them is often not acceded to. For this attitude of negation towards them, two circumstances are probably largely responsible. The spatial endowment of the retinal sense itself is of such pre-eminent and exquisite degree that it has seemed, especially under more recent investigations, a sufficient source in itself for almost every spatial attribute of vision. The likelihood, therefore, that adjuvant factors of non-retinal origin make any important contribution to visual space has seemed small. Again, the demonstrated existence of a wealth of afferent nerve-fibres in the eye-muscles is a discovery of comparatively recent date. At the time of the studies of visual space-perception by Wells, Panum, Lotze, Aubert, Hering, and others, the possession of muscular sense by the eye-muscles, although on general grounds probable, had no proven neurological basis.

Yet, that a sense-datum derived from the external muscles of the eyeball does furnish factors of importance in visual space, even in uniretinal vision, is, I think, demonstrable by extremely simple experiments. Recourse to certain old and often repeated observations seems sufficient

---

[1] Further experiments confirming the degeneration of the sensory endings in the extra-ocular muscles after section of the 3rd, 4th, and 6th nerves are reported by Tozer and Sherrington, *Proc. roy. Soc.*, 1910, **82B**, 450-457.

[2] Reprinted from *Brain*, 1918, **41**, 332-343.

to show this, if the findings be reconsidered from the proprioceptive stand-point.

An observation of such a kind is the following: With the head erect let three spots A, B, C be looked at directly in front—for instance, on a bare wall across the room. Let us suppose one eye only to be used, the other closed. Let the three spots be equally spaced and in one vertical; and suppose the middle one B the point of visual fixation, and at the level of the eye so that the eyeball is in the so-called " primary " position. Suppose A to lie above B and C below B. The spots are perceived as forming one vertical. How is their verticality recognised ? An answer often accepted is as follows: The spots stimulate three retinal points α, β, γ, the mental reactions attaching to which give sensual " verticality " as an attribute inherent in the perception of those points taken as a group. Let us test this statement. Without moving the head, let the eye be directed toward three similar spots A', B', C', on some other part of the wall, say higher and to the right and lying in one vertical, and let the middle one B' be fixated.

For strict demonstration the plane surface toward which the gaze is directed should, as in the strict demonstration of Listing's law, be per-pendicular to the line of vision, which it will not be if the wall is used for the secondary eye-posture as well as for the test. The well-known slight " perspective " deviation then complicates the Listing so-called " false " torsion. A flat screen set perpendicular to the direction of the visual line in the secondary posture chosen for the eye obviates this.

Then these three spots are perceived likewise as situate in one vertical. But Listing's law of the postures of the eyeball tells us, and its demonstration proves to us, that in this second case, although the spot B' stimulates the same retinal point β as did B, the spot A' does not stimulate the retinal point α as did A, but a retinal point α' lying to right of α, and the spot C does not stimulate retinal point γ, but a point γ' lying to left of γ.

We have therefore on the above-offered explanation a dilemma. The explanation says that an inherent quality attaching to the three retinal points α, β, γ gives them as a group verticality in visual space. It says the same of three retinal points α', β, γ' which lie in a retinal line inclined to and crossing at β the line formed by α, β, γ.

If it be doubted that the line of retinal points stimulated by spots A', B', C' is really oblique to and crossing the line of retinal points stimu-lated by A, B, C, we have only to obtain the after-images of A', B', C', and turn the fixation of the eye back to B. The projected after-image of A' then appears to the left of spot A, and the after-image of C' to the right of C, and the line connecting the after-images of A' and C' runs obliquely through B and appears no longer vertical but at an angle to the vertical. Though seen at vertical when the eyeball was in the secondary position— namely, gazing upwards and to the right—it is now, with the eyeball in the primary position, seen as if it had undergone an anti-clockwise rotation round its middle point. Conversely, if the after-images obtained in the primary ocular position from spots A, B, C are projected when spot B′ is fixated—that is, with the eyeball in the given secondary position—the line they form no longer appears vertical, but is seen as inclined to and crossing the vertical line formed by A′, B′, C′, as if it had suffered a clockwise rotation round its middle point.

Thus it is clear that verticality is no unalterable inherent sense-datum attaching to the retinal point-group α, β, γ as such; for, though in one position of the eyeball that group says inalienably " vertical," in another position of the eyeball it says " inclined to the vertical "—namely, in this particular case, upwards and to the right. And the like is conversely true of the other line of retinal points α', β', γ'. Indeed, as the ordinary after-image method for demonstration of Listing's law shows, there is no oblique posture of the eyeball in which the after-images belonging to A, B, C do appear truly vertical. When the gaze is upward to the left the row they form leans up to the left, when the gaze is downward to the right the row leans downward to the right, and when the gaze is down to the left the row leans downward to the left. The inclinations are in fact both in sense and degree those of the well-known findings that demonstrate Listing's law.

The spatial reference, therefore, of a rectilinear row of retinal points— e.g., α, β, γ—says " vertical " *conditionally*. What condition decides it to affirm verticality in some circumstances, non-verticality in others ? In other words, on what factors is based its decision discriminating between vertical and non-vertical ? For simplicity of statement the discussion may be restricted to the one experiment where, firstly, the vertical row of spots A, B, C is fixated, and, secondly, the gaze is then, without other movement than that of the eyeball, turned upward to the right for observing the projected after-images. The first stage of this experiment may be called obs. 1, the second obs. 2. What is the difference of sensual conditions obtaining between obs. 1 and obs. 2 respectively ?

Evidently the only essential difference between them is that the posture of the eyeball has changed. Unless we suppose that the eyeball-muscles, unlike all other striped muscles, are unprovided with muscular sense, the new posture which they have assumed, and given to the eyeball, must be registered and perceptible. And the presumption is high that these muscles are liberally endowed with muscular sense, for they are known to be supplied copiously with proprioceptive nerves—the very system of nerves which in other muscles is the basis of muscular sense. If in an entirely dark room we direct the eyeballs in this direction or in that, we, although without retinal guidance, are still aware of the directions given to the eyeball. And this is so even when the whole front of the eyeball and the inner surface of the lids have been rendered insentient by cocaine. The direction of the eyeball is then judged almost as accurately as with use of the retina in the undarkened room. Such appreciation of the posture of the eyeball must be attributed to muscular sense. The experiment under discussion may therefore be stated thus: In obs. 1 the sensation from the retinal point group α, β, γ is accompanied by a muscular-sense impression p from the extrinsic ocular muscles, an impression attributive to their postural state at that time—namely, to the so-called primary position of the eye. In obs. 2 the similarly evoked retinal sensation from the same retinal point group is accompanied by a muscular-sense impression from the eye-muscles which is not p but p', attributive to a different postural state obtaining in them—namely, that of the given so-called secondary position assumed by the eyeball in obs. 2. The sensual complex is different, and the resulting perception differs accordingly. Evidently what we might suppose at first acceptance to be a purely visual perception is, in fact, the result of a fusion of retinal sensation with eye-muscle posture-sensation.

Granting this, can there be distinguished in these perceptions, which we may still call visual, the spatial elements which are purely retinal from those to which muscular sense is adjuvant? Let us leave aside, as not germane to the present question, perspective and third-dimensional features, as far as any such attach to these observations, arranged as they are to be as stripped of them as practicable. The spatial features then attaching to the perceptions are briefly as follows: In obs. 1 (1) three spots of a certain size and shape; (2) situate equidistant; (3) on one rectilinear axis; (4) which axis is " vertical," and (5) directly in front of the observer. If any of these features persist from obs. 1 unaltered into obs. 2, we may infer securely that muscular sense of the eyeball-muscles is not involved in them. Of the above five features (1), (2), and (3) do continue unaltered in obs. 2; they are, therefore, space-attributes of purely retinal origin. But (4) and (5) have undergone modification in the perception belonging to obs. 2, as compared with that of obs. 1. The row of spots, as seen in obs. 2, is no longer vertical, as it was in obs. 1, but is inclined to the vertical. And in obs. 2 the row is seen not directly in front of the observer, as in obs. 1, but is seen above and to the right. Therefore (4) and (5) are based on fusions of retinal sense with ocular-muscle sense. They may be *called* visual because natively apprehended to be such, but their source is not purely retinal.

A tactual analogue may serve in illustration. Let three points—say the prong-tips of a trifid fork—be set against the skin—*e.g.*, of a finger—by some other person and with one's eyes closed. One can perceive tactually not only that the points are three, and that they lie equidistant in one straight line, but, with approximate correctness, the orientation of that line to the vertical—also, of course, the whereabouts in the field of reach of the hand at which the touch is met. In this case the contribution made to the spatial perception by the muscular sense is well known and no longer debated. The recognition of the whereabouts in the arm's field of reach is based on the muscular sense of the arm, which tells us the arm's posture —*e.g.*, whether outstretched or not, whether outstretched to right or left when the touch is met with, etc. So also with the recognition of the orientation to the vertical of the line of the three touches.   Thus, if the line of the prong-tips be set parallel with the finger's long axis, and the finger be vertical when the touches are received, we perceive the line of touches as " vertical."   The postural muscle-sense of the arm, including the finger, is here, of course, the factor which gives the touch-row verticality.   If the finger be horizontal when the same three skin-points are touched, the touches say " horizontal."   Although the touch-loci have not been changed, the concomitant muscle-sense datum—the finger posture—has changed, and the touches now report " horizontally," *e.g.*, of the line of prong-tips, where formerly they reported " vertical."

The analogy between the tactual and the visual results is obvious. Further, the tactual example makes perhaps more evident another sensual factor involved similarly both in its own and in the visual problem, a factor whose consideration was postponed for the time being in the above statement of the two cases.   The evaluation of the posture of the arm in relation to surrounding objects is based upon two sets of proprioceptive data.   The impulses from the proprioceptive nerves of the limb itself originate the sense-data concerning the posturing of the limb itself, the local posture as it has been termed.   But at the same time the proprioceptive nerves of the rest of the body, and especially those of the gravitational labyrinth, are registering the attitude of the whole body and its orientation to the vertical. Perception of the local posture of the limb—*e.g.*, whether its pose is flexion or extension—gives no definite knowledge of its orientation unless there is concurrent perception of the attitude and orientation to the vertical of the rest of the body of which that limb is an appendage.   If one leans the trunk to the right, extension of the right arm thrusts the hand toward the ground; if one leans the body to the left, extension of the arm thrusts the hand away from the ground.   To orientate, therefore, by a touch with the hand the position in which an object lies, the local muscular sense of the limb is not enough; there must be combined with it the proprioceptive perception of the posture and gravitational orientation of the rest of the body.   The previously made statement of the perceiving of the whereabouts of the fork-prongs relatively to oneself has to be amplified as to its factors. In addition to T, the three touches, with purely tactual local signature, and to the sense-datum given by the arm's, including the finger's, own posture, there is a third, P, the sense datum of the attitude and gravitational orientation of the rest of the body.   So similarly in perceiving whether the row of touches is in a vertical or a horizontal line.   The factor p, the local limb posture, says nothing decisive about verticality unless combined with factor P.   But in the instance cited above factor P remains unchanged throughout the observation, as also do the three skin-points touched.   The only change is p, the posture of the limb—*i.e.*, the finger; the line of the touches is perceived vertical when the finger is vertical, horizontal when the finger is horizontal.

Returning to the visual observations, a like explanation holds.   The sense-datum derived from eyeball-muscles gives the " local " posture of the eyeball—*i.e.*, the attitude of the eyeball in relation to the head. But in order to evaluate the direction in which the seen object appears the sense-datum p of the " local " posture of the eyeball in the head is not enough. With it must be combined the sense-datum P of the posture and gravitational orientation of the head itself. The sense-datum p is indecisive as to the " direction " from the seeing self of the thing seen, and about the relation of a seen line to verticality, unless it be linked to P. But throughout the instance of visual observation which was chosen for discussion P remained unchanged. The head was fixed and the direction of uniocular gaze was shifted only by shifting in the orbit the local posture of the globus. Also, as said above, the three retinal spots were throughout the observation the same spots. The difference of spatial attributes between the perceptions belonging to the two stages of the observation are therefore due to change in the factor p—*i.e.*, the sense-datum from the ocular muscles, the only factor which does change. The change observed in spatial attribute of the perception was twofold. In the first part of the observation the three spots appear directly in front of oneself, in the second part they appear to the right and above. In the first part they report the line they lie in to be vertical. In the second part they report it inclined—*i.e.*, obliquely upwards to the right. Muscular sense attributive to the extrinsic ocular muscles is therefore a source of certain of the space-attributes of visual perception. It contributes to perceptions of the direction of the regarded object as projected by the observer. It is also one of the factors deciding the apparent verticality of a visual line or of that line's degree of obliquity to the vertical.

Lotze, when introducing the now generally adopted term " local sign," wrote luminously, " By ' local sign ' I mean that the position of the stimulated sensual point acts on the mind." The term in its practical application today has come, however, to be employed for something more restricted than spatial reference as a pure generality. It is employed for spatial reference to a locus in that combined space-system composed from the so-called spatial senses—*e.g.*, vision, touch, muscular and labyrinthine senses. Indeed, it seems inappropriate to use it for spatial attributes not referred to that common system of, so to say, ordinary workaday sensual space. Henry Watt's theory of a spatial reference constituting the basis of tonal pitch conceives a space reference not orientated in the common workaday space-system of the other senses. In Watt's view tonal pitch is an ordinal arrangement of space-signs giving merely degrees of distance between sensations of auditory modality and so generating impressions of movement but wholly devoid of orientation of position in reference to space perceived by us through other senses. To call the spatial reference in such a case " local sign " seems inadvantageous.

But the space-reference of vision has always orientation in common sensual space. If the position of the stimulated sensual point acts, as

Lotze said, on the mind—*e.g.*, in the retina gives visual local sign—it may be expected that where muscular action determines, as with the retina, the position of the stimulated point, a muscular-sense factor will intrude itself into and be, so to say, contained in the " local sign."

Two degrees of visual localisation have been long discriminated: the one, localisation relative to the fixation point; the other, localisation of the fixation point in reference to the observer. The former is often termed " relative " localisation, the latter " absolute " localisation. The simple observations forming the theme of this paper argue that the principle underlying the difference between these two kinds of local sign in vision is that muscular sense is a factor in the one and not in the other. That muscular sense is not a factor in relative local sign is tantamount to a recognition that where the space-relation between one sensory point and another cannot be altered by a muscular act, that muscular act contributes nothing sensorial to the perception of the space-relation between the points. The extrinsic muscles of an eyeball move and posture that eyeball's retina as a whole and cannot alter the mutual space-relations between points composing it. In the observations adduced in this paper the sensual line of points retains its intrinsic pattern unmodified by the posturing of the eyeball. The relative local signature of those points is unaltered by altering the muscular sense concomitant in the perceptions. Such local signature may be termed " pure retinal " local signature, because able to be regarded as pertaining to the retina itself purely.

Lotze, it will be remembered, entered upon, indeed raised, the interesting question as to how the retina has come to be endowed with its " relative " or, as termed above, " pure " local signature. That question is no part of our problem. But the view he advanced does possibly affect the suitability of the term " pure retinal " signature as equivalent to " relative " local signature. It does so because Lotze attributed the genesis of relative local sign to central sensations of eye-movement and sensations of effort accompanying or forerunning those. He argued that in the retina the distance and direction from the fovea of a peripheral point has become established as a sense-attribute to that point owing to accumulated experience of the degree and kind of central motor discharge necessary for moving the fovea so as to receive the objective image previously received by the peripheral point. He supposed, in short, that the " relative local sign " attaching to a retinal point has its origin in a long history of experience of muscular sense—not muscular sense as now usually understood with the connotation of peripheral proprioceptive source, but muscular sense in that older and now less prevalent acceptation, implying a " central sensation " gauging the degree and direction of motor discharge. Lotze's view is adverted to here merely to make clear that its appeal to a kind of muscular sense in its attempt to explain the genetic history of " relative " local sign is not touched by the argument we are now following. Hering explicitly denied to muscular sense any share either in relative or in absolute

local sign. As regards relative local sign, apart from its possible past
genetic history, on which this paper has nothing to submit, the argument
of the present paper is in agreement with Hering.

But with regard to absolute local signatu᷄ ᷄ th᷄ case is different. The
principle emerged above that where a muscular act cannot alter the space-
relation between two receptive sensory points, its proprioceptive sensation
does not affect or enter into the perception of that space-relation. Conversely, where a muscular act does alter the space-relation between two
such points its sensation does enter into the perception of that space-
relation.

There is a spatial point in the head which Hering termed the " basal
point of vision." " The head, or more exactly the place where, with
reference to the object viewed, we imagine our head to be, forms the centre
of visual perception." The position of this point may be defined as corresponding with the centre of rotation of Hering's cyclopean eye, or, briefly
paraphrasing, the cyclopean point of outlook. Though a subjective point,
it corresponds with a material point; this latter, as Hering showed, lies in
the mid-sagittal plane of the head. And in that plane its position is where
that plane is intersected by a line joining the centres of rotation of the two
eyeballs right and left. The movements and postures executed by the
extrinsic ocular muscles affect the spatial relation between their retina and
this material point. Therefore, into the visual space-signature which refers
to spatial relation between the perceptual object and the point of visual
outlook, there will enter the muscular sense attribute of the movements
and postures executed by the extrinsic ocular muscles. Hence, in the
observations cited above, a change confined to alteration of the posture of
the eyeball brings a change in the " absolute " local signature, a change
in the spatial reference of the retinal point. The sensation pertaining to
the stimulated retinal point is projected to a locus in sensual space surrounding the subjective point of outlook, and that locus shifts with shift
in the eyeball's posture. The absolute local signature has therefore in it
a muscular sense factor derived from the extrinsic ocular muscles.

There remains obviously a further element in visual space-assignment.
Lotze says, were vision our sole sense our visual field would be an expanse
without upper or lower or right or left, and for the same reason that no
one in thinking of the universe as a whole regards it as being erect or
vertical or horizontal, inclined, etc. Yet, in visual perception, among the
seemingly elemental features of it are verticality, horizontality, etc. We
have to consider on what this orientated nature of visual space is based.
In the simple observations, the subject of this paper, when the retina has
passed from the primary visual posture to the oblique secondary, and by
so doing has arrived at a posture exhibiting the so-called " false-torsion "
of the authors, objective verticality is still perceived, although through
partly a new line of retinal points. The only other change in the condition
of the observations is the altered muscular state and altered muscular

sensation attaching to maintenance of the eyeball in its new posture—namely, the oblique secondary posture.

That is a proprioceptive factor. Now, obvious considerations urge that the main agency by which the environment impresses upon sense its orientation translated by the mind as right-side-upness or deviations therefrom, is gravitation—i.e., the direction of the line of gravity. This seems indeed the only direct environmental influence by which that orientation becomes an immediate sensual datum. It is the only one which in so far as concerns that orientation causes reflexes directly and *per se*. In some fields of musculature gravity undoubtedly affects physically the muscular reactions in considerable measure, although whether reflexes or sensations are thereby excited is as yet insufficiently known. But the muscles of the eyeball constitute a field of proprioception which gravity can hardly affect more than so slightly as to let one suppose its influence there must be of negligible degree. There is, however, an organ, the otic labyrinth, definitely reacting to gravity. We know that organ to be the source of postural reflexes employing the extrinsic eye-muscles. The proprioceptive mechanism of the eyeball-muscles is therefore yoked with that of the otic labyrinth in reflex action. Following the principle established in like cases, the inference is that the sense-impressions of the two are likewise associated. This means that the orientation of the retina in space in regard to the line of gravity, that is to say in the mind in regard to verticality, results from co-operation between the special gravity sense-organ and the muscular sense of the orbital muscles. The so-called primary position of the eyeball is therefore a posture in which the extrinsic ocular muscles co-operate with the otic labyrinth, and the perception of that posture is based on sense-data from both those sources. That posture, however, because it is sensed visually, is perceived by the mind not as a state of the eyeball, but as a state of the external world, of the world as seen; it is " projected."

It appears, so far as space orientation is concerned, as a direct perception of the orientation of the external world. In the observation above the verticality of the line seen by the three retinal points in the primary eye-posture has therefore an otic and an ocular muscle factor combined in it. That a change as regards verticality occurs for those same three retinal points when the eye-posture becomes a secondary oblique one, although the head and therefore the labyrinth posture remains unchanged, shows that in the visual perception of verticality the otic labyrinth datum is so bound up with the proprioceptive datum from the eye-muscles that the latter is a condition for the meaning of the former. Visual local signature as regards the spatial orientation connoted by verticality and deviations therefrom is therefore compounded of at least three factors—namely, retinal, proprioceptive from the extrinsic eye-muscles, and otic labyrinths. There is almost certainly a further, though probably minor, factor in it, and that a proprioceptive one, with its source in the muscles of the neck.

Recent experiments by de Kleijn (*Archives néerlandaises de Physiologie*, tome ii., p. 644, 1918) show that in the rabbit alterations in the posture of the neck, especially of the two uppermost segments, provoke and maintain definite postures of the eyeballs. These he determined after previous extirpation of the otic labyrinths. They resembled those provokable from the labyrinths themselves, and like those latter were, so to say, in the interest of retaining the retina in the position from which the altered posture of the head displaced it. Sensory impressions of neck-posture have therefore probably to be added to the factors implicated in visual perception of orientation as regards verticality and inclinations thereto.

The above simple observations have been confined to uniocular vision in order to render description and consideration of them more easily given and more clearly followed. But the instances cited, though individual cases only, are of widely applicable type. The upshot of similar binocular observations is similar and similarly explicable. In binocular observations the greater intrusion of the third dimension makes the problem more complex but at the same time enhances its interest. All, however, that is attempted here is to call attention to some simple yet cogent evidence of an important contribution made by the proprioceptive nerves of the external ocular muscles even to uniretinal space perception. It is not that such contribution is unexpected. On the contrary, it is but what on grounds of analogy with other organs—*e.g.*, the hand—we should expect. In so saying, the word "organ" seems preferable to the word "sense." If we state the analogy as one between visual perceptions and other specially endowed perceptions, such as tactual, we run a risk of possibly obscuring what is one of the objects of this short paper to make clear. For what the paper desires to insist upon is that the spatial perceptions under discussion are not purely visual, but are in fact, though such nomenclature would be cumbrous, visuo-musculo-labyrinthine, and their analogy is with tactuo-musculo-labyrinthine.

Finally, apart from subscribing or not subscribing to the general doctrine of psycho-physical parallelism, there is a conviction which the neurologist studying the taxis of the nervous system cannot but derive. If in the sensation or perception which belongs to a particular act analysis reveals components derived from nerves of two or more sensual species, the taxis, even though subconscious, of the muscles employed in that act, whether movement or posture, will likewise involve the co-operation of those same two or more species of afferent nerve. Hence, in the ocular reactions discussed, impairment of the muscular sense of the eye-muscles will impair not only the spatial perceptions, but also the taxis, the spatial reaction, even the subconscious and purely reflex taxis, of the eye-movements and eye-postures normally accompanying the perceptions. The proprioceptive afferents of the eye-muscles at their exit from the central nervous system are, unlike the proprioceptive afferents of most muscles, not separated from the motor fibres. This makes a difficulty for the experimental investigation of the influence which their destruction would have upon the movements and postures of the eye. They cannot for experiment be severed apart from the motor fibres themselves. But in tabes we have a disease which attacks systematically the proprioceptive afferents, and spares at least for long the motor fibres. For the problem touched in the present paper it seems significant that squints, often transient in character, are not infrequently an early feature of tabes.

THE INFLUENCE OF SENSORY NERVES UPON THE MOVEMENT AND NUTRITION OF THE LIMBS[1]

In the 14th of the *Leçons sur la physiologie et la pathologie du système nerveux*, Claude Bernard draws attention by experiments on the frog and on puppies to the degree of impairment in movement undergone by a limb that has been rendered insensitive by section of the sensory roots of its spinal nerves.

In a series of experiments carried out during the last eighteen months, we have examined the same thing in the monkey, using chiefly *Macacus rhesus*, and observing the animals for periods up to four months from the time of operation.[2] We propose to give here a brief account of the results obtained.

Our experiments deal separately with the lower limb and with the upper limb. The phenomena observed in the two limbs do not essentially differ, but are rather more marked and much more accessible to examination in the case of the upper limb.

On Movement

(1) *Effect of Section of the Whole Series of Sensory Roots belonging to the Limb.* —By the " whole series " is meant in the brachial region from the 4th cervical to the 4th thoracic inclusive; in the lumbar from the 2nd to the 10th post-thoracic inclusive.

From the time of performance of the section onwards, as long as the animal may be kept, the movements of the hand and foot are practically abolished; the movement of grasping, which is so frequent and useful to the monkey, both with the hand and foot, never occurs at all in our experience. On the other hand, the movements at the elbow and knee, and especially the movements at the shoulder and hip, are much less impaired. The fore-limb hangs from the shoulder partially flexed at the elbow; the hind-limb is flexed at hip and knee. As the animal runs about it does not attempt to use the leg; the fore-limb swings helplessly, with flexion at elbow and wrist and adduction at shoulder, in much the same position as if carried in a sling. The hind-limb looks as if it were being held up so as to be kept off the ground while the animal runs on three

---

[1] Published in *Proc. roy. Soc.*, 1894-5, **57**, 481, with F. W. Mott, under the above title.—ED.

[2] In all operations the animals have been deeply anæsthetised with chloroform and ether.

legs; we are inclined to think that this appearance is deceptive, and that the position results from an equilibrium of the action of the muscles, in which purposive action on the part of the animal does not play a rôle. When the animal is allowed to climb a rope or the side of the cage, the fore-limb swings more or less helplessly, and is not used for the climbing; similarly, the hind-limb is kept more or less flexed at the hip or knee, and is not used for the climbing. If the feeding-time be deferred, and an animal, in which the apæsthete[1] limb is an arm, be tested by offering it fruit after the sound arm has been secured behind the back, there is no attempt to use the apæsthete limb for reaching the food, but the neck is thrust forward in order for the mouth to seize it. If the fruit be placed in the hand of the apæsthete arm, the animal does not lift the hand, and appears quite unable to do so, even though encouraged. If, however, the hands of a tame normal monkey be secured behind its back, and, as it lies on the floor, fruit be placed near it, the fruit is usually taken at once with the foot; but if the leg is apæsthete the fruit cannot be taken, although in one monkey the attempt used to be made. The foot was rapidly thrust toward the fruit by extension of the hip and knee, but the foot missed its object widely—i.e., by several inches—and the digits were not moved, though the ankle appeared to be slightly plantar-flexed. The impairment of motility in the limb ensues immediately upon completion of the section— that is to say, directly the effects of the anæsthetic have passed off sufficiently to allow requisite examination of the animal's ability to move its limbs, the above-described inability is discoverable as fully developed as at any subsequent period. We have kept the animals alive for various periods up to and over three months, and there has been no obvious change in the condition, either in the direction of improvement or the reverse. In the case of the lower limb, after two or three months, the constant position of flexion of hip and knee, on two occasions, gradually induced a change in the muscles of the thigh, which prevented hip and knee being properly extended, even by passive stretching.

As to the nature of the disturbance of motility in the limbs, one feature— namely, its peculiar topographical distribution—is salient and constant. The defect in motility increases from the attached base to the free apex of the limb, so that, for instance, while comparatively slight at the hip, it is successively greater at knee and ankle, and greatest (amounting as regards volition to absolute loss) in the digits.

In this respect it curiously closely simulates the impairment of motility ensuing upon ablation of the limb region of the cortex cerebri; but it is, in the monkey, somewhat *more severe* than the impairment following cortical ablation.

We find, however, that forcible and rapid movements, even of the fine joints at the end of the limb, can be induced in the animals by causing

---

[1] " Deprived of sensation," in distinction from anæsthete, " devoid of sensation." We are indebted to Dr. Verrall, of Trinity College, Cambridge, for the suggestion of this term.

them to " struggle "; for instance, while recovering from ether inhalation, or while trying to free themselves on being held awkwardly, the whole limb at all its joints may exhibit movements; but even under these circumstances it is only once or twice that we have seen " grasping " movements of the digits, although sharp extension of the digits is not nearly so infrequent.

We are led from these and other considerations to conclude that *associated movements in the limb* (" Mitbewegungen ") *are comparatively little impaired* by loss of the sensation from the limb in which they occur; but that the independent and more delicately adjusted movements which employ preponderantly the smaller and more individual muscular masses of the hand and foot, and serve to move the digits, especially the hallux and the thumb—in fact, just *those movements which are represented most liberally in the limb area of the cortex—are extremely severely impaired, and, in some instances, are abolished*. We say " abolished " advisedly, because we are persuaded from our observations that, in the case of certain movements—*e.g.*, grasping movements of the hand and foot, opposition of pollex and hallux—the animal is rendered absolutely powerless to perform them, even under the strongest possible inducements. This conclusion has been gradually forced upon us. Although we are aware of the danger of introducing terms relating to consciousness into descriptions based almost solely on motor reactions, we believe that we cannot more lucidly state the condition of the animals than by saying that the volitional power for grasping with the hand, etc., had been absolutely abolished by the local loss of all forms of sensibility experimentally produced; further, that this volitional power was lost immediately from the time of operation and that there was not the slightest evidence of any recovery of it during the longest periods to which our observations extended (about four months).

This being so, it is natural to inquire what influence, if any, is exerted by the section of the posterior spinal nerve-roots of the limbs upon the reactions obtainable from the limb area of the cortex? That no diminution, but rather a slight increase of the excitability of the cortex, is the immediate result has been shown by one of us previously.[1]   But the question remained, What will be the result when, for many weeks, the severance of the roots has led (as above shown) to disappearance from the limb of those very movements which the cortex, when experimentally excited, is especially able to produce? We have answered this, both by electrically exciting the cortex and by giving absinthe intravenously to produce epilepsy. On exciting the cortex cerebri of the hemispheres in the appropriate regions for eliciting movements of the thumb, hallux, or digits, the responsive movements have been as easily elicited from the apæsthete limb as from the normal limb, and it has several times seemed to us rather more easily—that is to say, with a slightly less intensity of faradic current (the rate of interruption always remaining the same, $\frac{1}{50}$ second).

[1] C. S. Sherrington, *Philos. Trans.*, 1893, **184B**, 690, 691.

As to the absinthe epilepsy, it always affected the apæsthete limb in a manner not distinguishably different from the normal limb. Convulsions sometimes started in the normal and desensitised limb simultaneously, sometimes a little earlier in one or the other; but no indubitable predominance or preference was shown by either limb. In a very few of our experiments (three) no movement was obtained in the apæsthete limb on excitation of the cortex; this was found to be explained subsequently by naked-eye degeneration of the pyramidal tract as revealed after hardening in Müller's fluid. This degeneration was due to injury accidentally inflicted upon the lateral column of the cord by the operation. The spinal tonus in the muscles of the apæsthete limb is undoubtedly much diminished.

These observations seem to us to point to the profound difference existing between the production of the finer movements of the limb in volition on the one hand, and by experimental stimulation of the cortex on the other. The fundamental importance of sensation for those finer movements of the limb, which are so especially well represented in the cortex of the ape, has by no authority been more forcibly emphasised than by Dr. Bastian. We think these experiments go even further than his arguments in pointing to the influence of sensation upon voluntary movement, inasmuch as they indicate that not only the cortex, but the whole sensory path from periphery to the cortex cerebri, is in action during voluntary movement.

(2) *Effect of Section of a Single Sensory Root.*—In striking contradiction to the above-stated impairment of movement in the limb ensuing upon section of the whole series of its sensory nerve-roots stands the effect of section of any one of the sensory nerve-roots of the series singly and alone. In the latter case no impairment of movement at all results, or, at least, can with certainty be detected.

This is the case even when the largest and most important sensory root of the series is chosen for section—namely, in the upper limb the 8th cervical, and in the lower limb the 6th post-thoracic. (These are the nerves that supply the skin over the whole of the hand and foot respectively. It is to be remembered, however, that hand and foot respectively are each of them supplied with sensation by at least three sensory roots, the middle root covering the whole surface in each case.)

We attribute the fact that section of these large roots with their wide distribution over hand and foot produces so little appreciable effect to the fact that the distribution of all the spinal nerves in the skin is an overlapping one. The extent of overlapping is great enough to prevent the section of any one nerve, even of the largest, producing actual anæsthesia of the skin in any part.

We further find that even if a field of absolute anæsthesia be actually produced by section, for instance, of the 7th, 8th, and 9th post-thoracic roots, or, in some cases, by section of the 7th and 8th cervical and 1st and 2nd thoracic roots, the impairment of movement resulting in the limb is comparatively slight. This is the more remarkable when the region deprived of sensibility includes some of the most highly sensitive parts in the limb—namely, those of the palm.[1]

On Nutrition

In the experiments upon the lower limb we were at first led to suspect that section of the sensory roots caused trophic changes in the skin of the foot. After a time, varying from three weeks to three months, an ulcer appeared over the outer malleolus; the subsequent experiments on the upper limb, which never led to such a change, show, in our opinion, that the apparent trophic change in the lower limb may more justly be attributed to the liability to pressure and microbic infection. No change in the hand was ever noticed which in the least indicated trophic disturbance. Wounds accidentally inflicted by the animal itself or its companions on the apæsthete part healed readily when dressed.

As to the condition of the muscles in the apæsthete limb, which were themselves removed from all afferent connection with the central nervous system, the following points were noticed:

There was a certain degree of wasting, but no appreciable alteration of colour; and the muscles responded readily to the excitation of their motor nerves. In some instances it was found that on excitation of their motor nerves, after somatic death, muscular contractions were evoked for a longer period than in the normal side. The time of onset of *rigor mortis* was delayed in the apæsthete muscles, as one of us has already noted in the cat (p. 246).

[1] Further experiments involving partial sensory denervation of the hand and foot, and attempts to section roots which produced a loss of sensation predominantly in the muscles of the foot, or conversely in the skin of the foot, are reported. On account of the complexity of the factors concerned they are omitted here. The problem is discussed further in the last chapter (p. 512).—ED.

IV

ON THE SPINAL ANIMAL AND THE NATURE OF SPINAL REFLEX ACTIVITY

[Goltz and his pupil Freusberg had, at Strasbourg, studied the reactions of the spinal dog, and their papers in 1874 had described many reflexes as they are seen in the intact animal after spinal shock has passed off. They had observed inhibitory cessation of reflexes by appropriately timed strong stimulation of the skin. Sherrington made several long visits to Strasbourg between 1885 and 1895, and in this period began his study of spinal reflexes in monkey, dog, and cat at the Brown Institution, London. The spinal cord of the monkey survived transection badly, and his initial interest in spinal shock derives from this circumstance. It was shown, however, that the reflexes in the monkey were essentially the same as in the dog, and further studies were then chiefly made in the latter animal, which survives transection much better than the monkey or cat.

*The preliminary studies were directed to defining the principles of spread of reflex effects, demonstrating that the rigid laws of Pflüger (1853) did not hold for many reflex responses. Nor were spinal reflexes bound by anatomical segmentation. Many new reflex effects were described, and particular reflexes were then subjected to close analysis. The pattern of reflex arrangement and interaction gradually emerged, including the principle of reciprocal innervation and the demonstration of the postural reflexes.—*Ed.]

ON SPINAL SHOCK[1]

" Shock," like " collapse," is a term more used by the clinician than by the physiologist; the scope of both words is usually left ill-defined. In some forms of the clinical condition circulatory disturbance and inspissation of the blood play a part in " shock," but, as understood by the physiologist, " shock " is primarily a nervous condition. " If in a frog the spinal marrow be divided just below the occiput, there are for a very short time no diastaltic actions in the extremities. The diastaltic actions speedily return. This phenomenon is ' shock.' "[2] In this, as in previous papers, I myself mean by the term *the whole of that depression or suppression of nervous reaction which ensues forthwith upon a mechanical injury of some part of the nervous system, and is of temporary nature.* The best explicit account of the condition is contained in the papers of Goltz. By him temporary paralysis following injuries of the brain or cord are all classed as *Hemmungserscheinungen*, and

---

[1] From *Philos. Trans.*, 1898, **190B**, 133 (Croonian Lecture).
[2] Marshall Hall, *Synopsis of the Diastaltic Nervous System*, London, 1850.

these collectively may be considered to compose the phenomenon of "shock." Goltz's[1] descriptions of spinal shock are masterly, but they refer entirely to the dog, and to transection below the middle of the back. As it is in the monkey that the phenomenon appears at maximum, and especially consequently to high cervical transection, I shall give a description of it as so seen.

[2] There can hardly be witnessed a more striking phenomenon in the physiology of the nervous system. From the limp limbs, even if the knee jerks be elicitable, no responsive movement, beyond perhaps a feeble tremulous adduction or bending of the thumb or hallux, can be evoked even by insults of a character severe in the extreme. That which the delicate yellow spot is to the sensifacient sheet of the retina, may the thumb and index be said to constitute in the great sensifacient field of the limb. Nevertheless, a hot iron laid right across thumb, index, and palm remains an absolutely impotent excitant, or able only to evoke a faint flexion of the thumb; the crushing of a finger has no greater effect. A huge afferent nerve, such as the internal saphenous, containing some five thousand sensory nerve-fibres, when laid across the electrodes and subjected to currents absolutely unbearable upon the tongue, elicits no further response, and probably no movement whatsoever. To the whole popliteal nerve representing an area of sentient skin which includes the entire sole and much of the leg besides, intolerable faradisation can be applied and elicits no more, and often even less, response. A more impassable condition of block, or torpor, can hardly be imagined: its depth of negation resembles, to superficial examination, profound chloroform poisoning. The circulation is, however, approximately normal in these cases, and the respiration absolutely so. The skin, as above stated, is well warm, even to the tips of the hands and feet. Further, the fundamental distinction between the condition and that induced by any chemical nervous depressant is clear in the following two features. (1) The spinal motoneurones, though profoundly inaccessible to stimuli, applied via skin or afferent nerve-trunks, are perfectly open to any applied via the pyramidal paths: excitation of the pyramidal tract at the top of the cord evokes as readily as or more readily than ever, in both limbs, its usual variety of movements. (2) Excitation, mechanical or by weak currents quite imperceptible to the tongue, of the *central ends of the spinal posterior (dorsal, sensory) roots themselves, fairly readily evokes the usual reflex movements* elicitable—although enormously stronger stimuli fail absolutely when applied to the skin and afferent nerve-trunks. At first finding this, I supposed an explanation might lie in the fact that the roots contain large numbers of afferent fibres from muscles, while the peripheral nerve-trunks and surfaces tried are chiefly cutaneous; but excitation of the spinal end of the hamstring nerve, with its quantities of afferent nerve-fibres from muscle and deep structures, caused no more effect; caused, in fact, less effect than a pure cutaneous sensory trunk, such

[1] *Pflüg. Arch. ges. Physiol.*, 1874, **8**, 460, *Die functionen des Lendenmarkes des Hundes.* [2] *Ibid.*, p. 412.

as the long saphenous.[1] This condition, although most usual and striking in the monkey, and therefore here chiefly described in his case, is seen, to a certain extent, also in cat and dog. When, in them, the spinal depression is great, it is easily found to be more marked when examined by excitation of skin or peripheral nerves than when examined by excitation of the afferent spinal roots; the motor reactions, provokable from the former, are less ample and less numerous than from the latter. It is no question of escape of exciting current to the motor roots themselves.

[2]Whether the position of the severance be near the top or at the bottom of the thoracic region makes some, but no very great, difference to the general result, beyond of course increasing or reducing the *number* of spinal segments displaying the phenomenon. The "shock" appears to take effect in a *downward* direction only. Thus section below the brachial enlargement does not obviously disturb in any way the reactions of the upper limb, and this although we know by anatomy (Wallerian method) that the number of upward channels ruptured by such a section is enormous, and must think, therefore, that many co-ordinating ties between the upper and lower limbs are destroyed. Again, most striking instances of the absence of upward spread of the depression due to "shock" are afforded by transections abutting on the lower edge of the 5th cervical segment; these depress the respiratory activity of the phrenic motor neurons hardly at all, even momentarily (cat). The rhythmic action of the motoneurones (for the diaphragm) is not obviously interfered with, although on the lower side of the transection depression may be profound. Analogously, the sudden cutting off of that stream of subconscious centripetal impulses which must be continually pouring to the brain from tail, lower limbs and trunk seems to disturb the head and brain not at all. The animal immediately after the section will direct its attention to catching flies, or looking out of the window, taking no notice of nor apparent interest in its paralysed and insensitive parts. After section of the cord above the 1st cervical pair there is no obvious disturbance in the head; as the creatures lie quiet and watchful, the only and dubious sign of abnormality is a tendency to drop off rapidly and frequently into sleep. The pupils are equal and, of course, small.

If after transection above the 1st cervical level in the cat sufficient time be allowed for the first effects of shock to pass away, the condition of the reflexes in the limbs, both fore and hind, be examined, and if then the cord be a second time transected, and this time at the 6th thoracic level,

---

[1] Direct stimulation of a dorsal nerve-root is a more powerful stimulus in virtue of its containing many more pain fibres than a peripheral nerve. The effect of shock, therefore, would appear to be a quantitative one, and in later papers was attributed to a fall in the excitability of the motoneurones in the spinal cord, to some extent reversible by strychnine (Cooper, Denny-Brown, and Sherrington, *Proc. roy. Soc.*, 1926, **100B,** 456). If the fall in excitability be due to removal of a "subsidy" from the pyramidal, reticulo-spinal, vestibulo-spinal, and other descending tracts, the above observation of the remaining potency of stimulation of the pyramidal tract is the more understandable.—ED.   [2] *Ibid.*, p. 134.

the second section produces a shock effect but only on the aboral side of it. In the lower limb the skin reflexes, which may have been numerous and of sustained discharge, become few and brief—e.g., at the ankle, instead of an alternating discharge of dorsal and plantar flexors, the idiolateral reflex may be reduced to a simple dorsal flexion. In the fore-limbs, on the contrary, exaltation has occurred: the skin reflexes are more numerous and more sustained. The crossed reflex (in my experience rarely obtained) from one fore-limb to the other may become elicitable, although not so previously. Similarly, in front of the top section signs of exaltation are present. The surface seems hyperæsthetic; a single touch with a piece of paper on the snout elicits vigorous licking of the spot touched; the mere approach of a hot-water can (used to keep the animal warm) evokes screwing up of the eyes and of the mouth; salivation is profuse, as a rule; a touch on the vibrissæ evokes exaggerated facial movement; I have seen photophobia.

After transection at the top of the cord there appears to be more shock in the fore- than in the hind-limbs. Long path reflexes are less able to evoke movement from the fore-limbs than from the hind—e.g., stimulation of pinna of ear more easily evokes movement of foot than of hand. Also the reflex movements obtained from each limb by excitations incident on itself are movements less forcible than those elicitable from the hind-limb. Occasionally, stimuli applied to the fore-limb evoke no movement in itself, though a brisk movement in the fellow hind-limb. The reflexes obtained under these conditions from the fore-limb, especially of flexion of elbow, tend to be tonic rather than clonic, whereas clonic contractions are the rule in the hind-limb, but this may depend on something other than depression. The depression of reflex activity after high cervical transverse section might be supposed to be due to the fall in general arterial blood-pressure which must ensue. That this cannot be the chief part of the explanation of this shock is clear from the above considerations: (1) that the head does not participate in the " shock," although participating in the lowered blood-pressure; and (2) that when the transection is in lower dorsal region, the " shock " distal to the sections is about as severe as after cervical transection. Besides, Owsjannikow[1] pointed out that section of the splanchnics and its accompanying fall of blood-pressure does not cause shock, and that excitation of the peripheral ends of the cut splanchnics and the production of a good arterial pressure does not set it aside.

[2]The existence of spinal vasomotor centres subsidiary to the bulbar is asserted on the ground that it is still possible to obtain reflex alterations of blood-pressure when the cord has been transected at *calamus scriptorius* if strychnia be exhibited to heighten its reflex activity. To demonstrate the existence of potent vasomotor centres in the spinal cord does not, however, require the exhibition of strychnia. It is enough to allow the lapse of a few days or, better, weeks after transection of the cord in the cervical region.

[1] Ludwig's *Arbeiten*, 1874, p. 314.
[2] Extract from " On the Spinal Animal," *Med.-Chir. Trans.*, 1899, **82**, 470 *et seq.*

The blood-pressure will then be found to have in the carotid of the dog a mean value of something over 100 mm. of mercury. By stimulating the skin mechanically or by temperature changes, or by faradising the central end of the afferent nerve—e.g., of the foot—reflex increase of blood-pressure raising it 20 to 30 mm. of Hg is easily obtained.[1] It is only in the first few hours immediately succeeding the initial trauma of transection that the cord being in a condition of shock gives no reflex response by its vascular musculature any more than by its skeletal musculature. This visceral shock seems no more severe in the higher than in the lower verte-brata. It is as regards the performances of the skeletal musculature that great difference exists in regard to shock distinguishing between the spinal frog and spinal monkey. I have ventured to suggest that the spinal shock of the latter animal is connected with an isolation dystrophy such as occurs in cases where nerve-cells habitually actuated by other nerve-cells are suddenly and completely cut off from their influence. That the difference is very great and real between lower and higher types in this respect of spinal shock is shown by such instances as the following. The cat from which the Rolandic area of the cortex has been removed, so as to ablate the whole of the limb centres from one hemisphere, if some weeks later " decerebrate rigidity " be induced in its limbs, yields the rigidity without perceptible difference between the sides both right and left. But in the monkey similarly prepared, a great difference between the limbs of the two sides is apparent. The rigidity on the side crossed to the cerebral lesion is very much less than on the homonymous side. At the same time it must not be thought that the whole depression of function in the parts innervated behind the spinal transection is due to removal from them of merely cerebral influence. That that cannot be the case is shown by a fact that I have several times had opportunity to observe—namely, that the performance of a second spinal transection some weeks later, and some segments behind a former spinal transection, is followed by the recrudescence of many of the original symptoms of depression of function that had followed the original transection. It is significant that such a second transection behind a previous one causes a considerable increase in the descending spinal degeneration, showing that there descend from upper parts of the spinal cord many channels arising in those upper spinal regions and con-necting them with other spinal regions further back.

Whence comes the great difference existent between, on the one hand, ape and man, and, on the other, fish and frog, as regards the depression of the reactions of the skeletal musculature ensuent upon total transverse lesion of the spinal cord ?

Shock is not only more severe in the monkey than in the other laboratory types, but it is also more lasting, and its symptoms are more profound and prolonged than in any other animal I have observed. The symptoms of

[1] Figured in the original description. See also *Integrative Action*, 1906, Fig. 67, p. 242; *Proc. roy. Soc.*, 1900, **66**, 390, Schäfer's *Textbook*, 1900, **2**, p. 854, and this volume, pp. 214 and 223.—Ed.

shock, in many monkeys, persist for days instead of hours and minutes, as in cat and dog. It is important to note that in the monkey much of what we are, from observations upon the lower animal types, inclined to regard as temporary, and relegate to block or " shock," in Goltz's language " *Hemmungserscheinungen* "—not " *Ausfallserscheinungen* "—proves, under prolonged observation to be, I must admit, permanent—in fact, to be *true deficiency phenomenon*. Every histologist acquainted with the comparative structure of the spinal cord in the ape and in the dog must have been impressed with the far greater complexity obvious in the former. The above evidence is in accord with that, for it shows that the same trauma inflicted upon the cord leads, in the monkey, to much heavier permanent defect than in the dog; just as, in fact, ablations of the cortex cerebri are pregnant with far greater " *Ausfallserscheinungen* " in the monkey (Ferrier, H. Munk, Schäfer, Mott) than in the dog (Goltz). It is reasonable to argue still severer results in the case of the human spinal cord; of which, again, we know the minute structure to be yet more complex still. *The permanent damage done is therefore, as well as the initial shock, disproportionately greater in monkey than in cat and dog.*

My own experience leads me to think that the condition of a spinal cord isolated by a spinal transection is often more normal a few hours after the transection than it is when long periods of weeks and months are allowed to elapse. I am well aware that this is contrary to the opinion of Goltz and others. The advantage believed to accrue from waiting is that the phenomena of shock may have time to pass off as completely as possible. How long the phenomena of shock may last at longest is a question on which very different views are held. Goltz, to whose trenchant observations and bold system of experiment we owe so much of our knowledge of the physiology of the central nervous system, is the founder of a school which works in the belief that the phenomenon of shock may persist for months, even years. It is, as far as not, merely a matter of nomenclature, a question on which no definite decision seems as yet possible. I myself have gradually been driven to the belief that " shock " does not take long to pass off— *i.e.*, does not at longest persist for more than a few weeks. I am not considering here the complications arising out of long, badly healing and suppurative wounds, and the continual irritation they may produce if situate in the nervous system. But though shock passes off, the alterations produced in the isolated cord or piece of cord (by permanent withdrawal of the influences it has lived accustomed to receive from other portions of the central nervous system) progress, and are in a sense cumulative. The decreasing depression merges—at present inextricably for us—in the increasing onset of an " isolation-dystrophy." Much of what is called " shock," in regard to the mammalian cord, is, I believe, due to " isolation-dystrophy," and is really permanent—that is to say, would not pass away if the animal were to live healthily for any number of years. The most favourable time for the examination of the independent capabilities of the

spinal cord is that when the sum of " shock " and " isolation-dystrophy "
together is of smallest amount.   That time, compounded as it is of two
such variable factors, is itself extraordinarily variable.   In result of spinal
transection in monkey, I am sure that " shock " lasts longer, and that
" isolation-dystrophy " comes on earlier than in the other animal types
commonly observed in the laboratory.   It is the conjunction of the periods
of these two phenomena which renders so difficult and so largely defeats
attempts at observations on proper spinal reactions of the monkey.   If the
overlap of the two is great, then no spinal reflexes, or only the merest traces
of them, may be observable.   In man it is only natural to suppose—and
what clinical experience I have had access to strengthens me in the belief—
that even more than in monkey will " shock " be protracted, and " isolation-
dystrophy " speedy and severe.   The observations of Bastian,[1] Bowlby,[2]
and Bruns[3] teach us that the clinical picture of the effects of total transverse
lesions of the human spinal cord does not accord in the way that medical
textbooks have been wont to describe with the long known results obtained
from the transected cord by the physiologist.   Older physiological experiments are, however, not based on nervous systems so approximate to the
human as is that of Macacus, Cercocebus, etc.   Of these latter I would
say that their condition after spinal transection commonly resembles in its
features in the most striking manner the condition of spinal depression
observed after spinal translesion in man, and considered by Bastian to be
the typical status.[4]

   In the monkey in most cases—partly, perhaps, because the lesion is
more localised by experimental infliction than by accidental—the depression
is not so severe.   For instance, the knee jerk, which disappears almost
immediately after the transection, returns usually in a week or ten days—
often, however, not for three weeks; occasionally, on the other hand, in ten
minutes.

   The great motor organ—the skeletal musculature—is at the command
of the sense-organs.   Not only is it actuated by contact sensations evoked
in the neural system of the individual by the tangible quality of the circumambient environment; each light that causes the animal to move, each
sound, each odour, shows how the motor machine lies at the behest of the
great sense-organs of the head.   Now these latter are broadly distinguishable
from the sense-organs of the trunk inasmuch as they subserve sense possessing
the *quale* of " projection."   For each individual creature the material
universe is thus separated into two parts, the part that is " me," and the
part that is " not me."   I think it was Lotze who said that doubtless to
the trodden worm, of these two halves the trodden " me " shall surely

---

[1] *Med.-Chir. Trans.*, London, 1891.   [2] *Ibid.*   [3] *Neurologisches Centralblatt*, Berlin, 1893.
   [4] The human spinal cord was later shown to make ample recovery from spinal shock, as was
proven from verified spinal injuries of warfare (Holmes, *Brit. Med. Journ.*, 1915, **2**, 815, and
especially the detailed studies of Head and Riddoch, *Brain*, 1917, **40**, 188).   Though exceptionally the human spinal reflexes recover almost to the degree of those of the spinal dog, the
average amount of recovery appears to be rather less than that of the average spinal monkey.—ED.

appear the greater. By a high spinal transection the splendid motor machinery of the vertebrate is practically as a whole and at one stroke severed from all the universe except that fraction the " material me." The deeper depression of reaction into which the higher animal as contrasted with the lower sinks when made " spinal " appears to me significant of this, that in the higher types, more than in the lower, the great projecting senses actuate the motor organ and impel the motions of the individual. That deeper depression shows how, as the individual ascends the scale of being, the more percipient, the more cognisant does it become of the circumambient universe outside that is " not me "; and thus the latter acquires a more and more preponderant directive influence over those reflections, those expressions of the creature's neural states, its " doings."

ON THE RECOVERY OF SPINAL REFLEXES

In the monkey[1] in some instances three-quarters of an hour or so after transection below the region of the brachial enlargement, a *status* supervenes in which with cold hands and ears the animal lies down listless, and perhaps unconscious, with respiratory movements of the Cheyne-Stokes type. This state may persist twelve hours or so, and end either in gradual recovery or death. In most monkeys this condition does not occur. I have never met it consequent to similar operations in the cat or dog. It has nothing to do with the surgical progress of the wound, which is trifling in extent and heals readily. It is usual for the rectal temperature to fall a degree or more immediately after section of the cord in the thoracic region.

As regards the nervous reactions elicitable from the isolated length of cord, for about twenty minutes after the performance of the severance, neither by mechanical, thermal, nor electrical excitation of the skin inner-vated from below the point of severance, can any reflex movement at all be elicited. The one exception to this is occasionally the so-called crossed knee jerk. It may appear strange that a " crossed reflex " should be thus early among the reflexes to appear. I find on examination that the reflex is not in reality a " crossed reflex," a statement which is amplified below, p. 148. After the brief interval certain skin-reflexes begin to appear; almost always earliest is adduction-flexion of the hallux, elicitable by stimuli applied to the 3rd, 4th, or 5th digits (plantar surface or sides), or to the skin of the sole, especially of the fibular side. The movement obtained from the hallux is often tremulous. Similarly, after section above the brachial enlargement, the earliest skin-reflex to appear is usually flexion and adduction of the thumb on stimulation of the palmar surface, or sides of the little 4th or 3rd fingers, or of the palm, especially in its ulnar part. A little later, or equally soon in some instances, appears feeble movement (generally protrusion) of the anus in response to stimulation in the perineal

---

[1] From *Philos. Trans.*, 1898, **190B**, 136 *et seq.* See also Schäfer's *Textbook of Physiology*, 1900, **2**, 811 *et seq.*

region; also feeble abduction of the tail in response to stimulation in the perineal region, or of the ventral surface of the tail itself; also, further, movement (usually flexion, sometimes extension, sometimes abduction, especially of index) of the digits, in accompaniment to that of the hallux (or pollex) on excitation of the plantar (or palmar) surface, generally excluding, however, the skin of the hallux (or pollex) itself.

Usually somewhat later, a slight contraction of the hamstring or gracilis muscles—at first often of the inner hamstrings only—becomes elicitable by severe excitation of the sole, and generally of no other region than the sole. All this time the limbs hang limp and flaccid, without any sign of spasm, except not infrequently fine feeble irregular twitching of the hallux (or pollex), sometimes of the other digits as well. The foot is warm. In these experiments, when reflexes are to be evoked from the skin, care should always be taken to maintain the temperature of the skin. As to the knee jerk, this phenomenon, not truly reflex[1] yet intimately dependent on the reflex tonus of the *crureus* and *vastus internus*, in many instances is elicitable for a few seconds immediately following the severance of the cord, but then disappears, to reappear only in the course of days or even weeks.[2] In some monkeys, however, as in the cat and dog, the knee jerks are not even temporarily abolished by the section. I have seen them maintained both after section as high as the 1st cervical segment and as low as the 1st post-thoracic segment.

The reflex reactions may remain in the just-described condition of paucity and depression for many hours and for many days; in this a striking and significant contrast exists between the monkey on one hand, and the cat and dog upon the other. The sphincter ani, however, possesses some tone, and is not relaxed. There is no marked trouble with defæcation; but, after section at a low level, I have seen retention and dribbling overflow of urine, and the bladder may have to be evacuated by a catheter. In the course of time the action of the bladder, if lost at first, is regained, and further reflex movements usually become obtainable. A drawing up of the leg by the flexors of the hip and knee can generally be best evoked by pressing the foot or applying a cold sponge to the sole. A feeble wag of the tail can be obtained by pinching it. Flexion and adduction of the hallux become elicitable from a much wider area than formerly, from the whole foot, from the inside of the thigh, and from the end of the penis. The movement of hallux is usually associated with flexion of the other digits, also curiously often with extension of the other digits, an interesting movement which I have frequently obtained by excitation of the appropriate region of the cortex. The " cremaster " reflexes can be obtained.

In one young *M. sinicus* on the fourteenth day after the section a bilateral reflex appeared, and remained regularly elicitable for four months; on pinching the prepuce, both great toes were strongly flexed and adducted, both knees were slightly extended, and at the same time, by apparently

---

[1] 1898. Since shown to be undoubtedly reflex.—ED.   [2] *J. Physiol.*, 1892, **13**, 666-672.

a slight action of the flexors of the hips, thrust forward; the smaller digits were generally slightly flexed together with the hallux. I have seen a similar reflex from one other male, but only from one. I have never seen it in the female, the nearest approach being flexion of the hallux as an accompaniment of depression of the tail and protrusion of the anus in response to stimulation of the skin near the ventral commissure of the vagina. In the cat I have seen bilateral movement (sometimes extension, sometimes flexion) of the ankles in response to irritation of the labium.

Abduction of the tail from its median symmetrical position is easily obtained, generally from a large area including the perineum, back of sacrum, back of thigh, and even the soles of the feet. The abduction is not unfrequently in a direction away from the side stimulated—that is to say, crossed reflexes are not uncommon; this often happens in the sense that, after excitation of the left side of the perineum has evoked abduction of the tail toward the left, excitation of the right side of the perineum evokes similarly abduction toward the left. Sometimes the crossed movement is elicitable without any previous " bahnung " (facilitation).

As time goes on, the " drawing up " movement of the limb can be obtained from a larger area than at first; the calf, the outer side and back of the thigh, the skin lateral to the callosity and of the gluteal region near the root of the tail, not however as far inward as the median line, all yield it. The flexion of knee is not always carried out by the same muscles; thus, the inner hamstrings and often the gracilis seem to play a predominant part when the skin stimulated is of foot or leg, the outer hamstring when the middle or back of thigh. I have seen flexion of the knees with abduction of the thighs result from stimulation of the entrance to the vagina. Depression of the tail is elicitable from the skin above the ischial callosity. Defæcation can be sometimes induced by stimulation of the anal opening; it is accompanied by elevation of the tail and to-and-fro and side-to-side movement of it. A curving downward of the end of the tail is obtainable as an isolated movement from the skin of the ventral surface of the tail distal to the root. Protrusion of the anus is elicitable from a large field— i.e., from the perineum around the anus and along the side of the vaginal orifice, also from over the back of the sacrum up to, but not beyond, the position of my *dorsal axial line* of the limb, and from the extreme top of the inner aspect of the thigh, near the raphe and beside the pubic fold. There and along its lateral border this anal reflex field overlaps the reflex field of the hallux.

Flexion of the hip, apparently unaccompanied by flexion of the knee, comes to be elicitable from the femoral triangle, and, broadly speaking, from the whole front of the thigh; not infrequently associated with this *flexion of the hip* is adduction, and also adduction with slight *extension of the opposite* knee.

From the tibial side of the sole and hallux inversion of the foot, never, perhaps, as an isolated movement, generally associated to flexion of hallux with movement of the other digits, may be elicitable; from the fibular side of the sole, and from the small digits, eversion of the foot, never as an isolated movement, but generally associated to digital movement. Similarly, in the forearm, excitation of the skin of the little finger sometimes elicits some pronation with the flexion of elbow, while from the thumb some supination with the flexion of elbow is usual. Primary dorsal, more often than primary plantar, flexion of ankle accompanies flexion of knee. Flexion of hip, more often than extension of hip, goes with flexion of knee. Extension of knee is a movement of such rare occurrence as to be, as a local homonymous reflex,[1] hardly seen in most cats and monkeys in my experience. Adduction of the hip is much less uncommon, and among crossed reflexes is common; in one animal it was regularly elicitable without other movement, or with slight extension of knee, as a crossed reflex from the skin near the raphe and pubic fold. It is not unfrequent to find that from some part of the sole can be evoked flexion of the small digits even when from most of the sole extension of them (at the metatarso-phalangeal joints) is elicited; generally the area for flexion lies on the fibular side of the sole.

The above-stated degree and multiformity of reflex action having been attained, feeble and poverty-stricken as it is, I have never seen any further progress made in the monkey. The longest periods through which I have maintained individual experiment have been *six months* and *five months*. Not a little surprising is it to find that the movement which, on account of its being the most easily evoked and the one evoked alone when depression of reflex activity is great, may be called the primary spinal reflex of the limb, is the very movement which has been often urged to be *par excellence* the most eminently cortical one—namely, flexion-adduction of hallux. I have previously drawn attention to this significant fact.[2] Similarly, in the fore-limb, flexion-adduction of thumb, though often instanced as an action of peculiarly cortical nature, is really the most frequent and facile pure spinal reflex of the upper extremity. Its large and predominant representation in the cortex is concomitant with, rather than in contrast against, a large and predominant representation in the spinal cord. So also in the torticollis reflex obtainable from 5th cranial nerve, and especially from 2nd and 3rd cervical roots, the movement, a turning of the chin and neck (with some lateral rotation of the head) away from the side of excitation, we have another example of a movement preponderantly represented in wide regions of the cortex (Ferrier, from frontal cortex; Schäfer, from occipital cortex), also preponderantly represented in an extensive set of bulbo-spinal reflex mechanisms.

An almost invariable sequence to transection is eventually ulceration in the neighbourhood of the outer malleolus. The ulcers heal readily if dressed; but they recur: I find no evidence for believing them due to trophic disturbance. They seem the result of pressure during the paralytic con-

---

[1] *I.e.*, a reflex elicited by excitation of the limb itself.   [2] *J. Physiol.*, 1892, **13**, 621.

dition of the limb. Œdema of the foot also occurs. The muscles waste greatly, especially, I think, the quadriceps extensor of thigh.

A fact of importance is that if regularly repeated passive extensions be not undertaken and kept up, "*late rigidity*" "contracture" ultimately flexes the hips and knees. The onset of the rigidity is shown by resistance to movement in the direction toward which act the muscles antagonistic to those becoming rigid; this can be in some cases felt in two or three weeks. The atrophy is severest in the extensors of the knee—at least, that is my experience in the cat, dog, and monkey. I cannot confirm Freusberg[1] when he states there is to be found in the dog no alteration in the nutritive condition of any of the muscles. Myself, I find it affect both sets of muscles, flexor and extensor; much as Munk[2] describes after cortical ablations, when hemiplegic contracture occurs in the monkey. That the rigidity "*contracture*" affects in the lower limb the flexors in the monkey, rather than the extensors, as I am told is the case in man, may be due to extension of the limb being more predominant in the erect position than in the quadrupedal.

In some of the monkeys with hind-limbs insensitised by spinal transection, the animals attacked the insentient limb: they began to pull it literally to pieces with an air suggesting playful curiosity. In one case the great sciatic nerve at the hip was frayed out and through in the course of a fore-noon. In our research on the effect of rendering the limb insentient (apæsthete) by section of its afferent nerve-roots, Dr. Mott and myself met with a similar experience in some individual animals.[3] The ataxic and semi-paralytic condition of the limb evidently annoys the creature, although not causing it pain.

The amount of reflex movement elicitable, after spinal transection, varies much in different monkeys of the same species: also in one and the same individual from day to day. On some mornings mere vestiges of reflexes obtainable on the previous morning might be all that were possible. In most cases a few repetitions tire out the reflex reaction; after increasing somewhat for a few repetitions at the beginning of the examination, they begin to fade out, and do so unless a rest is allowed. To increase the intensity of the stimulation is not of much avail; *the reflex arc behaves somewhat like cardiac muscle in responding its approximate best or not at all if the stimulus applied be not subliminal.*

The *discontinuance* of a prolonged stimulation, especially when it is itself becoming inefficient, I have very often found provoke a fresh outburst of reflex activity. Head[4] and Freusberg[5] have pointed out the same thing. I have seen it with faradic and with mechanical stimuli. After stretching a muscle from its tendon steadily and then suddenly relaxing it, the relaxation often causes a sudden fresh outburst of movement, *a terminal discharge.*

In the dog, soon after the performance of transection, vigorous reflex movements can be easily obtained, especially in the hind-limbs and tail;

---

[1] *Pflüg. Arch. ges. Physiol.*, 1874, **9**, 358.   [2] H. Munk, *S. B. preuss. Akad. Wiss.*, 1894.
[3] *Proc. roy. Soc.*, 1895, **57**, 481.   [4] *J. Physiol.*, 1889, **10**, 1.   [5] *Loc. cit. sup.*

these have been known and their vigour and variety appreciated since the papers by Marshall Hall,[1] Longet,[2] Brachet,[3] Cayrade,[4] Goltz[5] and Freusberg, and especially by the papers of the two last-named observers. From my account above given of the monkey it will be seen, therefore, that there exists a difference between the condition of monkey and of cat and dog in regard to reflex play in the spinal cord after spinal transection. To meet so great a physiological contrast between these two mammalian types is surprising: the difference is distinctly great. I do not, however, believe it a really profound difference; it is, I think I shall show, quantitative rather than qualitative. But it is nevertheless great and significant. One may almost say the dog in this respect seems to differ less from the frog than does the Macaque from the dog, although the morphological gap between the two latter is so much less than between the former. In the dog and cat the spinal reflex movements are more forcible, more prolonged, more readily obtained, and less easily exhausted by fatigue. In the cat and dog it is not unusual to see the hind-quarters raise themselves reflexly—with superficial similitude to willed movement—from the sitting to the standing posture; this powerful reflex, described by Goltz, often occurs when the animal moves on being encouraged to stand up. In the monkey, on the other hand, the hind-limbs hang helpless, with a lethargy comparable to deep stupor. The few feeble abortive movements above described are difficult to arouse and sometimes not elicitable at all. It might, perhaps, have been anticipated that in the monkey, with its wealth of range and scope of limb movement, compared with which the hind-limbs of the dog are little more than props, the reflex spinal machinery would have exhibited conformably a more multiform and surpassing co-ordination than in the cat and dog. " Shock " once over, spinal reflexes might have been expected more various than those of other animals. Such a supposition is dispelled by actual experiment, as far as all cutaneous reflexes are concerned, although it is true that the variety of homonymous reflex about the knee of the monkey appears slightly greater than at knee in the other species.

On the other hand, the difference between the variety and even the extent of the spinal reflexes obtainable from cat and dog on the one part and from Macacus on the other, is much diminished when, instead of skin and nerve-trunk, the spinal roots proximal to their ganglia are stimulated. The direction and muscular composition of the primary movements elicitable by faradic excitations of the afferent spinal roots themselves are in cat, dog, and monkey, especially in the hind-limb region, almost the same for all three types. The spinal machinery for movement is therefore actually present in the monkey as in the other two, and indeed, as was expected, appears to be more complex. But it is more difficult to set in motion and to keep going.

---

[1] *Memoirs on the Nervous System*, London, 1837-1852.   [2] *Traité de Physiol.*, **2**, 241.
[3] *Recherches expérim. sur les Fonctions des Systém. Nerveux gang.*, Paris, 1839.
[4] *Le Mouvement Réflexe.* Thèse pour le doct. en méd., Paris, 1864.
[5] *Pflüg. Arch. ges. Physiol.*, 1874, **8,** 460.

THE FAILURE OF REGULATION OF TEMPERATURE[1]

In dogs long after complete subsidence of spinal shock as judged from usual post-transection reflexes, there persists in the region innervated from behind the transection marked failure of adjustment of the surface blood-supply (paws, pinnæ, nose) to changes of surrounding cold and warmth. The failure of this vascular adjustment, though not absolute, remains severe and without improvement. Along with it there is complete abeyance of sweating to heat, and in the muscles complete abeyance of shivering to cold. Diurnal fluctuation of 2° C. in the stall temperature affected conspicuously the vaginal temperature of cervical paraplegic dogs fully recovered from spinal shock.

In dogs all attempts, even by considerable exposure, to induce cold-shivering in the paraplegic region as a spinal reflex entirely failed.[2]

On cold immersion of the insentient paraplegic portion of the dog, shivering occurred headward of the spinal lesion even when the skin surface headward of the lesion still felt to the touch fully " warm." Shivering under these circumstances is, on older views of the nature of the adequate skin stimulus for " cold," difficult to explain as a reflex, but is yet not precluded from being reflex on the view propounded by Ebbecke[3] for the nature of the adequate skin-stimulus for " cold " sensation. Shivering under these circumstances may, on the other hand, be possibly of deep origin from direct cooling of a central (diencephalic) thermotaxic mechanism.

Shivering seems not to require the afferent nerves of the lung or of the shivering muscles. Shivering, reflex or " central," requires, like Richet's heat-polypnœa,[4] some central nervous mechanism anterior to the mid-brain.

Instances where, under severe but short-lasting changes of surrounding temperature, the body temperature (vaginal) of the dog fell to 32·3° C., or, on the other hand, rose to 42·5° C., were not productive of serious mischief, and after the animal's return to its stall at 27° to 28° C., the body temperature quickly regained its approximate normal. A rise of temperature (vaginal) reaching 43·2° C., productive of delirium, profuse salivation, and acute symptoms of distress, was yet rapidly recovered from on removal to cool surroundings. It would seem, therefore, that even in high paraplegia thermometry of somewhat frequent interval can, as Pembrey[5] has pointed out, notify over-stress of thermotaxis in ample time for the taking of successful measures of relief.

---

[1] From *J. Physiol.*, 1924, **58**, 405. Only the conclusions of the paper, which contains detailed observations and temperature charts, are presented here. See also pp. 210 and 216, this volume.

[2] Shivering is thus not regarded as a spinal reflex, in spite of a report by Freusberg (Goltz, *Pflüg. Arch. ges. Physiol.*, 1874, **8**, 496). See also Richet, *C. R. Soc. Biol.*, 1892, p. 896, and 1893, p. 33. Nor was sweating found as a spinal reflex in dogs, though it occurs as a reflex unrelated to heat in man (Head and Riddoch, *Brain*, 1917, **40**, 188).—ED.

[3] *Pflüg. Arch. ges. Physiol.*, 1917, **169**, 395.   [4] *Arch. Physiol. norm. path.*, 1893, **25**, 312.

[5] *Guy's Hosp. Rep.*, 1912, pp. 66, 87. See also Freund and Strassmann, *Arch. exp. Path. Pharmak.*, 1912, **69**, 12.

SEGMENTAL REFLEX EFFECTS[1]

The segmental arrangement of the spinal nerves in their gross anatomy does not, of course, necessarily carry with it any proof of the functional segmentation of the cord. That proof can be furnished only by analysis of the functional plan. A point of first importance for this question is the capacity of the fractionated spinal cord. Herbert Mayo[2] by his experiment showing the pupil reflex to be elicitable when but a single cranial segment remains, and Legallois[3] by his localisation of the respiratory centre in the bulb, had at the outset of the century laid the foundation of the segmental theory of the functions of the cord. Marshall Hall[4] and Grainger[5] further contributed experiments demonstrating the functional powers of spinal fractions.[6] The latter drew significant observations from the reflex movements of invertebrata. The study of the functions of the nerve-chain of invertebrata became later neglected, most unwisely. Quite recently such work has vigorously been resumed. An example of its fruitfulness for the present problem is furnished by the observations of Hyde[7] on Limulus made in the laboratory of Professor Loeb, of Chicago.

When in Limulus all that is analogous to the brain has been ablated, and indeed only the abdominal region of the spinal cord remains, the rhythmic respiratory movements of the abdominal segments still proceed regularly and co-ordinately. Even when a fraction of the nerve-cord, separated by transections in front and behind, is left corresponding with a single abdominal segment, the musculature of that segment continues its rhythmic action. Its rhythm is then no longer timed to that of the adjacent segments; its co-ordination with the rest is destroyed, but its activity is maintained. Its activity ceases only if the segmental fraction of the spinal cord is itself destroyed. This instance is paralleled by the sexual " clasp " reflex of the brachial segments of the male frog, maintained when all the rest of the central nervous system is destroyed.[8] Similarly in the cat and monkey, the reflex wagging of the tail persists when behind the spinal transection only the sacral region of the cord is left intact.

To judge how far the reactions of the spinal cord can be really considered as segmentally arranged, it is important to have a conception as clear as possible of the spatial relations of the spinal nerve-cells. The delineation of the spinal segment usually given presents its true extension very imperfectly.

[1] Extract from " On the Spinal Animal," *Med.-Chir. Trans.*, London, 1899, **82,** 449.
[2] *Physiol. Commentaries*, London, 1823.   [3] 1830.
[4] *Memoirs on the Nervous System*, London, 1838.   [5] *Functions of the Spinal Cord*, London, 1837.
[6] " Stephen Hales first proved the spinal cord to be a seat of ' reflection ' as against other places where nerves seem to unite (for example, the nerve plexuses). Grainger later indicated that in the spinal cord the grey matter is the seat of the reflection " (Schäfer's *Textbook of Physiology*, 1900, **2,** p. 784). For an historical account see *ibid.*, p. 786.—ED.
[7] *Journ. of Morphology*, 1894, **9.**
[8] Goltz, *Centralb. f. med. Wissensch.*, 1870.

The spinal segment[1] is often loosely, though arbitrarily, laid down to-be a fraction of spinal cord included between two imaginary frontal sections, placed one on each side of a nerve-pair, and each half-way between the next pair below and the next above. Neither morphologically nor physio-logically does this cylindroid mass of the cord merit the term "spinal segment." To take such a fraction as representing either a structural or a functional unit or spinal link, from a series of which the cord is built up by concatenation, is to ignore one of the most important characters of construction of the myelon. Overlapping and inlapping of segments exist in the segmental arrangement of the cord itself just as in the segmental arrangement of the neurones in the body-metameres outside. The "block" delimitation of the spinal segment is no longer defensible or useful. It omits structures which are essential components of every complete spinal segment; it includes much that is extraneous. It is applicable, probably, to one set only of the spinal neurones—namely, to the motoneurones—for, as I and A. S. Grünbaum[2] have shown, the spinal motor root is of strictly local origin.

The extent of intra-spinal attachment is very different in the two cases of the dorsal (afferent) and of the ventral (efferent) root respectively. The former overlaps a *series* of the latter. If, for mere convenience of statement, the *surface* attachment only of the roots is considered in the definition "segment" there remains, apart from the obvious artificiality of the postulate, still a difficulty with the dorsal (afferent) root. This difficulty lies in the frequency with which the filaments of dorsal roots trespass upon each other's territory, a filament from one root ganglion not uncommonly joining a filament from the next ganglion to plunge together with it into the postero-lateral fissure of the cord. Not very rarely a filament on issuing from the ganglion pursues an oblique course (generally in my experience *downward*) across a part or even the whole of the filaments from the next ganglion to enter the cord among or even subjacent to them.

Example.—I recollect noting in the human brachial enlargement a filament from the 7th cervical ganglion plunging into the cord half-way down the series of filaments from the 8th ganglion. I believe such variations are not found in the filaments of anterior roots. I have myself, with considerable opportunity for search, never yet found any.

The surface attachment of the dorsal (afferent) root is, therefore, just as its deep attachment, a less reliable segmental guide than that of the ventral (efferent) root. But the collection of cells composing the spinal ganglion is a segmental collection, just as the collection of the intraspinal neurones of the efferent root is a segmental group; indeed, the two are segmentally equivalent. To include in the "spinal segment" the cells of one root, and to omit those of the other, is obviously artificial and incon-

---

[1] Extract from *Philos. Trans.*, 1898, **190B**, 145.
[2] Sherrington, *J. Physiol.*, 1892, **13**, see p. 707, *ibid.*, 1893, **14**, footnote, p. 300; Grünbaum, *J. Physiol.*, 1894, **16**, 368.

sequent. The spinal segment is, therefore, in this paper understood to include the neurones of the spinal ganglion, as well as those of the corresponding ventral (efferent) root, and along with these all other intraspinal neurones whose cell-bodies lie between the same frontal levels as the neurones of the efferent root in question. I omit reference to the ganglia of the sympathetic, this paper not being immediately concerned with them.

[1]Just as the peripheral distribution of the afferent fibres of the spinal ganglia is an overlapping one, so also is their central intraspinal ramification. The central or stem-process of each afferent root-cell, after entering the cord, bifurcates, as was discovered by Frithjoff Nansen,[2] the explorer. The headward branch of division ascends in the case of many fibres to the grey " nuclei " of the dorsal columns in the bulb; the aboral branch descends only a short distance, one or at most a few spinal segments. Each of these branches gives off collaterals into the grey matter, especially into the grey matter of the same segmental level as the root ganglion, whence the root-fibre in question is itself derived. The intraspinal extent of the afferent root-cell is therefore far more expanded than is that of the efferent root-cell. The dendrites of the latter seem to be practically confined to the segment in which the cell-body lies; the processes of the afferent fibres, on the other hand, are traceable far into segments widely distant from that into which they plunge first on entering the cord. There is, therefore, a very extensive intraspinal overlap in the central distribution of the afferent fibres derived from each afferent root ganglion. Whether this applies equally to the afferent root-cells connected with the viscera as to other afferent root-cells is a question. The focal and circumspect character of the areas of tenderness and referred pain studied by Head in cases of visceral disorder, and their correspondence in situation with the skin areas of distribution of the individual spinal roots, suggests that the central end-distribution of these visceral afferent fibres is less diffuse and less extensive intraspinally and more concentrated within a single segment. On the limitations of intraspinal root-overlap the study of the reference of visceral irritations may give most valuable light. Regarding the existence of segmental boundaries to the intraspinal spread of impulses, observations such as the following illustrate the slightness of the evidence in support. If the central end of the afferent root of a thoracic nerve be carefully stimulated with gradually increasing strengths of stimulus, the musculature of the chest wall belonging to its own motor root is the first to reply, and all parts of it do not reply with equal readiness; certain portions are thrown into contraction more readily than others. The *intercostales* are rather late; as the intensity of the stimulus is increased, the effect, curiously enough, is not easily pushed across the median line; long before that passes, some of the musculature supplied by the next adjacent motor roots behind and in front comes into play. It is difficult to note a distinct step in the spread, and the spread passes often a little earlier to the segment behind than to that in front.

[1] From *Med.-Chir. Trans.*, 1899, **82,** 14.   [2] Bergen's Museum, 1887.

Yet the intraspinal resistance—to borrow electrical terminology—is for its own afferent path in the segment stimulated a little lower than in the adjoining. There is, therefore, some functional segmentation. But in the case of the limb muscles I could not obtain such evidence. Taking the flexion-adduction of the hallux of the monkey, this reflex could be obtained from each single one of a row of the rootlets of the three last roots of the limb-plexus.[1] When obtained from an afferent rootlet of the first sacral root it was obtained with equal facility, whichever of the motor roots supplying the short muscles of the hallux remained unsevered. There was thus no evidence of a segmental barrier of resistance between the spinal segments concerned with the innervation of this muscle. These segments in regard to this muscle seem to have become so welded together as to form a physiological unit.

[2]The above results possess points of interest, but it must not be forgotten the value of a reflex obtained by exciting the afferent spinal root, or one of its filaments, is but slight as regards the light thrown by it on the normal working of the spinal cord. It is only truly estimated when it is remembered that the mammalian spinal root is not a functional combination, but a morphological one. To stimulate the whole of one single afferent root by itself is to do what Nature never normally does. So also to stimulate one continuous half or fourth of such a root is to do what is never done naturally. The end of a penholder pressed upon the skin anywhere—at least, anywhere on the limbs—excites contemporaneously single nerve-fibres scattered through two consecutive (in many cases three consecutive) spinal afferent roots. Experiments on the roots are suitable at the commencement of an investigation of the spinal reflex actions, because the dorsal roots, more readily than the peripheral nerves, provoke reflexes, and the experiments are, therefore, easier to perform; but they are less valuable in their physiological results, because the accompanying conditions are less known and less controlled. The *root* reflexes, to be of use for the understanding of the working of the cord, must be considered in collation with peripheral nerve reflexes and with skin-spot reflexes.

THE REFLEX IS NOT LIMITED BY SEGMENTATION[3]

In the above instances centripetal impulses poured into one spinal segment evoke centrifugal impulses in adjacent segments without demonstrably greater difficulty than when confined to the actual segment into which they were themselves thrown. Irradiation appears to meet with no increase of resistance when passing from one segment to another in these cases. The solidarity of these parts of the essentially segmented cord must be extraordinarily complete. The connection between the endings of the

---

[1] Further examples of the reflexes from stimulating single roots in various regions of the cord and discussion of their significance will be found in the paper in *Philos. Trans.*, 1898, **190B**, 45-186.—Ed.   [2] From *Philos. Trans.*, 1898, **190B**, 133.   [3] *Ibid.*, p. 151.

afferent fibres and motor cells of other segments may be as close as between them and *any* of the neurones. It follows that, in many instances at least, excitation of their own segment applied in minimal or approximately minimal degree to a single afferent root or of a fraction of a single afferent root evokes pluri-segmental " motor " discharge. Now I have shown that the group of motoneurones innervating a limb muscle—*e.g.*, flexor brevis, hallucis, or pollicis—is composed of individual neurones, belonging not merely to one, but to two and three adjacent spinal segments. From the above it is clear that the rule of segmental proximity does not operate to the extent of making motoneurones belonging to one segment in the pluri-segmental motor nucleus greatly more accessible by its own afferent root than are by that root the motoneurones of the other segments composing the nucleus; in fact, they are only very slightly if in any degree more so. Here again facts lend no countenance to the assertion that the collection of fibres in each motor root represents one highly co-ordinate functional synergy. On the contrary, they indicate that not the whole motor root, but particular fractional combinations of several motor roots are, in spinal reflex actions, to be considered units. The afferent channels of the cord treat the pluri-segmental motor stations or nuclei of these limb muscles as entities of homogeneous structure, as in fact physiological units.

From the foregoing it follows naturally that the reflex centrifugal discharge of the spinal cord is pluri-segmental. The rule may be stated thus: *in response to excitation even approximately minimal of a single afferent root, or even of a single filament of a single afferent root, the spinal discharge of centrifugal impulses evoked tends to occur via more than one efferent root—i.e., is pluri-segmental.* It is interesting to note that this is more strongly the case in the limbs than in the thoracic region, where the segments are less commingled. The segmental arrangement of the motor cells of the spinal cord is said by Schwalbe[1] to be more obvious in the thoracic than in the limb regions. But in the limb region the arrangement, if existent, consists of cell groups quite confluent at the boundaries of segments. I look upon the solidarity of the limb as structurally expressed by the pluri-segmental character of the motor nuclei. Kaiser's[2] measurements lend no colour to Schwalbe's assertion of a segmental grouping of the motor cells. With care, the reflex discharge can, as above stated, be confined in the intercostal series to one segmental region, the spinal centrifugal discharge being then uni-segmental. This circumstance is in accord with the uni-segmental innervation of these muscles as compared with the pluri-segmental innervation of most limb muscles.

This serves to emphasise what I have frequently insisted on—namely, the physiological homogeneity of limb muscle and nerve-trunk, and the physiological heterogeneity, in spite of morphological unity, of the spinal nerve-root in the limb region; the spinal nerve-roots of the thoracic region are far less heterogeneous. The peripheral *nerve-trunk* is the *physiological*

---

[1] Schwalbe, *Lehrbuch der Neurol.*, 1881; also Lüderitz, *Arch. Anat. Physiol.*, 1881.
[2] *Ganglienzellen des Halsmarkes*, Haag, 1891.

collection of nerve-fibres—*e.g.*, flexors collected together, vaso-dilators included with motors to muscles, etc. The *nerve-root* is the *morphological* collection; it contains, commingled into one, such heterogeneities as adductors of great toe, protrusors of anus, and vaso-dilators of the penis. Similarly with the skin, the median nerve-trunk supplies a patch of the palm that has obviously functional unity, but 1st thoracic nerve-root supplies such incongruities as the back and front of the little finger and of half the annulus and the tip of the olecranon process. It is *the formation of functional collections of nerve-fibres (peripheral nerve-trunks) out of morphological collections (nerve-roots)* which *is the explanation*—the meaning—*of the existence of limb-plexuses*. The reply to the oft-asked question what is the meaning and explanation of the distribution of the brachial and pelvic limb spinal nerves by plexuses, while the spinal nerves of the trunk region are not distributed by plexuses is, in my opinion, as follows: In the trunk region the innervation of the muscles of the skin is, as regards the distribution in them of the segmental nerves, a system of comparatively slight overlap: the peripheral territory of each segmental nerve—especially each motor territory—is confluent with, but does not mingle nearly so widely with, the neighbour territories as in the limb regions. That is to say, in other words, each several area of skin and of muscle, especially of the latter, has in either of the limbs a more pluri-segmental spinal innervation than a comparable area in the trunk. The anatomical mode of innervating a definite area of tissue is, as we know, by means of collecting the nerve-fibres for the region into a nerve-trunk. Where the innervation is pluri-segmental the nerve-trunk will therefore naturally be combined from components of several segmental nerves; where several such areas coexist several pluri-segmental nerve-trunks will be formed and the separate segmental nerves will be split up into components, which become redistributed in the combinations which constitute the pluri-segmental nerve-trunks of the region—as, for instance, in the brachial region. The brachial and lumbo-sacral plexuses are an anatomical result of the greater degree of overlap, especially in the distribution of the motor part of their spinal nerves obtaining in the limbs as compared with other—*e.g.*, the trunk region of the body.

REFLEX DISCHARGE SELECTS CERTAIN GROUPS OF MUSCLES[1]

In a spinal segment of the limb region among the entire collection of its motor nerve-cells certain sub-groups are far less excitable in local spinal reflexes than are others. In other words, of the entire contraction produced by direct excitation of a whole motor root certain parts are elicitable by spinal reflex much less easily than other parts. Whereas, between **its own** afferent root fibres and some of the motoneurones of the segment connection is facile, resistance low, between its afferents and others of its motoneurones

[1] From *Philos. Trans.*, 1898, **190B**, 154.

connection is difficult, resistance high. Hence, under the conditions maintained in my experiments, the centrifugal discharge, although occurring contemporaneously in several segments, in each of the several segments engaged certain only among the motoneurones. The motor discharge, although pluri-segmental, is in each segment only fractional: certain neurones in the segment are selected, certain neglected. The nature of the selection recurs with a degree of constancy altogether remarkable, although not invariable.

Examples: Good contraction of supinator longus group in arm of Macacus, by excitation of dorsal (afferent) root 5th cervical nerve with Kronecker secondary coil at 15 k.s.; to evoke contemporaneous biceps action as well as supinator, secondary had to be brought up to 90 k.s. No contraction of triceps could be provoked contemporaneously with supinator longus.

In the cat, cerebrum and cerebellum above their crura having been ablated, and the cord transected above 2nd cervical nerve, a touch on the roof of the mouth causes wide opening of the mouth—i.e., depression of the mandible. The elevators of the jaw being much more powerful than the depressors, the afferent path (5th cranial) must have selected the motoneurones of digastric, mylo-hyoid, etc., and neglected comparatively or absolutely, or inhibited those of the elevator muscles.

The intercostal muscles cannot at all readily be reflexly excited via the lateral cutaneous branches of the corresponding spinal nerves, but the superficial muscles of the chest can be.

Excitation of the lateral cutaneous branch of the 2nd thoracic only with difficulty evokes any pupil reflex, the entire afferent root of 2nd thoracic evokes reflex dilatation fairly readily. In the same way lateral cutaneous branch of 2nd thoracic evokes retraction of shoulder very easily, but only with difficulty any contraction in the intercostal muscles.

Again, of the muscles of the front of the thigh, some tend to be brought into reflex play by the internal saphenous nerve—playing upon the spinal segments of those muscles via their own proper afferent roots—much more readily than others; the rectus femoris (its upper part especially), sartorius and fascialis much more readily than the crureus and vasti. Excitation of the central and of the nerve to one of the vasti evokes contraction of its own fellow vastus, and the associated crureus less easily than sartorius and a part of the rectus femoris.

Again, excitation of the central end of the nerve to one head of the gastrocnemius evokes contraction in the hamstring muscles more readily than in the *gastrocnemius itself* and the soleus.

Again, excitation of the plantar nerves evokes contraction more readily in the pre-tibial muscles than in the post-tibial group, though segmentally they belong rather to the post-tibial group than to the pre-tibial.

It can be said that of the movements of the limb some are easily provoked by spinal reflex action, some only rarely and with difficulty. Among those induced as primary spinal reflexes (the cord being transected above) are, in order of facility of production, in my experience:

In the *upper limb* :

  Retraction of upper arm.
  Flexion-adduction of thumb.
  Extension of wrist (especially in cat).
  Adduction at shoulder.
  Flexion of elbow.

Flexion (less often extension) of digits (always in accompaniment to flexion-
adduction of thumb).
Slight pronation of forearm (especially in cat).
Abduction at shoulder.
Extension of elbow (rare).
Less common is flexion and some pronation of wrist.

In the *lower limb* :

Flexion of hip.
Flexion of hallux.
Flexion of knee.
Adduction at hip.
Flexion (less often extension) of digits (always in accompaniment to flexion-
adduction of hallux).
Flexion—less commonly plantar flexion—of ankle.
Less common is extension of hip.
Abduction of hip (not common).
Extension of knee (rare).

The preponderance of the above movements over others in the limb is
exemplified in the following summary of movements, commonly evoked by
excitation of various peripheral nerves in the limbs. The transection of
the cord had, in most of the cases on which the summary is based, been made
from a few days up to six months prior to the observation.

Internal saphenous nerve in highest third of thigh (monkey) evoked flexion of hip;
flexion of knee.

Internal saphenous nerve just above knee (monkey; cord cut at 6th thoracic level
five months previously) evoked flexion of hip, adduction of thigh, slight flexion of knee,
movement of tail to the homonymous side.

Internal saphenous nerve at knee (dog), flexion of hip, with some feeble flexion of
knee (cat); flexion of hip, especially due to fascialis and upper part of sartorius of quadriceps,
with some flexion of knee, and usually some dorsi-flexion at ankle.

Internal saphenous nerve at the ankle (monkey), flexion of hip, with slight flexion
at knee.

External saphenous nerve near ankle evoked flexion of knee, flexion of hallux and
toes, depression of tail, sometimes abduction of tail.

The most lateral digital branch from the musculo-cutaneous on the dorsum of the foot
evoked flexion of hip, slight action of hamstring muscles, slight dorsal flexion of ankle.

Internal plantar at heel (monkey) evoked dorsi-flexion of ankle, flexion of hallux
(less easily flexion of short digits as well), flexion of knee, slight flexion of hip.

Internal plantar at heel (cat), dorsi-flexion of ankle and flexion of knee.

External plantar at heel (monkey) evoked dorsi-flexion of ankle, flexion of hallux
and digits, flexion of knee, and some flexion of hip; (cat) dorsi-flexion of ankle, with slighter
flexion of knee.

Cutaneous branch of musculo-cutaneous at annular ligament: dorsi-flexion of ankle,
with some inversion of foot; slight flexion at hip and knee.

Hamstring nerve evokes flexion at knee and hip, with generally crossed extension of
knee and ankle, including contraction of extensors of knee and relaxation (inhibition) of
the hamstring muscles.

Nerve to outer head of gastrocnemius (cat) evokes usually contraction of the dorsal
flexors of ankle, less usually contraction in gastrocnemius itself, and very usually contraction
in the flexors of the knee.

Peroneal nerve at knee (monkey) evokes flexion of knee and hip, dorsal flexion of ankle, and flexion of digits; abduction of tail.

Peroneal nerve at knee (cat), flexion of knee, hip, and dorso-flexion of ankle.

Popliteal nerve at knee (monkey) evokes flexion of knee; tail abduction; adduction of both thighs.

Popliteal nerve at knee (cat), flexion of hip and knee, generally extension of opposite knee.

Dorsal branch of ulnar on hand evokes flexion of digits, extension of wrist, pronation (slight) of forearm, flexion of elbow, some retraction at shoulder, and extension of opposite elbow.

To these may be added the root-reflexes.

It is very obvious from the above that in these spinal reflexes of the limb certain limb movements are of very preponderant occurrence; in other words, certain functional groups of motor neurones are less easily excited than others by the incoming local impulses. Sanders-Ezn,[1] Schloesser,[2] and Lombard[3] have pointed out how difficult it is to evoke extension of the knee as a spinal reflex movement. In a previous paper I noted that in the monkey the representations of movement in the cord, as tested by excitation of the ventral spinal root and of the dorsal (afferent) root, do not coincide—in fact, by no means coincide. Sanders-Ezn, Lombard, and myself[4] have pointed out that the movement elicited by excitation of the afferent root is often widely different, or even the converse, of that evoked by excitation of the efferent root corresponding.

Motor Cells in the Same Segment which exhibit Marked Inequality of Accessibility to Afferent Stimulation are those which innervate Antagonistic Muscles[5]

Of the functional groups of motor neurones in the cord some, in view of the actions of the muscles they innervate, may be termed *synergetic* with some, *antergetic* to this or that other. Those of the flexors of knee may thus be said to act in synergy with those of the flexors of the hip, but in antergy to those of extensors of knee, also in a certain measure to those of extensors of hip. These last are in synergy with the extensors of the knee, but in antergy to flexors of hip, also in certain measure to those of knee. *The groups of motor neurones which in one and the same spinal segment exhibit marked inequality of local reflex excitability innervate antergetic muscles.* So much is this the case that in reflex movements of local spinal origin it is the rule for only one set of an antagonistic couple of muscles to be thrown into contraction, and especially for only one group of antagonistic groups to be contracting at the same time. I have already alluded to this, and pointed it out in a previous paper,[6] but will add here further illustrations.

Flexion of ankle by dorsal flexors, the post-tibial and crural muscles remaining absolutely without contraction, in response to excitation of internal plantar nerve (or external plantar, or cutaneous of musculo-cutaneous generally).

[1] Ludwig's *Arbeiten*, 1867.   [2] *Arch. Anat. Physiol. Lpz., Physiol. Abt.*, 1880, p. 303.
[3] *Ibid.*, 1885, p. 408.   [4] *J. Physiol.*, 1892, **13**, 621.
[5] From *Philos. Trans.*, 1898, **190B**, 161.   [6] *J. Physiol.*, 1892, **13**, 621.

Contraction of those parts of quadriceps extensor (rectus internus and fascialis) which flex the hip, while the part that extends the knee remains absolutely without contraction, in response to excitation of long saphenous nerve. Contraction of flexors of elbow, the triceps remaining quite flaccid, except for a part which retracts the arm without extending the elbow.

Contraction of the triceps of the arm, while biceps and brachialis remain absolutely without contraction, in response to excitation of the afferent root of the 8th cervical nerve.

Contraction of the extensors of the wrist, the flexors remaining absolutely without contraction, in response to touching the fore-pad of the cat.

Contraction of the flexors of the elbow, the extensors remaining absolutely without contraction, in response to thermal stimulation of the palm (cat).

Contraction of the adductors (pector. maj. and latiss. dorsi) at shoulder, the abductors remaining quite slack (deltoid).

In dealing with rules of irradiation in spinal reflexes, I have mentioned reasons for believing the groups of motor neurones innervating small pieces of musculature, acting synergetically upon the selfsame joint, to be commonly treated by the spinal action as entities, and employed as units in these spinal reflexes. From that and the foregoing it follows that in adjoining spinal segments the groups of motor nerve-cells contemporaneously selected for excitation by spinal reflex action are synergetic, not antergetic. This is, of course, the reverse of what since Winslow[1] and Duchenne[2] has been common belief concerning the co-ordination of " willed " movements of man, but it agrees with the co-ordination which I have proved to take place in the frog.[3] I have shown that in the limb, while for muscles antergetic at the distal joints the groups of motor neurones largely overlap each other in segmental position, the groups of muscles antergetic at the proximal joints of the limb do not so largely segmentally overlap. Hence the reflex spinal discrimination between motor neurone groups for the antagonistic musculature of the proximal limb-joints involves a field wider than merely three adjoining segments.

But not only are certain of the movements about a single joint opposed to each other, certain movements at one joint are opposed to certain movements at neighbouring joints. Thus the extensors of the knee may be called antergetic not only to the flexors of the knee, but also to the flexors of the hip. In such cases the rule above given still holds. The groups of motor neurones selected by the reflex action as it irradiates over spinal segments lying apart in the limb series are still those of synergetic muscles. For instance, while the reflex movement evoked by excitation of the 4th post-thoracic afferent root, or that responsive to the long saphenous nerve, usually primarily contracts the flexors of the hip, it involves next, not the antergetic muscles in the nearest spinal segments (e.g., vasti and crureus), but neglects these and embouches into the synergetic of more distant segments—e.g., the hamstring muscles. *In this way the reflex action, by its " spread," develops a combined movement, synthesises a harmony.* Broadly put,

---

[1] *An Anatomical Exposition of the Structure of the Human Body*, London, 1749.
[2] *Physiologie des Mouvements*, Paris, 1867.   [3] *J. Physiol.*, 1892, **13**, 621.

there is elicitable as a pure spinal reflex from the lumbo-sacral region, but one movement of the limb as a whole. This movement is a combined movement of general advance and flexion of the limb. It is combined of flexions of hip, knee, ankle (dorsi-flexion), and digits. These components of the combined movement appear in accordance with the rule of segmental proximity to be each rather more readily elicitable via afferent roots of the segmental locality of their own motoneurones than via roots belonging elsewhere. Nevertheless each, when the excitation is pushed, tends to have associated with it more or less of the rest of the general movement of flexion. It is hardly too much to say that there is in this limb-region of the cord of, for instance, the dog, from the point of approach of the local afferent channels, but one motor centre, and this the one which produces general flexion of the limb. Into it at one point or another lead all and each of the afferent channels which provoke movement of the limb at all; and the outcome is therefore, broadly stated, monotonously flexion. Similarly, with the fore-limb, the combined movement of flexion at elbow, extension at wrist, and flexion (*i.e.*, retraction) at shoulder, is *the* movement elicitable from the limb as its local homonymous spinal reflex action. There is, however, it is true, *emphasis* on or predominance of this or that detail, according as this or that particular nerve-root or nerve-trunk affords the particular channel of approach. The arrangement of the intraspinal resistance is such as to make certain functional groups of the motor neurones especially easy of access to, broadly speaking, all the afferent channels of the limb. Inasmuch as the motor groups thus found to be especially easy of access are such as, when synchronously active, give one harmonious movement of the whole limb—*e.g.*, drawing it upward and forward by co-operative flexion at the various joints—these groups can be considered to constitute one large functionally connected nucleus, which itself may constitute an entity in the co-ordination of the limb in the movements of the body taken as a whole. It is conceivable that such a nucleus is dealt with as a whole, especially when the long cerebro-spinal arcs—ruptured in my experiments—remain intact.

THE UNIFORMITY OF RESPONSE DESPITE SPATIAL VARIETY OF PROVOCATION

From the above we are led almost as a corollary to a *rule of uniformity of response despite spatial variety of provocation*, for it is obvious that excitation of any one of a large number of afferent channels will evoke approximately the same movement in reflex response.[1]

---

[1] The response of the limb to nociceptive stimulation in any part, over a wide area, is withdrawal (flexion). This response takes precedence over other reflex effects; it is *prepotent* (see pp. 150 and 178, and *Integrative Action*, 1906, p. 228). The principle as applied here to the nociceptive flexion-reflex is nevertheless applicable to reflexes in general. Each has an area from any part of which it can be elicited with uniformity of outcome.—ED.

Examples.—The digital nerves of foot or hand separately excited evoke the same movement, although their segmental value and root composition is severally very different, varying from 5+6 to 7+6 in the foot, and from 6+7 (+8) to 1+8 in the hand. The same result occurs when, instead of the nerve-trunks, various points of the skin of hand and foot are excited.

Again : If, in the cat, the cord is divided at 11th thoracic level, and the afferent roots of 3rd, 4th, 5th, 6th, 8th, 9th, and 10th right post-thoracic nerves cut, the field of æsthesia of the right limb is that of the 7th post-thoracic nerve. The reflex movements elicitable from this field is then studied with special regard to difference of movement in result of difference of locality of stimulation. The field of remaining æsthesia includes whole of foot, the outer and (less) the inner aspect of the ankle, the outer aspect of the lower half of the leg, and the calf nearly up to the popliteal space. A slight pinch of the skin at any point within the whole of this area elicits a contraction in the hamstring muscles and in the median half of the gracilis; this contraction is accompanied by flexion of the ankle, and by some spreading of the toes when the pinch is applied to the dorsum pedis or planta, especially the pad. The contraction in the hamstring muscles is chiefly in the inner hamstrings when the inner side of the foot, chiefly in outer hamstrings when the outer side of the foot, is the place of provocation. A deep reflex—*e.g.*, a pinch of the tibialis anticus tendons—elicits the same contraction of medial half of gracilis as do the skin reflexes. A crossed reflex, exciting the crossed quadriceps extensor cruris, was obtainable from the whole of the skin area.

Again : If the afferent roots of the limb-region of the dog are split up into a series of filaments, twenty-five in number, all fairly equal in size (I have prepared the filaments as follows: 9th post-thoracic, one filament; 8th post-thoracic, four filaments; 7th post-thoracic, six filaments; 6th post-thoracic, five filaments; 5th post-thoracic, three filaments; 4th post-thoracic, two filaments; 3rd post-thoracic, two filaments; 2nd post-thoracic, one filament), excitation of each of these, except the first and sometimes the twenty-fifth, usually readily evokes flexion of the knee, and from the uppermost twenty flexion of hip can usually be obtained. Sometimes each of the whole series of twenty-five will evoke flexion of knee.

Again : From the cervical afferent roots of the monkey, by individual excitation in descending series, contraction of supinator longus muscle is obtainable from each in succession from 3rd cervical to 8th cervical, though not usually inclusive of the latter.

A very striking character of the reflexes elicitable from the isolated mammalian cord is the machine-like want of variation with which, on repeating the stimulation, the movement is repeated. Of this fatality, temporal monotony, or monotonous repetition, it is not necessary to give further example than the flexion of thumb or hallux that follows uniformly each time the little finger or toe is pinched. It is true that after the first few repetitions a slighter pinch than that required at first generally becomes adequate ("facilitation" or "bahnung"), or the reply from the same degree of stimulus becomes more extensive, and that after twenty or thirty repetitions an interval may ensue during which the movement becomes less, and may even be scarcely perceptible; then it returns again gradually, as it were, from fatigue. The *breakdown due to fatigue appears to involve the afferent rather than the efferent apparatus*, at least to affect it *earlier*, for, if *another* finger or toe be excited, the movement is at once elicited from it, in accordance with the rule of spatial monotony. Among the deep reflexes a good example of monotony of repetition is contraction of the median part of the gracilis muscle, which occurs each time one of the two tendons of the tibialis anticus muscle is nipped above the annular ligament (cat).

The " March " in the Development of Spinal Reflexes as Stimulation is Continued

The reflex movements elicitable from the mammalian spinal cord after cross-section are often extremely brief—surprisingly so; in fact, as Fick[1] has pointed out in dealing with the dorsal nerves of the frog, often like simple motor twitches. The movements have seemed to me most brief when least vigorous and most limited in extent, more so in the monkey in its early condition subsequent to cord-section than in the cat and dog under similar conditions. Stimuli that at first elicit only a single movement of a single joint later elicit frequently a short sequence of movements about a series of joints; the capacity for developing a sequence is much earlier regained by the isolated cord of cat or dog than by that of monkey.

For the sequence of movements in a spinal reflex the term which Hughlings Jackson's writings on epilepsy introduced and have rendered classical will here be used—" the march." As instances of " the march " in spinal reflex movements may be given the following:

Excitation of afferent root of 8th post-thoracic (monkey) gave flexion of hallux, with some adduction of it, followed by plantar flexion of ankle, followed by movement of tail.

Pinching the back of the thigh towards its medial side high up elicited (monkey) flexion and adduction of hallux, followed by flexion of knee, followed by movement of tail, accompanied by protrusion of anus.

Touching the skin at the side of the vaginal orifice (monkey) evoked depression of tail, accompanied by protrusion of anus, followed by flexion of knee, with some abduction of thigh, followed by flexion of hallux.

A long-continued pinch of the pad will in the cat sometimes induce a short series of alternating flexions and extensions of both hind-limbs, or simply a series of alternating flexions of the two ankles. In the rabbit similarly a series of flexions of the ankles are sometimes elicitable, but—in accordance with the hopping progression of the animal— are not alternately, but bilaterally, symmetrical. These reflexes can sometimes be evoked by merely holding the animal up so that the paralytic hind-limbs hang.

Touching the pad of the fore-paw evokes (cat) flexion of all digits, then extension of wrist and pronation of forearm, then flexion of elbow and retraction of shoulder.

Pinching the outer edge of the sole (Macacus) evoked adduction and flexion of the hallux, accompanied by extension of the other digits at metatarso-phalangeal joints, followed by eversion of foot, with dorsi-flexion at ankle, followed by flexion at knee and hip, accompanied by adduction toward opposite thigh, and, finally, slight depression of tail and adduction of opposite thigh itself.

Pinching the inner edge of the sole (Macacus) evoked adduction-flexion of hallux, accompanied by extension of the other digits at metatarso-phalangeal joints, followed by inversion of foot, followed by flexion of knee, in which the inner hamstrings were chiefly concerned.

Pressure close in front of heel (Macacus) gave flexion of hallux and other digits, followed

[1] *Pflüg. Arch. ges. Physiol.*, 1870, **3**, 326.

by plantar flexion of ankle, followed by flexion at knee. In one monkey, stroking or blowing upon the hair of one flank evoked flexion of hip, followed by flexion of knee, followed by flexion of ankle and digits.

From a spot in the perineum the following sequence was obtainable: protrusion of anus, followed at once by elevation of tail, succeeded by lateral wagging of tail, continued for about thirty seconds; evacuation of fæces sometimes followed (Macacus).

In the monkey after spinal transection it is quite rare for a moderate stimulus to provoke discharge of successive opposite movements at one and the same joint—e.g., those of lateral wagging of tail or alternating flexions and extensions of limb-joints. This is consonant with the rule that the groups of motoneurones most readily combined in action by spinal reflexes are those which are synergetic, not antergetic. In cats and dogs, in whom the depression of spinal reflex action is not so severe as in Macacus, the spinal reflexes in their march do combine and discharge, especially in the hind-limbs—where depression is less than in fore-limbs—antergetic groups of neurones in the course of their march, but not (my own experience is never) contemporaneously, though often successively. Hence the *alternating discharges*, which, though very rare in Macacus, are common and characteristic of the reflexes of the hind-limbs and tail of cat and dog and of the guinea-pig and rabbit. In these alternating discharges only one group of an antagonistic couple is discharged at a time. These alternating discharges are especially prone to appear when the stimulation is prolonged. An excellent illustration of this is given by cat or dog when one of the hind-paws is pressed between finger and thumb, and continued to be held even after the flexion of ankle, knee, and hip which results; alternating extensions and flexions of the limb then occur, giving exactly an appearance of the limb struggling to get itself free. Freusberg's[1] "beating-time" reflex (dog), which can also be studied in the cat, is another example. The "tail-wagging" reflex, even in isolated tail cord, which I have seen also in the monkey, is another. The flicking backwards and forwards of the ear in the cat is another. I would distinguish carefully between these reflexes with "alternating discharge" in antagonistic muscles and the discharge which is merely clonic in character.

The nerve-cells for the extensors of the knee, rarely as they initiate—i.e., are *primary*—in any spinal reflex, are frequently involved in the later progress of the march. Thus flexion of the knee, combined with flexion of hip and ankle, is frequently followed by and gives way to extension of knee, hip, and ankle; extension at hip is perhaps the most frequent of these extensions. It is noteworthy that in cat, as I previously pointed out in frog, the extension is rapid in onset, short in duration, and rapid in disappearance—a kick, in fact—as compared with the contraction in the flexors.

For instance, following flexion of the knee, extension frequently occurs in the march of the spinal reflex, started from a pinch of the ipsilateral foot; similarly, it may rapidly follow extension of the hip; or, as a crossed

[1] *Pflüg. Arch. ges. Physiol.*, 1874, **9**, 358.

reflex, it may follow and accompany flexion of hip and knee of the opposite side, and in this last case may initiate an alternating " extension-flexion " reflex in the limb of its own side. The relation between the neurones of extensors and flexors at elbow is much the same as between those of extensors and flexors at knee, the flexors of elbow corresponding with flexors at knee. But the difference between flexors and extensors at elbow does not seem to be quite so pronounced as between flexors and extensors at knee. In its behaviour in spinal reflexes, the brachial triceps resembles the extensors of the knee, also in its crossed relation with the flexors of the opposite elbow. In the cat, contraction of the triceps brachii, as a primary idiolateral local reflex, is rare, but it is quite usually occurrent as the primary contraction of the *crossed* fore-limb, while contraction of the flexors of elbow is the primary contraction in the homonymous fore-limb. But I have seen flexion of the opposite elbow occur on rare occasion in response to strong excitation of the fore-paw of one side in the cat.

In the rabbit, extension of the knee is still rarer as the primary movement of a spinal reflex than even in cat and dog, but, on account of the relatively slight depression caused by spinal transection in the rabbit, it is a very frequent movement in the course of the " march " of a spinal reflex. It does not, however, occur nearly so frequently—in fact, I have never yet seen it occur as the initial movement of the crossed side in the rabbit—for in rabbit, flexion of the knee and hip seem the primary crossed just as they are the primary ipsilateral reflexes. This is in obvious relation to the mode of progression of the animal. Thus, in rabbit, a pinch of the tail will cause symmetrically bilateral flexions, followed by extensions of the hind-limbs, although in the fore-limbs flexion of one fore-limb occurs with extension of the opposite fore-limb. Pinch of one foot will evoke *flexion* of the knees and hips of both sides, instead of flexion of ipsilateral and extension of contralateral knee, as is usual in the cat.[1]

VARIOUS COMMON REFLEX RESPONSES

Crossed Spinal Reflexes

By " crossed reflex " is understood a reflex involving travel of nervous impulses across the median plane of the cord. The need for the definition will be obvious in what follows.

The second of Pflüger's[2] " laws " of spinal reflexion—that termed the " law of symmetry of bilateral reflexes "—states that if to idiolateral

---

[1] In the original description a chapter on " reflexes of long intraspinal path " follows. These are reflexes linking a fore-limb with the hind-limbs, and *vice versa*, pinna with the limbs, the limbs and tail, etc. (*Philos. Trans.*, 1898, **190B**, 169-173) (some of these are described below, p. 204). Interesting as these effects are, and important in demonstrating the inapplicability of the " Laws " of Pflüger (*Über die sensorische Functionen des Rückenmarkes*, Berlin, 1853) which had dominated the theory of spinal reflexes up to the time of this paper, they are omitted here owing to lack of space.—ED.   [2] *Über d. Sensorische Funct. d. Rückenm.*, Berlin, 1853.

movement there be added, in the course of a spinal reflex, contralateral, the latter is symmetrical with the former. The cat and monkey afford several examples of this.

Bilateral adduction of thighs (Macacus).

Bilateral extension of hips, on stimulation of skin of abdomen (cat).

Bilateral abduction of hips, with some extension.

Stimulus to fore-limb of cat; very similar extension and abduction of thighs by stimulating 2nd cervical root.

Bilateral protrusion of anus by stimulating one side of the perineum.

Bilateral extension of elbows and retraction of shoulders by stimulating pinna (cat).

Bilateral flexion of elbows with some supination of both forearms and a forward adduction of both fore-limbs, so that the paws cross each other in front of the chest, from stimulation of one fore-pad embrace reflex.

Bilateral retraction of abdomen on stimulating the side of the chest or upper part of abdomen.

Bilateral flexion of hips and knees on excitation of skin above an ischial tuberosity in the cat.

Bilateral protraction of " whiskers " on excitation of skin of the face.

But there are many and important instances which do not conform to the " law." A most important crossed reflex of progression elicitable from hind-limb of cat and dog does not conform to it. Under deep but not very profound anæsthesia, it is a common thing in these animals for alternating flexion of the two hind-limbs to take place. In the rabbit the flexion of the two hind-limbs, which occurs under similar conditions, is synchronous, not alternate. After spinal transection at the top of the lumbar region the same alternating flexion and extension often is started by merely lifting the animal so that the hind-quarters hang. If, when the movement thus started has ceased and the limbs hang inactive, one hind-paw is pressed, the leg is drawn up, and if the pressure be discontinued, or if the reflex activity is slight, the limb is let down again slowly. If the pressure be, however, continued or the reflex activity brisk, the drawing up of the limb is succeeded by movement of the opposite limb; this crossed movement is usually extension of the knee, generally accompanied by extension of ankle (plantar-flexion), and slight extension at hip. That is to say, the flexors of the knee, so inaccessible, as stated above, to the local ipsilateral excitation, are delicately sensitive to contralateral. The same result often follows electric excitation of either of the plantar nerves, of the cutaneous division of musculo-cutaneous nerve, and of the popliteal and hamstring nerves themselves—i.e., ipsilateral flexion of knee, contralateral extension of knee. Sometimes bilateral flexion is obtained, and in the rabbit, in my experience, crossed flexion instead of crossed extension is the rule.

Again, excitation of 6th and of 7th post-thoracic roots evokes flexion of ipsilateral knee, hip, and ankle, but extension of contralateral knee. Excitation of the perineal skin I have seen give the same. In this reflex there is produced on the crossed side not only excitation of the extensor muscles, but *inhibition* of their antagonists.   In dog and cat, when the flexion of one hip and knee—*e.g.*, right—has been evoked and is in progress, contra-lateral excitation appropriately timed often relaxes the contracted flexors of the right limb.   Similarly, when after ablation of the hemispheres (cat, rabbit) the extensor tonus, which I termed *decerebrate rigidity*, has set in, excitation of the hind-foot of one side inhibits the contraction of the same side extensors of knee, but increases the contraction of the extensors of the opposite knee.   And in the same way, at elbow, the triceps of the crossed side is increased in its contraction, while triceps of the same side elbow is inhibited even to the extent of reaching its *post-mortem* length.   Graphic records show that with the contraction of triceps occurs active relaxation of biceps, with the contraction of biceps occurs active relaxation of triceps, and similarly with the antagonistic muscles of the knee-joint.   Similarly, excitation of the side of the superior vermis or of funiculus cuneatus (*e.g.*, at calamus scriptorius) causes, during the state of decerebrate rigidity, relaxation of the same side triceps brachii with contraction of the same side flexors of elbow, and at the same time still further relaxation in the opposite biceps and increase of contraction in the opposite triceps.   The case of the antagonistic muscles at knee-joint I have similarly examined from superior vermis and funiculus gracilis with similar result, except in rabbit, where flexion of both knees seems the rule.

In a monkey with mid-thoracic spinal transection in the course of months flexion of hip as a crossed reflex developed. It was much easier to obtain this in one limb than in the other, and was obtained more readily as an ipsilateral reflex on that side on which it was the easier as a contralateral reflex. Late rigidity affects in the monkey flexors of hip; I do not therefore lay stress on this instance, but it deserves mention.

The asymmetry of the crossed reflexes of the legs is important because obviously connected with the co-ordination of progression.

The ipsilateral flexion reflex is *prepotent and inhibits* the crossed extension —*e.g.*, stimulation of both feet together causes drawing up of both, so also at elbows. Semisection above the lesion makes the crossed reflex more easily evoked from the side of the semisection. Splitting lengthwise, from top of 5th lumbar to bottom of 7th, destroys the crossed, but not the idio-lateral. Again, contralateral flexion is apt to accompany ipsilateral flexion when the stimulation is strong.

In the monkey the ipsilateral flexion of hallux, knee, and hip excited by an excitation of the foot is often followed in the opposite hind-limb by adduction of thigh.   In the same animal dorsi-flexion of the ankle elicited from the 7th (afferent) post-thoracic root is often followed by plantar flexion of the contralateral ankle. Similarly, in the cat, when 3rd, 4th, 5th, 6th, 8th, 9th, and 10th post-thoracic afferent roots have been severed after spinal transection at 11th thoracic level, a pinch on sole or dorsum pedis, or lateral aspect of lower region of leg and calf, evokes ipsilateral flexion of toes, ankle, and knee with some contraction in the ipsilateral gracilis, but contralateral plantar flexion of ankle. Again, the reflex that

I call the *torticollis reflex* (see p. 130) breaks this " second law " of Pflüger, because it employs muscles on both sides of the median plane, and the muscles on the crossed side are not symmetrical with those on the uncrossed.

Pflüger's third law states that if a spinal reflex is bilateral, the movements on the side opposite to that stimulated is much weaker than the ipsilateral. This is the so-called law of unequal intensity of bilateral reflexes. The experiments in cat, dog, and monkey afford instances of it.

When from one fore-paw bilateral movement of the fore-limbs is excited the movement is less forcible on the crossed side, and also less ample.

When excitation of one pinna evokes bilateral movement in the hind-limbs, as described above, the crossed movement is the weaker.

When bilateral retraction of abdomen is excited from the chest wall the crossed retraction is much the less extreme.

In the above-described asymmetrical progression reflex the crossed movement is much the less vigorous.

In the bilateral " whisker reflex " the crossed movement is the less ample.

But some reflexes controvert the law.

Both in the monkey and in the cat and dog a touch on the side of the tail at its root usually evokes abduction from the median line and away from the side stimulated. This recalls Luchsinger's reflex from the tail of the newt. The same crossed action is obtainable from the dorsal (afferent) roots of coccygeal nerves. Again, a pinch of little toe or a pin-prick at the inner edge of the ischial callosity in monkey often elicits a similar switch of the tail *from* the idiolateral side. This reflex not only breaks the third law, but also first law, which lays down that if a movement caused by a spinal reflex is unilateral it occurs always on the same side as the application of the stimulus. Caudal lateral movement of reflex spinal origin is, however, not always abduction from the side stimulated.

Conduction across the median sagittal plane of the cord is certainly very unequally facile at different spinal levels. I have found it curiously difficult to drive irradiation across in the thoracic region from a thoracic afferent root so as to elicit bilateral action of intercostal muscles. It is easier in cat, dog, and monkey to obtain cross-reflex from one hind-limb to the other than from one fore-limb to the other. It is easier to obtain in these species cross-reflex from one hind-limb to the other than from a hind-limb up to a fore-limb. It is, however, easier to obtain a reflex from fore-limb to ipsilateral hind-limb than from fore-limb to fore-limb. In the hind-limb of cat and dog, the extensor neurones of knee, hip, and ankle have more facile communication with the crossed side of the cord than have the flexor neurones, but this does not seem the case with the hind-limb of the rabbit.

Reflexes elicited by Percussion

A tap on the ischial callosity (tuber ischii) in the monkey elicits excellently a bilateral adduction of the thighs.

A tap upon the spinal column (skin removed) at the level of the iliac crests evokes rotation outward of both thighs with slight extension of both knees. This must be similar to a reflex mentioned by Sternberg[1] as of clinical importance: it involves action of the *glutei*.

A tap upon the articular surface of the lower end of femur evokes contraction in the adductors of both thighs: the contraction is bilaterally symmetrical, or more often greater on the contralateral side.

A tap on lower end of femur, or on insertion of tendo patellæ, usually excites dorso-flexion of ankle with slight inversion of foot. This seems to be "Erb's *tibialis anticus* reflex" of clinicians; in my experiments *extensor longus digitorum* replies more amply than does *tibialis anticus*. The tap generally elicits dorsi-flexion of the contralateral as well as of the ipsilateral ankle.

I am not inclined to consider any of the above to be true cross-reflexes. The so-called *cross knee-jerk* and perhaps the *cross adductor* reflex are not cross-reflexes. That they are reflexes seems certain from the length of their latent period estimated by the time-measurements of Burckhardt,[2] recently repeated with a similar result by Gotch.[3] The former is contralateral and reflex, but not a cross-reflex, for I find it persist *after complete longitudinal splitting of the cord* from a lumbar transection above to the coccygeal nerves below. It must be excited by jar as suggested by Waller and Prevost.[4] And other "jar" reflexes are flexion of hip, protrusion of anus, protrusion of vaginal orifice, all readily excited by a tap on an unyielding part. All the "jar" reflexes implicate parts easily moved by reflex action, and are cut out by section of the appropriate sensory roots on their own side—*i.e.*, the contralateral to application of blow, and not by section of the sensory roots on the side of the blow given. At first sight, inasmuch as they are bilaterally symmetrical, they appear as cross-reflexes, which support Pflüger's "Law of Reflex Symmetry." I would apply Waller and Prevost's explanation of excitation by transmission of mechanical vibration to them as to the so-called cross knee-jerk. I would differ from Waller and Prevost, however, in so far that if I understood their meaning aright, they consider the vibration acts as a direct stimulus to the muscle or its motor nerve. I think, on the other hand, the jar excites the afferent nerve-fibres of the nerve-roots corresponding with the muscles, and excites them at or just peripheral to the ganglion. It is remarkable how distinctly even a slight tap upon the end of one femur is felt by holding the lower end of the other femur, particularly in some positions of the thigh, especially, I think, when the thighs are somewhat abducted.

Some Features of the Muscular Contractions occurring in Spinal Reflexes

When spinal depression is great and the reflex movements difficult to evoke they are usually characterised by the following features: feebleness, restriction of scope, minute tremor, and brevity of duration. As they

---

[1] *Die Sehnenreflexe*, Vienna, 1893.   [2] *Über Sehnenreflexe*, Bern, 1877.
[3] *J. Physiol.*, 1896, **20**, 322.   [4] *Revue Médicale de la Suisse Romande*, 1881.

improve they become more ample, more vigorous, less tremulant or quite steady, and of longer duration. Many of them when quite vigorous are nevertheless clonic; for instance, the abduction of thighs with flexion of toes obtainable in the hind-limb by exciting the fore-paw is in the cat nearly always clonic. Some are long—*i.e.*, persist for nearly a minute—exhibiting steady contraction all along with a final access. This I have seen especially in flexion of knee and in flexion of elbow. Finally, as the reflexes become more active," " march " develops, taking courses as above described. A feature frequent in thoroughly active spinal reflexes is *alternating discharge of antagonistic muscles*, especially, perhaps, at ankle and at wrist. The alternations may recur many times over. The reflex contractions of one of the alternating groups are usually much shorter than of the other: thus at ankle and wrist the plantar flexion and the dorsal extension are shorter, sharper than the return movements.

Inhibition in Spinal Reflexes

It has been shown by Goltz and Freusberg[1] that in the dog spinal reflexes can be inhibited by appropriately timed strong excitations of the skin. Thus, pinching of the tail stops the " beating time " reflex of the dog. They found, too, that a cord tied round a leg may, in the dog as in the frog, make all reflexes inelicitable from the limb for a time. Nipping the tail sometimes succeeds in interrupting micturition in the monkey—spinal transection of mid-thoracic region. The local homonymous leg reflex will inhibit the crossed.

My own observations lead me to believe that *inhibito-motor* spinal reflexes occur *quite habitually and concurrently* with many of the excito-motor described in this paper. In graphic records of the reflex limb movements of the frog the sudden and absolute relaxation of the muscles of one group at the very moment (to a 0·05 second) of the onset of contraction in the antergetic group[2] suggests this. Again, after spinal transection in dog or cat the flexion-reflex being obtained in the ipsilateral limb by pressing the foot, if while that limb is drawn up by the reflex the other foot is squeezed, not only is the squeezed leg drawn up, but the limb previously flexed is, very usually, let down, relaxation of the flexors occurring concurrently with contraction of the extensors. This co-ordination I term " *reciprocal innervation*."

That when the flexors of knee and hip are reflexly thrown into action the extensors are inhibited seems proved by the *impossibility* of obtaining the crossed reflex in the extensors when the foot of the crossed side is pinched.

Again, on two occasions, once in cat and once in Macacus, the leg lying at the time in a state of rigidity due to tonic spasm of the extensor muscles

[1] *Pflüg. Arch. ges. Physiol.*, 1874, **8**, 460; 1874, **9**, 358.
[2] Sherrington, *J. Physiol.*, 1892, **13**, 722, Plate XXIII.

of hip and knee, gentle excitation of the central end of a twig of the internal saphenous nerve at the ankle at once produced *relaxation* of the extensors, and at the same time some contraction of the flexors. In each case the phenomenon is one of regular occurrence so long as the conditions are regularly repeated. The carrying out of a movement by the overpowering of the active contraction of one muscle-group by the active contraction of another muscle-group is throughout my experience *foreign to the tactical mechanism of the spinal cord*. This experience harmonises in part with an idea put forth some years ago by H. Munk,[1] and made the subject of a research undertaken at his instigation by Schlösser.[2] In short, my observations prove the existence of " reciprocal innervation " of antagonistic muscles as part of the machinery of spinal reflexes, and point to it as possibly a widely extensive part of that machinery. It not only affects contrasted muscle-groups, but also contrasted parts of one and the same muscle, as in quadriceps ext. fem. and in triceps brachii.

PHASIC VARIATION IN THE REFLEX ACTIVITY OF THE CORD

Although, as the " rule of monotonous repetition " above states, absence of variation of the movement elicited by repetitions of a particular stimulus is a striking character of spinal reflexes in the mammal and lends to them a machine-like quality of regularity, there does occur a curious variety of result when they are examined in the same individual from day to day. The very spot of skin that one day evokes constantly flexion of all the toes may the following day evoke nothing but flexion of hallux and extension of the other toes, and the day following may evoke nothing, or, again, only the movement obtained three days before. A stimulus usually eliciting dorso-flexion at ankle may on some days elicit in the same individual plantar flexion of ankle. As a broad rule, it is certain that spinal reflexes are more easily elicited when a well-nourished animal is hungry and expectant of food, and less easily after a heavy meal.[3] Altogether apart, however, from feeding time on some days hardly a reflex can be elicited from the very animals that on other days yield a variety with readiness. Conditions of individual age, and especially of general nutrition, influence, as Freusberg points out for the lumbo-sacral reflexes of the dog, the facility of reflexes very greatly indeed.

[1] *Verhandlungen der Berliner Physiologischen Gesellschaft*, October, 1881.
[2] *Arch. Anat. Physiol. Lpz., Physiol. Abt.*, 1880, p. 303.
[3] See also observations on the enhancement of reflexes by rise of temperature, *J. Physiol.*, 1924, **58**, 420.—ED.

V

ON SOME PARTICULAR FEATURES OF SPINAL AND BULBAR REFLEXES

1. THE INFLUENCE OF PRE-EXISTING POSTURE[1]

[*The outcome of a spinal reflex is influenced in some degree by the posture present at the time of the application of the stimulus.*]

MACHINE-LIKE regularity and fatality of reaction, although characteristic of spinal reflexes, is yet not exemplified by them to such extent that similar stimuli will always elicit from the spinal animal similar responses. This want of certainty as to response is an interesting difficulty attending the study of spinal reactions. The variation in the responses of the skeletal musculature manifests itself not only in regard to the extent of the movement, but also in regard to the direction of the movement.

Some of the factors determining the character of the reactions are factors contained within the stimulus. Important among these is the " *locus* of the stimulus." Thus it has long been known that the direction and other characters of the reflex movement are influenced by the mere location of the stimulus. Nevertheless, stimuli identical in all respects, including locality, may evoke reflex movements of widely different, even of absolutely opposite, character. Such differences of response must be referred to differences obtaining at the time in the spinal organ itself. One cause for such differences seems indicated by the following observations:

The most usual, indeed the almost invariable, primary reflex movement of the hind-limb of the spinal dog (and cat), when spinal transection has been performed in the cervical or upper thoracic region, is flexion at hip, knee, and ankle; the limb is " drawn up." This movement can be well obtained by, among other stimuli, the pressing of the pads of the digits upward so as to extend the toe-joints, a stimulus that in some measure imitates the effect upon those joints of the bearing of the foot upon the ground under the animal's weight. Extension as a reflex result from this stimulus is, in my experience, never met with in the homonymous limb in the early time after transection. When a certain period has elapsed, three weeks or more after transection, and shock has largely subsided, it becomes possible to, at times, obtain extension at hip as the primary movement in the homonymous limb. The pressing of the toe-pads upwards, spreading

---

[1] Published as " On the Innervation of Antagonistic Muscles. Sixth Note." *Proc. roy. Soc.*, 1900, **66**, 66, 67.

and extending the digits, elicits a sharp movement of extension at the hip, if at the time the initial posture of hip and knee be flexion. If the initial posture of hip and knee be extension, the primary reflex movement excited is, in my experience, invariably flexion. The reflex movement is, it is true, not unfrequently flexion, even when the initial posture is one of flexion; but it is, on the other hand, very frequently, and especially preponderantly in certain individual animals, extension. The passive assumption of a flexed posture at hip and knee seems to favour the reflex movement at those joints taking the form of extension. The influence of the posture of the ankle-joint upon the reflex movement at the hip seems negligible, for I have often remarked the reaction at the hip to be unaltered, whether the ankle were flexed or extended, at the time of excitation.

In some dogs, when the spinal transection has been made at the hinder end of the thoracic region, stimulation of the skin of the limb evokes the usual primary flexion at hip and knee wherever the *locus* of the stimulus, except it be in the upper three-fourths of the front of the thigh. Applied in this latter region the stimulus, if the limb be midway between extension and flexion, not unfrequently evokes reflex extension at hip and knee; it does not evoke extension if the initial posture of the limb be extension; but if the limb be, at the time of application of the stimulus, well flexed at hip and knee, reflex extension, instead of reflex flexion, becomes the rule.

In the spinal frog, as in the spinal dog, flexion at hip and knee is the regular reflex response of the musculature of the homonymous hind-limb to skin stimuli applied at any part of the surface of that limb. This being true when the initial posture of the limb is, as when pendent, one of extension at hip, knee, and ankle, a difference becomes evident when the initial posture is one of flexion at those joints. In the latter case excitation of the skin within a small gluteal and pubic area, lateral and somewhat ventral to the cloacal orifice, causes extremely frequently not flexion at hip, but extension at that joint. Stimuli (mechanical and chemical) to that area which evoke flexion at the hip-joint when the initial posture of the limb involves extension at that joint, evoke, when the initial posture is flexion, reflex extension at the joint.

These instances seem to indicate distinctly that the direction which a spinal reflex movement elicited by stimuli similar in all respects, including "locality," may take, is in part determined by the posture already obtaining in the limb at the time of the application of the stimulus.

The reaction described above for the spinal frog holds good after previous removal of all the skin from both hind-limbs, with the exception of the small gluteal piece necessary for application of the skin stimulus. It would appear, therefore, that the influence of the posture of the limb upon the spinal condition and reaction is not traceable to the nerves of the cutaneous sense-organs of the limbs. There still remain the afferent nerves subserving muscular sense, and connected with the sense-organs in muscles, tendons, and joints. These, as is well known, are largely affected by the various postures of the limb, even by such postures as are passively induced.

2. SELECTIVITY FOR A CERTAIN QUALITY OF STIMULUS

[*Qualitative difference of spinal reflex corresponding with qualitative difference of cutaneous stimulus.*[1]]

Qualitative differences between spinal reflexes provoked from the skin are usually distinguished only in so far as dependent on differences in the regional *locus* of their initiation. The experimentalist has in general to be content to tacitly treat these skin reflexes as of a single kind. But the variety of species of sensation elicitable from the skin suggests that possibly different reflex motor reactions attach to the different species of end-organs undoubtedly coexisting in one and the same skin-field. The different kinds of end-organ belonging to one and the same cutaneous region may possess reflex spinal connections differing *inter se*. That this is really the case is indicated by the following observations undertaken in examination of the question.

1. In the " spinal " dog (*e.g.*, after exsection of a short piece, a segment, from the posterior cervical region of the cord), if the skin underneath and between the toe-pads and cushion of the hind-foot be pressed or stretched, a sudden forcible extension of the limb is evoked. This is especially the case if at the time of stimulation the limb be resting flexed at hip and knee. I have called this reflex the " direct extension reflex."[2] The extensor movement is brief and ample, and resembles the sharp extension of the spinal frog's leg, of which tracings were furnished in a previous paper.[3]

It is obvious that such a movement, helpful as contributory to progression, would on the contrary be harmful in response to certain other possible stimuli to the foot. Suppose a thorn lying below the foot and applied so as to prick it underneath. If there then ensued the extensor movement that as above described ensues when broad pressure is applied, the consequence would be a further wounding of the foot by the reflex movement of the leg itself. The foot would be driven forcibly upon the offending point. Observation shows that, in fact, a prick of the pad-region evokes not extension but flexion of the limb. And the reflex effect of the prick is typical of the reflex effect produced by application to the *planta* of *harmful* stimuli in general. In result the foot is withdrawn from the offending stimulus. Instead of wounding itself further it escapes from the threatened wounding.

Thus in the case of the under-surface of the hind-foot two stimuli of different quality evoke respectively two movements of exactly opposite sense. Two different sets of efferent nerves belonging to this part must therefore be directly connected with respectively two opposed elements of the muscular organisation of the part. Or probably it would be a truer expression of the relation to say that each of the two sets of efferents is connected with both flexor and extensor musculature, but that the one set

---

[1] Published under this title in *J. Physiol.*, 1903, **30**, 39.

[2] *Proc. roy. Soc.*, 1899, **66**, 66; and *J. Physiol.*, 1903, **29**, 67 (later called " extensor thrust," see pp. 183 and 208).

[3] *J. Physiol.*, 1892, **13**, Plate XXIII., Figs. 4 and 5.

primarily acts in a pressor manner upon extensor neurones, and in an inhibitory manner on flexor neurones, while the other set acts conversely in
a pressor manner upon flexor neurones, and in an inhibitory on extensor
neurones.

As to the quality of the nerve-endings involved in each case, the nerve-
endings stimulated by the prick lie undoubtedly superficially, for a light
prick suffices.   Neither mere touch nor cold nor warmth (unless amounting
to injurious heat) evokes the reaction.   Heat sufficient to threaten injury
to the skin does, however, quickly and regularly, like the prick, evoke the
flexor movement.   It is fair to infer that the species of nerve-ending excited
is that which may be termed the nocicipient, and certainly that division
of it which lies in the more superficial layers of the skin.

I have elsewhere put forward a view that there has been evolved in the skin " a
special sense of its own injuries."[1]   There is considerable evidence that the skin is provided
with a set of nerve-endings whose specific office it is to be amenable to stimuli that do the
skin injury, stimuli that in continuing to act would injure it still further.   These nerve-
endings when still connected with the sensorium (using that term simply to mean the
neural machinery to which consciousness is adjunct) on excitation evoke skin pain.   They
are in that respect algesic.   After their disconnection from the sensorium by spinal
transection they still possess spinal connection with large fields of musculature.   The
reactions they then evoke being devoid of psychical feature, the term algesic becomes
inappropriate for them.   But harmfulness still remains the characteristic of the stimuli
by which they are provocable.   For physiological reference, therefore, they are, it seems
to me, both on this ground and on others which need not be entered upon here, preferably
termed nocicipient, a name which has the advantage of greater objectivity.

The other species of nerve-ending—namely, that excited by the broad
pressure about the pads and cushion and eliciting the " direct extension
reflex "—is more difficult to identify.   Separation of the toe-pads one from
another or from the plantar cushion so as to stretch or squeeze one or the
other is often a very effective mode of stimulation.   The reflex very often
ensues on *removal* of such pressure or tension.   Although sometimes the
pressure or tension applied must affect the small tendons, ligaments, or
joints of the foot, I feel satisfied that the reflex often ensues when the application of the stimulus is really confined to the skin, including, however, the
deepest layers of that organ.   The pressure and tension requisite in this
stimulus seem to resemble what must occur when the limb supports the
weight of the animal as it steps.   The *relief* of this pressure and tension,
often even more than the application of it, appears to excite the reflex.
This suggests that the reflex normally ensues on some change of pressure and
tension in the *planta* occurring towards the latter part of the performance
of a step in locomotion.

Applications of either cold, warmth, heat, or of chemical reagents are
ineffectual *per se* to evoke the reflex: nocuous mechanical stimuli are also
inefficient.   But the form of stimulus adequate is nevertheless of mechanical
quality, of a kind that may fairly be described as pressure and tension

[1] " Skin and Common Sensation," article in *Textbook of Physiology*, edited by Schäfer, 1900, 2.

rather deeply applied. Of terms in ordinary use, "*deep touch*" might be the least inappropriate.

Applied therefore to the dog's *planta*, broad harmless pressure on the one hand and surface damage on the other both readily evoke reflex movements of the whole limb, and the movement evoked in the one case is totally different from the movement evoked in the other.

2. One of the most striking reflexes in the " spinal " dog is the " scratch " reflex. This is a " skin reflex "—*i.e.*, it is excited by stimulation of the skin. It is, however, not every stimulus to the skin that can provoke it. In the large reflexigenous field of skin whence it can be evoked[1] various kinds of stimuli can be applied without eliciting any trace of the reflex.

To examine evidence to this effect it is best to work with the skin carefully and cleanly shaved. It is on the shaved skin only that some of the following points can be demonstrated. The application of certain forms of stimuli experimentally through the hairy coat is unsatisfactory. But the existence of a hairy coat in no way essentially alters the problem or the argument.

The finger-tips or the whole hand can be applied to the skin, pitting it, exerting strong pressure upon it and doubtless applying mechanical stimulation to the nerve-endings in it throughout its depth, and yet no scratch-reflex is produced. The skin thus firmly pressed upon can be moved to and fro over the subcutaneous tissue and its deep surface thus rubbed over and against underlying structures soft or hard, and yet this fails to evoke the reflex. If a fold of skin either thin or thick be gathered up between thumb and fingers and then the two layers composing the fold be compressed and, further still, be rubbed freely against one another by their deep opposed surfaces, the scratch-reflex is nevertheless not evoked. Not only is mechanical stimulation in these conditions applied to the deep layer of the skin, but the stimulation is applied successively to adjacent fresh areas of the deep layers, and, as can be shown otherwise, successive spatial summation is an adjuvant of great potency in regard to stimuli exciting the scratch-reflex.

But the reflex is obtained at once if a finger-tip be lightly moved along the skin surface. To draw a pencil point along the surface is even more effective. These stimuli that effectively evoke the reflex press so lightly as to cause very little deformation at all of the skin surface. The difference between the character and efficacy of these stimuli and those mentioned in the previous paragraph is demonstrable in various striking ways. Two may be sufficient to cite here. A rigid ring, such as a bracelet or a large curtain-pole-ring, is applied to the skin, pressed on it, and while pressed upon it moved freely, carrying with it the skin over the subcutaneous tissue; no trace of the scratch-reflex is evoked. But let pencil point or finger-tip be moved over the surface of the skin surrounded by the ring, the scratch-reflex is then provoked forthwith. Again, while the fingers by rubbing

---

[1] See pp. 165 and 205 this volume, and *J. Physiol.*, 1906, **34**, 1.

over the surface of the skin are exciting a vigorous scratch-reflex, let them be pressed more against its surface; they then cease to move over its surface, but instead press into it, squeeze all its layers and carry the area to which they are immediately applied with them, rubbing its deep surface over underlying tissue, stretching the skin immediately behind and wrinkling that immediately in front. On this change from superficial to deep stimulation the scratch-reflex at once ceases.

That the nerve-endings which evoke this reflex lie therefore exclusively quite close to the skin surface seems clear. I find further that ablation of the surface of the skin to a depth of 0·6 mm. abolishes the reflex from the area so treated. The ablated sheet of skin need not include the deepest ends of the hair follicles in order to secure this abolition of the reflex.

When such a surface is made it is obvious that the nerve-fibres belonging to the removed *nerve-endings* must remain, and must, when the surface is fresh, lie exposed. It is noteworthy that of all the stimuli applied none is able to excite the reflex *through* these. The same phenomenon is met in the case of the deep moving pressures on the skin which, as mentioned above, fail to excite the reflex. In such cases, as explained above, the surface stimulation is not a moving one, but the deep stimulation is, and must, one would think, affect the nerve-fibres passing downward from the overlying surface end-organs that under moving " touches " excite the reflex. Yet no reflex is evoked. Both phenomena, though paradoxical in appearance, remarkably confirm the rule insisted on by Marshall Hall, that spinal reflexes are far more easily excited by stimulation of end-organs than by stimulation of the nerve-fibres conducting from the end-organs.

As to the form of stimulation adequate for these end-organs exciting the scratch-reflex, the observations just mentioned show that mechanical stimuli are competent. Such mechanical stimuli as these would, we can hardly doubt, did the condition of the animal allow—that is, were consciousness still adjunct to this region of its skin—provoke psychical " touches." I feel similar stimuli applied to my own skin as " moving touches." Hence it seems fair to conclude that among the species of cutaneous end-organs competent to evoke this reflex in the dog are those of " surface touch," the analogue of those that psychologically examined in man yield evidence of " stereognostic touch."

This set of end-organs, provoking the scratch-reflex in response to purely tactual stimuli, is distributed in close relation to hairs. Evidence of this is as follows: (1) Punctiform stimuli on the shaven skin applied at a hair or hair group—the hairs frequently lie in triads—or just " windward " of a hair, excite the reflex, while elsewhere they fail or are less effective. (2) The threshold value of the stimulus in a given skin area rises after shaving it. This rise is of twofold character: (*a*) *immediate*, (*b*) *late*. The threshold value for a stigmatic touch exciting the reflex by a v. Frey bristle being, *e.g.*, 60 mg. prior to cutting the hairs rises to, *e.g.*, 520 mg. directly after the shaving, although the mechanical stimulation of the shaving itself favours and facilitates (*bahnung*) the reflex. This is the "immediate" blunting. If the skin area be kept shaven, gradually in the course of a few weeks ensues a further rise of the threshold values. The difference of facility of the reflex from a shoulder shaved for the first time and that kept shaven for three weeks is marked: the reflex is much less easy to obtain in the latter. The presence of these tactual levers, harbouring no doubt some parasitic life, and constantly subjecting their particular nerve-endings to some stimulation or another, seems necessary for the maintenance of the full *biotonus*—to use Verworn's expressive term—of the reflex arcs which execute the scratch-reflex. (3) The peculiar efficacy of the moving touch as compared with the stationary touch in the provocation of the reflex applies both to the shaven and to the unshaven skin. The finger-tip simply pressed on the skin hardly evokes the reflex, but does so directly it moves along the skin. The moving touch acts more effectively on the hairs and hair stumps; and movement *against* the hairs is somewhat more effective than movement with the hairs. (4) *Depilation* of a skin area practically abolishes the capacity of the area to initiate the scratch-reflex. In the process of depilation the plucking out of a hair not unfrequently itself excites the reflex.

It is noteworthy, however, that to pull on a hair, or even on a little group of hairs, usually fails to excite the scratch-reflex. That mode of stimulation of the hair-nerves is of course not "normal." It is not improbable that the *tactual* apparatus of the hair follicle is not excitable by that kind of application of stimulus. Also it must be remembered that the nerve-endings associated with the hair follicles are considered by some observers to yield sensations *sui generis*, and distinct from tactual proper. The peculiar tickling sensations evoked by light stimulation of the hairlets of the human skin were by Noischewski and Ossipow,[1] working in Bechterew's clinique, found to be well developed in various skin areas where "touch" was not especially fine. The neck, shoulder, back and sides of the trunk— namely, a region corresponding with that which is reflexigenous for the dog's scratch-reflex—are specially mentioned by these observers as yielding strong tickling sensations *sui generis* under light mechanical stimuli applied to the hairlets. V. Frey[2] has, as is well known, demonstrated the great lowering of threshold for mechanical stimuli to the skin which the hairlets effect.

On the other hand, the foregoing shows that the *deep* skin nerve-endings are incompetent to evoke the scratch-reflex. Next arises the question, "Among the superficial cutaneous nerve-endings are those peculiar to the hairs the only species efficient?" I have tried various "*warm*" and "*cold*" stimuli and find them ineffective for the purpose. I conclude that neither

---

[1] Noischewski, *Gesellschaft der Aerzte*, Dünaburg (Dwinsk), April 2 and November 23, 1896; Ossipow and Noischewski, *Gesellschaft der Aerzte*, Petersburg, March, 1898; Bechterew, *Neurolog. Centralblatt*, **22**, 1032, November, 1898.

[2] "Beitr. z. Sinnesphysiol. d. Haut," *Ber. d. k. Sächs. Gesells. d. Wissensch. z. Leipzig. Math.-phys. Classe*, 1894, 1895.

warmth nor cold are *per se* adequate. But early in the investigation I was struck by the efficacy of dragging along the surface a *scratching* point. This stimulus seems often more effective than the areally far larger stimulus of a moving finger-tip; it is obvious that the former's efficacy may be due to its having not only tangible but noxious quality. It may stimulate *nocicipient* endings as well as purely *tangocipient*. Repeated light pricks seem similarly more effective than repeated simple stigmatic touches.

To test this possibility I have had recourse to combination of noxious stimulation with stimulation otherwise *per se* insufficient. Thus, as has been shown above, a steady pressure applied on one skin area, even large, does not evoke the reflex, even though it be severe. But if a small fold of skin be severely compressed, a short outburst of the reflex may be evoked. The mechanical stimulus is then of obviously noxious kind, and that the reflex is excited through nocicipient end-organs is indicated by its non-appearance when the same mechanical stimulus is applied with intensity insufficient to make it acutely harmful. Again, a warm metal plate one centimetre square and one millimetre thick applied to the skin evokes no trace of the scratch-reflex if applied with a temperature of 65° or less. But let it have when applied a temperature of 85° or more and the reflex is at once vigorously evoked. In order to altogether eradicate tangible quality from the stimulus I have also employed the heat beam as in previous observations. The radiation from a good source appropriately collected and applied focally to the skin of the reflexigenous area suffices, if not merely " warm " but " hot " (to the hand), at once to provoke the scratch-reflex. I conclude therefore that among the superficial nerve-endings in the skin the *nocicipient* as well as those merely of the hairs are competent to elicit the reflex, but that the " cold " and " warmth " end-organs are not competent.

Over a large area therefore *hair nerve-endings and nocicipient nerve-endings of the skin-surface* are *physiologically* distinguished from the pure " cold " and " warmth " endings and from all the deep cutaneous end-organs by the fact that the two former sets, in contradistinction to all the latter, are spinally so connected with the musculature as to induce under irritation (simulating that caused by parasites) a movement of grooming of the skin itself and of its hairy coat.[1]

Conclusion

The foregoing observations demonstrate that in the dog different kinds of nerve-endings situate in one and the same cutaneous field possess reflex spinal connections differing wholly *inter se*. For discrimination between certain sets of end-organs in the skin there are, in fact, available not only psychological criteria involving processes of sense, but data purely physiological with characteristics given in tensions of the musculature.

[1] The scratch-reflex was later subjected to a complete analysis, the results of which are reported in *J. Physiol.*, 1906, **35**, 1-50, and *Quart. J. exp. Physiol.*, 1910, **3**, 213. See also *Integrative Action of the Nervous System*, 1906.—ED.

3. ON THE CO-ORDINATION OF MUSCLES TAKING PART IN THE FLEXION-REFLEX[1]

(1) In the spinal cat and dog as in the spinal frog the reflex movement of the limb most readily evoked by stimulation of the skin of the limb or of its afferent nerves is flexion. This reflex may be termed the " flexion-reflex of the limb." In the hind-limb the flexion is of hip, knee, and ankle, in the fore-limb of elbow, shoulder, and wrist.[2]

This reflex is obtained from the decerebrate preparation as regularly as from the spinal. By the decerebrate preparation is understood one in which the whole brain in front of the posterior colliculi has been removed. The decerebrate preparation offers in some respects a better field for the examination of the reflex than does the spinal preparation. For that reason the reflex as obtained in the decerebrate preparation will be described first.

(2) It was sought to ascertain at outset which of the several muscles of the limb are actually employed in the execution of this reflex. The sample reflex taken for examination was excited from one particular afferent nerve only—namely, from the cutaneous branch of the musculo-cutaneous division of *n. peroneus*, at a point close above the annular ligament of the ankle (cat, dog). There the nerve was severed, tied, and its central stump faradised or stimulated mechanically by tightening on it a thread previously looped loosely. The experiments showed that, elicited in this way, the reflex brings into contraction certain only of the muscles of the limb. However intense the stimulation the distribution of this reflex effect did not spread in the limb musculature beyond those particular muscles. The muscles which the reflex causes to contract are the following:

TABLE I (*Cf.* Fig. 40, A, on p. 277)

Ilio-psoas.	Semitendinosus.
Pectineus (slight).	Posterior part of biceps femoris.
Sartorius, (?) the part inserted into patella.	Tenuissimus.
Tensor fasciæ femoris (weak).	Tibialis anticus.
Rectus femoris.	Peroneus longus.
Gracilis.	Extensor longus digitorum.

The extensor brevis digitorum contracts very slightly if at all.

When the reflex is elicited in the decapitate[3] preparation the same muscles contract and only those. In neither preparation does increase of the stimulus make the reflex contraction spread to limb muscles additional to the above. The threshold of stimulus for the reflex is nearly the same for all the muscles which contract.

---

[1] Extract from *J. Physiol.*, 1910, **40**, 28-35.
[2] See also *Integrative Action of the Nervous System*, 1906, p. 28.
[3] *Cf.* Sherrington, *J. Physiol.*, 1909, **38**, 375.

Thus: faradisation of central end of cutaneous branch of musculo-cutaneous division of *n. peroneus*; Berne inductorium, interruptor in primary circuit vibrating 30 p. s. resistance box of 100,000 ohms in secondary circuit.

At 8 Kronecker units contraction just obvious in tibialis anticus.
,, 10 ,, ,, ,, ,, tensor fasciæ femoris longus.
,, 10 ,, ,, ,, ,, ,, ,, ,,
,, 10 ,, ,, ,, ,, semitendinosus.
,, 14 ,, ,, ,, ,, psoas magnus.
,, 50 ,, ,, ,, very strong in tibialis anticus and semitendinosus and stronger than before in tensor fasciæ femoris and psoas, but no contraction in semimembranosus or gluteus maximus.

At 125 Kronecker units contractions as before.
,, 6,000 ,, ,, ,, ,,
Again: stimulation of central end of *n. internus saphenus* half-way up thigh.

At 15 Kronecker units contraction just obvious in gracilis.
,, 18 ,, ,, ,, ,, ,, tensor fasciæ femoris.
,, 20 ,, ,, ,, ,, ,, psoas magnus pectineus, semitendinosus and psoas parvus.

At 50 Kronecker units contraction strong in all the above muscles.
,, 150 ,, ,, ,, very strong in all the above muscles, but no trace of contraction in semimembranosus, or anterior part of biceps or gluteus maximus.

At 5,000 Kronecker units contraction same result as with 150 units.

In these observations the muscles stated as contracting or not contracting are merely those definitely prepared for observation in the particular experiment, the other limb muscles being paralysed by nerve-section or actually excised. The observations do not mean that other muscles than those specifically mentioned would not have been excited had the observations extended to them. The question of spread of reflex was tested in these observations simply on the muscles mentioned as a sample of the musculature. But a number of such experiments were made; those quoted instance the kind of result always reached.

The above list (Table I) embraces all the muscles which contract, but the reflex effect is not restricted to contraction. In certain other muscles the reflex result is relaxation of contraction. To detect this it is necessary to observe the muscle at a time when some degree of contraction is already at work for the inhibitory influence to show upon. A background of contraction against which the inhibitory relaxation can show up is generally absent in the decapitated preparation. In my experience the best chance of it is offered during the first forty minutes after decapitation. A background can, however, easily be produced at any time by faradisation of an afferent nerve of the opposite fellow-limb. This evokes reflex contraction in the required muscles, and this reflex contraction is readily seen to be inhibited by stimulation of the ipsilateral musculo-cutaneous nerve.

The necessary background of contraction is more conveniently obtained by simply using the decerebrate preparation, not the decapitate. On decerebration there ensues a tonic rigidity[1] of the limb muscles. Each relaxation of them is then easily seen and felt or recorded graphically.[2] Another way, presenting certain advantages, is to obtain a rebound

---

[1] Sherrington, *J. Physiol.*, 1898, **22**, 319.   [2] *Cf.* Fig. 1B, *Proc. roy. Soc.*, 1905, **76B**, 273.

contraction and then to reapply the original stimulus during the rebound contraction; the contraction is then seen to relax immediately under the reflex inhibition. In the flexion-reflex the muscles thus observed to relax are as follows.

TABLE II

Vastus lateralis.	Anterior part of biceps femoris.
Vastus medialis.	Flexor longus digitorum (?).
Crureus.	Quadratus femoris.
Gastrocnemius.	Adductor minor.
Soleus.	Adductor magnus (a part).
Semimembranosus (both parts).	

These muscles are the same as those observed by the other method to relax in the decapitate preparation. The muscles which contract and the muscles which relax are therefore the same in the decerebrate as in the decapitate preparation.

Increase of intensity of the stimulus does not change the inhibitory result; it merely accentuates the sharpness and extent of the relaxation; it does not cause the inhibitory effect to spread to other muscles in the limb than those mentioned above. The limits of the field of inhibition in the musculature of the limb seem as fixed as are those of the field of excitation.

Those limb muscles which the reflex excites and those which it inhibits if put together are seen not to cover all the items of musculature of the limb. Some of the muscles, the reflex does not so far as I have seen affect at all. Among these are gluteus medius, gluteus maximus, gluteus quartus, peroneus brevis, peroneus tertius, and tibialis posticus. However intense the stimulus its reflex effect does not appear to reach the motoneurones of these muscles.

(3) The reflex as thus elicited from this cutaneous nerve of the dorsum of the foot is typical of the reflex elicitable, by stimuli of like quality, from the limb generally. It can be evoked from the skin as well as from the cutaneous nerve itself, and in the former case has the same features as in the latter.

The term " *receptive field* "[1] may be conveniently applied to designate the total assemblage of receptive points whence by suitable stimuli a particular reflex movement can be evoked. Thus the scratch-reflex of the hind-limb of the spinal dog can be evoked from series of points in a saddle-shaped area of skin of the shoulder, back and loin.[2] The collective area of distribution of these points constitutes the receptive field of the scratch-reflex. For the flexion-reflex of the hind-limb the receptive field includes the skin of the whole limb as far up as the groin in front, the perineum medially and the ischial region behind. The stimuli best effective for the reflex are of mechanical, especially if nocuous, quality and electrical—

---

[1] Sherrington, *Integrative Action of the Nervous System*, 1906, p. 126.
[2] Sherrington, *Proc. Physiol. Soc.*, 1904, p. xvii (*J. Physiol.*, **31**), and *ibid.*, 1906, **34**, 1. *Cf.* also Graham Brown, *Quart. J. exp. Physiol.*, 1909, **2,** 243.

e.g., faradic. In working over the field with mechanical stimuli an impression is received that the reflex is provoked more readily from the foot than elsewhere. Electric stimuli are more easily measurable in intensity, and these substantiate the impression given by the mechanical. For electrical stimulation I used a small silver entomological pin as stigmatic electrode inserted about 2 mm. into the skin, the diffuse electrode being a wide copper plate bandaged to the shaven and well-moistened skin of one of the fore-limbs. A resistance box of 100,000 ohms was placed in the secondary circuit to minimise differences in conductivity of the skin, etc. The observations show that from the skin of the distal end of the foot, the digits and the plantar cushion the reflex is provoked by weaker faradisation than from the skin higher up the limb. The surface of the foot on the whole excites the reflex more easily than the limb surface elsewhere.

Illustrative instances from the spinal dog after thoracic transection are the following:

Situation of Electrode.	Intensity of Stimulus in Units of the Berne Coil.		
	Exp. i.	*Exp. ii.*	*Exp. iii.*
Outermost toe-pad	20	30	25
Innermost ,, ...	25	30	30
Plantar cushion	25	30	70
Between toe-pads and cushion ..	150	175	275
Outer malleolus	220	300	1,000
Close below patella	400	600	750
Half-way up front of thigh	400	600	1,000
Ischial skin	600	800	1,000
Calf	1,500	1,500	1,600

The receptive field of the skin for this reflex has so to say its focus at the free apex of the limb. This fact is of assistance in attempting to decipher the functional significance of the reflex. In that connection it will be referred to later.

From all parts of this receptive field the reflex movement as evoked by the above-mentioned stimuli presents characters so closely similar that the observer at once recognises that it constitutes a single " type-reflex."[1] That is, the individual reflexes produced from the several points of the field are all examples of one reflex which is broadly speaking the same from whatever point of the field it be provoked. This uniformity of the reflex movement excited from the various skin-points of the limb harmonises with the results of observations on the distribution of the reflex effect on the limb musculature when the reflex is elicited from the several cutaneous nerves of the limb.[2]

The results of the observations confirm the inference drawn by inspection from the actual skin-reflexes—namely, that whatever the cutaneous nerve-trunk stimulated in the limb the reflex effect is broadly the same in its

[1] *Integrative Action of the Nervous System*, 1906, p. 127.
[2] In the original paper analytical tables of the reflex effect of each of the various peripheral nerves in the limb upon each of the muscles of the limb are given here.—ED.

distribution in the limb musculature. Though broadly the same, it is not fully the same when nerve by nerve the whole series of afferent trunks are examined; differences in detail appear but are small; the general effect throughout is excitation of the motoneurones of flexors and inhibition of the motoneurones of extensors.

That is the effect as regards the skin and the skin-nerves of the limb proper. Other cutaneous nerves near to but not actually within the limb proper yield reflexes of other type. Where the limb surface abuts on regions inguinal, perineal and gluteal its afferent nerves tend to evoke reflex extension instead of limb-flexion. Their reflexes do not come within the great " flexion-reflex " of the limb.

The uniformity of the reflex effect of the various afferents of the limb extends beyond the category of the skin-afferents. It pertains to the deep afferents likewise. It is clear that the reflex effect in its distribution in the limb musculature is broadly the same for all the deep afferents examined. Also that the reflex effect of these afferents is practically the same as that of the skin-afferents and the skin itself. The receptive field of the flexion-reflex of the limb is therefore not merely an area of surface, a skin-field, but is musculo-articular as well and includes the whole thickness of the limb as well as its surface. In this respect the receptive field of the flexion-reflex differs fundamentally from a receptive field such as that of the scratch-reflex, which is wholly cutaneous.

It is not surprising, therefore, to find that when the various large afferent nerve-trunks of the limb are themselves examined in regard to the reflex effect they each evoke, the effect found for all of them is flexion, and that the reflex given by each of them is practically the same. In these large nerve-trunks the afferent fibres are of course mixed in origin, cutaneous, fascial, muscular, articular, etc. Yet when the mingled collection of each trunk is thus stimulated the reflex result is regular and harmonious; it is always, in fact, the flexion-reflex.

(4) This makes clear how it is that when the afferent spinal roots themselves are stimulated each root of the whole series belonging to the limb evokes in the limb simply the same reflex movement; and how it is that that movement is flexion.

Whichever of the roots is stimulated the movement obtained in the limb is flexion at its larger joints. Flexion of ankle is less marked with the more anterior of the roots of the series and flexion at hip less marked with the most posterior, but a general flexion of the limb is the reflex result from each root. The heterogeneity of the afferent fibre constitution of each of these large roots is very great. The uniform result which they regularly produce in their reflex effect becomes, however, intelligible in light of the flexion-reflex being practically the one reflex obtained by direct stimulation (mechanical and electrical) of each and all the afferent nerves of the limb.

(5) Taken together the results of examination of various afferent nerves can be summarised in the following condensed statements.

The afferent nerves of the limb—apart from n. lumbo-inguinalis (genito-crural), n. cutaneus clunis, and n. pudendus inferior, which are from groin, perineum, and buttock rather than from limb proper—all excite a limb reflex of the same type characterised by flexion at hip, knee, and ankle.   This reflex may be called the *flexion-reflex of the limb*, understanding by that a type-reflex[1] —*i.e.*, a group of reflexes of almost identical form which when concurrent combine in harmonious action on the same final common paths.

Though the individual reflex obtainable from any one of the various afferents of the limb conforms fully to this type-reflex, and is a " flexion-reflex," it is not necessarily wholly like that produced from some among the other afferents of the limb which also provoke the flexion-reflex.   That is, the individual reflexes as provoked from nerve to nerve differ one from another to some extent though all conform to the type " flexion-reflex." The differences consist chiefly in the reflex contraction excited by one nerve extending less to certain muscles of the flexor group than it does when excited from some other nerve.   The contraction in all cases is limited to the flexor group, but each afferent does not in all cases cause contraction of the entire group, and the muscles omitted are not entirely the same for one nerve as for another.   Differences in detail of effect are thus detectable between different afferent nerves.   Thus, semitendinosus contracts more powerfully in reflex response to the cutaneous foot nerves than to branches of external cutaneous or internal saphenous nerves; tensor fasciæ femoris contracts little or not at all from the plantar nerves but strongly from internal saphenous or external cutaneous.   Such differences seem to reach their maximum in the divergence between external cutaneous and hamstring nerve.   The former causes reflex contraction in tensor fasciæ femoris, pectineus, rectus femoris, and gluteus minimus, and these muscles the latter nerve does not reflexly reach; and the latter nerve causes contraction in tenuissimus and biceps femoris' posterior part while the former nerve does not; both, however, alike cause contraction of psoas, sartorius, tibialis anticus and semitendinosus.   The difference between the segmental origins of n. cutaneus externus and hamstring nerve is greater than between almost any other of the limb nerves.   Similarly skin-points whose nerve-supplies lie segmentally distant one from another tend to exhibit flexion-reflexes less closely similar than do skin-points segmentally near together.   Thus there comes to be some accentuation of movement at this joint or that according as the skin-point stimulated lies in this limb-region or that.   Excitation of outer edge of planta (spinal monkey) causes together with the flexion at ankle some eversion of foot; but excitation of inner edge of planta gives some inversion of foot along with the ankle flexion.[2]

---

[1] See *Integrative Action of the Nervous System*, 1906, p. 127.

[2] " This influence of the location of the stimulus upon the character of the movement . . . furnishes a large part of the direct evidence of the so-called ' purposive ' character of spinal reflexes. The physiological study of reflexes must be objective, and from this point of view it is preferable perhaps to adopt the expression ' local sign ' . . . to denote a quality in virtue of which the character of the resulting movement is partly determined by the spatial position of the reflexo-

Apart from these differences in detail the reflex provocable from the limb is the same reflex from whatsoever part of the limb it is produced (by the stimuli mentioned above). The whole limb, therefore, except for some part of its attached base, forms one receptive field whence the reflex provocable is the flexion-reflex, and this field is not merely skin-deep but includes muscles, joints, fasciæ, and other deep structures of the limb.

[1]Analysis of the muscular effect of the flexion-reflex shows this reaction to exhibit certain features in its co-ordinate handling of the musculature. Co-ordination is a wide term and embraces the management of muscles both in their simultaneous and successive employment. The simultaneous co-ordination of muscles in a reflex effect is conveniently spoken of as the " reflex-figure."[2] The form assumed by the reflex figure in the case of the flexion-reflex of the hind-limb exhibits the following features.

The reflex does not in many cases treat as entities muscles regarded as such by anatomical nomenclature. Thus the reflex throws into contraction that part of biceps femoris—i.e., posterior part—which is inserted below the knee while it inhibits that part—i.e., anterior part—which is inserted above knee. The latter portion is an extensor of hip, the former flexes knee. Again, the reflex in dealing with quadriceps extensor causes that part which flexes hip (rectus femoris) to contract while it inhibits that part (vastocrureus) which extends knee.[3] Similarly in fore-limb, the flexion-reflex inhibits the humeral heads of triceps and at the same time excites to contraction the scapular head: this last is a flexor at shoulder, the former are extensors of elbow. Again, in the sartorius its medial band and the upper part of its lateral band contract in the reflex, but the lower part of the lateral band does not appear to contract. This latter part tends to extend knee, the rest of the muscle flexes knee and hip. In regard to quadriceps extensor cruris and triceps brachii the taxis shown in the reflex is similar to that observed by H. Hering and myself[4] under cortical stimulation; we did not particularly examine the other muscles here mentioned.

Those muscles which the reflex excites to contract and those which by inhibition it relaxes or restrains from contraction form two functional groups broadly describable as flexor and extensor respectively. Thus there are excited by the reflex, psoas magnus, sartorius, gluteus minimus,

---

genous area whence initiated. In the spinal dog (cervical transection) the hind-foot is with fair accuracy brought to scratch the spot on the shoulder under irritation, although that spot lie behind the spinal lesion. The centripetal impulses from the spot—although they can yield no sensation—possess, therefore, in the above sense ' local sign' " (Sherrington, in Schäfer's *Textbook of Physiology*, 1900, **2**, 832). The variations in the flexion-reflex here described show the effect of local sign in the afferent stimulus in modifying the withdrawal of the limb in a purposive manner.—ED.

[1] Extract from *J. Physiol.*, 1910, **40**, 45-49.

[2] *Integrative Action of the Nervous System*, 1906, p. 161.

[3] *Cf.* for independence of rectus from rest of quadriceps in man, Beevor, *Ergebn. d. Physiolog.*, Jahrg. 8, 1909.   [4] *Proc. roy. Soc.*, 1897, **62**, 183 (p. 259 this volume).

tensor fasciæ femoris and rectus femoris, flexors at hip; and inhibited are semimembranosus, biceps femoris, adductor minor, and quadratus femoris, extensors of hip. Excited are semitendinosus, biceps femoris posterior, sartorius,[1] and gracilis, flexors at knee; inhibited are vastus medialis, vastus lateralis and crureus, extensors at knee. Excited are tibialis anticus and extensor longus digitorum, flexors at ankle; inhibited are gastrocnemius, plantaris and soleus, extensors at ankle. It is clear that reciprocal innervation of antagonistic muscles is a principle observed in the nervous taxis of the reflex. The reflex application of the principle seems especially to muscular antagonism such that were both muscles to contract at the same time the main action of one muscle would impede the main action of the other.

But among the " flexor " group excited by the reflex to contract are semitendinosus, biceps femoris posterior, and gracilis, muscles which though flexors of knee are extensors of hip. These are therefore to some extent antagonists of the hip flexors, yet the reflex throws them into contraction along with the hip flexors. Their possible extension-effect at hip is completely prevented during the reflex by the concomitant contraction of the hip flexors. This is a case comparable with the well-known concomitance of contraction of the long flexor of the fingers and the extensors of the wrist. In the execution of the grasp contraction of the extensors of the wrist accompanies contraction of flexor longus digitorum (Duchenne,[2] H. E. Hering,[3] Beevor[4]). This latter muscle besides flexing fingers flexes wrist; but its action at wrist is prevented by concurrent contraction of extensors of wrist. The action of flexor longus digitorum is less at wrist than fingers; its effect, therefore, which is suppressed by an antagonist, is its subsidiary one; and that suppression increases its other and main effect —namely, flexion of fingers. So also with semitendinosus, biceps femoris posterior, and gracilis. Their main effect is flexion at knee, their subsidiary extension at hip. The suppression of this latter by the hip-flexors enhances the main effect, flexion at knee. And it was experimentally shown that in the actual reflex the contraction of merely one of the hip flexors—*i.e.*, sartorius—is perfectly able to produce this suppression, and thus while flexing hip and knee by its own direct action indirectly reinforces that action on knee by means of its pseudo-antagonists biceps femoris posterior and semitendinosus.

Again, extensor longus digitorum is by virtue of its femoral tendon a slight extensor of knee as well as a flexor of ankle and extensor of toes. By concurrent contraction of the great knee flexors the reflex prevents

---

[1] Sartorius evidently by its reflex contraction along with biceps femoris posterior and semitendinosus suppresses their action at hip and enhances their action at knee—*i.e.*, these pseudo-antagonists under identical innervation act harmoniously and with mutual advantage as flexors although two of them are as judged by their attachments extensors at hip.

[2] *Physiologie des Mouvements*, p. 154, Paris, 1867.

[3] *Pflüg. Arch. ges. Physiol.*, 1898, **70**, 559.

[4] Beevor, Croonian Lectures, *Roy. Coll. of Physicians*, London, 1904, p. 11.

extensor longus digitorum from extending knee, and by flexing knee in its despite enhances its action as an ankle-flexor and toe-extensor.

Similarly with the lateral band of sartorius. This band flexes hip but tends to extend knee. The reflex by concurrent contraction of the strong knee flexors prevents the band from extending knee and turns its whole power into flexing hip.

These cases may be summarised thus. A muscle A acts at a joint a and with less ample effect at another joint b; a muscle B opposes A's action at b but by doing so exalts it at a. The co-ordinative relation observed between the two in neural taxis employing both is not reciprocal innervation—the one is not inhibited when the other is excited, but both are excited together or inhibited together. In other words the taxis treats the two muscles not as antagonists but as adjuvants. And this holds whether A's action at the two joints is in similar sense—e.g., flexor longus digitorum at fingers and wrist—or in opposite senses—e.g., semitendinosus flexing at knee, extending at hip.

It is evident that the reflex uses certain muscles as protagonists (Winslow's[1] " principal movers," Beevor's[2] " prime movers ") and certain as fixators (Beevor's[3] " synergics," H. E. Hering's[4] pseudo-antagonists) and that it commonly employs at one and the same time one and the same muscle in both these capacities. Thus it uses the hip-flexors not only to flex hip but at the same time to serve as fixation muscles for knee-flexors which would extend hip were the hip not kept from extending. Similarly the reflex employs semitendinosus, biceps femoris posterior, and gracilis as protagonists to flex knee and at the same time also as fixation muscles for certain flexors of hip—namely, rectus femoris and lateral band of sartorius—which were the knee not kept flexed would extend it and thereby lose part of their efficiency for flexing hip. In these actions the reflex employs flexors which are prime movers of a joint as fixation muscles at that joint for flexors which act as prime movers at another joint. In the reflex taxis, therefore, flexors are used as fixators for flexors.

The concurrent contraction of flexors with flexors so that prime movers serve also as fixators is an extension of a principle well shown by the musculature of the frog's hind-limb and there studied particularly by Lombard and Abbott.[5] Flexors of one joint even when the flexors of other joints of the limb are inactive flex those other joints as well as their own. Thus in Lombard's model the frog's hip flexor when it flexes that joint flexes also knee and ankle. This results from the mere mechanical attachments of the knee and ankle flexors. Similarly in cat and dog contraction of tibialis anticus or extensor longus digitorum not only flexes ankle but flexes knee, in virtue of the attachments of gastrocnemius. By flexing ankle it draws down the heel so that the gastrocnemius even when toneless and paralysed by nerve-section flexes the knee in virtue of its upper insertion at femur.

[1] Structure of the Human Body, Douglas' transl., 4th ed., 1756, 1, Sect. iii, p. 159.
[2] Loc. cit., 1904, p. 71.   [3] Ibid.   [4] Z. Heilkunde, 1895, 16.   [5] Amer. J. Physiol., 1907, 20, 1.

So again in cat and dog contraction of a hip-flexor produces in consequence of the attachments of semitendinosus and biceps femoris posterior flexion of knee even when these muscles have been paralysed by nerve-section. Now, in the actual reflex these muscles enter into contraction along with the hip-flexors; the taxis of the reflex therefore uses and extends the principle indicated in the mere non-contractile mechanics of the part.[1]

The details of the participation of the adductor group in the flexion-reflex I have found difficult to observe. Pectineus contracts, adductor minor undergoes inhibitory relaxation. My observations suggest that those parts of the adductor mass which flex hip as well as adduct contract in the reflex, and those parts which would extend hip as well as adduct do not contract and in part at least are relaxed by inhibition. The circumstance pointed out by Lombard[2] in his study of the frog's hip muscles that some lateral muscles—e.g., adductors, abductors—flex when the limb is in one position and extend when it is in another has to be reckoned with and perhaps introduces lack of apparent uniformity in the reflex results.

On certain muscles of the limb the reflex exerts, so far as my observations go, no influence either of excitation or inhibition. These muscles are gluteus maximus, gluteus medius, gluteus quartus, tibialis posticus, peroneus brevis, and peroneus tertius.

The reflex evoked by the deep afferents of the limb presents no obvious difference from that evoked by the cutaneous. Head, Rivers, and Sherren[3] have shown that deep afferents (of forearm) evoke sensations broadly resembling the tactual evoked from the overlying skin. The deep afferents furnish a sort of " deep " touch with qualities differing from and yet entirely harmonious and complemental with the sensations of superjacent skin. Along with this conformity between the surface and deep sensual reactions there coexists a conformity between the surface and deep reflexes. The adequate stimulus for the deep afferents appears to be mechanical in kind; its source lies in movements active and passive of the limb, itself producing changes in shape and tension of muscles, etc. In other words the deep afferents belong to the " proprioceptive " system. The relation in which their stimuli stand to stimuli given by the environment is a secondary one. The secondary character of the relationship argues that the reactions evoked by the deep afferents will be auxiliary and adjuvant to those evoked by the afferents of the surface. Experimental observation supports this argument, and one item of the support is the just mentioned similarity of reflex effect yielded by deep and surface afferents respectively.[4]

[1] For further analysis of the reflex effect of muscles with action at two joints the reader is referred to the original paper.—ED.

[2] *Loc. cit.*   [3] *Brain*, 1905, **28**, 99.

[4] The electrical and mechanical stimulation of the deep nerves used in this analysis would not discriminate between afferent fibres from nociceptors and those from stretch receptors. The latter are the more selective and variable in their effect (see below and Chapter VIII). The deep nociceptive field appears to be prepotent in its reflex effect of flexion of the limb.—ED.

From observations such as those given above on p. 164 it appears that the difference between a flexion-reflex that is stronger—*e.g.*, owing to more intense reflex stimulus—and one that is weaker (its stimulus being weaker) does not lie in the latter's employing few muscles the former many. Both employ approximately, probably exactly, the same muscles, but the contraction of each muscle is in the stronger reflex stronger, in the weaker reflex weaker.

Although the afferent nerves from the large area which forms almost the whole surface of the limb yield as their reflex effect pure flexion of the limb, a few afferents belonging to the attached base of the limb excite, instead of flexion, extension of the knee. Among these afferents are n. lumbo inguinalis (spermaticus externus), n. cutaneus femoris posterior, a small branch from 3rd lumbar to skin of groin, and certain perineal nerve-branches.

(i) *N. lumbo inguinalis (spermaticus externus, genito-crural)*. From this nerve the reflex obtainable as regards contralateral knee is always contraction of the extensors; on the ipsilateral knee the effect is sometimes contraction, sometimes relaxation. Examination of the reflex in fourteen individuals yielded contraction of the ipsilateral knee-extensor in all, but complicated in two individuals by occasional replacement of the contraction by distinct inhibitory relaxation. The inhibitory relaxation seemed favoured by faradic stimulation instead of mechanical. Among the afferent fibres of the nerve some therefore excite reflex extension of ipsilateral knee and others excite flexion of it. This holds of both the inguinal and the spermatic branches of the nerve. The field of distribution of the nerve includes the inguinal mamma and a pad of fat covering the medial part of the groin. Manipulation of the groin of the spinal dog not unfrequently evokes reflex extension of the ipsilateral knee. The extension which the nerve provokes may be movement unflexing the limb to allow the young better access to the inguinal mammilla, as in suckling. The reflex effect of the nerve is, however, in my experience the same in the male as in the female. The sense of the movement is compatible with a sexual significance. Beck and Bikeles[1] have recently reported a somewhat similar reflex movement elicitable in the spinal dog by stimulation of the skin of the scrotum.

(ii) The small branch from the 3rd lumbar nerve to the skin of the groin enters that region between the external cutaneus and the spermaticus externus. It causes reflex contraction of the ipsilateral vastocrureus muscle extending the knee.

(iii) *Ischial and perineal nerves*. From the skin over tuber ischii and from that of the perineum broad touches excite extension of the ipsilateral knee as well as of the contralateral. The vasti and crurei of both limbs are seen to contract. The crossed reflex is the more powerful and the root of the tail is deflected toward the crossed side. N. cutaneus femoris posterior bared, severed, and proximally stimulated mechanically by ligation yields usually

[1] *Pflüg. Arch. ges. Physiol.*, 1909, **129**, 416.

a similar reflex result; so also do the afferent nerves of the perineal skin. Yet this result is not regular in regard to the contraction of ipsilateral knee-extensor, sometimes the contraction is replaced by inhibitory relaxation. Similarly the ischial and perineal skin sometimes yields flexion instead of extension of ipsilateral knee.   Flexion is the result when the skin is pinched or pricked: extension when merely touched or stroked.   Ischial skin, therefore, resembles plantar in so far that it yields reflex extension of ipsilateral limb when stimulated by harmless pressure, but yields flexion in response to stimuli whose character is hurtful.   The irregularity of result from the ischial nerve-trunks may mean that it contains afferents some of which excite ipsilateral extension, others ipsilateral flexion.   Faradisation seems more effective for the latter, mechanical stimuli for the former.

Apart from the usual but not invariable extension elicited by these afferents of perineal skin, buttock and groin, and apart from the extensor thrust elicited by broad pressure on the planta, the reflex elicited from the limb is uniformly flexion—the flexion-reflex.   It has to be remembered, however, in thus summarising the above observations that in them the excitation of the deep afferents was unavoidably very artificial in character —namely, by faradism or gross mechanical stimuli.

4. REFLEX MOVEMENTS ACCESSORY TO THE FLEXION-REFLEX THE REFLEX OF CROSSED EXTENSION[1]

The stimulus which evokes the flexion-reflex in the stimulated limb commonly evokes at the same time certain reflex movements elsewhere. In the fellow-limb of the crossed side the movement is almost invariably extension.   In the other pair of limbs it usually provokes extension and retraction of the homonymous limb and flexion with protraction of the crossed limb.   Thus, when the seat of stimulation is a hind-limb the reflex effect is extension at knee, hip, and ankle of the crossed hind-limb; extension at elbow, shoulder, and wrist of the ipsilateral fore-limb with retraction; flexion at elbow, shoulder, and wrist of the crossed fore-limb with protraction. When the stimulus is applied to a fore-limb the flexion-reflex in that limb itself and in the other limbs extension of elbow, shoulder, and wrist of the crossed fore-limb, extension at hip, elbow, and ankle in the ipsilateral hind-limb and flexion at knee, hip, and ankle in the crossed hind-limb.[2]

These reflexes are accessory to the flexion-reflex rather than parts with it of one integral reflex.   Though often linked with it they are separable from it.   The flexion-reflex of the stimulated limb itself is of such constancy that given the stimulus the ensuing flexion is a matter of practical certainty. But the reflex results extending to the other limbs are not so.   The most constant of them is the crossed extension in the contralateral fellow-limb. The least constant is in my experience the flexion of the limb diagonal to the limb stimulated.   Here the effect is usually flexion, but is not rarely

[1] Extract from *J. Physiol.*, 1910, **40**, 55-57.   [2] See Fig. 51, p. 324, this volume.

extension. The effect does not oscillate from one form to the other in the course of any one experiment; but in some experiments it is flexion, in others extension. Occasionally in the course of the same experiment it suddenly changes from flexion to extension, but I have not seen it then change back again. When reflex extension replaces the more usual flexion, the total result of the reflex is extension of all the limbs outside the stimulated limb itself. This variability of the accessory reflexes separates them from the reflex of the stimulated limb itself. Even the crossed extension-reflex of the twin limb has a variability which indicates that it is adjunct to rather than part and parcel of the reflex of the stimulated limb itself. The threshold stimulus for the crossed extension-reflex may differ considerably from that of the ipsilateral flexion-reflex itself; often it is practically the same for both, but often that of the crossed reflex is markedly the higher. In some instances the crossed reflex is unobtainable though the ipsilateral is obtained readily. The crossed reflex is clearly separable from though usually adjunct to the ipsilateral flexion-reflex. Ether and chloroform narcosis also commonly dissociates these reflexes by suppressing crossed extension-reflex earlier and longer than ipsilateral flexion-reflex. So also does spinal shock.

Crossed Extension-Reflex

(i) So commonly is the crossed extension-reflex an accompaniment of the ipsilateral flexion that serial analysis of its muscular composition does not involve great expenditure of material. The limb muscles which contract in it are found to be the following (Fig. 40, B, p. 277, shows these muscles by the broken lines and numerals):

vastus medialis,	quadratus femoris,
vastus lateralis,	gastrocnemius,
crureus,	soleus,
adductor minor,	semimembranosus,
adductor major (a part),	anterior biceps femoris,
sartorius (part inserted into patella),	flexor longus digitorum (late).

On the other hand certain muscles relax in it. Amongst these are:

semitendinosus,	sartorius medial band,
biceps femoris posterior,	sartorius lateral band in proximal part.
tibialis anticus,	

Probably the other flexors relax also, but only those observed by actual isolation are entered on this list. In the fore-limb the reflex excites contraction in supra-spinatus and humeral heads of triceps, and relaxes by inhibition brachialis anticus. Other muscles as well are excited and inhibited in fore-limb, but those actually observed by isolation are the above.

(ii) In its handling of the limb musculature this reflex exhibits the same principles of simultaneous co-ordination noted above in the flexion reflex. It illustrates them further. Muscles regarded as units by anatomical nomenclature—e.g., biceps femoris, triceps brachii, quadriceps extensor—

are not so treated by the reflex. The reflex handles each of these as compounded of antagonistic parts; in each it inhibits and restrains the contraction of one part while it excites that of the other.

As in the flexion-reflex so in this extension-reflex muscles which are antagonistic, in the sense that one as a prime mover would oppose the other as a prime mover, are dealt with by reciprocal innervation. But in this reflex all of the muscles which are excited to contract are muscles which in the flexion-reflex are inhibited and restrained from contraction. Conversely in this extension-reflex the muscles inhibited are those which in the flexion-reflex contract. Reciprocal innervation though exercised in this reflex equally with the flexion-reflex is exercised in exactly the reverse direction.

This reflex like the flexion-reflex employs at one and the same joint one and the same muscle both as prime mover of the joint and fixator of the joint for muscles which are prime movers at other joints. Thus it employs vastocrureus to extend knee and gastrocnemius to extend ankle: but gastrocnemius of itself would flex knee as well as extend ankle; its former action is prevented by the concurrent contraction of vastocrureus and this the reflex provides. And by prevention of the knee flexion the action of gastrocnemius as an extensor of ankle is enhanced. Again, the lateral band of sartorius at its distal end contracts in this reflex. It is an extensor of knee but also a flexor of hip. Experiment shows that when all other muscles of hip and knee are paralysed including medial band of sartorius itself the lateral band as excited by the crossed extension reflex does actually flex hip as well as extend knee. But in the crossed reflex when the other hip muscles are intact concurrent contractions of the extensors of hip prevent the hip flexion and the whole power of the lateral sartorius so far as excited in the reflex is devoted to extending knee. In the flexion-reflex flexors at one joint act as fixators for flexors at the next joint. In the extension reflex extensors at one joint act as fixators for extensors at the next joint. In the extension-reflex, as in the flexion-reflex, where muscle A acts at joints a and b, and muscle B opposes A's action at b but by so doing exalts it at a, the neural taxis does not treat A and B by reciprocal innervation: it excites them together or inhibits them together; it treats them not as antagonistic but as adjuvant each to the other.

5. THE NOCICEPTIVE FLEXION-REFLEX[1]

The flexion-reflex is elicitable from the skin of the limb and with especial facility from the skin of the foot. The stimuli especially effective are of nocuous quality. The flexion-movement provoked lifts and withdraws the foot. If the stimulus be continued the reflex holds the limb even for minutes at a time flexed under the body as though out of harm's way. If the stimulus be strong and the reflex condition brisk the first flexion which results may be quickly followed by a brief active extension as if to shake

[1] Extract from *J. Physiol.*, 1910, **40**, 71-85.

off the irritation.[1] This secondary extension is always short and followed by immediate return to flexion, this latter occasionally to be broken by a brief extension and the manœuvre repeated a few times before unbroken flexion ensues. This result occurs even when a small spring clip affixed to the foot is used as stimulus, and when therefore the mechanical stimulus is constant. It is of interest as showing the reflex in the form of alternating flexion and extension although the alternation is irregular, repeated only a few times and then subsides into steady flexion. The more usual form of the reflex is maintained flexion unbroken by active extension even from the first. The description given is for the hind-limb (cat) but applies to the fore-limb also; there also not unfrequently the flexion is broken at first by a few brief irregular extensions especially at elbow.

Under these stimuli and in these forms the flexion-reflex is evidently protective. It is often accompanied by stepping of the crossed hind-limb and, though less commonly, of the other limbs as well, but not of the limb itself stimulated. The irritated foot is withdrawn from harm and the other legs run away. The protective reflex is associated with a flight-reflex. The dog kept under observation by Goltz subsequent to ablation almost entire of both cerebral hemispheres was noted after incidental injury to one hind-foot to keep the injured foot off the ground and run on three legs. Goltz's interpretation of that " behaviour " as largely reflex is borne out by the above-mentioned less complete yet broadly analogous reaction in

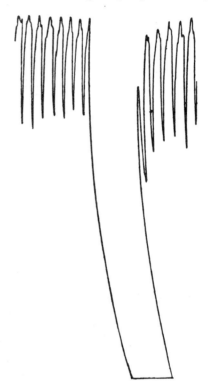

FIG. 23.—REFLEX STEPPING OF HIND-LIMB INTERRUPTED BY A NOCICEPTIVE STIMULUS TO SKIN OF FOOT EVOKING A NOCICEPTIVE FLEXION-REFLEX

Decapitate preparation (cat); descent of lever= flexion

the decapitate preparation (cat). The decerebrate rabbit shows a similar reaction, except that in the rabbit while the stimulated limb is kept flexed the other three legs show the hopping movement more usual to the natural progression of that animal. In the decerebrate preparation (cat) the reaction shows, in addition to the limb movements, a turning sideways and backward of the head, an opening of the mouth, retraction of the lips, and occasionally vocalisation. The significance of this pseudo-affective reflex is clearly

[1] Cf. in the donkey, Chauveau, Brain, 1891, **14**, 173.

related to the nocuous quality of the stimulus.   There is a reflex combination of movements of protection signifying both flight and preparation for defence.

This reflex is elicitable from all points of a large area of the limb surface and also though less easily from the deep structures as well.   But from the deep structures of the limb certain stimuli which are not nocuous can evoke reflex flexion.   This latter reflex flexion is not a movement of withdrawal of the limb out of harm's way but is the flexion phase of the alternating reflex act of stepping.   The above-described maintained flexion-reflex excited by nocuous stimuli applied to the limb itself is therefore not the only form of flexion-reflex exhibited by the limb.   And its sub-variety mentioned above as showing some brief and irregular discontinuity in the flexion is of interest as indicating a transitional form toward the rhythmic flexion-reflex of the step.   But the nociceptive flexion-reflex of the limb and the rhythmic locomotor flexion-reflex of the limb are, as is obvious from their significance to the individual reactions, mutually incompatible.   Hence the nociceptive flexion-reflex can interfere with, break through and interrupt the rhythmic locomotor flexion-reflex (Fig. 23).   The peculiar character, in fact the " adequacy," of its stimulus lies in intensity.[1]   It is prepotent when pitted against the locomotor reflex: and this is a further mark of its nociceptive character, since nociceptive reflexes like painful sensations are habitually " dominant " in competition against others.

6. SPINAL STEPPING

From the decapitated preparation (cat) reflex stepping of the limb can be readily evoked.   As to the reflex being really that of stepping there is no doubt, and other facts known of stepping as a reflex act make it not surprising that the decapitate preparation should exhibit it.   After spinal transection in the thoracic region when the period of shock is passed the hind-limbs of the dog execute stepping movements strikingly complete.   Photographic kinetoscope analysis of the outward character of these movements establishes the fidelity of their resemblance to those of the natural step (Philippson).[2]   Usually the spinal stepping is that of walk or trot, sometimes it is that of the gallop (Philippson).[3]   Occasionally the decapitate cat also shows the gallop; the decapitate rabbit does so more frequently.

The ordinary stepping movement of hind-limb may be briefly described as exhibiting two phases.   In one the limb suspended from pelvis is brought forward above the ground to a new point of support in front of that which it last used.   In this phase the limb carries its own weight only, and even for that, conditions non-vital — e.g., atmospheric pressure on hip-joint (Weber)—largely obviate the strain from falling upon muscle.   Then follows a phase in which, while the foot presses on the ground, the limb is extended,

---

[1] *Integrative Action oj Nervous System*, 1906, p. 231.
[2] *Trav. Lab. Physiol., Instituts Solvay, Bruxelles*, 1905, **7**, 2, 5.   [3] *Ibid.*

carrying its own weight and a share of the superincumbent body weight, and finally aids the advance of the body by a propulsive thrust from the ground. Thus the stepping in each limb is a rhythmic movement of alternating flexion and extension. The salient features of this movement in the walk and trot (cat, dog) may be summarised thus.[1]

(i) Flexion phase, during which the anterior angle between thigh and ilio-ischial[2] line continually decreases owing to flexion at hip. During the earlier two-thirds of this phase flexion at knee and ankle proceeds along with the hip-flexion. In the latest third the angles at knee and ankle begin to open. During part of this phase the toes are somewhat spread and extended (dorsal flexion) on metatarsus. During the whole of this phase the foot is off the ground.

(ii) Extension phase, during which the anterior angle between thigh and ilio-ischial line gradually opens, and the angles at knee and ankle also open (except for a transient yield under the weight of the body in the earliest third of the phase). During this phase, except at its extreme end, the foot is on the ground; at the extreme end of the phase, after the foot leaves the ground, the toes are adducted together and plantar-flexed on metatarsus.

(iii) At end of flexion phase there is an anterior turning point when hip flexing changes to hip extending. At end of extension phase there is a posterior turning point when extension of limb changes to flexion.

(iv) Synchronism of extension phase in one limb with flexion phase in opposite fellow-limb; in other words, synchronism of anterior turning point of one limb with posterior turning point of the other.

These main features of the normal step of the hind-limb characterise also the reflex stepping of the limb in the spinal preparation. They are main items calling for examination in the analysis of the neural taxis of the reflex step.

Stimuli for Stepping-Reflex

Remote.—Among the stimulations which excite stepping movement of the limb in the decapitate preparation are certain of cutaneous application and nociceptive character. The most effective *loci* for these are as follows: perineum especially at scrotum or near vulva; a foot, not that of the limb itself exhibiting the stepping movement; neck or back, tail, and pinna when this has been preserved in performing the decapitation. The stimulus may be simply rubbing or squeezing the skin, or the affixing to it of a small clip, or the faradisation or ligation of an exposed nerve. Although cutaneous stimulation of that limb which itself exhibits the stepping is not provocative of the reflex in that limb during the stimulation, on the cessation of the stimulus reflex stepping of that limb may follow. And occasionally stimulation of the skin of the limb near its base excites stepping in it. The

---

[1] *Cf.* the kinematograms from Prof. Marey's Station physiologique, Paris, published in Philippson's paper, *op. cit.*, 1905.   [2] Defined in original paper, p. 42.

stepping evoked by stimulation of perineum or of pubic skin just in front of vulva is always bipedal. It might be thought that this stepping is bipedal because stimuli applied to the mid line of body may excite both right and left nerve-afferents together at their overlap in mid-ventral line. But the reflex is still bipedal when the stimulus is shifted well to one side of the mid line, and also when the afferent nerves of one side have been severed. Under these latter circumstances the reflex stepping begins with flexion in ipsilateral limb and with extension in contralateral. In all cases the stepping of the two limbs is synchronous in tempo and of opposite phase in right and left limbs.

But stimuli to the skin of the limb itself elsewhere than at its extreme base excite unipedal stepping of the crossed limb and in the stimulated limb itself the maintained flexion reflex, and when the limb is already stepping a stimulus to its own skin actually stops the stepping, replacing it by maintained flexion (the nociceptive reflex) (Fig. 23). The cutaneous nociceptive stimuli which excite stepping are as regards their seat of application " remote "—*i.e.*, situate outside the limb itself. And in their case the significance of the reflex stepping is clearly protective, the protective act being flight.

Intrinsic.—But other stimuli which are non-nocuous and have their seat in the limb itself can evoke reflex stepping of the limb. And, in fact, in using the spinal limb itself for starting and controlling its stepping the observer has recourse not to skin stimuli but to passive movements. A sure way of eliciting the reflex stepping of the spinal hind-limbs (dog, " late spinal " preparation) is the lifting of the animal from the ground with spine vertical and hind-limbs pendent. The reflex stepping immediately sets in and continues for long periods at a time. This manœuvre evokes the reflex even so soon as a couple of weeks after thoracic spinal transection. Later when the reflex is better developed it occurs with spine horizontal as well as with spine vertical. Extension at both hips is a condition favouring the reflex and the passive hip-extension is greater with spine vertical. With spine vertical when one limb—*e.g.*, right—hangs freely under its own weight and the other, left, is supported by the observer's finger with hip semi-flexed, both limbs usually remain quiet and there is no stepping. On then removing the support and allowing the left thigh to drop into passive extension a transient active extension seems to ensue with the falling of the limb, and on the limb's reaching its fuller extension there follows an active flexion at hip, knee, and ankle. This is succeeded by extension partially active, to be followed again by active flexion, and so on. Thus the stepping-reflex commences and proceeds. But it is at once arrested by passively supporting one thigh in semiflexion.

The reflex stepping thus proprioceptively excited is bilateral. At the first dropping of the limb (left) reflex flexion sets in in the opposite hip; and this occurs so immediately that the left limb has not nearly reached its full extension when active flexion is obvious at the right hip. And when the left limb after its extension flexes, right limb having completed its flexion extends. The reflex is therefore bilateral with opposite phase in the opposite limbs.

In this experiment the passive extension of hip and knee under the limb's own weight evidently provides the stimulus. Passive extension of ankle or knee alone or together but without hip does not suffice to start the stepping, although frequently exciting extension of contralateral knee without hip. Passive full extension of one hip alone, knee and ankle being even flexed, evokes reflex extension of opposite hip and limb. Stretching psoas muscle in the decerebrate preparation sometimes evokes extension of crossed knee. The inference is that in starting the reflex stepping by allowing one limb to drop under its own weight the stimulus is mainly due to extension of hip.

Evidently passive movements of the limb can excite from it its reflex step or at least can initiate that reflex. And the reflex when once started either by a passive movement or by one of the remote skin stimuli above mentioned shows like the scratch-reflex a tendency to continue, as if the movement of the stepping or scratching limb constituted to some extent an intrinsic stimulus in the limb itself further promoting and maintaining the reflex. Reinforcements of action in this way is not uncommon in complex reflex acts. Thus in the scratch-reflex the neck stimulus not only causes a flexion of ipsilateral hip but a turning of neck to ipsilateral side, and this turning of neck itself excites reflex-flexion of ipsilateral hip. Local proprioceptive stimulation as a factor in the reflex is further shown by the prompt arrest of the reflex by gentle restraint applied to the moving limb itself.

What are the receptors in the limb which movements of the limb excite ? The limb receptors belong to the two categories, exteroceptive and proprioceptive. The former are broadly speaking those of the skin, the latter belong broadly speaking to musculo-articular and deep fascial structures.

It might have been supposed that the main stimulus for the reflex step would arise in the planta from contact with the ground. Facts argue, however, against this somewhat natural suggestion.

A light harmless stimulus, a touch, on the planta does it is true evoke in the spinal hind-limb a lifting and slight spreading of the toes and slight dorso-flexion of ankle. But this movement of the toes and ankle is often a conspicuous feature of the reflex step when the dog is supported free from the ground with the reflex stepping of the spinal hind-limbs taking place in the air. Moreover, in the intact animal (cat, dog), severance of all the nerve-trunks directly distributed to all four of the feet up to and above the wrists and ankles impairs walking so little as to make it highly unlikely that the loss of receptivity of the feet destroys any large factor in the reflex basis of these acts.[1]

[1] These animals were demonstrated to the Physiological Society, 1910, walking accurately on a ladder laid horizontally.—ED.

For the denervation of the feet the following nerves have been severed: in hind-limb the anterior and posterior tibials, musculo-cutaneous and external saphenous about 5 cm. above ankle, and internal saphenous above knee. In the fore-limb the severed nerves have been musculo-cutaneous, radial, median and dorsal and palmar divisions of ulnar about 4 cm. above wrist. It makes no obvious difference to the result whether these sections are made all at one time or seriatim. The section of anterior and posterior tibial, and of median and ulnar paralyses, of course, the intrinsic muscles of the feet. Yet in some cases hardly any noticeable disturbance follows. More often, however, the following defect appears in one or more of the feet. The animal is apt to stand with the toes of one or more of the feet doubled up underneath the planta. And although it may not do this in standing, on taking a few steps the toes of one or other foot are apt to double under in that manner. The way in which this occurs is that in the advance movement of the step the toes instead of just clearing the ground brush against it and are passively turned under the foot, and when the foot is set down at the anterior turning-point of the step the toes lie under it, and no correction of the malposition is made, the animal seeming unaware of it.

It might be thought that this defect was due to motor paralysis of the short extensor of the toes which of necessity follows severance of anterior tibial nerve. But section of that nerve alone does not produce the underturning. Moreover, a similar defect appears in fore-foot where there is no short extensor of the toes. In some cases this disturbance is transient. Slight increase of the lift of the foot in the advance phase of the step would obviate it. Hence it occurs less when the walk is quick than when it is slow. The desensitised foot later in some cases shows an abnormally high lift in stepping.

Apart from this defect in the management of the toes the natural standing and walking of the animal appears little affected by this denervation of the feet. In regarding the feet as denervated by the above nerve-sections it must be remembered that long tendons which enter the foot proceed from a number of leg muscles situate far above the ankle, and the fleshy parts and musculo-tendinous regions of these muscles contain many deep receptors, whose afferent nerves enter high up and never approach the foot directly, and are therefore not severed in the above experiments. But the fact remains that in so far as contribution to the reflex taxis of the step is made by receptors from the foot the contribution concerns merely the posture and movements of the digits of the foot. With the actual reflex execution of the step by the rest of the limb these receptors seem to have little or nothing to do. Reflex stepping excited by any of the stimuli mentioned above as competent in the decapitate or spinal preparations is evoked as easily and perfectly from the limbs with denervated feet as from the limbs with foot-nerves intact. Moreover, in those preparations the reflex stepping starts and continues well when the preparation is laid on its side, the feet not touching the floor, or when, as mentioned above, the preparation is supported freely above the ground so that the feet hang merely in the air.

Nor is the reflex stepping annulled or even obviously impaired by section of all the various cutaneous nerves of the limb. When in addition to the foot-nerves the external cutaneous, ilioinguinal, internal saphenous, small gluteal, and postero-external cutaneous in both hind-limbs are severed, no obvious impairment results in the reflex stepping.

A prominent skin-fold (dog) extends along the outer edge of the groin. Stroking the anterior part of this fold or the skin in front of it often evokes reflex stepping of the spinal hind-limbs, and this is accentuated if the skin right and left be stroked alternately. This stepping opens with flexion of ipsilateral knee and hip and ankle. It seemed that stretching of this skin might occur when the limb extends fully as at end of the extension phase of the step. Yet stretching of the skin with the fingers fails to give the limb reflex. Also cocainisation of this skin region makes no obvious difference to the reflex stepping.

There is one reflex from the planta which appears in several ways suited to play a part in the reflex step. Broad innocuous pressure on the planta spreading the digital pads and cushion excites a vigorous brief extension of the whole limb. This is the " extensor thrust."[1] It is practically annulled by severance of the two plantar nerves. The movement amounts to a vigorous thrust of the foot downward and backward. Were the foot on the ground this extensor thrust would propel the body forward and upward. The mode of its elicitation suggests that the weight of the animal applied through the foot against the ground probably excites it in the natural course of the step. When first describing[2] the reflex I regarded it as likely to supply the looked for stimulus of direct extension of the stepping limb. Philippson[3] has allotted this rôle to the reflex in his description of the reflex mechanism of the trot.

Further acquaintance with this reflex leads me to doubt whether it plays an important part in the stepping of the walk and trot. Section of the nerves of the foot annuls this reflex, but does not seriously impair reflex stepping. The ipsilateral extension which the reflex gives is usually synchronously accompanied by crossed extension, the form of extension of the crossed limb being a brisk vigorous thrust backward like that of the ipsilateral limb itself. The stimulus evokes, in fact, a bilateral thrust backward symmetrically executed by both hind-limbs. Such a movement is incompatible with walk or trot. It is, however, perfectly accordant with the movement of the gallop. This latter significance for the reflex is strengthened by a further observation. In a dog, in which spinal transection had been carried out between 6th and 7th cervical nerves and the animal kept under examination 132 days subsequently, the " extensor thrust " was easily obtained from either hind-foot. The elicitation of the thrust in either hind-foot was accompanied by a synchronous sharp extension not only of the fellow hind-limb, but of both fore-limbs as well. Elbows and wrists were extended and thrown forward at the same time that hind-limbs were extended and thrust back. The movement obviously resembled a phase of the gallop. The observation supports Philippson's view of the reflex as contributory to the gallop. If, however, it plays any part in the walk or trot it can only do so in some weakened form in which it is unaccompanied by its collateral effects on crossed hind-limb and ipsilateral fore-limb. Moreover, reflex stepping, even in the shape of the gallop, continues in

[1] *Integrative Action of the Nervous System*, 1906, p. 67.   [2] *J. Physiol.*, 1903, **29**, 58.
[3] *Op. cit.*

spinal dog, as Philippson has shown, when the animal is supported in the air and therefore in absence of all pressure stimuli to the feet. The extensor thrust cannot therefore be an indispensable factor in the reflex step. The possibility, however, remains that, under conditions appropriate to it, it is a contributory factor, though not an indispensable one.

Extension of the limb can also be obtained as a reflex result of stimulation of certain superficial afferents of the inguinal, ischial and perineal regions. Grounds were adduced above for regarding these reflexes as not concerned with progression, but as more probably sexual, etc. The extension they evoke in their own limb is accompanied by synchronous extension of the crossed fellow limb, a movement incompatible with walk or trot.

The intrinsic stimuli for reflex stepping of the limb do not therefore appear referable to any part of the skin of the limb. Movement of the limb as an excitant of stepping in it appears to act in virtue of deep receptors of the limb. Supporting this latter possibility are the following data. (i) Artificial stimuli, both mechanical and electrical, applied to the afferent nerves of the limb muscles uniformly evoke reflex flexion of their own limb and reflex extension of the fellow limb. (ii) Passive stretch of the knee extensor excites reflex relaxation of that muscle[1] and reflex contraction of the crossed fellow muscle,[2] and this reflex is excited through the afferent nerve of the extensor muscle itself.[3] (iii) Passive, and also active, shortening of the knee extensor excites contraction of that muscle and sometimes, though not regularly, reflex relaxation of the crossed fellow muscle;[4] and here again the afferent nerve is that of the knee extensor itself. (iv) A gentle brief passive extension of the limb in the decapitate preparation is often immediately followed by active flexion of the limb. Of the muscles engaged in spinal stepping, one of the most active is the sartorius. With this muscle the following observation can usually be obtained in the decapitate preparation (cat). The peroneal, popliteal, small sciatic and obturator nerves are severed, also internal saphenous at groin and the nerve of quadriceps extensor. Sartorius in that limb is rapidly resected from its insertions and separated from all lateral and deep connections, so that it lies free and retracted on the front of the thigh, retaining, however, its nerve and blood supply. The knee is then lightly held with one hand and somewhat quickly extended by means of the foot held in the other hand. As this is done the sartorius is seen to contract, especially when the extension of knee reaches completion. This reflex contraction of sartorius occurs chiefly in the medial band of the muscle. That band is pre-eminently a flexor of knee. This reflex can be obtained many times in fairly rapid succession. Conversely on passively flexing the knee a reflex contraction usually occurs, also in sartorius, but pre-eminently in the lateral band of the muscle. This band is especially in its distal part an extensor of knee. Adduction and abduction of thigh under these circumstances and also when obturator nerve has been left

---

[1] Sherrington, *Quart. J. exp. Physiol.*, 1909, **2**, 109. [2] Philippson, *op. cit.*, p. 31.
[3] Sherrington, *loc. cit.*, reprinted here, p. 329. [4] Sherrington, *ibid.*

unsevered does not in my experience cause contraction in sartorius. Extension of hip does do so occasionally and then the contraction is chiefly of the proximal part of lateral band; that part is a flexor of hip.

Similar observations can be obtained from semitendinosus, biceps femoris posterior, tenuissimus and gracilis. Passive extension of knee and ankle or of either of these joints alone excites contraction in those muscles when they have been completely detached from their insertions at knee. The passive extension still excites the reflex when internal and external saphenous nerves and musculo-cutaneous of peroneal and posterior tibial close above ankle have been severed and the foot thus far deafferented is used for manipulating the limb in the movement. The reflex contraction is a brief one, the stimulus seeming to consist therefore in the movement of extension and not in the extended posture when once assumed.

(v) An important stimulus in the reflex step lies at the attached base of the limb and is produced by extension of hip. Exteroceptive stimuli having been excluded it seems natural to relate that stimulus to changes in form and tension of muscles and fasciæ. The muscular sense-perceptions of the limb are finer for its proximal joints than for its distal (Goldscheider).[1] Magnus[2] has shown that in regard to the influence of initial posture upon the direction of the reflex movement of the limb, the influence of hip is greater than knee and of knee than ankle. The flexion-reflex, as an exteroceptive reaction, is most potently excited from the free apex of the limb. The stepping reflex, as regards deep stimuli situate in the limb itself, seems most excitable by stimuli at its attached base. This is as would be expected if the latter reflex is as regards its afferent source in the limb itself a proprioceptive reaction.

Flexion Phase of the Spinal Step

The flexion movement evinced in the reflex step differs in several particulars from that seen in the scratch-reflex. But with the flexion movement of the nociceptive flexion-reflex it agrees singularly closely. The main difference is that in the flexion phase of the step the flexion is not maintained and flexion at knee and ankle ceases somewhat earlier than does the flexion at hip, whereas in the nociceptive reflex flexion at all three joints is maintained. But when the reflex step is not vigorous in the spinal preparation the flexion at all three joints tends to cease at the same time. The stepping reflex then has the character to which its earliest observer, Freusberg,[3] probably alluded when he termed it the " mark-time " reflex, for it then fails to properly advance the limb over the ground. The other differences between the flexion of nociceptive flexion-reflex and that of the reflex step are that in the former the flexion is greater, and is succeeded by extension only after the stimulus is withdrawn, whereas in the step-reflex it is succeeded by extension during the continuance of the stimulus.

[1] *Arch. Anat. Physiol. Lpz., Physiol. Abtg.*, 1889, pp. 369, 540.
[2] *Pflüg. Arch. ges. Physiol.*, 1909, **130**, 219.
[3] *Ibid.*, 1874, **9**, 358.

Under analysis of the musculature at work in the two reflexes the similarity between the flexion of the flexion-reflex and that of the flexion phase of the step is again significantly close. By appropriate isolation of the muscles of the limb and by then exciting the stepping-reflex it is possible from a series of experiments to draw up a list of the muscles which contract and relax in the flexion phase of the spinal step. The list can hardly hope to be complete, since the procedure for isolating the individual muscles is necessarily severe and heightens the reflex threshold. The interference with the reflex which the requisite severance of a number of muscular nerves in the limb causes is greater than in the case of the nociceptive flexion-reflex. This is of itself suggestive of the proprioceptive nature of the former reflex. Often when the necessary isolation of a particular muscle has been completed the reflex, although previously regular and vigorous, is obtainable no longer.

In the series of experiments performed the muscles actually observed to contract in the flexion phase of the reflex step have been as follows (see Fig. 40, A, p. 277):

Psoas magnus	Semitendinosus
Sartorius median band	Tibialis anticus
Sartorius lateral band, upper part	Extensor longus digitorum
	Tensor fasciæ femoris brevis
Rectus femoris	Peroneus longus
Gracilis	Gluteus minimus
Biceps femoris, posterior part	Tenuissimus
	Extensor brevis digitorum.

These are all of them muscles which contract in the flexion of the nociceptive flexion-reflex. In the latter certain other muscles (psoas parvus, pectineus, tensor fasciæ femoris longus) were ascertained to contract also. In the flexion phase of the spinal step I have not been able to assure myself that they do, but it would be hazardous to say that they do not when the step is well developed.

In addition to the above which contract the experiments show that certain other muscles relax in the flexion phase of the reflex step. These are:

Semimembranosus	Adductor minor
Vastus lateralis	Gastrocnemius
Vastus medialis	Soleus
Crureus	Biceps femoris anterior.

These also are all of them muscles which relax in the flexion of the nociceptive flexion-reflex. In the latter there were also ascertained to relax part of adductor major, and distal part of lateral band of sartorius. These may relax also in the flexion phase of the reflex step, but I have not been able to assure myself that they do.

Extension Phase of the Spinal Step

Just as flexion phase of the reflex step resembles the flexion-reflex in its play on the musculature of the limb, so the step's extension phase resembles similarly the crossed extension reflex of the limb. Observations by the same method show that in the extension phase of the step muscles which contract are:

Quadratus femoris	
Vastus lateralis	Biceps femoris, anterior part
Crureus	Gastrocnemius
Sartorius (part of lateral band)	
Vastus medialis	Soleus
Adductor minor	Flexor longus digitorum.

The muscles observed to relax are:

Psoas magnus	Biceps femoris, posterior part
Sartorius, medial band	Gluteus minimus
Rectus femoris	Tibialis anticus
Gracilis	Extensor longus digitorum.
Semitendinosus	

The muscles which contract are muscles which contract in the crossed extension reflex and those which relax are muscles which relax in that reflex. Flexor longus digitorum in the crossed extension reflex certainly contracts late; its contraction appears to come late also in extension phase of step.

The " Simultaneous Co-ordination " Exhibited

Analysis of the behaviour of the individual muscles confirms, therefore, the similarity between flexion phase of step and the flexion-reflex of the limb and between extension phase of step and the crossed extension reflex of the limb. The principles of neural taxis and co-ordinative handling of the muscles exemplified in the nociceptive flexion-reflex and the crossed extension reflex therefore apply also to the reflex step.

Just as the nociceptive flexion-reflex does not exhibit fully the same form when excited from widely different small afferent nerves of the limb, so in the decapitate preparation the step-reflex varies somewhat in character as excited from this or that afferent source. When elicited in the decapitate preparation from perineal region or tail the stepping movement includes less flexion at hip than when elicited from a fore-limb or from the neck. In the dog the stepping when it first emerges after spinal transection in the thoracic region is often almost exclusively a rhythmic flexion at hips. The most usual imperfection in the step executed as a purely spinal reflex is in regard to the extension and flexion of the digits. The digits may even slightly passively flex when the ankle dorso-flexes, indicating that extensor brevis digitorum is not acting and that extensor longus digitorum is not acting strongly. Movement of the digits is often practically absent when the spinal stepping is feeble, though strikingly present in the vigorous reflex stepping of the spinal preparation after full recovery from shock.   These variations in form and completeness of the spinal step suggest that as regards any source which it has in the afferents of the limb itself that source is multiple, and though predominantly connected with the hip has also contributory channels from other regions of the limb.   The remote source is often single, but the intrinsic source is probably commonly multiple.

Conclusions as to the Nature of Factors underlying the Alternating Co-ordination of the Step[1]

The successive co-ordination of the reflex taxis of the spinal step may be summarised thus.   It is a rhythmic reflex which may be excited by continuous stimuli applied either to various peripheral points outside the limb or to the cross-section of the spinal cord itself.   In stepping a pair of antagonistic reflexes, E and F, alternately operate; the stimulus which generates and maintains the action is, however, not intermittent but continuous. The production of this intermittent reflex response from a continuous stimulus occurs in the following way.   The primary generating stimulus excites its reflex movement of the limb.   The reflex thus excited constitutes the opening phase of the step and is E or F according to the locus of the primary stimulus.   The active movement thus executed excites in the limb a proprioceptive reflex diametrically antagonistic to that of the primary stimulus. If the primary stimulus evoke E, this secondary reflex is F.   Three main factors combine to produce the secondary reflex which interrupts the primary one: (i) centripetal impulses from the deep structures passively moved by the primary reflex, (ii) centripetal impulses from the muscles actively used by the primary reflex, (iii) the central change underlying rebound in the spinal limb-centres reciprocally excited and inhibited by the primary stimulus.   " Umkehr " has also to be reckoned with as an accessory factor, also perhaps under certain circumstances the " extensor thrust."   When the secondary reflex is F the factor (i) is especially marked; when the secondary reflex is E the factor (iii) is especially marked.   Where the limb has been largely or completely deafferented by severance of its afferent roots factors (i) and (ii) fall out, but factor (iii) remains, and there remain crossed effects of factors (i) and (ii) from the stepping fellow limb.

When both limbs are engaged in reflex stepping the extensor phase of the step in one limb is reinforced by a crossed extension reflex whose stimulus arises in the flexion of the other limb; and similarly the flexion phase is reinforced by a crossed flexion-reflex derived from the other limb.   The influence of the fore and aft limb-pairs on each other is less.   The observations indicate that in natural stepping the excitatory influence descending from the brain to the spinal limb-centres is not intermittent but is continuous, although it results in rhythmic alternating movement of the limb.

[1] Extract from *J. Physiol.*, 1910, **40**, 102-3, following a lengthy discussion of the mechanical and nervous mechanism of the step.

7. REFLEXES ELICITABLE FROM THE PINNA, VIBRISSÆ, AND JAWS IN THE CAT[1]

REFLEXES OF THE PINNA

The aural pinna of the cat, sensitive and mobile as it is, yields a number of reflexes. One of them has been briefly referred to by me before:[2] I know no other reference to them, although doubtless they have been met by other observers. For the following experimental examination of them the animal was deeply chloroformed and then decerebrated with the decerebrator.[3,4] The decerebrator was so adjusted that the head was removed inclusive of fore-brain and mid-brain, the transection passing close behind the posterior colliculi and close in front of the Gasserian ganglia and the third divisions of the trigeminal nerves. By drawing the pinnæ well back when the head is guillotined these can be left attached to the carcase and their reflexes then examined. The narcosis being relaxed, the examination of the reflexes was begun usually about an hour later.

In this way the reflex movements elicitable from the pinna are found to be in the main five in number. These, to distinguish them, may be termed (1) the retraction reflex, (2) the folding reflex, (3) the head-shake reflex, (4) the cover reflex, (5) the scratch reflex, this last being the already-studied reflex in which the ipsilateral hind-foot is brought forward to scratch the stimulated part.[5]

Interrelations of the Pinnal Reflexes

Certain of these pinnal reflexes, though each under a moderately brief and circumscript stimulus commonly occurs alone, tend to occur together,

[1] Published with the above title, *J. Physiol.*, 1917, **51**, 404-431.
[2] C. S. Sherrington, *Proc. roy. Soc.*, 1893, **53**, 409, and *Integrative Action*, 1906.
[3] F. R. Miller and C. S. Sherrington, *Quart. J. exp. Physiol.*, 1915, **9**, 147.
[4] *Physiol. Soc. Proc.*, *J. Physiol.*, 1915, **49**, lii.
[5] These reflexes are described in detail, with illustrations of the receptive areas concerned, in the original paper. Their chief characteristics might here be summarised:

The Retraction Reflex.—The swinging backward of the pinna when it is touched—*e.g.*, as when a fly settles on it. The receptive field is nearly the whole inner and outer surface of the pinna, but not the meatus, and a small strip of scalp and neck.

The Back-folding Reflex.—A folding of the upper part of pinna backward and downward in response to strong tactile stimulation on the pinna itself.

The Head-shake Reflex.—Alternate right and left rotations of the head about its long axis in response to a drop of water, or mechanical stimulus in external auditory meatus. Afferent roots vagus and part of mandibular root of 5th n. Respiration not disturbed. Receptive field includes small part of concavity of concha.

The Cover Reflex.—A forward rotation of the pinna, elicited by mechanical stimuli from the concavity of the concha of higher intensity than for the head-shake reflex. Has analogies with the gill-slit cover response, but is without interference with respiration.

The Scratch Reflex.—The postural and rhythmic effect in the trunk and limbs is as for the reflex when elicited from the neck (see p. 159), but the head is lowered and rotated sideways in addition. The receptive field in the cat extends within the concavity of the concha and the meatus, and runs into the neck and scalp, but does not include the distal part of the pinna or the cheek. The response can be elicited by unipolar faradisation of the descending spinal root of the fifth nerve, in section of the bulb (Graham Brown and Sherrington, *Quart J. exp. Physiol.*, 1911, **4**, 202).—ED.

making a compound reflex response to a single stimulus. The retraction reflex and folding reflex are in this sense rather closely linked, so also the cover reflex with the head-shake. A strong stimulus evoking the head-shake sometimes evokes the scratch reflex also; and then occasionally it seems that there is inco-ordination, for the hind-limb appears to move towards the head and make scratching movement while the head itself instead of being steadily turned back toward the advancing limb, is still upturned and executing the rotational movement of the shake.

The retraction, folding, and cover reflexes of right and left sides are strikingly independent of each other. It is as easy to obtain them from the pinna of one side while that of the other side is itself exhibiting one of the reflexes as when the fellow ear is quiet. This is in marked contrast to the close interrelation, usually inhibitory, between right and left reflexes of the neck and limbs.

Comparison of the Receptive Fields of the Pinnal Reflexes with the Skin-fields of the Cranio-spinal Nerves of the Pinna Region

Study of these reflexes gives opportunity for seeing how far the functional unity of a receptive field conforms with, or represents, the morphological unity of a segmental root-field. Comparison of the receptive fields of the respective reflexes with the skin-fields of the several nerve-roots, cranial and spinal, distributed to pinna-region shows clearly that the factor which decides the central reflex connections of the afferent fibres of each root is the functional position of each portion of the skin the root supplies, rather than any primitive morphological entity which each respective cranial or spinal nerve may be supposed to represent. This is evidenced plainly if the extents and borders of the reflex-fields are contrasted with the root-fields.[1] No single root-field is identical with any single reflex-field; nor is any single reflex-field identical with any group of root-fields. There is not even approximate agreement between them. Even the vagus skin-field,[1] confined entirely to the concave face of the pinna, contributes to the head-shake and cover reflex below in the concha, but to the retraction and folding reflexes above where it extends over part of the scapha. Similarly trigeminus, where it is distributed over the cheek in front of tragus, intertragus, and posttragus, contributes fibres to the head-shake reflex and to the scratch reflex. Again, the 1st cervical nerve where it spreads into the concha supplies afferents for the head-shake, cover, and scratch reflexes, and where it spreads over the scapha and back of the pinna supplies afferents for the retraction reflex and the folding reflex. The functional topography of the skin of this region is evidently not governed by the limits of the ancient root supply.

---

[1] In the original paper the reflex-fields and nerve-root innervation are illustrated by drawings. The innervation of the meatus by the vagus was demonstrated by its reflex effects (*ibid.*, pp. 415, 417). No afferents for *e.g.* cover reflex are supplied by the geniculate ganglion.—Ed.

Vibrissal Reflexes

The long vibrissæ of the cat's face are arranged in two groups, the one on the upper part of the muzzle above the mouth, the other superciliary. From the former in my experience no reflexes are clearly elicitable. From the latter reflex-closure of the eyelids is easily obtainable. In the decerebrate preparation a light touch on a superciliary vibrissa, displacing it even slightly, is often a sufficient stimulus.

As to the muzzle-vibrissæ, although in my experience reflexes are not readily or regularly evocable from them, movements of them not rarely accompany the retraction and folding reflexes of the pinna evoked, as above, from the pinnal region itself.

Jaw Reflexes

1. *Jaw-closing Reflex*

Reflex closing of the jaw accompanies the reflex swallow which is so readily obtainable in the decerebrate preparation by putting a little fluid into the mouth.[1] Reflex jaw-closing is also evoked as a movement by mechanical stimulation—*e.g.*, by stroking with a feather the dorsum of the tongue near its tip. The tongue tip is curved slightly upward and somewhat retracted, and at the same time the mandible is raised and the mouth rather deliberately closed and in the decerebrate preparation tends to remain so. This slow movement leads to no reverse action of opposite phase in the antagonistic muscles employed; it thus offers striking contrast to the jaw-opening reflex described below with its quick movement tending to be followed by strong reversal.

2. *Jaw-opening Reflex*

In the decerebrate preparation the jaw maintains a closed posture.[2] This is in harmony with the rule[3] that decerebration brings all the antigravity muscles into steady reflex postural activity. With this steady posture as a background, stimuli applied to a rather restricted receptive surface evoke regularly in the decerebrate preparation the opening of the jaw. The surface in question is that of the gum bordering the teeth both of the upper and lower jaws, also the front part of the hard palate.

The reflex movement is quick and is followed immediately on withdrawal of the stimulus by a quick return to the previous closed posture. So quick and sudden is the opening and so sharply followed by active return of closure that, under electrical elicitation, the phenomenon at first suggests escape of the stimulating current to the motor nerve of the jaw-opening muscles. That the reaction is truly reflex can, however, be easily

---

[1] Miller and Sherrington, *loc. cit.*, p. 189.   [2] *Integrative Action of the Nervous System*, 1906.
[3] *J. Physiol.*, 1910, **40**, 104.

proved. (1) The induction currents cease to evoke it from the gum of the upper jaw as soon as the afferent nerve of that jaw (superior maxillary of trigeminus) has been cut, and from the gum of the lower jaw when the inferior dental nerve is cut. (2) The reaction is evocable by mechanical stimuli to the gum or teeth either of upper or lower jaw, and these stimuli likewise cease to evoke it after severance of the above afferent nerves. (3) In the freshly killed animal strong faradisation (unipolar or bipolar) of the gum upper or lower often produces strong closing of the jaw, but never opening of it. Current-escape therefore in this situation tends, as one would expect, to excite the near adjacent closing muscles and closure, not opening, is the result. The reflexly excited jaw movement is accompanied by some retraction of the cheek and angle of the mouth, as if to keep the border of these out of the way of the bite.

Receptive-field and the Stimuli.—Blunt pressure, as for instance with the shaft-end of a small feather, on the gum bordering the crown of a tooth evokes the reflex. So also pressure on the tooth-crown often markedly evokes the reflex. These mechanical stimuli have to be much heavier than those sufficing for the pinnal reflexes. The gum border is not equally responsive for the reflex all along its length. It seems in my experience most responsive near the 2nd premolar teeth and least so at the canines. Faradisation evokes the reflex well. I have used this by the unipolar method. The stigmatic electrode excites the reflex not only when applied to the gum bordering the teeth but also when applied actually to a tooth. Here again the stimulus has acted best at the premolars, but even at the tip of a canine it will also often evoke a good reflex. Faradism also excites the reflex from points in the front part of the hard palate. Stimulation of the central stump of the severed superior dental branch of superior maxillary nerve likewise elicits the reflex.

After separating the halves of the mandible at the symphysis it is possible to see how far the reflex movement evoked, say from the premolars of one side, is bilateral or unilateral. The reflex is then found to be practically unilateral. Mechanical or faradic stimulation of the gum or teeth of the right side produces its reflex effect on the muscles of that one half of the mandible, and not unless the stimulus is quite strong is the other half involved as well. Even then the reflex effect on the contralateral musculature is feeble.

The opening muscles of the jaw—*e.g.*, digastric—when exposed can be seen to contract in the reflex. This observation becomes particularly clear in these muscles after their detachment from the jaw in front. And if after their detachment, the head being prone and the split half of mandible still closed against the maxilla by reason of the decerebrate rigidity, the stimulus be applied—*e.g.*, the stigmatic electrode brought to touch a premolar—the ipsilateral half of the mandible is seen immediately to drop. This occurs by reason of the reflex central inhibition of the jaw-closers: *temporalis, masseter*, etc. It can be ascertained in other positions of the head by light pressure against the mandible with the finger. The reflex therefore strikingly exhibits reciprocal innervation in its taxis of the antagonist muscles.

The reflex further exhibits strikingly the phenomenon of rebound[1] met with especially as a post-inhibitory reaction in the extensor muscles of the fore- and hind-limbs. On withdrawal of the stimulus—e.g., faradic—to the maxillary gum the temporarily relaxed jaw-closers immediately enter into a strong contraction relifting the split half of the mandible and shutting it tight, often with a powerful snap. It is to be noted that here, just as in the fore- and hind-limb, the rebound-contraction is exhibited by anti-gravity muscles, the extensors—e.g., supraspinatus, vastocrureus, gastrocnemius—being anti-gravity muscles in the limb in the same sense as are temporalis and masseter at the jaw. When the stimulus is strong the rebound appears to predominate and contraction of the closers may ensue earlier in the reflex.

This jaw reflex as thus evoked from gum, teeth, or hard palate is therefore, like the ipsilateral flexion-reflex of a limb, a diphasic reflex. The first phase, as excited at least by weak or medium strength stimuli, is opening of the jaw; the second, which tends of itself to follow on the first, is closure of the jaw. The ipsilateral flexion-reflex of the limb in decerebrate rigidity and under slowly repetitive stimulations gives a stepping movement, the flexion phases of the stepping occurring with each stimulation, the extensor phases occurring by rebound between the successive stimulations. Similarly, the jaw reflex under a series of repetitive stimulations results in a masticatory movement, the openings of the jaw occurring with the stimulations, the closings by strong rebounds between the stimulations. From the prominence in this reflex of reflex central inhibition and the central rebound ensuent on that it would seem that in the rhythmic act of mastication in so far as concerns all the large part of it which it executed reflexly, and subject to the same reservations,[2] just as in the rhythmic act of stepping, the rhythmic alternation of two active reflex phases is obtainable by the mere alternate recurrence and lapse of one single mode of stimulus. On the mouth's seizing a morsel the mandible, when it has closed—e.g., voluntarily—upon whatever is between the jaws pressing it against the gums and teeth and hard palate, by so doing, as is clear from observation of the reflex, produces a stimulus which tends reflexly to reopen the jaws. That done the central rebound of the previously reflexly inhibited jaw-closing muscles, or rather of their motoneurones, for the inhibition is central, sets in and tends to powerfully reclose the jaws again. The reclosure brings into operation once again the jaw-opening stimulus. And so, after being started by a first bite, a rhythmic masticatory reflex tends to keep itself going so long as there is something biteable between the jaws.

[1] C. S. Sherrington, J. Physiol., 1907, 36, 135; Proc. roy. Soc., 1908, 80B, 53; and A. Forbes, Quart. J. exp. Physiol., 1912, 5, 149.

[2] J. Physiol., 1913, 47, 196, and see T. Graham Brown, Proc. roy. Soc., 1911, 84B, 319, and J. Physiol., 1914, 48, 18.

NARCOTICS AND THE REFLEXES

The pinna reflexes emerge very early from the shock of decerebration and are submerged very late in chloroform or ether narcosis. They disappear often much later under chloroform than does the conjunctival reflex. Their suppression serves as a good index to complete chloroform narcosis, and I have been accustomed for a long time past to use them as such in the laboratory, thus obviating the necessity of removing the chloroform apparatus from the face in order to test the conjunctiva.

The jaw reflexes in my experience take longer to emerge from the shock of decerebration; but they can generally be elicited soon after the conjunctival reflex has appeared.

All the above reflexes can be demonstrated easily in the normal—*i.e.*, not decerebrate—animal under various degrees of chloroform or ether narcosis. For the jaw-opening reflex faradisation of the gum is then more efficient than is mechanical stimulation (pressure, etc.).

REPRESENTATION IN THE CORTEX CEREBRI OF THE MOVEMENTS

Recalling previous experience of stimulating the cerebral cortex in the cat and other animals, I could not remember having there met with the pinnal movements seen in the above reflexes of the decerebrate preparation. Nor on referring to the literature of the cortex do I find record of any such. I have therefore explored the cat's cortex again with special reference to them. The hemisphere was exposed under deep chloroformisation, and the surface then gone over point for point by unipolar faradisation. This was done in six animals. The various usual responses were obtained: flexion of fore-limb and of hind-limb, rotation of neck, retraction of angle of mouth, closure of contralateral eye, twisting of the nostril, opening of mouth, retraction of tongue, etc. The only movement of the pinna obtained was a slight protraction, a " pricking," not like any of the pinnal movements obtained as reflexes in the decerebrate preparation. This cortical movement was obtained from the coronal gyrus near the junction of that with supra-sylvian and close against the anterior supra-sylvian sulcus of Langley.[1] This is the position originally noted by Ferrier[2] to yield in the cat " a drawing forwards and downwards of the ear." The movement was also, though irregularly, obtained from somewhat further lateral—namely, from a part of gyrus sylviacus anterior of Langley. The movement was one which protracted the pinna as a whole, not involving any separate movement of the tip or other parts. Of the reflex movements of pinna the one to which it bore some though not close semblance was that of the cover reflex, but the twisting and eversion of the bursella characteristic of this latter was not present in the cortical movement, nor was there the flattening of the scapha. This negative result was somewhat strengthened as evidence by the fact

---

[1] *J. Physiol.*, 1884, **4**, 253.   [2] *Functions of the Brain*, London, 1876.

that the degree of etherisation which permits motor responses from the cortex permits also elicitation of the pinnal reflexes by stimulation of the pinna, so that these—*e.g.*, retraction and folding reflex—remained elicitable by mechanical stimuli of the pinna during the faradic exploration of the cortex. That the slight protraction movement obtained from the cortex had nothing to do with these reflexes was further shown by evoking a pinnal reflex and while that was in progress evoking the cortical movement of the pinna. The result was that the retracted and folded pinna was simply shifted forward as a whole, without either increase or diminution of the reflex engaging it. Nor did the occurrence of the reflex interfere with the obtaining of this cortical response.

The evidence is negative, but so far as it goes it asserts that the group of reflex movements above described, elicitable so readily from the de-cerebrate preparation and also (*v. infra*) from the normal animal, are not represented in the cortex cerebri. As a rule movements of the skeletal musculature readily obtainable as spinal or cranial reflexes are also ob-tainable by excitation of the cortex, and are, indeed, preponderant among the cortical responses. A negative result in this respect is therefore not without interest.

The scratch reaction was also looked for in the cortex, and not found. From the hind-limb area of the cortex rhythmic flexion of the contralateral hind-limb including flexion of ankle was sometimes evoked, and on some occasions bore some resemblance to a feebly developed scratch-reflex response, but the characteristic flexion of the toes accompanying ankle-flexion was wanting, and the rhythm was too slow. Similar rhythmic alternate flexions and extensions of the fore-limb could at the same period of the experiment be evoked by shifting the electrode to the fore-limb area; these were evidently stepping movements. The inference was therefore that the hind-limb movement also was " stepping," and this was borne out by the movement being evoked in fore- and hind-limb together, and then flexion in one was seen to follow that in the other, although agreeing in frequency. The exploration failed, therefore, to find the scratch reflex represented in the cortex.

But although the pinnal reflexes including the scratch could not be found, the movement of eye-closure as elicited from the superciliary vibrissæ, and of jaw-opening as elicited in the jaw reflex, were easily evocable from the cortex; and both are of course well known among cortical reactions, the situation of their foci in the cat having been determined first by Ferrier.[1] As elicited from the cortex the movement of opening of the jaw tends to be smartly followed by jaw closure as it is also in the decerebrate reflex. Also, just as after the mandibular symphysis has been split the reflex is found to be practically unilateral, so is the reaction as provoked from the cortex, though in the latter case the muscular effect is of course contralateral, in the former ipsilateral. There are, however, some evident differences between

[1] *Loc. cit.*

the cortical and the reflex reactions in the cat in regard to their muscular taxis. As obtained from the cortex the jaw opening is accompanied by retraction of tongue and it is often not easy to dissociate the two reactions. As obtained in the decerebrate reflex the jaw opening is not accompanied or is accompanied little and rarely by movement of the tongue. Again, the cortical reaction of jaw-opening, especially as obtained from low down in the anterior composite gyrus of Langley, tends to be the first phase of a rhythmic act of alternating openings and closings of the jaw (mastication). But the decerebrate reflex, although it tends to produce a sharp closure ensuent on the opening, does not under simple continuance of its stimulus develop a rhythmic succession of alternating movements. In other words, the reflex tends to exhibit a single complete bite, the cortical reaction a performance of mastication.

COMPARISON OF THE REFLEXES WITH REACTIONS IN THE NORMAL ANIMAL

After study of the above reflexes in the decerebrate preparation it was of interest to examine the normal cat's behaviour when touches, etc., were applied at various parts of the ear. With the animal comfortably seated on an assistant's lap the touches were applied with the ordinary æsthesio-meter or with a small camel's hair paint brush. The stimuli evoked from the points touched the same movements as those described above in the purely reflex preparation; and they evoked no others, except that the animal at times became impatient and restless, though for the most part it remained quiet, often purring. It would continue purring even when the attitude of the ear temporarily assumed was that indicative of anger as in the figure furnished by Darwin.[1]

Summarising the results, they were as follows: The retraction and the folding reactions were evoked about as readily as in favourable reflex experiments—that is, the threshold of excitation seemed as low, certainly no higher. They were evoked much more readily than in many of the reflex experiments. To apply touches isolatedly to some of the points in the ear one had to work with the ear cleanly and completely shaven. On several occasions, then, the touches evoked the retraction reaction when applied to concha below the crescent, a region lower than had been ob-served to yield the reaction in the reflex preparation. The shake reaction was likewise evoked about as readily as in favourable reflex experiments; the limits of its receptive field seemed exactly the same as that delimited in the reflex preparation. A puff of air or a droplet of water evoked it with about the same readiness as under pure reflex conditions. The reaction, however, was usually more violent and more prolonged than for corre-sponding intensities of stimulus in the reflex preparation. It also had

---

[1] C. Darwin, *Expression of the Emotions*, London, 1873, Fig. 9, p. 58, furnishes a figure of the retraction of the ear as a characteristic expression of emotion in a cat threatened by a dog.

frequently a much longer latency. The cover reaction seemed the least readily induced. The scratch reaction was readily excited by its appropriate stimuli and from both divisions of its receptive field—*i.e.*, both from the front and from the back of the pinna. A prolonged touch by a blunt pencil on the concha of the shaven ear provoked it well, so also pressure with a wad of cotton-wool. Just as in the reflex preparation there was a tendency for some of the several reactions to occur together in response to a single stimulus. Thus retraction and folding reactions were often conjoined, and the head-shake along with the cover. Sometimes retraction reaction or folding reaction occurred along with the head-shake, the latter following on the former. Occasionally the scratch reaction and the head-shake were coupled together, but always in sequence, the sequence being head-shake, scratch, and then head-shake again. The posturing of the head in the scratch reaction is antagonistic to—*i.e.*, incompatible with—the movement it makes in the head-shake. Touching the superciliary vibrissæ caused closure of the eyelids as in the reflex preparation.

Differences noted between the reactions in the normal animal and those in the reflex preparation were the following: In the normal animal the receptive field of the retraction and folding reactions extended somewhat further into concha. The shake-reaction was frequently slow in appearing, as though the animal were not disposed to make it. The head-shake was usually a much more prolonged movement than in the reflex preparation. Occasionally when the cat, at a break in the examination, was placed on the floor to walk about, the first thing it did was to give the head-shake, although just before while lying in the assistant's lap it had not given any response to a droplet of water placed in the concha; the reaction had then presumably been for the time being suppressed, but was permitted when the cat was set down on its feet in freedom. The scratch reaction often showed a very long latency, the cat seeming indisposed to permit it to ensue. When the movement appeared it was much more perfect and prolonged than in the reflex preparation. The two middle toes were put actually within the concha, whereas in the reflex preparation the foot very rarely actually reaches the head, commonly beating in the air several centimetres away from the pinna. In the normal cat a touch upon the muzzle-vibrissæ usually caused turning of the head toward the side touched, whereas in the reflex preparation very rarely is any movement at all evoked. In the normal cat a sound coming from the adjoining room would sometimes excite a slight lifting of both ears, a cocking of both pinnæ; this movement was quite different from any of the reflex ear movements met with in the decerebrate preparation; but from the cortex as Ferrier noted it is elicitable, though then in my experiments (*v.s.*) it appeared in one pinna only, the contralateral.

Any endeavour to elicit the jaw reflexes from the normal cat promised so little likelihood of reaching an unconfused result, owing to the requisite faradisation, etc., of the gum making the animal fractious, that I did not attempt it. Remembering, however, that the mucosa of the human cheek is practically devoid of nociceptors in the region of the second upper premolar,[1] I tried on myself faradisation of that spot and its neighbourhood, by the unipolar method, with the stigmatic electrode on the mucous surface. When one does this with a fairly strong current one experiences an almost uncontrollable impulse to open the jaw wider. A form of electrode suitable for the purpose is that previously described for work with the central nervous system (Fig. 35, p. 229), because the wire is sheathed with ebonite up to its tip, while the free end of the platinum being fused to a little bead and the platinum itself carried by a light spiral spring, the mucosa, though easily steadily pressed on, cannot be pricked. A convenient way of making the observation is with one hand to bring the tip of this electrode through the open mouth to the gum and then, while the interrupter of the inductorium is running and the secondary circuit unbridged, to dip the other hand in a basin of salt water in which the diffuse electrode has been placed.

Nature of the Adequate Stimuli and the Sensations

Of questions raised by these reflexes one concerns the intimate nature of their adequate stimuli. For human touch-spots the progress of research has gradually traced the nature of the adequate stimulus to be local deformation of the skin surface. This analytic result can answer obviously for those stimuli of the cat's pinna or vibrissæ which move the hairs or hairlets, or consist in mechanical touches by the æsthesiometer, etc. But it is difficult to apply it to explain the operation of such stimuli as a faint puff of air directed upon the cleanly shaven skin, or into the hairless concha; or to such as a droplet of oil or water gently placed practically without impact upon them.

Yet if these latter act as thermal stimuli the thermal receptivity must be extremely acute, for they still act when warm at a temperature imperceptible to one's own finger and ear, though of course one cannot be sure that the temperature of these latter and of the cat's pinna in the experiment are the same. The problem recalls one that is raised by the swallowing reflex.[2] There a few drops of water warmed to the temperature of the tongue and placed on the back of the dorsum in quantities as small as 0·2 c.c. excite in the decerebrate preparation the swallow reflex from a mucous surface already wet with saliva. There also it was shown that the stimulus, whatever its intimate mode of operation, is of mechanical quality.

Another question raised is the species of sensation excited by the stimuli adequate for these reflexes when applied not in the decerebrate but in the sentient animal, in short the modality or modalities of sensation which is or are adjunct to these reflexes. For the human skin four species of sense

---

[1] Kiesow, *Philos. Stud.*, **9**, 540; **14**, 567.
[2] Miller and Sherrington, *Quart. J. exp. Physiol.*, 1915, **9**, 147.

are recognised: touch, warmth, cold, and pain. Of these it is well known that pain is closely bound up with bulbar and spinal reflexes, touch hardly at all. " Pains " are, so to say, " subcortical "; " touches," " cortical." The stimuli adequate for these pinna reflexes do not resemble the stimuli adequate for nociceptors (pain receptors), but do resemble and are practically identical with those adequate for human touch. In the cat's pinna there seems therefore to be a group of touch reflexes, bulbar and spinal. But touch on the general surface of the cat's body—except for the scratch-reflex zone—is as impotent to excite spinal reflexes as it is in man. If one applies to one's own pinna the stimuli adequate for the cat's pinnal reflexes one notes that the sensations they evoke, although tactual, are tactual of a distinctive kind, quite apart from local signature, etc. They are not of neutral affective tone, which is to say, devoid of affective tone; they are all of markedly negative affective tone, which is to say, all distinctly dis- agreeable. The inference is therefore that in the cat among the modalities of cutaneous sense and among the species of skin receptors there is one intermediate between pain and touch, between nociceptive and tango- ceptive, probably nearer to touch than to pain. It might be termed " affective touch." As regards the stimuli adequate for this intermediate species, its receptors resemble the tangoceptors not nociceptors, yet like nociceptors they are closely and potently attached centrally to motor mechanisms in the bulb and cord; yet they are not, as nociceptors are, closely attached to the bulbar vasomotor and respiratory centres. Whether this intermediate form in the cutaneous series amounts actually to a separate species and modality further research must decide; it is partly a matter of name; receptivity suggests no, the reflex connections suggest yes, and the sensual experience tends to support the latter.

Conclusions

A number of reflexes are elicitable from the pinna of the cat. The decerebrate preparation gives facility for observing these as pure reflexes. Their movements are protective of the pinna: some, the retraction and folding reflexes, seem directed against irritant touches—e.g., the settling of flies, etc., or against exposure to injury in fighting; others, the cover and head-shake and scratch reflexes, against the ingress of foreign matter, including water, dust, or insects, into the meatus and its ampulla.

The threshold of the mechanical stimuli exciting these reflexes is ex- tremely low; on the other hand, the reflexes with the exception of the scratch reflex are excited with difficulty and uncertainty by electrical stimuli. The reflexes although connected eminently with the hairs are connected also with other skin receptors separate from the hairs. Some of the stimuli may be thermal.

The constancy of response and the low threshold obtainable in these pinnal reflexes allow minuter observations which tend to question the probability that the intimate nature of the mechanical stimuli " adequate " for them can, as is generally accepted for human " touch," be subsumed under the rubric " local deformation of skin surface." The modality of sense attaching to them in the normal—*i.e.*, sentient—animal is probably best stated as " affective touch."

The afferent nerve-fibres concerned with each of these reflexes are supplied from several segmental nerve-roots, among them the vagus. The afferent nerve-roots of the reflexes taken as a group are those of trigeminus, vagus, and 1st, 2nd, and 3rd cervical nerves.

The afferent nerve-trunks respectively involved evoke the retraction and the folding reflexes better when stimulated mechanically than when stimulated electrically.

No one of the reflex receptive fields is identical with the skin-field of any one of the segmental nerves carrying its afferent fibres.

The superciliary vibrissæ evoke reflex closure of the eye; the maxillary vibrissæ evoke no reflex in the decerebrate preparation.

Mechanical and electrical stimuli applied to the gum, or teeth, both of the maxilla and mandible, or to the front part of the hard palate, evoke reflex opening of the jaws followed by rebound closure; the reflex is preponderantly unilateral.

Exploration of the cortex cerebri finds large representation of the jaw-opening reflex and of the superciliary reflex but no evidence of any cortical representation of the group of pinnal reflex movements.

All the reflexes are easily obtained under narcosis. The pinnal and superciliary reflexes are also readily elicitable in the normal animal, their threshold of excitation by the adequate stimuli being then somewhat lower than in most, though not than in all decerebrate preparations.

VI

ON THE ANATOMICAL COURSE OF
REFLEX CONNECTIONS IN THE SPINAL CORD

1. DESCENDING REFLEX PATHWAYS[1]

[By making a second partial section of the isolated lower segment of the spinal cord, at a long interval after the first complete transection, it is possible to trace by degeneration nervous pathways linking the various segments and transmitting intersegmental reflexes.]

INTRODUCTION. PREVIOUS OBSERVATIONS

IN experiments upon paths of nervous conduction in the mammalian spinal cord, departures, both numerous and wide, from the " Fourth Law " of Pflüger have been recorded by one of us.[2] Pflüger's " Fourth Law " runs: " Reflex irradiation in the spinal cord spreads upwards or anteriorly—*i.e.*, towards the medulla oblongata."[3] Contrary to this statement, there certainly exist many spinal paths by which the activity aroused in spinal segments situate nearer the head is communicated to segments lying further backward. The present paper results from search for more detailed evidence regarding aborally-running reflex spinal paths.

The above-quoted " law " of Pflüger is usually accepted and endorsed without comment, but physiological literature records here and there examples of spinal reflexes irradiating aborally. Thus: the " trab reflex " (Luchsinger[4]) in goat and cat; the " scratching " reflex (Haycraft,[5] Goltz[6]) in dog and rat; the " shake " reflex, mentioned by Goltz and Ewald,[7] in the dog; reflexes radiating from the pinna (skin supplied by 2nd cervical nerve) to neck, to fore-limb, to hind-limb, and to tail (Sherrington[8]) in cat, dog, and monkey, and numerous similar instances furnished by the last named.

Regarding the demonstration of intraspinal nerve-fibres disposed

---

[1] Published with E. E. Laslett under the title " Observations on Some Spinal Reflexes and the Interconnection of Spinal Segments," *J. Physiol.*, 1903, **29**, 58-96. The protocols of seventeen experiments are cited, of which only seven are reprinted here. The list on p. 209 gives the site of section of the remaining experiments reported in the original.—ED.

[2] Croonian Lecture, *Philos. Trans.*, 1898, **190B**, 171.

[3] " Reflex-Irradiation in dem Rückenmarke nach oben, resp. vorn. gerichtet ist; also gegen die *Medulla Oblongata.*" *Die sensorischen Functionen des Rückenmarks d. Wirbelthiere, nebst einer neuen Lehre über die Leitungsgesetze der Reflexionen*, p. 73, Berlin, 1853.

[4] *Pflüg. Arch. ges. Physiol.*, 1882, **28**, 65.   [5] *Brain*, 1890, **12**, 516.

[6] *Pflüg. Arch. ges. Physiol.*, 1892, **51**, 570.   [7] *Ibid.*, 1896, **63**, 362.

[8] *Philos. Trans.*, 1898, **190**, 170.

suitably for such conduction—*i.e.*, to be intermediary between receptive " centres " headward and motor root-cells several segments further back— the definite information is very scanty. By the Golgi method, axis-cylinder processes from cells in the spinal grey matter have been traced to enter all the white columns (*cellules des cordons*, Ramón,[1] van Gehuchten; *Strangzellen*, Kölliker), especially the ventro-lateral. To discover in which direction these then run—*i.e.*, whether headward or backward—is difficult. Von Lenhossek[2] writes that he could not from his preparations decide which way they went. Ramón[3] and van Gehuchten[4] say that for the most part the neuraxons bifurcate at once into an ascending and a descending nerve-fibre, but that some without division turn upward, others similarly downward, and that in some instances the neuraxon divides into three fibres which all turn upward or all turn downward. It is impossible to see to what distance the fibres run along the length of the cord—*i.e.*, what segmental interval they bridge.

Pathological material indicates existence of some slender aborally-running tracts in the dorsal column. These have received various names in various regions of the cord: the " comma-bundle " (Bastian,[5] Pick,[6] Schultze[7]) in the brachial region; the cornu-commissural (P. Marie,[8] including the " triangle of Gombault and Philippe "[9]) in the lumbo-sacral region; the septo-marginal tract of Bruce and Muir[10] (including probably Flechsig's " oval centre " and the " dorso-median sacral bundle of Obersteiner "[11]) in the lumbo-sacral region. Both the " comma-bundle " and the " septo-marginal tract " have been shown[12] to exist also in the thoracic region. It has been a question whether these tracts may not consist of the descending stems of afferent root-fibres (Schültze, Schaffer, Ramón y Cajal, Redlich, Flatau, and others); that they come largely from intraspinal nerve cells (Marie, Margulies, Pick, Bruce, Pineles, Wallenburg, and others) is supported by (i.) degeneration in them subsequent to necrosis of the grey matter of the lumbo-sacral region (Ehrlich and Brieger,[13] Singer and Münzer,[14] Rothmann[15]); and by (ii.) the fact that the tabetic decay largely spares them though it affects the afferent root system, while conversely syringomyelia,[16] which destroys the grey matter, often causes degeneration of these tracts. Barker[17] appropriately groups these intrinsic tracts together as the *fasciculus dorsalis proprius*.

[1] *Nuevas observaciones sobre la estructura d. l. médula espinal d. l. mamiferos*, Barcelona, 1890, p. 6.
[2] *Der feinere Bau d. Nervensystems*, Berlin, 1893.
[3] *Nuevo concepto d. l. Histolgia d. l. Centros nerviosos*, Barcelona, 1893.
[4] *Système nerveux*, Louvain, 1897, p. 323, etc.   [5] *Med.-Chir. Trans.*, 1867, p. 429.
[6] *Archiv. Psychiat. Nervenkr.*, 1880, p. 179.   [7] *Ibid.*, 1883, p. 359.
[8] *La Semaine Médicale*, 1894.   [9] *Arch. Méd. Exp.*, 1894, p. 377.
[10] *Brain*, 1896, **19**, 333; and Bruce, *ibid.*, 1897, **20**, 261.
[11] *Nervöse Centralorgane*, Vienna, 2nd edit., 1891, p. 264.
[12] Hoche, *Neur. Centralbl.*, 1896, p. 155, and others later.
[13] *Zeit. klin. Med.*, 1884, **7**, Suppl. Band.   [14] *Arch. exp. Path.*, 1895, **35.**
[15] *Arch. Anat. Physiol. Lpz.*, *Physiol. Abt.*, 1899, p. 120.
[16] Schlesinger, *Obersteiner's Arbeiten*, Wien, 1895.   [17] *The Nervous System*, New York, 1899.

In the ventro-lateral column the "sulco-marginal bundle" of Marie undergoes some descending degeneration and is regarded as intraspinal in origin. Various observers[1] have noted that descending lateral degeneration after spinal translesion exceeds the utmost degeneration consequent on cortical lesions however extensive. That this excess is in some measure due to the degeneration of additional fibres of spinal origin has been really established in an ingenious experiment by Münzer and Wiener[2] (1895). After semi-section of the cord of a newborn rabbit at the last thoracic segment total transection at the 2nd lumbar segment was performed when the animal was full grown. Behind the later section " as many fibres degenerated on the semi-section side as on the intact." Fibres therefore arising in the 1st lumbar segment course backward thence. In a recent paper, Münzer and Wiener,[3] referring again to the same experiment, furnish a figure illustrating the position of the fibres in a cross-section in the lumbar region. This important experiment still remains a single one, and deals only with the lumbar region of the cord, but its authors announce that they will give its full publication later in a paper dealing systematically with endogenous spinal fibres. Rothmann[4] has noted that embolism of the lumbar spinal arteries produces descending degeneration in the region of the pyramidal tract, and argues that the fibres involved arise in spinal nerve-cells.

METHODS EMPLOYED

Our own observations have been on the dog and cat. The spinal lesions have in every instance been made under deep $CHCl_3$ narcosis. The resulting conditions have been examined and tested altogether subsequent to the surgical procedure. Where the tracing of intraspinal paths by the microscope has been among our aims we have employed the Wallerian degeneration in a special way to meet the conditions required. For our purpose the degeneration following a simple translesion in the spinal cord is inadequate. The degeneration then produced in the cord behind the lesion befalls alike all nerve-fibres with perikarya headward of the translesion, whether those perikarya be cerebral, cerebellar, bulbar, or spinal. It is then impossible to identify which, if any, of the degenerate fibres have origin in cord-segments, the special object of inquiry.

To obviate this difficulty we have had recourse to a method which may be termed that of "successive degeneration." Two or more degenerations are evoked successively with allowance of an interval of time between them. The interval allowed is sufficient for all evidence of the earlier degeneration, as examined by Marchi's method, to have disappeared from the region of the cord in which degeneration due to the second lesion is to

---

[1] Bouchard, *Arch. générales de Méd.*, 1866, **6**, sér. vii., p. 272, etc.; N. Löwenthal, *Dissert. Genève*, 1885; Sherrington, *J. Physiol.*, 1885, **6**, 177; v. Monakow, *Archiv für Psych.*, 1890, **22**, 1; and others.
[2] *Prag. med. Wochenschr.*, 1895, p. 481.   [3] *Monatschr. f. Psych. u. Neurolog.*, 1902, **12**, 241.
[4] *Loc. cit.*

be traced.   An interval of 260 days in the cord of the dog suffices according to our experience for this period.   Periods tried by us and found insufficient have been 90 days, 130, 150, 180, and 200 days.   Two hundred days subsequent to the translesion of the cord in the posterior cervical region there are still traces of degenerative *débris* in the anterior thoracic segments.   But the amount of *débris* then persisting is quite small, constituting only sparse traces in the cross-sections.   An observation which especially fortified our confidence in a period of 260 days for disembarrassment of the cord from all fatty *débris* is given in the protocol quoted in our paper as Exp. 6.   In that experiment we exsected the 12th thoracic segment 260 days after exsecting the 1st thoracic.   The exsected 12th thoracic segment, carefully hardened and stained by Marchi's process, when examined in serial preparations, revealed to the microscope no myelin *débris* in its cross-sections.   The " scar " of the degeneration was obvious enough, but the fatty *débris*, for which Marchi's reaction is specific, had disappeared in the interval allowed between the two surgical operations.   The numerous other experiments that we have made have never given any reason to suspect that in the dog's cord for the lesions studied by us 260 days is insufficient for clearing up the fatty *débris* of the spinal degeneration.

Our experiments were begun in 1897.   Several of the experiments individually extended over a twelvemonth.   We communicated a brief note on our earlier results to the Liverpool Medical Institution in 1900 (*British Med. J.*, Feb. 15, **1**, 446).   These results were also mentioned in an article on the Spinal Cord, Schäfer's *Textbook of Physiology*, vol. ii., p. 805, 1900, and Allchin's *Manual of Medicine*, vol. iii., Physiological Introduction, p. 16, also a figure, Pl. II.   A short summary of our later results was communicated to the Royal Society, November, 1902 (*Proc. roy. Soc.* 1902, **71**, 115).   Preparations illustrating the degenerations were demonstrated at the Meeting of the Physiological Society, November 8, 1902.

RESULTS

Before proceeding to protocols of experiments it is necessary to state what we employ certain terms to mean.   The spinal cord may, in its relation to the sensifacient surface and the skeletal musculature, be considered divisible into right and left lateral halves, each subdivisible into regions of neck (cervical) including pinna; fore-limb (brachial); trunk (thoracic); hind-limb (crural); and tail (caudal).   " A reflex action in which the stimulus applied to a reflexigenous area in one of the above regions evokes a reaction in the musculature of another of the regions is conveniently called a *long spinal* reflex.   A reflex reaction in which the muscular reply occurs in the same region as the *locus* of the stimulus is conveniently termed a ' *short spinal* ' reflex."   We have used the terms " long " and " short " reflex in this sense.

Long Reflexes

Of " long " spinal reflexes, those specially useful to this research have been four.   Brief general remarks concerning these save repetition in the subjoined extracts from protocols.

(i) Stimulation of the mid-dorsal skin of the " spinal " dog near the shoulder sometimes elicits simultaneous movement in all the limbs: the pair of hind-limbs are moved symmetrically, so also the fore-limbs. With the cord severed in the mid-brachial region, the movement in the fore-limbs is retraction at shoulder, extension at elbow, in the hind-limbs flexion at hips and knees. From the skin in the mid-ventral line at the same zonal level, a similar reflex can more rarely be evoked. The hind-limb portion of this reflex obviously employs " long " spinal paths passing aborally.

(ii) The " shake " reflex (mentioned by Goltz and Ewald[1]) evoked by rubbing the skin at or near the mid-dorsum, especially between the shoulders, or in the loin, or over the sacrum. The movement resembles the " shake " given by a dog when it comes out of water, but in our spinal animals it was mainly confined to the rump and tail. If started from the skin well to one side of the mid-line of the back it can be seen that the first movement carries the rump toward that side, the spine curving concavely to that side. It appears to be an " alternating " movement of muscles symmetrically disposed to right and left of the mid-plane. With dogs in which the spinal transection has been cervical the " shake " is sometimes, when the stimulus is applied at the junction of the æsthetic with the " spinal " skin-field, evoked contemporaneously in the neck and in the trunk and rump: it is then wholly reflex in the spinal part of the animal and reflexo-conscient in the intact part of the animal. This seems to show that the " purpose " of the reflex is really the same as is that of the " shaking " (e.g., to get rid of certain skin stimuli) in the perfect animal. The shake-reflex sometimes succeeds micturition and defæcation in the spinal animal.

(iii) The " scratching " reflex. *Stimulus*; rubbing or scratching the skin: *movement*; rapidly alternating flexion and extension at knee and ankle, and less at hip. The reflex movement usually begins with plantar flexion of the digits so that the foot becomes claw-shaped, and with flexion and protraction at hip; some flexion at hip and digits is more or less maintained throughout the duration of the reflex. Goltz,[2] Haycraft,[3] and Goltz and Ewald[4] have called attention to this reflex. The field of skin whence it can be initiated in dogs with mid-cervical transection includes the hind-part of the back of the neck, a zone of skin round the front of the chest, the surface over the scapula, the side of the chest, the axillary fold over the triceps, the loin and the flank, meaning by the latter the dorso-lateral abdominal wall nearly down to the hip. The frequency of the rhythm of the scratching movement little if at all depends on the rate of the scratchings of the stimulus, but the frequency seems greater when the reflex is strongly elicited than when feebly. If instead of a rubbing or moving (intermittent) stimulus one steady touch or pinch is employed the reflex movement elicited is usually a short series (2-6) of " scratching " flexions and extensions. Thus it is only the outset of the constant stimulus that is effective, although the

[1] *Pflüg. Arch. ges. Physiol.*, 1896, **63**, 362.   [2] *Verrichtungen des Grosshirns*, Strassburg, 1881, p. 98.
[3] *Brain*, 1890, **12**, 516.   [4] *Pflüg. Arch. ges. Physiol.*, 1896, **63**, 362.

reflex movement excited evidently tends to repeat itself when once it has been started. The reflex is uncrossed—*i.e.*, rubbing the right scapular region throws the right hind-limb, not the left, into " scratching " movement. The unilaterality is so marked that rubbing the skin just to the right of the mid-dorsum having thrown the right leg into " scratching," a shifting of the application of the stimulus by 3 per cent. so as to lie just the other side of the mid-line stops the right leg and starts the left one.   Bilateral rubbing of the scapular or other parts of the field does not in our experience succeed in evoking the reflex bilaterally, the reflex remaining unilateral, but shifting from time to time from one side to the other and back again. The reflex of the crossed side seems regularly cut short by the stimulus that evokes the uncrossed reflex.   This indicates that part of the reflex is some maintained posturing of the crossed hind-limb, which inhibits a scratching movement there or prevents access to it of the impulses eliciting the scratching movements.   This would be an instance of the same kind as the throwing out of action of one group of muscles coincidently with the establishment of activity in another correlated group such as has been studied in the reciprocal innervation of antagonistic muscles.

In spinal dogs this reflex is enormously exaggerated, vigorous, and facile. In one dog we found it elicitable by application close behind either shoulder of a hair-æsthesiometer (v. Frey) of the value of 0·02 grm.   It is common where such dogs are kept to hear a rhythmic hammering noise in the stalls: a chance stimulus (straw, some shifting of the animal as it feeds, etc.) initiates the reflex, and the rhythmically acting limb, which generally falls short of the trunk in its range of excursion, beats the floor or a side of the stall.   The place to which the paw of the scratching limb is brought near by the reflex movement distinctly varies with the " locus " of application of the stimulus: the paw is carried further forward when the stimulus is further forward; the paw is carried further dorsally when the stimulus is applied more dorsally.   This influence of the " locus " of the stimulus, which has long been studied in the " spinal " frog, is thus demonstrable in the " spinal " mammal.

The reflex once initiated will generally continue of itself long after cessation of the cutaneous stimulus that called it forth.   It continues with about the same frequency of rhythm as that obtaining during the skin stimulation. We have timed it to continue three and a half minutes after the skin stimulus ceased.   If continuance occurs when the limb is so placed that in the execution of the movement it touches neither another part of the body nor any other object—*e.g.*, when the hip is kept, as it often is, very little moved by the scratching, but only steadily flexed and protracted, the skin of the trunk adjacent to the hip is really little moved or otherwise influenced by the movement. Yet the reflex continues to be " self-supporting." This is suggestive in connection with the following fact.   The reflex is rapidly stilled by gently confining the movement of the limb; the excursions at once begin to dwindle and rapidly the movement ceases.   It may therefore well be that this " alternating " movement is kept up reflexly by mechanical stimulation of the afferent nerves of muscles and joints involved in the movement. Inasmuch as the reflex is a rapidly alternating one of antagonistic muscles the play of reciprocal innervation would go far to account for the phenomenon. The same afferent impulses that excited the extensor muscle would depress the flexor action; the subsequent stretch of the flexor by the active extensor would lead to temporary inhibition of the extensor's activity, accompanied by incitement to action of the flexor itself. The automatic continuance of the " scratch " reflex seems in fact just the phenomenon that observations by one of us on the reciprocal correlation of antagonistic muscles would suggest.

This reflex does not usually emerge from the " shock " following cervical transection for several days. We have, however, sometimes met with it within twenty-four hours after the transection, especially in quite young puppies, and once in an oldish dog habitually scratching itself prior to operation because suffering from eczema of the skin.

On certain occasions we have noted that rubbing skin in the neck innervated from spinal nerves indubitably headward of the spinal transection produced scratching movements in the hind-limb. In all such observations we have been able to detect that the rubbing in front of the " spinal " field of skin obviously caused considerable to and fro displacement of the soft parts and skin in the " spinal " field. Hence in our opinion the scratch reflex. We mention this as it probably elucidates some of the phenomena of extreme zigzag conduction along the spinal cord of the dog as argued by Osawa from his triple contralateral lesions.[1]

(iv) " Hand-foot " reflex. With spinal transection far forward enough to include the fore-paw in the spinal region, stimulation of the fore-paw elicits movement in the hind-limb. The movement in the hind-limb usually is flexion at hip, knee, and ankle, the limb being raised and brought forward as though to take a step.[2] There is usually with this a movement of the crossed hind-limb as well, but feebler and opposite in character —namely, retraction and extension. The stimulus to the fore-paw excites movement in the fore-limb itself; this movement with the translesion at the 6th or 7th cervical segment is retraction at shoulder, extension at elbow, and sometimes plantar flexion at wrist. The reflex rarely irradiates to the crossed fore-limb. The above remarks apply to the reflex in the dog. In the cat we have studied it less, but found it possess the same general features. In regard to whether the path of conduction from the fore-paw to the crossed hind-paw is blocked or not blocked by spinal semi-section at the hind-end of the thoracic on the same side as the fore-paw stimulated, in our observations the path is not altogether blocked; this is somewhat contrary to Luchsinger's observation[3] on the cat, but agrees with his observation on the goat.

[1] *Inaug. Dissert.*, Strassburg, 1882, and comment, Schäfer's *Textbook of Physiology*, 1900, **2**, 866.
[2] Sherrington, *J. Physiol.*, 1897, **22**, 319.　　　　[3] *Pflüg. Arch. ges. Physiol.*, 1882, **28**, 61.

Short Reflexes

In our observations the " short " reflexes of the hind-limbs were of interest chiefly as indicating the presence or absence of " shock " in the " crural " centres of the cord. They are therefore frequently mentioned in the observations, and it saves tedious repetition to indicate each by a name and simply record its presence, its absence, or its condition. The following are the " short " reflexes thus dealt with: (1) The " flexion " reflex, noted by Freusberg[1] and others, a flexion at ankle, knee, and hip in response to stimulation of the hind-foot of the same leg. (2) " Crossed extension " reflex, noted by Freusberg,[2] extension at knee and hip in response to stimulation of the opposite hind-foot; when it occurs it is almost always or always in the accompaniment to (1). (3) " Direct extension " reflex, noted by one of us,[3] obtained by gentle pressure between the pads of the hind-paw. The limb itself being at the time passively flexed at hip and knee, the stimulus excites a rapid, powerful, short-lasting extension at both these joints (" extensor thrust "). (4) " Marking time " reflex, noted by Freusberg;[4] when the dog is held up by the shoulders so that the hind-limbs hang down, those limbs begin to make " walking " movements, flexion in one leg accompanying extension in the other. (5) " Tail-wagging " reflex,[5] excited by pinching side of tail or holding tip of tail, or in succession to defæcation or micturition. (6) " Depression of tail "[6] reflex, induced by touching skin of under surface of tail or of perineum, especially in neighbourhood of anus or vulva. (7) " Lifting of tail " reflex,[7] induced by stimulation of mucosa inside anus, by defæcation and micturition (in the female). (8) Spinal defæcation; for an account of this in the dog see Schäfer's *Textbook*, vol. ii., p. 850, to which we would only add the following: Vertebral muscles which flex the lumbo-sacral region of the spine ventrally are in strong continuous action; the tail is, however, raised and flexed dorsally; towards the completion of the act of evacuation a sudden forcible bilateral and short-lasting contraction of the great part of the ventral abdominal muscles ensues, which often finishes the evacuation: the evacuation is followed by spinal extension of both the hind-limbs (previously held in the bent everted posture described by Freusberg) and waving of the tail: micturition, if imminent when defæcation sets in, is postponed. (9) Spinal micturition; see Goltz and Freusberg.[8] We would add that in our animals this act has usually been evoked by hand-pressure on the abdomen, and that it is easier to evoke the act thus and to expel the urine thus in dogs

[1] *Pflüg. Arch. ges. Physiol.*, 1874, **9,** 358.   [2] *Ibid.*
[3] Sherrington, *Proc. roy. Soc.*, 1900, **66,** 66 (p. 155 this vol.). Later called " extensor thrust " (*Integrative Action,* 1906).   [4] *Loc. cit.*
[5] Freusberg, *ibid.*; see also L. Merzbacher, *Pflüg. Arch. ges. Physiol.*, 1902, **92,** 585.
[6] V. Ducceschi, *Riv. Patol. nerv. ment.*, 1898, **3,** 241; L. Merzbacher, *Pflüg. Arch., loc. cit.*
[7] Ott, *J. Physiol.*, 1879, **2,** 54; Bickel, *Rev. Med. d. l. Suisse romande*, 1897; V. Ducceschi, *Riv. di Patol. nerv. ment., loc. cit.*; Sherrington, Schäfer's *Textbook of Physiol.*, **2,** 850; L. Merzbacher, *loc. cit.*
[8] *Pflüg. Arch. ges. Physiol.*, 1874, **8,** 478, and 1874, **9,** 360.

with lumbar transection than in dogs with cervical or high thoracic transection. The ease with which the bladder can be emptied by hand-pressure on the abdomen serves as some guide to degree of shock after spinal transection.

Summaries and Extracts from Protocols of Some Experiments

The figures illustrating the protocols are all of them camera lucida drawings to one and the same scale. They were drawn on squared paper and the squares made to correspond with squares in an engraved microscope-ocular; this allows contiguous fields under a higher magnification to be accurately conjoined in the same map. In dealing with the lesions the drawing has been made from the section where the lesion had greatest transverse extent, and then there has been added the extreme limits of the lesion from the particular sections in which in various directions those limits happened to lie. To give the limits of the lesion at any *one* level is, of course, to underestimate in nearly every case the real

Table of Experiments Cited in Original Paper

(Only 1, 2, 3, 4, 5, 7, 13, *reprinted here*)

	L.R.			L.R.			L.R.
Exp. 1	$+ T_1$		Exp. 7	$+ T_2$		Exp. 13	$+ C_8$
	$\vdash L_4$			$\vdash T_{11}$			$\vdash T_3$
,, 2	$+ L_{1\text{-}2}$		,, 8	$+ C_7$		,, 14	$+ C_6$
	$\vdash L_3$			$\vdash T_{10}$			$\vdash T_{10}$
,, 3	$+ T_{13}$		,, 10	$+ C_7$		,, 15	$+ C_5$
	$\vdash L_2$			$\vdash T_{12}$			$\vdash T_{10}$
,, 4	$+ T_1$		,, 11	$+ T_2$		,, 16	$\dashv C_4$
	$\dashv T_{12}$			$\vdash T_9$			$+ T_4$
,, 5	$+ C_8$		,, 12	$+ T_5$		,, 17	$\vdash C_6$
	$\vdash T_{13}$			$\dashv T_7$			$+ C_8$
,, 6	$+ T_1$						
	$+ T_{12}$						

Total translesion	$= +$	C = cervical
Partial ,,	(left) = $\vdash$	T = thoracic
,, ,,	(right) = $\dashv$	L = lumbar

The small numerals indicate the regional number of the segments.

transverse extent of the lesion. The dots in the figures signify degenerate nerve-fibres, but the number of dots does not, of course, represent the absolute number of degenerate fibres, but falls far short of that. Extreme care has been taken to make the number of the dots bear accurately the same general proportion in one drawing as in another to the density of the degeneration. In the reproduction of the drawings for this paper the reduction has been to one-quarter the original size.

EXPERIMENT I.—Terrier ♀.

First lesion: exsection of 1st thoracic segment for the posterior half of its length.

Two hundred and fifty days later: knee jerks very brisk and usually clonic; " *short* " *reflexes* of hind-limbs all very vigorous and facile; " flexion " reflex, " direct extension " reflex, " crossed extension " reflex, " marking time " reflex. Also " wagging " tail and depression of tail, and anal and vulval reflexes. Urine evacuated daily by hand-pressure on abdomen; defæcation usually accompanies micturition. Membrane nictitantes protruded, pupils small. Temperature not maintained in rooms at ordinary temperature, but more controlled than formerly (room is always warmed to 82° to 88° F.). "*Long*" reflexes: " scratch " and " shake " brisk.

Second lesion: right semi-section in 4th lumbar segment. Exact limits determined post-mortem in microscopic serial preparations—result mapped in Fig. 24, IV. L. Immediately on recovery from CHCl₃ narcosis right knee jerk not elicitable, left with great uncertainty and feebly. Right leg hung less flexed at hip and knee than left. No reflexes, either long or short, in either hind-limb.

Two days later: knee jerk absent on right side, but brisk left side, though not so brisk as prior to second lesion. Right limb now the more flexed at hip and knee. Stimuli

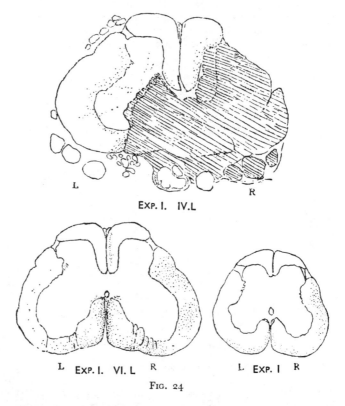

Exp. I. IV.L

L Exp. I. VI. L R   L Exp. I R

Fig. 24

(squeezing, pinching, rubbing, faradising) to right foot elicit no muscular response in the right limb, but evoke slight dorsi-flexion at crossed ankle. A tap on the right knee extensor tendon evokes crossed adductor action, and often crossed dorsi-flexion of ankle, but no response on right side. Stimuli to the left foot elicit dorsi-flexion of left ankle and slight flexion of left knee, but no crossed movements.

Twenty-one days after second operation condition was much the same as on the second day, except that by stimuli to left foot more vigorous flexion-reflex of left leg was obtained. By stimuli to the right hind-foot and knee good reflexes were elicitable from the left limb; but the motor response was confined to the crossed side. By stimuli to the left hind-foot motor responses were obtained in the left leg, but no crossed ones in the right leg. On holding the dog up by shoulders the left leg marked time feebly, but the right did not. The scratch reflex was elicitable from the left shoulder-skin in the left leg, but

from the right shoulder no scratch reflex was elicited in the right leg.   Bladder less easily
emptied than before second lesion.

Degenerations.—Fig. 24.   Behind the second lesion, at IV. L, a copious degeneration
was found in the lateral and ventral columns; this involved fibres especially numerous in
the lip of the ventral fissure, in the dorso-lateral part of the lateral column, and near the
exit of the ventral root-fibres.   Close to the lesion it involved many fibres near the grey
matter, as well as a considerable number along the free periphery of the white columns.
The degenerate fibres diminished in number rapidly through the lowest lumbar and
upper sacral segments, but even in the caudal region the degenerate fibres were numerous.
In the segments behind the 1st sacral the region of the white matter abutting on the grey
was comparatively free from degenerate fibres.   At no level did the ventral column
degeneration become separated from that of the lateral column by a distinct intervening
width of white matter free from degeneration; but in the lower sacral and coccygeal
segments the degeneration was more sparse in the ventro-lateral angle of the column
than elsewhere in the cross-area.

In the dorsal column of the right side a narrow field of degeneration near the median
septum was traceable, gradually diminishing in amount, as far back as the 2nd caudal
segment—*i.e.*, through seven segments.

EXPERIMENT 2.—Terrier ♀.

First lesion: total exsection of the posterior part of the 1st lumbar and of the anterior
part of the 2nd lumbar segment.

Condition 270 days later: knee jerks very brisk, often clonic; short reflexes very active—
e.g., " marking time " reflex, " flexion " reflex, " extension " reflex, " tail-wagging "

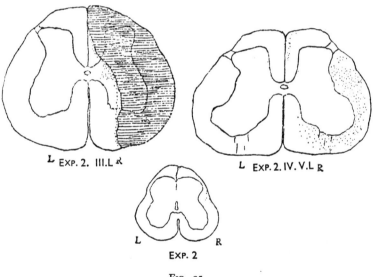

L EXP. 2. III.L ℛ   L EXP. 2. IV. V.L R

L   R

EXP. 2

FIG. 25

reflex.   Bladder easily emptied by hand-pressure on abdomen.   Micturition and defæcation accompanied by the usual reflexes in tail and hind-limbs.   Second operation then
proceeded with; a partial transverse lesion in the posterior part of the right lateral half
of the 3rd lumbar segment.   The exact extent of the lesion as ultimately determined in
serial sections is shown in Fig. 25, III. L.   The day following the second lesion the knee
jerk was good and about equal on either side, the " flexion " reflex and the " extension "

reflex were obtainable and about equally strong in either leg; the " marking time " reflex was as vigorous as before in the left leg, but much less extensive in the right. " Tail-wagging " reflex as before. Eight days later the " marking time " reflex is still imperfect on the right side; crossed extension is equally well obtained from either side; other reflexes as before. Twelve days after the second lesion " flexion " reflex was obtainable on application to either foot of a v. Frey hair equal to 20 milligrams; the application was to the skin between the toes. Animal sacrificed thirty days after the second lesion—*i.e.*, 300 days after the first lesion.

The degeneration examined by the Marchi method was traceable behind the second lesion throughout the length of the cord in the lateral column. Its distribution in the cross-area of the cord is shown in Fig. 25, IV., V. L, one full segment below the second lesion. As traced backward it rapidly diminished in the lumbo-sacral enlargement, and came to occupy more and more a peripheral position. Far back in the caudal region it is seen (Fig. 25) only in the dorso-lateral part of the edge of the lateral column, a position free from degenerate fibres in the mid-lumbar region. A small well-marked band of degeneration extends along the right dorsal column (Fig. 25, V. L), and as traced back comes to lie in the dorso-median angle of the dorsal column. No degeneration was found anywhere in the side of the cord opposite to the lesion.

EXPERIMENT 3.—Dog, terrier, ♀.

First lesion: total exsection of the posterior half of the 13th thoracic segment.

Two hundred and sixty-eight days later the condition was: knee jerks brisk, and often clonic; " short " reflexes all extremely vigorous and elicitable, covered by description given in Experiment 2. The second lesion established—namely, partial transection on the

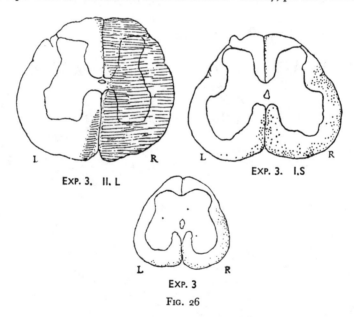

EXP. 3. II. L

EXP. 3. I.S

EXP. 3

FIG. 26

right side in the posterior part of the 2nd lumbar segment. The limits of the lesion as subsequently determined by microscopic examination of serial sections of the cord are given in Fig. 26, II. L. After the semi-section the " direct extension " reflex was obtained from the leg of the same side as the semi-section. The afternoon of the day of the second lesion the reflexes were as before the second lesion, except that (i) the right knee jerk was slightly less brisk than the left, (ii) the " flexion " reflex was impaired on the right side, (iii) the " marking time " reflex was much feebler with the right than with the left leg. One week later the knee jerks were equal and brisk, the " extension " reflex was about equally good right as left, the " marking time " reflex was less vigorous right than left, and did not continue so long. The " crossed extension " reflex of left knee was obtained from right foot better than that of right knee from left foot, and the " flexion " reflex of right leg was less than that of left leg. The animal remained in this condition and was sacrificed on the twenty-second day after the second lesion, and at that time the " marking time " reflex was still less vigorous right than left.

Degeneration.—In the whole length of the cord behind the second lesion degenerate fibres existed in both ventral columns, and in the right lateral and dorsal columns. The degeneration diminished much in amount in passing through the lumbo-sacral enlargement of the cord, and came to occupy a more and more peripheral position in the ventro-lateral columns (Fig. 26, I. S). The posterior sacral and caudal region revealed the degenerate fibres grouped mainly along the ventral part of the lips of the ventral fissure, and in the dorso-lateral part of the lateral column of the right side except in the region abutting on the dorsal root and apex of the dorsal grey horn. The degeneration in the dorsal column agreed closely with that described and figured in Experiment 2. The topography of the degeneration in the caudal region is shown in Fig. 26.

EXPERIMENT 4.—Dog ♀.

First lesion: total transection midway between 8th cervical and 1st thoracic nerve-roots.

Second lesion: 100 days after the former lesion, a partial semi-section on the left side in the 12th thoracic segment; the exact transverse extent of this lesion is shown in Fig. 27, XII. T, as determined by subsequent microscopic examination of serial sections. The condition just prior to the second operation: " short " reflexes of the hind-limbs all vigorous and easily obtained. " Long " reflexes: " scratch " obtainable equally well either side, " shake " reflex obtainable, but not so readily. Evacuation of bladder by pressure on abdomen gives the usual reflexes. Second operation performed in the afternoon under

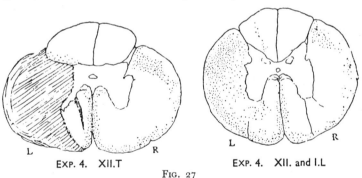

EXP. 4.   XII.T   EXP. 4.   XII. and I.L

FIG. 27

anæsthesia. Examination the same afternoon showed the knee jerks equal and brisk, perhaps even more brisk than before, the " flexion " reflex good each side. Next morning early: extension reflex from pad well obtained from right leg, poorly obtained from left. " Marking time " reflex less strong in left leg than right. " Flexion " reflex and " crossed extension " reflex good both right and left. " Scratch " reflex elicited in right and left (?) legs from right shoulder, but in neither leg from left shoulder.

Twelve days later: same condition as above; further details observed have been: pinching skin in mid-ventral line near umbilicus elicited bilateral flexion of hips and knees; the " extension " reflex from right leg is sometimes accompanied by flexion of left leg at hip and knee; the scratch reflex is easily obtained by rubbing anywhere in a large area of skin over and behind the right shoulder, and the scratching movement appears to implicate sometimes the musculature of the left as well as the right leg; but from the similar skin area of the left side nowhere has scratching ever been elicited since the second operation. The shake reflex is obtainable by rubbing skin between the shoulders. The blood-pressure in the femoral, which had been frequently estimated by Hill's sphygmomanometer at about 120 mm. Hg, was not obviously affected in any way by the second lesion.

Animal sacrificed thirty days after second operation—*i.e.*, 130 days after the first operation. Blood-pressure in carotid measured and recorded by kymograph and varied between 118 mm. Hg and 146 mm. Hg. under anæsthesia. After curare it rose to a mean value of 168 mm. Hg. The two vagi were cut. Good reflex heightenings of the carotid blood-pressure were elicited by stimulating branches of the internal saphenous and other nerves. A total transection through the 3rd thoracic segment caused a temporary rise of carotid pressure followed by a fall of only 6 mm. Hg below where it had previously stood, and that fall was in six minutes recovered from, so that the pressure was as before the fresh transection. The reflex rises of carotid pressure were also obtainable as well after as before the transection at 3rd thoracic.

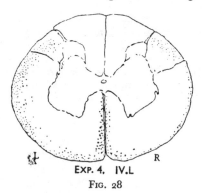

EXP. 4.   IV.L

FIG. 28

Degeneration.—Behind the second lesion the degeneration found was far heavier in the left half of the cord than in the right. It was found that the degeneration caused by the total transection in the cervical region was still very evident throughout the cord. But the excess of degenerate fibres in the left half of the cord as compared with the right throughout the region posterior to the second lesion demonstrates the existence of numbers of fibres arising in the anterior twelve thoracic segments which pass backward thence throughout the lumbo-sacral and caudal regions. These fibres rapidly diminish in number as they pass through the lumbo-sacral region. In the left dorsal column a small curved area shows degenerate fibres in the 13th thoracic segment (Fig. 27, I. L) and traces of the same tract can be followed to the 3rd lumbar segment. The dorsal columns were not actually trespassed upon by the second lesion anywhere; the left dorsal column descending degeneration must therefore have sprung from cells in the grey matter of the left half of the 12th thoracic segment.

EXPERIMENT 5.—Dog, rather old, ♀.

First lesion: total exsection of a slice at the posterior end of the 8th cervical segment.

Second lesion: right semi-section close behind the 13th right thoracic nerve-root; the transverse extent of the lesion as determined by subsequent microscopic examination in serial sections is mapped in Fig. 29, XIII. T; it was found to be very nearly an absolutely accurate semi-section. The condition of the animal as regards reflexes, etc., just prior to the second operation was so similar to that already mentioned in Experiment 4 that no particular record of it seems necessary except that the " tail-wagging " reflex was extraordinarily active in this animal. Also noteworthy was that the scratch reflex elicitable from the skin of shoulder and actuating the muscles of homonymous hind-limb was obtainable as early as twenty-four hours after the cervical translesion. The " scratch" reflex was elicitable from a large region of skin extending from over the shoulder right down to the flank; the " shake " reflex was similarly elicitable, but only from skin near the mid-dorsal line. Immediately—*i.e.*, ten minutes—after the second lesion the knee jerks right and left were as brisk as before, and the right perhaps even more brisk. Three hours later the " short " leg reflexes were as before the second operation, except that the " extension " reflex was not good on the right side. The "scratch" reflex could not be elicited from the right shoulder or from the right side of the chest or upper loin, but was easily elicited from the right lower loin and flank. The scratch reflex was elicitable as before from the left shoulder, left chest, left loin and flank. The shake reflex also was not obtainable from the right dorsal region, though from the left as before. These conditions remained unaltered to end of experiment. Twenty-eight days after the second operation the animal was chloroformed, the carotid blood-pressure measured and found to be 120 to 136 mm. Hg

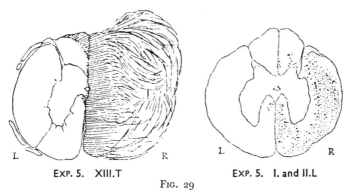

EXP. 5.   XIII.T   EXP. 5.   I. and II.L

FIG. 29

under curare. Good reflex elevations of blood-pressure were obtained by stimulation of various afferent nerves from hind-limbs, etc. Total transection of the cord at the 4th thoracic level caused a rise of blood-pressure followed by a very slight (10 mm. Hg) fall of transient duration (140"). Good reflex elevations of carotid pressure were evoked by excitation of afferent nerves from the hind-limbs after the fresh total transection at the 4th thoracic level. Both vagi had been cut prior to the blood-pressure experiment.

Degeneration.—In the right half of the cord behind the second lesion the degenerate fibres are found in the ventro-lateral columns the whole length of the cord and for a shorter

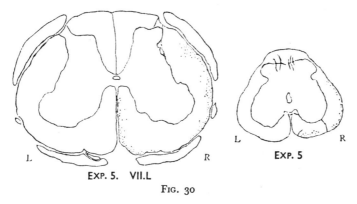

EXP. 5.   VII.L   EXP. 5

FIG. 30

distance in the dorsal column. Many of the degenerate fibres are even in the foremost lumbar segments at the periphery of the ventro-lateral columns (Fig. 29, I. L). The degenerate fibres rapidly decrease in number in their course along the lumbo-sacral region. At the posterior part of the lumbar and the anterior part of the sacral region they exist as two distinct groups, a lateral along the free edge of the lateral column and a ventral along the medio-ventral edge of the ventral column (Fig. 30, VII. L). In the caudal region the ventral group lies less in the lip of the ventral fissure, and the ventral and lateral groups of degenerate fibres are less separated by an intervening undegenerate piece of the periphery. Noteworthy is that, although the dorso-median piece of the left dorsal column was divided by the second lesion, no descending tract of degeneration is evident in that column. There are two small descending tracts of degeneration traceable in the right dorsal column from close behind the lesion in the 13th thoracic segment back to the 5th lumbar segment.

The left half of the cord is practically quite free from degeneration if a few fibres near the ventral white commissure in the neighbourhood of the lesion be excepted. The descending axons of the neurones of the thoracic segments as examined behind the thoracic region itself appears none of them therefore to decussate.

EXPERIMENT 7.—An oldish dog ♀.

First lesion: total exsection of about half the length of the 2nd thoracic segment.

Second lesion: liberal right semi-section just behind 11th right thoracic root, 270 days after the total transection of 2nd thoracic. The condition of the animal prior to the second operation was much like that above mentioned for the dogs with total translesion at the front of the thoracic region. The " short " reflexes of the hind-limbs and the tail, the actions of micturition and defæcation, the " long " reflexes of " scratch " and " shake " were all present and often very active; the knee jerks were very brisk. Less control over temperature was seen in this dog than in others with front thoracic or posterior cervical translesion. The animal shivered with the musculature in front of the total translesion only—i.e., when shivering either after cold bath or in cold air; the musculature innervated from behind the total translesion was never seen to participate in the shivering; the diaphragm seemed to shiver. This animal showed rutting in the spring, and shed its coat then as usual.

The exact transverse limits of the second lesion are mapped in Fig. 31, XI. T, as determined subsequently by microscopic examination of serial microtomed preparations. One hour after the second operation the right leg drooped at hip and knee more than the left when the animal was supported from the shoulders. " Flexion " reflex with crossed extension was easily obtained from either leg; extension reflex was not obtained either side, but not very persistently sought. The scratch reflex was easily obtained from the left shoulder and left chest, upper and lower, and elsewhere, exciting the muscles of the left leg; but from the right side nowhere could the scratch reflex either in the right or left leg be elicited. The bladder offered much greater opposition to evacuation than before the operation. Knee jerks both sides very brisk.

Next morning: both knee jerks very brisk, but right seems slightly the more so. " Extension " reflex easily obtainable in either leg. " Marking time " reflex slower and less vigorous in right than left leg. Scratch reflex only obtainable on left side. Bladder evacuated less easily than formerly.

In the following twenty-eight days during which the animal was observed the condition remained as above, with slight modification as follows: the evacuation of the bladder by pressure became easier; the " extension " reflex became more facile, and easy right and left; a slow extension, chiefly at knee, could be developed by handling the skin below and outside the anterior superior iliac spine; the vigour and facility of the left scratch reflex seemed to be increased more than ever, so that once started it often continued for three and four minutes at a time, and was often started by some active or passive movement of the animal as it lay in its cage; slight traces of a scratch reflex on the right side became regularly elicitable, but always were feeble and difficult to evoke; the rhythm of the alternating movement of foot and hip was much slower than on the opposite side, and the movement much less extensive. This trace of the right " scratch " reflex was obtainable from the skin behind the right shoulder, also from the skin of the right loin— i.e., probably behind the second (semi-section) lesion. It was often noted that the execution of the left " scratch " reflex could coexist with the execution of the " marking time " reflex on the right side. The scratch reflex, even when violent, could almost at once be cut short by gently restraining the limb. It could also be cut short usually by pinching the shin below the tuber ischii or, less efficiently, the tail.

Animal sacrificed on the three-hundredth day after establishment of the first lesion.

Degeneration.—In the whole length of the cord behind the second lesion are degenerate fibres in the right lateral and both ventral columns. These decrease in number rapidly in the lumbar region. In the posterior lumbar and sacral regions, those of them remaining

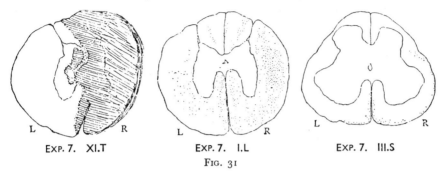

EXP. 7. XI.T   EXP. 7. I.L   EXP. 7. III.S

FIG. 31

exist as ventral groups and lateral groups, and this is so also in the front part of the caudal region (Fig. 31, III. S), where it is also notable that practically all the fibres lie near the periphery of the cord. The topography of the degenerate axons at their entrance into the lumbar region is mapped in Fig. 31, I. L. There is absence at that level of degenerate fibres in much of the margin of the lip of the ventral fissure. Two pairs of degenerate descending tracts are revealed in the dorsal columns, the right hand of these traceable backward along the cord as far as the 6th lumbar segment.

EXPERIMENT 13.—Dog ♀.

First lesion: exsection of the middle part of the length of the 8th cervical segment.

Second lesion: liberal left semi-section in the front half of the 3rd thoracic segment. The extent of this lesion transversely is shown in Fig. 32, III. T; the whole of the left

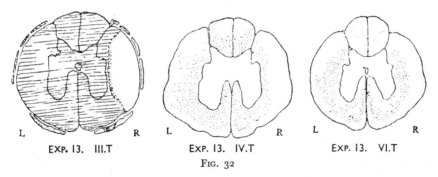

EXP. 13. III.T   EXP. 13. IV.T   EXP. 13. VI.T

FIG. 32

side was severed and the part indicated on the right. The second lesion was practised 568 days subsequent to the first lesion. The condition of the animal as regards reflexes, etc., was, prior to the second operation, so similar to that mentioned above of dogs with total spinal transection at the front of the thoracic region as not to require further description here. The hind-limb reflexes, short and long, were present and very brisk. The animal shivered only with the musculature in front of the spinal lesion and with the diaphragm. The animal showed rut, and shed its hair in two successive springs. The second lesion caused little or no obvious interference with the short reflexes of the hind-limbs. The animal was sacrificed twenty-one days after the second lesion—*i.e.*, 589 days subsequent to exsection of the 8th cervical segment.

Degeneration.—Behind the second lesion in the left lateral and in both ventral columns degenerate fibres can be traced throughout the entire length of the cord. These fibres diminish considerably in number in coursing along the thoracic region, and many cease in the five anterior lumbar segments, especially, I think, in the 3rd, 4th, and 5th. In these latter segments these fibres lie in two groups—a ventral and a lateral on either side.

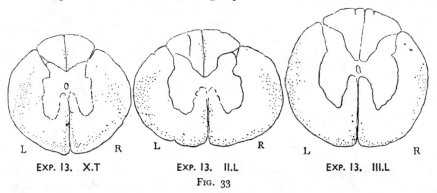

L   EXP. 13. X.T   R   L   EXP. 13. II.L   R   L   EXP. 13. III.L   R

Fig. 33

In the caudal region degenerate fibres cannot be traced as far backward in the right lateral column as in the left lateral or in either ventral column, showing that among the fibres in the outer lateral part of the lateral column at the 3rd thoracic level are some which arise not further headward than the 1st thoracic segment and extend backward into the posterior part of the caudal region of the cord. The maps (Figs. 32, 33, 34) furnish the features

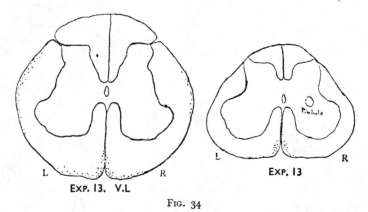

L   EXP. 13. V.L   R   L   EXP. 13   R

Fig. 34

of the relative distribution of the fibres at various levels of the cord more clearly than verbal description, which can therefore be omitted. In the dorsal columns two pairs of symmetrical areas of degeneration exist to the level of the 7th thoracic (Fig. 32); further back than that, a single pair of areas is traceable into the front end of the lumbar region; in the 3rd lumbar section no trace of degeneration is distinct in the dorsal columns. In the caudal region degenerate fibres are present in the left lateral column, but not in the right lateral.

REMARKS

The foregoing studies show that the neurones afferent from the great cervico-thoracic skin-field, which starts the "scratch" reflex in the muscles of the dog's hind-limb, owe their connection with lumbo-sacral moto-neurones to a path that, wholly uncrossed, descends the lateral white column (Exps. 4, 5, 7, 8, 10, 11, 12, 14, 15). No essential part of the path lies in either dorsal or ventral column, nor in the extreme dorsal or median part of the lateral column itself (Exps. 11, 12). Considering the large extent of the reflexigenous surface concerned, and the multi-segmental embouchure of the afferent neurones therefrom (*e.g.*, 3rd to 5th cervical inclusive, and 2nd to 13th thoracic inclusive), the internuncial path must be composed of quite a system of aborally-directed conduction lines; and these must reach motoneurones scattered from at least the 2nd lumbar to the 1st sacral segments (inclusive), since the movement evoked employs the activity both of the flexors of the digits and of the hip. In this required position and extent within the cord our other experiments demonstrate the presence of "long spinal" fibres arising in cervical and thoracic segments and running backward to terminate in lumbo-sacral segments (Exps. 4, 5, 6, 7, 11, 12, 13, 16, 17). These fibres suggest themselves as the lines of conduction active in the "scratch" reflex. These fibres, as we show, do not decussate, and the reflex we show to be likewise strictly "ipsilateral." The linkage between cervical and sacral segments being thus *mononeuronic* —*i.e.*, made of one long neurone, and not of a series of short neurones— it is possible that the "scratch" reflex—and probably others of the "long" reflexes discussed above, especially their uncrossed portions—require but a *trineuronic* arc, composed of (α) afferent root-cell, (β) "long spinal" neurone, and (γ) efferent root-cell. This internuncial "long spinal" neurone may perhaps be regarded as a special development of the "Schaltzelle" which some authorities (v. Monakow, v. Lenhossek) argue is intercalated, in even the shortest spinal arcs, between afferent and efferent root-cell.

The nervous arc for the "scratch" reflex, which reacts so readily and infallibly in the "spinal" dog, does not of course exhibit the same fatality of response in the normal animal. A normal dog when rubbed behind the shoulder may scratch or it may not. In both of our two dogs with cervical lateral semi-lesions (Exps. 16, 17), the "scratch" reflex was ob-tained from the shoulder on the side of the lesion about as readily and certainly as in a "spinal" dog. Evidently the reflex arc was on that side cut off from controlling mechanisms, which must therefore lie further headward. The dogs could, when standing, often be actually thrown off their feet by simply rubbing the shoulder on the same side as the semi-section. This loss of control over the reflex persisted undiminished. It seems due to section of the lateral column, for in one of the experiments the ventral column remained uninjured. It may be that the control is exerted via the pyramidal tract. The reflex was shown by Goltz to become more facile after extensive lesions of the *cortex cerebri*.[1]

It is clear from the experiments that each of the spinal segments examined gives off many nerve-fibres connecting it with spinal segments lying further backward. So numerous are these aborally-directed fibres that those arising even in a single segment can be traced backward, diminishing in number but recognisable throughout the length of the cord. At least this is shown for 2nd lumbar, 1st lumbar, 6th thoracic and 7th cervical segments (Exps. 2, 3, 12, 17), the four instances in which singly isolated segments were dealt with. It is also shown to be true of the fibres from the 1st and 2nd thoracic segments taken together (Exp. 13).

The number of these backward-running association fibres lessens progressively as traced further and further from their segment of origin, and the decrease seems more rapid near to that segment than at a considerable segmental distance from it; in other words, the ties of the segment are preponderantly with those segments adjoining itself.

If, as referred to above, spinal reflexes be classified as " short " and " long," the aboral association fibres of a spinal segment are usefully classified as " short " and " long." " Short " fibres are those which do not pass beyond the boundaries of the region (brachial, crural, caudal, etc.) in which they arise, while " long " fibres run from one spinal region into another—*e.g.*, from brachial region to crural region, from cervical to caudal, etc. In each of these main categories there can be distinguished, of course, fibres of sub-variety of length.

According to their topography in the cross-section of the cord we can distinguish in each of these two main categories of fibres three sets or tracts —fibres belonging to both of the above categories situate in the lateral column, in the ventral column, and in the dorsal column. It is true a fibre may have exactly the same functional significance whether it run in the lateral, ventral, or dorsal column of the cord, and fibres in the lateral, ventral, and dorsal column respectively may all be of exactly analogous function. Yet in absence of better criteria it is handy for descriptive purposes to distinguish among the aboral association fibres their lateral, ventral, and dorsal sets or tracts. The distinction between lateral and ventral tracts is even morphologically somewhat artificial, for there exists often, especially in the category of " short " fibres, no distinct gap between the ventral and lateral fields of the fibres in the transverse area of the cord.

We arrive therefore at the following tracts of *aborally-running endogenous* fibres in the spinal cord: (i) *lateral short association* tract, (ii) *ventral short association* tract, (iii) *dorsal short association* tract, (iv) *lateral long association* tract, (v) *ventral long association* tract, (vi) *dorsal long association* tract.

The features of the topography of these tracts, also their relative size and longitudinal extent, can be gathered better from the foregoing figures than from any even lengthy textual description. To them must be chiefly

---

[1] *Verrichtungen des Grosshirns*, p. 138, Strassburg, 1881.

attributed the progressive backward decrease in areal size of the ventro-lateral column, shown in the curves constructed by Woroschiloff[1] from Stilling's data. Both in these curves and in our degenerations the progressive decrease is less rapid in the trunk region than in the limb regions of the cord. The tracts may be regarded as units of the system that finds highest expression in the pyramidal tracts of the prosencephalic segments.

It is in the lateral column that the greatest number of the descending association fibres lie. Hence perhaps the pre-eminent importance of that column for the " long " reflexes studied in this paper. It must, however, be remembered that that column it is which constitutes at least a half of all the white matter of the cord. Relatively to its area, the ventral column seems to contain an even larger proportion of the aboral association fibres than does the lateral column. Certainly it is the dorsal column which contains both absolutely and relatively least of them; this fact is the more striking in that the dorsal column is the only column in which pathological material has furnished much evidence of their existence.

Speaking generally, the arrangement of the fibres as seen at cross-levels taken successively further and further from their origin is as follows: At first they are seen in a zone closely surrounding the grey matter; that zone becomes broader; then the fibres come to form a zone separated by a gradually increasing interval from the grey matter; then, distinctly diminished in number, they lie chiefly in a band, narrow in the ventral column, wider in the lateral, separated from the free surface of cord, except at the deep end of the ventral sulcus, by a zone clear of degeneration. Gradually diminishing, they encroach more and more on the peripheral layer of the white matter, finally enter that and descend in it grouped, especially about the ventral end of the lip of the ventral sulcus and about the junction of the middle and dorsal thirds of the free surface of the lateral column. The figures given above will amplify and correct the impressions conveyed by this bald statement; those of Exps. 5, 6, 7, 11, 12, 17, and especially 13, give successive levels that illustrate the course of the fibres best. In sections containing only fibres that have already traversed a considerable distance, these are found to lie almost exclusively near the surface of the cord. Their arrangement thus extends the rule, exemplified well in ascending fibres, that in the cord the longest fibres lie most remote from the grey matter (Schiefferdecker, Singer and Münzer, Sherrington, Hoche, Flatau). Hence in our experiments an asymmetrical lesion, although it causes a degeneration which in the segments near behind is obviously asymmetrical, may produce in segments still further backward a degeneration which presents little trace of the asymmetry (Exp. 13, Figs. 32, 33, 34).

In the ventral and lateral columns some of the " long " fibres are very long; thus some arising in the 7th cervical segment extend into the caudal region, bridging a spinal interval of more than twenty-five segments (Exp. 17). Again, some arising in the 1st thoracic segment extend also

[1] *Ludwig's Arbeiten*, Leipzig, 1874.

into the caudal region (Exp. 13). The existence of spinal nerve-cells with axons which on entering the white matter bifurcate each into a headward and tailward fibre (Ramón, van Gehuchten) makes it possible that some of the intrinsic spinal fibres demonstrated in our experiments connect segments even more distant than those we have accredited to them. It is only the backward-running arm of such T-shaped stem-fibres whose length is actually measured by our observations. In the light of our present experiments it is probable that in the "pinna-tail" reflex of the cat long association neurones directly bridge a spinal interval thirty or more segments in length.

In the dorsal column the endogenous fibres are in our observations none of them so long; thus those arising in the 7th cervical segment we fail to trace further back than the 10th thoracic (Exp. 17); those arising in the 1st and 2nd thoracic segment we lose sight of at the 3rd lumbar segment (Exp. 13). Moreover, these long associational fibres of the dorsal column are far less numerous than those of the lateral and ventral columns. Our experiments demonstrate them as slender tracts arising not merely in the cervical and anterior thoracic regions, but also in the posterior thoracic (Exp. 8) and anterior lumbar regions (Exp. 3), and descending thence into the caudal region. It has been a matter of surprise to us that they have not been so clear in certain of our experiments (*e.g.*, Exps. 4, 5) as other of our experiments would lead us to expect. It may be that they are subject to individual variation. The topography in the dorsal column agrees for the most part with the "septo-marginal tract" of Bruce and Muir (and Obersteiner's dorso-median sacral bundle) in man, a tract already shown to exist also in the thoracic region (Hoche).

It is interesting that Exp. 13 indicates that the long associational fibres from the anterior part (1st thoracic segment) of the isolated piece of cord extend further backward into the sacro-caudal region than do the similar fibres from the posterior part (anterior end of 3rd thoracic segment) of the isolated cord. The anterior part of the isolated piece contains largely brachial (limb) mechanisms, the posterior part does not. The fibres coming from the anterior (brachial) part have largely escaped on the right side, but have been cut on the left (Fig. 32, III. T); and in Fig. 34 the degeneration is seen to have correspondingly ceased further forward in the right lateral column than in the left.

In regard to the "long" fibres, we find in all the regions examined no evidence of decussation of these tracts. All our evidence is consentient that these axons nowhere cross from the white matter of one half of the cord into the white matter of the other. This does not exclude the possibility that the collaterals or fine ultimate terminals of these fibres may in some cases penetrate the grey matter to synapses in the grey matter of the crossed side. Also it is possible that the dendrites of the cells of origin of these fibres may have ramifications in the grey matter of the side opposite to that in which the axon-fibre itself descends. That the cells (perikarya) themselves, whence the fibres spring, lie in the grey matter of the same half of the cord as that in the white columns of which the fibres run is plainly indicated by the unilaterality of the distribution of the degenerate fibres after unilateral destruction of the grey matter (Exps. 2, 3, 5, 11).

We find the same true, broadly speaking, of the " short " tracts, thus confirming Münzer and Wiener's statement.[1] It is certain for the great majority of the " short " fibres; it may be true of all, but we hesitate to positively affirm that. If any of these fibres do decussate—and Fig. 29, II. L, Exp. 5, illustrates an appearance that suggests that a few of them do so in the ventral commissure—the number is small in the regions in which our lesions have injured the grey matter.

The experiments have allowed certain observations upon " spinal shock." Salient points noted were the following:

(i) The recovery of arterial blood-pressure after total transection in the posterior cervical region; this has been noted by one of us previously,[2] and in the above experiments the carotid pressure and the aortic pressure through the carotid were several times actually instrumentally measured and recorded, and found not inferior to the normal. The recovery appears to take place in a period varying from six days to about three weeks. At the end of that time good spinal reflexes upon the bloodvessels can be usually obtained by stimulation of the skin or the central end of afferent nerves belonging to the body-region behind the total translesion of the cord. The reflex effect upon the general arterial blood-pressure is usually in the direction of increase of the blood-pressure. The reflex activity of these spinal vaso-motor centres is heightened by curare in moderate dose. The subsequent lesions of the cord practised behind the original total transection did not appear to cause any recrudescence or recurrence of the vascular shock induced by the original transection.

(ii) Some degree of " depression " of the short reflexes of the hind-limb followed the establishment of a second lesion in the thoracic region subsequent to an original total transection in the cervical region. When the second lesion was a semi-section, this depression was evidenced on the same side as the lesion (Exps. 4, 5, 7, 11, 12). This " shock " was observed chiefly in the " marking time " reflex and in the " direct extension " reflex. The brachio-thoracic segments must play some part in or exert some influence favourable to the " marking time " reflex of the hind-limb, for the movement of that limb, on the homonymous side, is subsequent to semi-section slower on rhythm and less in excursion; and it remained so as long as the observations were continued (Exps. 2, 3, 4, 7, 11, 12). The channel for this association lies in the lateral column—e.g., Exp. 11. There was sometimes a depression of the knee jerk on the homonymous side, but it

---

[1] *Prag. med. Wochenschrift*, 1895, *loc. cit.*

[2] *Proc. roy. Soc.*, 1900, **66**, 390; *Med.-Chir. Trans. Lond.*, 1899, **82**, 449; and *Integrative Action*, 1906 —each giving tracings. See p. 124 of this volume.

was very transient, and was followed by some slight but lasting exaggeration of the jerk on that side.

We would infer from these observations concerning the shock that the fibres descending from posterior cervical and anterior and middle thoracic segments to spinal segments behind those of their origin make connections with " centres " for the skeletal muscles of the hind-limb (especially perhaps the hip) of their own side much more than with any spinal vaso-motor centres.

Conclusions

1. Pflüger's " Fourth Law " of spinal conduction does not hold good in the mammalian (dog, cat) spinal cord.

2. Afferent channels from the skin of the shoulder are freely connected with afferent channels to the muscles of hip, knee and ankle by an uncrossed path descending the lateral column.

3. Each spinal segment (in the dog) possesses a wealth of neurones with backward-running axons connecting it with practically all the spinal segments behind itself.

4. These association fibres may be grouped as

i.	lateral tracts	}	short—*i.e.*, confined to the spinal region (brachial, etc.) in which they arise.
ii.	ventral ,,		
iii.	dorsal ,,		
iv.	lateral ,,	}	long—*i.e.*, extending beyond the spinal region (brachial, etc.) in which they arise.
v.	ventral ,,		
vi.	dorsal ,,		

Of these the lateral tracts are largest; the dorsal are smallest, and not so long as either the lateral or ventral.

5. A small fraction of the fibres of the " short " tracts *may* decussate, but the great majority do not. The " long " tracts do not decussate.

6. There is agreement between the spinal path followed in the dog's " scratching " reflex and the course of the lateral long association tract. There is also agreement between that tract and the " hand-foot " reflex and the " marking time " reflex. These " long " reflexes may therefore employ conduction chains of no more than three links length. " Long " uncrossed spinal reflexes may therefore only require *trineuronic* arcs.

7. Certain of the spinal reflexes observed—*e.g.*, " scratching " reflex— though started by a stimulus of segmentally distant application, tend to maintain themselves by local automatic excitation; these show markedly " alternating " character explicable as outcome of " reciprocal innervation."

8. There is some evidence that the spinal association tracts descend to spinal mechanisms for skeletal musculature; none that they influence vaso-motor reactions.

9. Good vaso-motor reflexes can, by exciting afferent nerves or skin, be obtained from the spinal cord after cervical transection, if time has been allowed for subsidence of "shock." Nothing is then necessary to reveal the spinal vaso-motor reactions; but curare favours them.

2. REFLEXES ELICITED FROM THE DORSAL COLUMNS[1]

[*The Reflex Effect of the Collaterals of the Fibres of the Dorsal Columns of the Spinal Cord.*]

In a paper presented to the Society last year,[2] I drew attention to some striking instances of "long conduction" through the bulbo-spinal cord, and among others to the following singular one: If after transection above the bulbo-spinal axis the *funiculus gracilis* be excited—*e.g.*, at the *calamus scriptorius*—the excitation evokes movement (contraction, relaxation) in the ipsilateral hind-limb. If instead of *f. gracilis* the *funiculus cuneatus* be excited the movement (contraction, relaxation) is in the ipsilateral fore-limb. The movement in the hind-limb is in the monkey usually adduction and flexion of hallux; in the cat flexion of knee, hip, or ankle. In the monkey the fore-limb movement is usually flexion and adduction of pollex, often with extension of the other digits; in the cat, more usually flexion of elbow with protraction of the shoulder. The movements which occur are, however, various, and I will here only add that those from the *f. gracilis* include the vaginal and anal orifices, the tail, and the abdominal muscles; those from *f. cuneatus* the diaphragm; but that neither from *f. gracilis* nor *f. cuneatus* have I obtained ipsilateral extension of elbow or of knee.

In my former paper this phenomenon was recorded under the head of "long bulbo-spinal conductions." I did not offer any explanation of it, for it appeared to particularly require further investigation. I have, since communicating the above paper, taken various opportunities of examining the reaction further. My enquiry has elicited the subjoined results:

The movements evoked in the perineum or hind-limb by excitation of the *f. gracilis* after transection of the bulb are obtainable from that column, after its isolation, by freeing it above and from its ventro-lateral connections for a length of 3 cm., and then suspending its upper end from a thread. The reaction is therefore hardly due to escape of the stimulating currents used, so that they reach the lateral columns and the descending tracts there contained. The currents employed have been induced, and of an intensity imperceptible, or barely perceptible, to the tongue-tip. The electrodes have been bright steel needles, placed about 1 mm. apart, and laid on the surfaces of the cord or bulb.

The reaction is obtainable when the transection has been made altogether below the *nuclei graciles et cuneati*. It therefore does not necessarily involve the cells of those nuclei.

---

[1] Reprinted from *Proc. roy. Soc.*, 1897, **61**, 243-246.   [2] *Philos. Trans.*, 1898, **190B**, 45.

The reaction is not prevented by complete bilateral transverse severance of the ventro-lateral columns and grey matter of the cord at the:

5th cervical root level,
nor at the 8th   ,,   ,,
,,   5th thoracic   ,,
,,   1st lumbar   ,,
,,   5th   ,,   ,,   (cat).

The reaction is at once annulled on severance of the dorsal columns at any one of the above levels, although at the same time the ventro-lateral columns and the grey matter remain intact.

The reaction from the left *f. gracilis* is annulled by severance of the left dorsal column, that of the right by the severance of the right.

The reaction can almost always be obtained, although incompletely, by mechanical excitation—*e.g.*, by compression with ivory forceps, often even by a mere touching with the forceps.

That the conduction involved in the reaction does not implicate the fibres of the pyramidal tract—which at first instance suggest themselves as a source of fallacy—seems clear in light of the above. That supposition is also, and I think finally, excluded by the following observation: I have found the " long intraspinal reflexes " like decerebrate rigidity locally abolished or greatly depressed by total severance of the sensory spinal roots belonging to their own region of terminal discharge. Thus, to take an instance given in my former paper, if the right fore-paw be stimulated, the paths of " short spinal conduction " from it lead to discharge of its own flexors of elbow, extensors of wrist, etc., as specified in the paper; and the paths of " long spinal conduction " from it lead to discharge of the muscles of the ipsilateral hind-limb. To evoke from the fore-paw movement of the contra-lateral hind-limb is relatively difficult; this contralateral movement is less commonly and less easily obtained, and when obtained less vigorous, less prolonged, and usually commences later than the ipsilateral. But if, in the instance taken, the series of afferent spinal roots belonging to the right hind-limb be severed, and stimulation of the fore-paw (right) be then repeated, the movement induced in the hind-limbs is contralateral—*i.e.*, a *crossed* one. In the ipsilateral limb it is extremely difficult, often impossible, to then obtain by this facile long spinal path any discharge at all on the side of the transected afferent roots, although that side is usually peculiarly accessible. I find that similarly severance of the dorsal (afferent) roots in their extra-spinal course greatly impairs the reaction from the *f. graciles* and *f. cuneati*. Thus, if when flexion of right knee or right hallux is being regularly evoked by excitation of *f. gracilis* at the top of the cord, the extraspinal dorsal (afferent) roots of the right pelvic limb be severed, the reaction, until then regularly obtained, disappears or almost disappears. The section of right-hand roots annuls the right-hand reaction, but not the left hand, and conversely. On the other hand, the flexion of knee, or of hallux, or of elbow obtained by excitation of the Rolandic cortex or of the lateral column (pyramidal tract fibres) is, as has been shown in a previous number of these *Proceedings*[1] by Dr. Mott and myself, not impaired after the root severance; indeed, often appears, on the contrary, to be facilitated. In this respect, therefore, the reaction obtainable by direct excitation of *f. graciles* and *f. cuneati* is shown to be curiously different from that obtainable from the pyramidal tract fibres and Rolandic cortex. On the other hand, it is seen to resemble in this respect to a remarkable degree the " long spinal reflexes " as defined above.

What, then, is the nature of this reaction obtainable from the *f. graciles* and *cuneati*? The reaction is evidently one which involves each dorsal column of the cord as a conducting path, in many cases as a " long "—in not a few as a remarkably long—conducting path, even employing its whole length. In light of the evidence given above, I infer that although certainly, as has been long established, the dorsal column is, with the single exception of its short, scanty, and deeply placed ground-bundle, a functionally purely *upward* path, consisting of nothing else than sensory root-fibres, the vast majority of which fibres—and all the longest of which—are ascendant; the conduction along it in these experiments is *downward*, even extending its whole length. That is to say, the conduction must be downward and cellulipetal along ascending axons which function in a cellulifugal direction; that is to say, the propagation of the impulses artificially started in my observations must have been *antidrome* instead of *orthodrome*. The motor discharges evoked I refer to the spread of the excited condition into the collaterals of the axons excited to antidrome conduction, their collaterals impinging upon motor neurones.

The direction of propagation occurs, therefore, in opposition to the law of the "*polarisation dynamique des nevrons*" put forward by Ramon y Cajal[2] and V. Gehuchten.[3] It offers, however, no contradiction to what James[4] has termed " the law of forward direction "; it only emphasises that that law predicates the existence of at least two links in its conduction gear.

The reaction is therefore, in my view, an extreme illustration of double (antidrome, *doppelsinnige*) nervous conduction. After du Bois' fundamental observation with frog's sciatic and the electrical sign, it has been Kühne's *sartorius* experiment,[5] and Babuchin's[6] reversed discharge in the electric organ nerve-fibre, which have laid a satisfactory foundation for double conduction in peripheral nerves. But between those experiments and these, the subject of this note, there are, it is true, differences. In the latter (a) propagation occurs over relatively huge distances, and (β) the reaction occurs within the field of the central nervous system. These differences

[1] *Proc. roy. Soc.*, 1895, **57**, 481, extract here on pp. 115-119.

[2] *Medicina practica*, 1889; *Revista de Ciencias Medicas de Barcelona*, Nos. 21 and 22, 1891.

[3] *La Cellule*, 1891, **7**, 101.   [4] *Psychology*, and *cf.* Waller, *Science Progress*, 1895, **3**, 186.

[5] *Arch. Anat. Physiol. Lpz., Physiol. Abt.*, 1859, p. 595.   [6] *Ibid.*, 1877, p. 66.

need not, however, negative the relationship of the phenomena. They render it the more instructive.

It is obvious that there must be opportunity for detection of antidrome conduction in parts of the central nervous system besides the dorsal spinal columns. Thus, on exciting, especially with electric currents, the mammalian metencephalon (*vermis cerebelli*) and *isthmus rhombencephali*,[1] subsequent to ablation of the parts above, I have seen movements produced in the limbs and trunk, and also inhibitions occur. Thus, in instance of the latter, inhibition of the tonic extensor spasm of the fore- and hind-limbs combined with contraction of the flexors of knee and elbow, such as is seen under local spinal reflex action.[2] It will have to be determined whether in such cases as the former we have not before us instances of antidrome conduction along ascending paths. The antidrome phenomenon, while of valuable assistance when recognised, may, if unrecognised, give rise to very misleading inferences. Its methodic use should place in our hands a fresh instrument of value for neurological research.

3. AN ASCENDING PATHWAY IN THE LATERAL COLUMNS[3]

The condition of muscular rigidity consequent upon decerebration, described by one of us previously in this Journal,[4] forms, as was then shown, an excellent field for the examination of some phenomena of inhibition. We have in the present work attempted to trace the path of nervous conduction involved in some of the inhibitions that can be evoked under " decerebrate rigidity."

Method.—Our observations have been chiefly upon the cat, also on the dog and the Macaque monkey. The preliminary operation and the decerebration were always carried out under complete anæsthesia—deep chloroform and ether narcosis. Severe loss of blood was guarded against by thread loops placed round the carotids, controlling those arteries if necessary. The cerebrum was removed completely, and with it was taken the whole nervous axis in front of a transection midway down the anterior corpora quadrigemina. Artificial respiration was only occasionally found necessary, and then for no long time. The animal was after decerebration freely slung with its vertebral axis horizontal; its temperature was maintained by careful adjustment of hot-water tins. After decerebration the administration of chloroform was discontinued.

Electrical Stimulation of the Spinal Cord

I. A portion of the hinder thoracic or of the lumbo-sacral region of the cord was exposed in the vertebral canal. The spinal roots of the exposed portion were severed outside the dura mater; this was done to avoid local

---

[1] Sherrington, *Proc. roy. Soc.*, 1896-7, **60**, 414, reprinted on p. 256, this volume.
[2] Sherrington, *ibid.*
[3] Published with A. Fröhlich, as " Path of Impulses for Inhibition under Decerebrate Rigidity," *J. Physiol.*, 1902, **28**, 14-19.   [4] *J. Physiol.*, 1898, **22**, 319. Reprinted here on p. 314.

reflexes. The dural sheath was then opened freely and the cord transected cleanly with a very sharp knife. The previous severance of the adjacent two or three pairs of nerve-roots next above allowed the free end of the cord to be lifted up from the canal with its cut face tilted upward free from fluid and surrounding tissues and bare to the experimenter. It was lightly fixed in that position. For stimulation we employed the unipolar method with an electrode similar to that devised by one of us for localisation experiments on the cortex cerebri.

This electrode (Fig. 35) consists essentially of a fine platinum wire soldered to a piece of thin German silver wire, which latter is coiled spirally into a delicate spring before joining ordinary copper wire sheathed for insulation. The free end of the piece of platinum wire is fused to a minute bead. The tip of the electrode can be kept held steadily against a point of

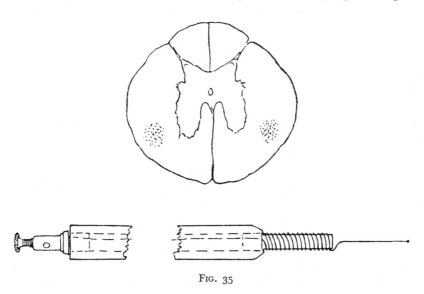

Fig. 35

the cut surface of the cord without risk of its either slipping as the animal moves under respiration, or of its piercing the nervous tissue of the cord. It is advantageous to have an ebonite projection from the handle of the electrode run up within the spiral spring, keeping the spring from moving laterally. The tip of the electrode is easily sterilised in flame. The handle of the electrode is hollow and the ordinary wire is threaded through it to a binding screw at the bottom.

A large copper plate strapped to the shaved thigh over a pad wetted with strong solution of sodium chloride served as the other electrode. Induced currents from an inductorium of Prof. Kronecker's pattern were used for excitation. The currents employed were very feeble, since we desired to restrict and localise the application of the stimulus as far as possible. The currents were usually just perceptible to the tongue-tip.

To judge by the resultant movements, etc., we obtained considerably more minute localisation than in experiments in which for purpose of control we resorted to the ordinary double-point electrodes.

The spinal operation was carried nearly to completion before decerebration. The spinal transection practised after the decerebration at once annulled the decerebrate rigidity in parts innervated behind the transection. The muscular regions headward of that level remained rigid—*e.g.*, fore-limbs and neck extended, jaw clenched.

Observations.—With the small pointed electrode the cut face of the upper piece of the transected cord was explored for effects upon the musculature of the fore-limbs, neck and head. The application of the electrode to the grey matter never produced obvious effects; neither did usually its application to the region of the pyramidal tract, to most of the area of the ventral white column, nor to the marginal area of the cord near the region of exit of the ventral root bundles. From the region of the direct cerebellar tract effects were frequently seen, usually an increase in the rigidity of the homonymous fore-limb. From the dorsal column effects were usually obtained, generally increase of rigidity of the homonymous fore-limb, with sometimes an increase of that of the crossed fore-limb also, but slighter.

From a small area, shown in the accompanying figure (Fig. 35), was obtained an effect much more constant and regular than any of the above. There the application of the electrode evoked marked inhibition of the rigidity of the homonymous fore-limb, often accompanied by a slighter inhibition on the crossed side. Sometimes the inhibition of the crossed fore-limb seemed as marked as that of the homonymous. Inhibition of the crossed fore-limb without inhibition of the homonymous was never met with. In the inhibition the triceps muscle was felt to relax. Not infrequently the relaxation of the extensors of the elbow was accompanied or followed by contraction of the flexors, and this by retraction of the upper arm; also by bending of the neck toward the side of the flexed fore-limb and rotation of the head so as to lower the ear of the homonymous side.

The situation of the little area yielding this result is figured as met at the 10th thoracic level in the cat. In the lower lumbar levels it lay somewhat more ventral in the spinal cross-section. All the species examined by us exhibited the same inhibitory spot, and the same resulting inhibition and related movement. The levels of cord at which we have found the inhibitory spot have extended from the 6th lumbar forward to the 5th thoracic.

The following may serve as a type of such observations:

July 8, 1901. Cat: chloroform and ether narcosis. Ligatures looped round carotids. Spinal cord exposed. Decerebration. Rigidity of right fore-limb less marked than of left. Cord transected between 5th and 6th lumbar nerve-roots.

Excitation. Left side: increase of rigidity of left fore-limb from the dorsal column. From ventral column, some inhibition of fore-limb. From ventro-lateral neighbourhood of ventral horn, weak inhibition of left fore-limb.

Right side: increase of rigidity of right fore-limb from dorsal column. From most parts of ventro-lateral column no effect, except on stimulation of the ventro-lateral neighbourhood of ventral horn; from that spot marked inhibition of right fore-limb.

Cord transected midway between 4th and 5th lumbar roots; result of excitation as before.

Cord transected midway between 3rd and 4th lumbar roots; result of excitation as before, except that inhibition from ventro-lateral neighbourhood of ventral horn is now well marked.

In two experiments we found that section of the two last thoracic and of the 1st lumbar root proximal to their ganglia fourteen days prior to the excitation of the transverse area of the cord did not render the inhibitory effect of the stimulation of the inhibitory spot of the cord unequal on the two sides. In a third experiment the inhibitory spot right and left was stimulated at the 12th thoracic level twelve days after complete spinal transection at the 3rd lumbar level; the inhibition effect was still obtained, but was not so marked as usual; it was not obtained at all in this experiment at the level of the 2nd lumbar segment.

II. We next enquired into the effect upon the rigidity of the fore-limb of excitation of separate peripheral nerve-trunks in the hind-limb. The effects from the different trunks were not all similar. Excitation of the central end of *n. cutan. femor. internus* lessened the rigidity of the homonymous fore-limb and increased that of the opposite fore-limb. Excitation of the central end of the plantar nerve, on the contrary, reinforced the rigidity of the homonymous fore-limb and decreased that of the crossed fore-limb.

EXPERIMENT.—June 18, 1901. Cat. Carotids guarded by ligatures. Tracheotomy. Decerebration. Three nerves in right hind-limb prepared. Decerebrate rigidity well developed and about equally in both fore-limbs. Nerves ligated and severed.

1. Right *n. cutan. fem. intern.*: excitation causes complete inhibition of rigidity of right fore-limb, with increase of rigidity of left. Head turned to opposite side.

2. Right *n. tibial. postic.* near ankle: excitation causes complete inhibition of rigidity of crossed fore-limb, with increased rigidity of homonymous. Head turned to same side.

3. Hamstring nerve: excitation causes increased rigidity of crossed fore-limb usually, but not always.

Our experiments have been on this point definite as far as they go, but are not sufficiently numerous to establish rules of relationship.

III. Applications of stimuli more nearly resembling those of natural life than do those applied to spinal roots and of the larger nerve-trunks of the limb are the stimulations of circumscript areas of skin surface. We found that application to the shaved skin of a pledget of cotton-wool soaked with hot water excited effects varying to some extent with the *locus* of application of the stimulus. When applied to the postero-external aspect of the thigh not far below the *tuber ischii*, extension was evoked at hip and knee, without obvious effect upon the extensor rigidity of the fore-limb. Similar stimulation of the skin of the top of the front of the thigh evoked extension at hip, and with it an increased rigidity of the homonymous fore-limb and turning of the head to the opposite side. The pledget applied to the skin over the gluteal muscles evoked flexion at hip. Applied to the hind-paw it always inhibited the extensor rigidity of the limb itself and increased that of the fellow hind-limb; hot water applied directly to hind-paw excited the same effect, and usually affected the rigidity of the fore-limbs by increasing that of the homonymous and decreasing that of the crossed fore-limb, but occasionally this effect was reversed. Stimulation of the tail often caused inhibition of the rigidity of both fore-limbs.

IV. The fact that while excitation of the hind-paw or of the plantar nerve caused inhibition of the extensor rigidity of the crossed fore-limb, on the other hand stimulation of the cross-section of the lateral spinal column in the lumbar region inhibits the homonymous fore-limb, suggests that the path of conduction involved for the inhibition of the fore-limb from the hind-foot may cross soon after its entry into the cord. With this suggestion in mind we examined the effect of transection of the right lateral half of the cord at the 1st lumbar segment upon the inhibitory influence of the left hind-paw upon the extensors of the right elbow. Although in one experiment this inhibitory influence failed completely after the semi-section, in another experiment it was not extinguished, although decidedly diminished.

Conclusions.—Inhibitory effects under decerebrate rigidity are evoked by electric stimulation of a small fairly-limited area of the cross-section of the cord (*vide* Fig. 35). These effects, studied mainly in relaxation of the triceps muscle, are combined with pressor effects in other muscles. The effect is more marked on the side homonymous with that of stimulation.

Electric stimulation of the central end of certain peripheral nerves in the hind-limb yields the same relaxation of the *m. triceps*. Stimulation of the *n. cutan. femor. intern.* was followed by relaxation of the triceps on the homonymous side. Similar stimulation of central end of the plantar nerve was followed by relaxation of the *m. triceps* of the crossed side. On the whole the predominant effect from the hind-limb seemed to be relaxation of the triceps of the crossed fore-limb.

The path of inhibition in ventro-lateral white column may be connected with the afferent nerves from the crossed hind-foot.

4. THE ASCENDING PATHWAY FOR NOCICEPTIVE REACTIONS[1]

[*A reflex effect in the decerebrate state is described which is identical with the reaction of the intact animal to pain. This mimetic " pseudaffective " response was used to assess the effect of various semi-sections of the spinal cord in determining the pathway of ascending nociceptive impulses.*]

If in the cat under deep chloroform narcosis the cerebral hemispheres and thalamencephalon be carefully ablated, and the body temperature maintained, on relaxing the depth of chloroformisation a number of motor

[1] Published with R. S. Woodworth as " A Pseudaffective Reflex and its Spinal Path," *J. Physiol.*, 1904, **31**, 234-238. The protocols of twenty experiments, with diagrams of section, at the end of the paper have been omitted here.

reactions can be observed against the background of " decerebrate rigidity." Among these reactions are some mimetic movements simulating expression of certain affective states. These " *pseudaffective* " reflexes we have endeavoured to utilise for elucidation of the spinal path conducting those impulses that, were the brain intact, would, we may presume, evoke " pain." The search for such a path is as regards channels from skin a search for a path as specific as those of the special senses. The truncation of the brain at the mesencephalon annihilates the neural mechanism to which the affective psychosis is adjunct. But it leaves fairly intact the reflex motor machinery whose concurrent action is habitually taken as outward expression of an inward feeling. When the expression occurs it may be assumed that had the brain been present the feeling would have occurred. A spinal translesion which prevents occurrence of the expression in response to a stimulus that previously excited the expression has therefore been regarded by us in the following experiments to be such as would, were the brain present, induce *analgesia* in regard to that stimulus.

Apart from that assumption, it is clear that such a lesion can be used for determining the path of a *nociceptive* reaction (see p. 158, Chapter V). That a reflex action should exhibit purpose is no longer considered evidence that any psychical process attaches to it, let alone any dictate of " choice " or " will." By the Darwinian hypothesis, of no less value in physiology than in morphology, every reflex must be purposive. But the assignment of a particular purpose to a particular reflex is often difficult and hazardous. The difficulty is in inverse degree to the amplitude of field covered by the reflex effect. Thus, a slight movement confined to a single limb, or a transient rise of blood-pressure observed alone, is open to many interpretations and admits of no security of significance; it is a fractional reaction that may belong to any of many general reactions of varied aim. The reflex effects studied in this paper have possessed sufficient width of co-ordination to be hardly equivocal. The spinal path concerned with the forward transmission of their impulses can therefore be designated, not merely a headward path, but, having regard to the character of the reaction, the headward path for *nociceptive* reactions.

The reflex effect observed has presented the following elements: diagonal alternating movements of the limbs as in progression (sometimes producing progression), turning of head and neck toward the point stimulated; opening of the mouth, retraction of the lips and tongue, movement of the vibrissæ, snapping of the jaws; lowering of the head; opening of the eyelids, dilatation of the pupils; vocalisation angry in tone (snarling), sometimes plaintive; and with these a transient increase of arterial blood-pressure.[1]

[1] This " pseudaffective " response to nociceptive stimuli is to be distinguished from the reflex mimesis of anger studied by Graham Brown and Sherrington (*Quart. J. exp. Physiol.*, 1911, **4**, 193-205). The pseudaffective response simulating anger, including side-to-side lashing of the tip of the tail, a pilomotor reaction, and a great rise of blood-pressure, was shown to be obtainable from a stimulation of a small descending tract in mid-brain and spinal cord. It could be obtained reflexly by certain acoustic stimuli in the cat after intercollicular section by Forbes and Sherrington

These reactions appeared not only in combination, but sometimes singly or in small combinations. The readiest to elicit were movements of the vibrissæ, opening of the mouth with retraction of the tongue, and lowering of the head.   In some cases the movements were vigorous and prompt, but they never amounted to an effective action of attack or escape.   A character-istic feature of their ineffectiveness was their brief duration.   The movement, even when most vigorous and prompt, died away rapidly, to be succeeded in some cases by a few weaker repetitions, each in succession weaker and more transient than the last.   Thus the movements of the head might recur three or four times in response to a single stimulus, or the vocalisations be repeated in a diminishing series for a minute or so.

Our method has been to compare by means of the above reaction the effect of two stimuli symmetrically applied on opposite sides of the body, after a semi-section or other lesion of the spinal cord headward of the entrance of the nerve-fibres stimulated.

After semi-section at the 13th thoracic level the pseudaffective reaction was obtained by stimulation of either sciatic trunk, but more vigorously and promptly from the nerve of the side of the semi-section; from this nerve also the reaction was evoked by weaker faradisation. This indicates that the headward pathway taken by the impulses eliciting the vocal and other pseudaffective reactions is from the hind-limb, both crossed and uncrossed, but is more largely crossed. Our other experiments have all given the same result; sometimes not much difference was observable between the reactions obtainable from the two sciatics respectively, but usually there was a distinct difference, and this was always in the sense that the nerve of the same side as the semi-section evoked the stronger reaction. Both purely cutaneous (internal saphenous) and purely muscular (hamstring) nerves were examined and the pathway found not appreciably different in the two.

After semi-section in the anterior cervical region (3rd to 4th cervical), stimulation of the brachial nerves on the same side as the spinal semi-section gave the pseudaffective reaction decidedly more strongly than did the nerves of the opposite side. Ulnar, median, a muscular branch of median, and the internal cutaneous nerves all gave this same result. The difference was more marked than between the two sides of the body in the hind-limb region. The lesion lay less far forward from the brachial region than did the lesion at 13th thoracic from the crural region. Sometimes it was difficult to obtain the reaction at all from the brachial nerves of the side opposite to the cervical semi-section. The headward nociceptive (or algesic) path from the arm is therefore in the anterior cervical region mainly crossed.

(*Amer. J. Physiol.*, 1914, **35**, 368), and therefore appears to have sensori-motor co-ordination at or below this level. Not only could these pseudaffective responses be obtained in the absence of cerebrum, but the converse of patent emotion without visceral or other bodily concomitants was described in the dog after high spinal and vagal transection (Sherrington, *Proc. roy. Soc.*, 1900, **66**, 390, and *Integrative Action*, p. 259).—ED.

When examined by a high *cervical* semi-section, the nociceptive (algesic) path from the hind-limbs is still, as at the 13th thoracic level, partly crossed, partly uncrossed, and rather more crossed than uncrossed.

The pseudaffective reaction is easily obtained from the splanchnic nerve. Mechanical or electrical excitation of the nerve branches connecting the semilunar ganglion with the sympathetic chain elicits the reaction promptly. Semi-section in the anterior cervical region interferes with the reaction from these sympathetic nerves on the same side as the semi-section hardly obviously, but lessens the reaction from the nerves of the crossed side rather more. The headward path of the impulses evoking the pseudaffective reaction under excitation of these visceral nerves is therefore in the anterior cervical region both crossed and uncrossed, but more crossed than uncrossed.

From all these unilateral regions the afferent nociceptive (algesic) path in the spinal cord is therefore bilateral—that is, divided between the two sides of the cord—the larger share belonging to the crossed side. The crossing appears in the anterior cervical region to be more preponderant for the brachial limb than for nerves of the other regions examined.

As regards the question which of the columns of the cord carry the headward path of the impulses evoking the vocal and other pseudaffective reactions, we are able to exclude the dorsal columns. Section of both of these made no appreciable difference in the reaction to the stimulus; neither did faradisation of them evoke the reaction. The median portion of the ventral column has sometimes been trespassed on in making the semi-section of the opposite side; this extension of the lesion has not prevented the reaction from occurring. In one case the whole grey matter of both halves of the cord was found on autopsy to be heavily infiltrated and ploughed up with extravasated blood at the level of the semi-section, and for several millimetres both ahead and behind it. It must have been largely, if not completely, thrown out of function. Yet the pseudaffective reaction was very briskly obtained.

If, therefore, neither the dorsal nor ventral column nor the grey matter affords the pathway for the nociceptive (algesic) impulses, the lateral column alone is left to them. This conclusion is confirmed by direct experiment. After transection of one lateral column alone the pseudaffective reaction is elicited from either lateral half of the body behind the lesion; after further section of the opposite lateral column, all pseudaffective reaction at once ceases to be elicitable from either half of the body behind the lesion. It is probable that in the posterior thoracic and lumbar segments this headward path is that already described above by A. Fröhlich and one of us as inhibiting, under direct faradisation, the rigidity of the *triceps brachii* in the decerebrate cat.

We conclude (1) that the *lateral* column furnishes the headward path in the spinal cord for *nociceptive* (algesic) arcs; (2) that each lateral column conveys such impulses from *both* lateral halves of the body, and somewhat preponderantly those from the crossed half; and (3) that this is true for these arcs, whether they be traced from *skin, muscle* or *viscus*.

It is noteworthy that the " chloroform " or " ether cry," that peculiar vocalisation emitted by men and animals during certain stages of anæsthetisation, was often uttered by decerebrate cats during continued administration of the anæsthetic to them after decerebration. This vocalisation, therefore, does not necessarily mean that the higher cerebral centres are still imperfectly anæsthetised, since in our animals the whole cerebrum and the thalamencephalon had been ablated and yet the administration of the vapour evoked the vocalisation typically.

Regarding *decerebrate rigidity* it was seen that after semi-section of the cord in the anterior cervical region the rigidity resulting from decerebration was much less in the elbow and knee of the semi-sected side. In some instances this freedom from rigidity persisted; in some it passed off, so that a few hours after the operation both elbows and both knees were about equally rigid. The pathway from the mid-brain to the limb by which the rigidity is kept up descends, therefore, probably in both lateral halves of the cord, though mostly on the same side as the muscles affected.

As regards the bilaterality of the headward path of the pseudaffective reflex, on several occasions it was observed that the turning of the head and neck was after semi-section still correctly toward the locus of stimulus, whether the stimulus was crossed or uncrossed in regard to the semi-section. Evidently, therefore, " local sign " was implicate in the impulses of each lateral half of the bilateral headward path.

VII

ON RECIPROCAL INNERVATION

THE CO-ORDINATION OF ANTAGONISTS

[Descartes (1662) had seen the necessity for some function governing the action of antagonistic muscles and had supposed the mechanism to lie in peripheral structures. Charles Bell (1823) had suggested the possibility of a " nervous bond " which would cause muscles to " conspire in relaxation as well as to combine in contraction." He also had in mind a peripheral structure.[1] In a long series of papers, some of which are presented here, Sherrington demonstrated and unravelled the reflex (central) *arrangement by which inhibition is harnessed with excitation to secure co-ordination of antagonists. The principle of this reflex nervous co-ordination, thus established and subjected to experimental analysis by him, was called " reciprocal innervation."*

*The action of the vagus in inhibiting the heart had been discovered by the Webers in 1846. Inhibition had also been postulated to account for many general nervous effects such as inhibitory cessation of movement by skin stimulation in the spinal dog (Goltz, 1874), and relaxation of skeletal muscle, as an ill-defined effect, by stimulation of the cerebral cortex (Bubnoff and Heidenhain, 1881). The discovery of reciprocal innervation allowed, and was followed by, the first quantitative estimation and isolation of inhibition as an active nervous process.—*Ed.]

1. THE KNEE JERK AND ANTAGONISTIC MUSCLES[2]

[The nature of the " knee jerk." The response is influenced profoundly by the condition of the antagonistic hamstring muscles. The effect is a reflex depression resulting from stimulation of afferents from the hamstring muscles.]

THE muscular reaction known as the knee jerk is notoriously affected by conditions obtaining in what is often described as a reflex arc, consisting of afferent and efferent paths, and a centre situate in the lumbar portion of the spinal cord. I recently[3] described experiments determining more particularly than hitherto the locality of the muscular and nervous mechanism on which the jerk depends. I showed that the muscular portion of this mechanism consists mainly of the *vastus internus* and part of the *crureus* divisions of the great quadriceps extensor muscle of the thigh. The *spinal centre* was found located in the 5th and 4th lumbar segments of the cord of the *Rhesus* monkey (4th and 3rd lumbar of man). The *efferent* path was found

---

[1] See Sherrington, *Integrative Action*, 1906, p. 287.

[2] Published as " Note on the Knee Jerk and the Correlation of Action of Antagonistic Muscles," *Proc. roy. Soc.*, 1892-3, **52**, 556.   [3] *J. Physiol.*, 1892, **13**, 666.

on the anterior roots of the 5th and 4th lumbar nerves, and was traceable along the anterior crural nerve into those of the muscular branches of that trunk which supply the above-mentioned portions of the quadriceps extensor max. The efferent side of the path corresponds accurately with the course of the motor nerve-fibres to the muscles in question, and there is little reason to doubt that it consists of nothing more or less than of those motor fibres themselves. The *afferent* path was found to lie in the posterior root of the 5th lumbar of *Rhesus* (4th of man, 6th of cat), and was not usually demonstrable at all in the posterior root of the 4th lumbar, but a small portion of it may, perhaps, lie within that root.

The posterior root, in which exists the afferent path on which the jerk is dependent, receives afferent fibres from the obturator and anterior crural nerves, and from the external and internal popliteal nerves, and sometimes from the division of the great sciatic, which may be called the hamstring nerve, because distributed to the hamstring muscles. Of the fibres entering the root from these various sources, those on which the " jerk " depends are not from any except the anterior crural nerve. Further, in the anterior crural nerve they are those fibres of the nerve which issue from the vastus internus and crureus muscles. Thus the afferent fibres on which the jerk depends seem to arise within muscles, and from exactly those muscles to which belong the efferent fibres with which the " jerk " is concerned.

The rapid abolition of the jerk produced by severing the posterior root of the 5th lumbar of *Rhesus* may conceivably be due less to mere interruption of an afferent path than to excitation of an afferent path by the " current of injury " set up in the injured fibres (" demarcation current ") of it. This doubt has frequently been strengthened in my mind by the fact that section of one half the root often suffices to abolish the " jerk," although the remaining half can, when tested, still be shown able to conduct centripetal impulses from the skin; and, further, by the fact that it appears immaterial whether the anterior or the posterior part of the posterior root be selected for the section. The " jerk " I have seen then abolished in a manner not obviously different from that in which section of the whole root abolishes it. Against such an explanation is, however, the permanence of the effect upon the " jerk " produced by section of the whole root, for the effect continues at least for many days. Regarding the permanence of the effect of section of half the root I have no observation.

I have repeated the observation, substituting for severance other modes of destruction of the conductivity of the root. The root is a fairly long one, longer in the monkey than in the cat, and it is not difficult to apply reagents to it. I find the jerk immediately abolished by cooling the root to near the freezing point. To do this I pass under the posterior root, well lifted from the anterior, one end of a copper strip, the other end of which lies in an ice and salt mixture. The application of CO_2 vapour to the root has a similar effect, and on removing the vapour the " jerk " returns. The vapour I have applied through a thin-walled india-rubber tube, made to enclose the root. Cocain I have also applied, and found it abolish the jerk in about 70 seconds, when used as a 1 per cent. solution in 0·6 per cent. sodium chloride solution. I place under the root, before applying the cocain, a thin strip of india-rubber sheeting, and apply the solution with a fine camel's-hair brush by painting on the filaments of the root.

There seems, therefore, no doubt that abolition of the jerk can be produced by lowering the conductivity of the fibres of this posterior root. Whatever the nature of these afferent fibres which thus come up from part of the quadriceps extensor of the thigh, and keep the " knee jerk " going, facts show that they are less hardy under experimental interference than are those from the skin which carry centripetal impulses subserving tactile sensation. A very little interference with this posterior root abolishes the knee jerk; a very great deal will often not obviously impair cutaneous reflexes elicited through it. To lift the posterior root by a thread passed under it will often suffice to interrupt the afferent fibres for " the jerk," but at the same time leaves the afferents of tactile sense not obviously impaired. Probably the former fibres are much the smaller and more delicate.

The irritation of this root, when cut, by its own demarcation current does not cause inhibition of the jerk. I have tried on three occasions to recover the " jerk," after its disappearance on section of this root, by electrical excitation of the central end of the divided root. The excitation, when too feeble to elicit any reflex contraction of the muscles, did not obviously influence the briskness of the jerk in either direction. The excitation very readily, however, causes contraction of the *hamstring* muscles, which so alters the position of the knee that the condition of the " jerk " can no longer be satisfactorily compared with what it was before.

Excitation of the central end of the divided hamstring nerve does at once abolish, or greatly reduce, the briskness of the " jerk." I have elsewhere[1] described a curious fact concerning the " jerk "—namely, that it can be rendered brisk by section of afferent or of efferent spinal roots immediately below that one on which the jerk itself depends. I added, with regard to it, " its explanation appears to lie in the abolition of the tone of the hamstring muscles by section of the afferent roots belonging to them." I wish now to support, and somewhat enlarge, the explanation then offered.

Severance of the great sciatic trunk produces, as Tschiriew[2] has pointed out in the cat, an increased briskness of the " jerk." This I find to depend scarcely at all, if indeed at all, on section of the external or internal popliteal divisions of the trunk, either singly or together; but to depend upon the cutting that portion of the trunk which is destined for the hamstring muscles —the portion referred to in my previous paper as " the hamstring nerve." In *Macacus* this " hamstring " division of the sciatic sends afferent fibres into the spinal cord by the posterior roots of the 8th, 7th, and 6th subthoracic nerves. In cat, the 8th and 7th posterior roots are those in question.

---

[1] *J. Physiol.*, loc. cit.　　　　[2] *Arch. Psychiat. Nervenkr.*, 1878, **8**, 689.

On severance of these afferent roots the " tonus " of the hamstring muscles is broken, and the " jerk " becomes more brisk; sometimes there is a short interval of depression immediately succeeding the operation. The motor fibres of the hamstring muscles leave the cord by the anterior roots, correspondent with the above-mentioned posterior. Severance of these anterior roots causes immediate increase in the briskness of the jerk.

As to the manner in which the loss of tonus of the hamstring muscles gives rise to increase of the knee jerk, two possibilities at once present themselves. One is purely mechanical; the other is of a physiological nature. The loss of tension accompanying the loss of " tone " will leave the leg more free to swing at the knee joint. It is for that reason that the posture of limb usually employed as the most favourable when the jerk is to be elicited is with the hamstrings relaxed and the leg at a right angle with the thigh. In this way the points of bony attachment of the hamstring muscles are approximated, and the knee can swing through a greater arc to that point at which it is cut short by the mechanical check of the flexor muscles passively tightened by the movement. The extensor movement during the " jerk " has, in this way, further scope before the hamstrings break it. As far as this explanation goes, the above-mentioned increase of the jerk would occur even if the hamstring muscles were replaced by india-rubber cords, the effect produced by severance of the hamstring nerve being equivalent to any arrangement which rendered those india-rubber cords less tight.

I should have considered this simple explanation sufficient had it not been for certain additional facts. During experiments on the effects of stimulating the motor spinal roots of the lumbo-sacral nerves there is much risk of being deceived by escape of the exciting current to other motor roots besides the one to which the electrodes are applied. When stimulating the motor root of the 7th lumbar, I frequently observed contraction of the extensor muscles of the knee as well as of the flexors, and imagining that the phenomenon must be due to escape of the exciting current to the 5th lumbar root, I was accustomed to reduce the strength of the exciting current until the contraction of the extensors of the knee no longer occurred. To avoid this supposed escape of current it was necessary to reduce the strength of stimulus sometimes to very slightly indeed above minimal efficiency for the motor fibres to which the electrodes were applied. The use of such weak currents has serious disadvantages, and was extremely embarrassing for the experiment. It was not until I had discarded a number of experiments on the ground of escape of current that three points concerning the contraction of the extensor muscles produced by stimulating the motor nerve to the flexors attracted my attention. (1) If for the excitation of the motor root to the flexors a series of induced currents are employed, succeeding each other at a rate slow enough to produce, not perfect tetanisation, but tremulant contraction of the muscles, the contraction obtained in the extensor muscles coincidently was, nevertheless, perfectly steady and tetanic, although not vigorous. (2) If the flexor muscles are severed from connection with the knee joint, so that their contraction cannot affect the joint, and if the " knee jerk " be elicited before, during, and after stimulation of the motor root to the flexor muscles, *during the excitation*, when those flexor muscles were contracting, the knee jerk, brisk previously and brisk later, disappeared, or almost disappeared. (3) If the sensory spinal roots

belonging to the hamstring nerve are severed, the stimulation of a motor root to the hamstring muscles is no longer accompanied by contraction of the extensor muscles of the knee, even when strong stimulation is employed.

One next observed the effect on the extensors of the knee of excitation of the central end of the nerve to the hamstring muscles after that nerve had been ligated and cut through. It was found that excitation with currents just perceptible at the tip of the tongue causes immediate *disappearance* or diminution of the " knee jerk." " Exaltation" of the jerk follows the depression by the excitation. If the excitation be continuously maintained for a time, the jerk tends to return in spite of the continuance of the stimulation. By use of stronger currents the extensors are immediately thrown into a tonic contraction, lasting so long as the stimulus is continued. The same effects on the knee jerk and on the activity of the extensor muscles are elicited by exciting the

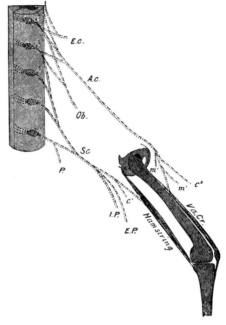

FIG. 36

E.c. External cutaneous nerve-trunk
A.c. Anterior crural nerve-trunk, with c, cutaneous, and m', muscular, branches
Ob. Obturator nerve-trunk
Sc. Sciatic nerve-trunk, with I.P., internal popliteal, E.P., external popliteal, divisions, and the division going to the hamstring muscles, which gives a cutaneous branch, c'
Va.Cr. The vasti and the crureus muscles, the internal portion being especially referred to

central ends of the divided posterior roots of the 7th or 8th subthoracic nerve.

I then attempted to determine if mere tension of the hamstring muscles could give the same result as electrical excitation of the central ends of their nerves. It is, of course, essential that the production of increased tension in the muscles should not alter the position of the knee joint or affect it mechanically. This precaution was observed by isolating the two inner hamstrings from their attachments, except at their origin, from the *tuber ischii,* and simultaneously cutting through all nerve branches to the outer hamstrings and to the adductor muscles. The nerves to the inner hamstrings were carefully preserved, although the muscles were otherwise dissected out. It was found that by pulling on the inner hamstring muscles sufficiently to stretch them out of the doubled-up shape they assumed after being freed from their lower attachments, the knee jerk, previously brisk, was at once *abolished or greatly diminished*, and on relaxing the strain on the hamstring muscles at once reappeared, and was apparently somewhat more brisk than before the diminution. It is often sufficient to merely compress the hamstring muscles, as they lie flaccid on the hand, between fingers and thumb. A kneading of the muscle as in *massage* has the same effect. On two occasions, at the end of an experiment, when the muscles had suffered from exposure, I have seen the curious phenomenon that excitation of a motor root supplying them of strength insufficient to throw the injured muscles into obvious contraction, yet suffices to at once cut out the " knee jerk," although before and after the excitation the " jerk " was very brisk indeed. The effect was obtained several times in succession, and immediately disappeared on dividing the sensory roots coming in from the exposed muscles. The current of injury in the muscles must have been considerable, and this suggests that the mere negative variation of the current of injury in the muscles might originate centripetal impulses. Certainly there was on neither occasion any obvious contraction in the muscles.

The most efficient mode of excitation of the afferent fibres from these muscles appears to be the mechanical above described—*i.e.*, the *myotatic* (Gowers).[1]

Excitation of the central end of the divided popliteal or peroneal nerves does not produce this effect upon the jerk. Neither does stretching of the sural triceps by pulling on the tendo Achillis, nor stretching of the rectus femoris muscle. Stretching of the rectus femoris can easily be employed without interference to the movement of the knee joint. It appears to me neither to increase nor to diminish the jerk. Excitation of the central end of the divided nerve to the rectus femoris exerts likewise no obvious influence on the jerk; nor does excitation of the central end of the cutaneous divisions of the anterior crural—viz., the internal saphenous and the internal and middle cutaneous nerves of the thigh. Excitation of the central end of the cutaneous branch of the hamstring nerve itself also appears without effect upon the jerk.

Tension produced in the sural triceps muscle by pulling on the Achilles tendon does not appear to influence the brisk flexor movement of the ankle joint evoked by tapping the subcutaneous face of the tibia, and related chiefly to the 6th lumbar spinal segment of Macacus and to the 7th lumbar segment of the cat.

It would thus seem clear that the exaggeration of the knee jerk produced by severance of the branches given from the great sciatic nerve to the

[1] *Diagnosis of Diseases of the Spinal Cord*, 2nd ed., 1881, p. 29. See also the same author's *Diseases of the Nervous System*, 2nd ed., 1892, **1**, p. 21; also pp. 202-205, 428, 429.

hamstring muscles is not due to the fact that the resulting relaxation of those muscles simply leaves the joint mechanically more free to move. The exaggeration would seem due rather to the severance of the nerves in question interrupting a stream of centripetal impulses that passes up from the hamstring muscles and enters the spinal cord by certain afferent roots, and in the cord exerts a depressing or restraining influence on the jerk. It further appears that a stream of impulses similarly efficient can be set up by moderate electrical excitation of the central ends of the divided nerves of the hamstring muscles; or by simply stretching or kneading those muscles when they are released from one of their fixed points; or, finally, by simply throwing those muscles into contraction through excitation of motor roots supplying them, so long as the sensory roots remain intact. The physician, when he, in order the better to elicit the jerk, flexes the knee and reduces the strain in the flexor muscles, by doing so removes, with relaxation of the flexors, a physiological depression which the tension of those muscles normally exerts upon the jerk obtainable from their antagonistic group.

Further, it would seem that at the knee joint excitation of the afferent fibres coming from one set of the antagonistic muscles induces reflex tonic contraction of the opposing set with extreme facility, despite the fact that the opponent muscles are not innervated from the same spinal segments. The reflex is obtainable with extraordinary facility, even across intervening segments of the cord.

Thus the degree of tension in one muscle of an antagonistic couple intimately affects the degree of " tonus " in its opponent, not only mechanically, but also reflexly, through afferent and efferent channels and the spinal cord.

It is obvious that the correlation of action thus existing between the antagonistic muscular groups of the thigh and knee may be not widely different from that originally pointed out by Hering and Breuer as regulative of the movements of respiration. One is tempted to institute a comparison also between it and the physiological arrangement studied by Biedermann in the antagonism of the muscles of the forceps of *Astacus*. I would, however, reserve further details until I have been able to perform a larger number of experiments. Anatomical evidence is at present so scanty regarding afferent nerve-fibres from muscle that investigation of their anatomical relation seems absolutely requisite for examining the problem further.

[Just as the lumbo-sacral region of the cord may be split along the median plane without interference to the jerk of either side,[1] so the same may be done without hindering the above ascending reflex abolition of the jerk. Extinction of the jerk by exciting the central end of the 8th root (from hamstrings) affects the jerk four segments higher without in that distance spreading over to the opposite side. But the excitation affects the jerk of the opposite side if the scope of a considerable length of cord be allowed

[1] Sherrington, *J. Physiol.*, 1892, **13**, 666.

it. If in the cat the cord be transversely divided at the 11th thoracic segment, excitation of the afferent fibres from a hamstring muscle of one side (*e.g.*, right) applies chiefly to the jerk on the same side (right), but also to the jerk on the opposite. If, however, in the cat (in which jerk belongs to the 6th and 5th lumbar segments) the cord be transversely cut at or below the 3rd, the extinction from the hamstring nerve is confined to the same side only. In other words, the presence of additional higher segments seems requisite before the passage of the impulses in question across the median plane of the cord, a fact in curious harmony with an observation by Hallstén[1] regarding the elicitation of " crossed reflexes " in the frog. The median posterior column between the 8th and 4th lumbar levels can be removed *in toto* without impairing the influence of the hamstring nerve on the jerk. It is clear also that those fibres of the posterior root which pass to Clarke's column cannot be the requisite afferents, either from the extensor or flexor thigh muscles, because the jerk and the above-described extinction of it are unaffected in the cat by transverse section of the cord just below the 4th lumbar segment—*i.e.*, the segment where Clarke's column stops short.— *February* 8, 1893.]

2. THE APPROPRIATE RELAXATION OF ANTAGONISTS[2]

[*Further observations on the inhibition of the knee jerk. Stretching of an extra-ocular muscle has reflex effects. Conjugate lateral movement of the eyes, when elicited by appropriate stimulation of the cerebral cortex, still occurs in some degree when the motor nerve to an internal rectus muscle of one side has been severed. In this case the intact external rectus muscle must relax by a process of inhibition. This, with other instances of the appropriate relaxation of antagonists, is discussed.*]

Appropriate excitation of the afferent nerves from the flexor muscles of the knee joint so alters, as I have shown, the condition of the extensor muscles of that joint that the reaction called the " knee jerk " becomes no longer elicitable. I have endeavoured to examine the quality of the alteration which thus restrains or abolishes the " jerk."

It must be remembered that there is some variance of opinion as to the nature of the jerk itself. In the opinion of some authorities the jerk is of reflex nature (Bowditch, Lombard, Senator, Warren); in the opinion of others it is not truly reflex, but is a direct muscular reaction, intimately dependent, however, on a reflex tonus in the muscle (Tschiriew), or on a spinal influence reflexly exerted, but not necessarily identical with " tonus " nor necessarily measurable by tonicity (Waller).

On the reflex theory of the " jerk," its disappearance or decrease under excitation of the sensory nerve from its antagonistic muscles tallies with phenomena of the mutual interference of spinal activities such as are

---

[1] *Archiv. Anat. Physiol., Lpg., Physiol. Abt.*, 1885, 167.

[2] Published as " Further Experimental Note on the Correlation of Action of Antagonistic Muscles," *Proc. roy. Soc.*, 1893, **53**, 407.

exemplified perhaps most clearly by those experiments of Goltz, in which, after section of the spinal cord in the thoracic region, the act of micturition could be cut short by strong stimulation of the skin of the tail. On the view that the jerk is not itself reflex, but depends on a reflex tonus, the abeyance of the phenomenon under excitation of the afferent fibres of the hamstring nerve might be owing to decrease thus induced in the tonus of the vasto-crureus muscle, just as on the same view abolition of the jerk by cutting the sensory roots of the crural nerve is due to the impairment thus produced in the tonicity.

As a step toward determining between these two possibilities, I have attempted to discover whether afferent impulses ascending from the hamstring muscles affect to any considerable extent the tonus of the antagonistic quadriceps extensor. Complete abeyance of the "jerk" under excitation of the hamstring nerve cannot, so far as I have seen, be long maintained. After a longer or shorter interval the jerk returns. Soon after discontinuance of the stimulation the jerk not only returns, but becomes markedly exaggerated. Though abolition or decrease of the jerk is thus temporary, exaltation conversely produced by severance of the hamstring nerve is permanent, lasting at least for some weeks. On the tonicity hypothesis concerning the jerk, exaltation of the jerk by section of the hamstring nerve should be accompanied by a concurrent increase in the tonus of the vasto-crureus muscle.

It is not easy to judge *slight* differences in tonus of muscles even where of the fellow muscles of the two sides of the body one normal muscle is available as standard for comparison. Yet any decided difference of tonus must, if multiplied into a sufficient time, amount to a not inconsiderable difference in the chemical condition of the muscle. I have therefore sought to test what influence, if any, section of the hamstring nerve exerts on the extensor muscle of the joint as judged of by the development of rigor mortis in that muscle.

In muscles paralysed by section of their nerves, onset of post-mortem rigidity is delayed (Kölliker,[1] Brown-Séquard[2]). Bierfreund[3] has found that after semi-section of the spinal cord made a few hours before death the onset of rigor in the limbs on the side of section is considerably later than on the opposite side. Inasmuch as depression of tonus is an alteration in the direction of this paralysis, I hoped that time of onset of rigor mortis might serve to indicate whether, *cæteris paribus*, decrease or increase of tonus had obtained in the muscle for the period immediately preceding death. A few experiments on the influence of nerve section upon speed of onset of rigor mortis gave results accordant with the original by Brown-Séquard and Kölliker. I then turned to the division of, instead of muscular nerves, the anterior roots supplying the muscles. Experiments made on the hind-limb of the cat showed the effect of section of the anterior roots

[1] *Virchows Arch.*, 1856, **10**, 242.   [2] *Gaz. Méd. Paris*, No. 42, 1857.
[3] *Pflüg. Arch. ges. Physiol.*, 1888, **42**, 195.

to be a marked delay in the onset of rigor in the muscles supplied by them. The effect was clear, even if the roots were cut only five minutes before killing the animal. I then experimented on division of the posterior roots. The posterior roots of the 6th, 7th, and 8th post-thoracic nerves of one side were severed. In result the hamstring muscles of the corresponding side became rigid later than did those of the opposite side, even in an experiment in which the animal was killed only a quarter of an hour after section of the roots. The effect of section of these sensory roots after previous severance of the cord at the 1st lumbar segment was then examined. The severance of the cord, as was to be expected, deferred considerably the onset of rigor mortis in both of the hind-limbs. It appeared also to decidedly reduce the difference between the time of onset of the rigor in the two hind-limbs; but still, in each case, the hamstring muscles on the side corresponding to the section of the posterior roots entered rigidity later than in the fellow limb. The effect of section of the hamstring branch of the sciatic trunk upon the time of onset of rigor in the extensors of the knee, the cord having been previously divided at the 1st lumbar segment, was then proceeded to. Twelve experiments were made, but the results obtained were conflicting. In seven of these experiments rigor commenced in the extensor of the side on which the nerve had not been cut before it did in the extensor of the opposite side. In three rigor commenced indubitably rather earlier on the side of nerve section than on the opposite. In two I could not detect that there was any difference between the two sides in the time of onset of the rigor. A point noted in nine of these experiments (it was not looked for in the remaining three) may be mentioned. When death is induced by hæmorrhage, the cord having a short time previously been severed at the top of the lumbar region, various reflexes can be elicited from the hind-limbs and tail for some little time after respiratory spasms and all reflexes have vanished from the body in front of the level of the section. There is in the cat an ear reflex which generally outlasts others under chloroform or ether administration, and often outlasts them by a considerable time. Indeed, so soon as this reflex has disappeared, the respiratory movements are reduced to a dangerous extent. It consists in a laying back of the pinna of the ear, the pinna being frequently twitched several times; it is elicited by sharply twisting the tip of the pinna. The corneal reflex and still more the knee jerk are both extinguished by chloroform and ether for some time before this ear reflex disappears. This reflex may in the cat, like Dastre's reflex from the gum of the upper jaw in the dog, be termed the reflexus ultimus. But when death is induced in the manner above mentioned, the knee jerk outlasts the ear reflex by as long in some experiments as four or five minutes; and in the limb in which the hamstring nerve has been divided the jerk persists longer than in the fellow limb.

Finally, I examined the effect of bandaging one knee in full extension, the other in full flexion, after previously severing the cord at the 1st lumbar segment. The bandages after an interval were removed. The jerk on each side was then found to be good, and rather brisker in the knee that had been flexed than in that which had been extended. Death was induced by hæmorrhage. No difference between the time of disappearance of the jerk on the two sides was detected. In each of five experiments performed the quadriceps extensor and the crural muscles became rigid later on the side that had been flexed than on the other side, but the hamstring muscles became rigid earlier in the leg that had been flexed than in the other. This is not what might have been expected in view of Wundt's observation that tension in a muscle hastens rigor in it. It must be remembered that Wundt's statement is not based on muscle *in situ*, intact and connected with the spinal cord. The observed fact harmonises with the existence of an augmentation of tonus of extensors in result of excitation of the afferent nerves from their opponent group.

The experiments so far therefore seem to indicate that the direction of the change induced in the extensor muscles by afferent impulses ascending from the flexors is in the direction of increased tonicity, and to strengthen the supposition that the interference with the "jerk" is located in the spinal mechanism of the "jerk."

The marked influence exerted reflexly by the flexors of the knee upon the extensors of that joint suggested search for instances of analogous correlation elsewhere. The delicately correlated muscles of the eyeball offer an experimental advantage in that even slight alterations of their length can be readily observed by inspection. I therefore exposed the inferior oblique muscle (cat and monkey), completely detached it from the globus, and then observed the effect of lightly drawing upon it, so as to stretch it between the end held and the end attached to the bony floor of the orbit. Reflex actions were in this way easily obtained, but were inconstant in character; the eyeballs were generally moved, perhaps most frequently conjugately, toward the side corresponding to the stretched muscle. I watched especially to see whether the globes were turned upward or downward, but those movements were far less frequent than movements apparently purely lateral. Sometimes the reflex obtained did not affect the eyes at all; the movement was often a pricking of the ear, either with movement of the eyes or apart from eye movement. Twice the muscle was detached altogether with careful avoidance of injury to its nerve and bloodvessel; held between two ivory-tipped forceps, it was then gently stretched. The results were the same as when its one end retained the natural attachment. In all cases section of the nerve which enters its posterior border to supply it immediately abolished all reply. This nerve is relatively long and easily isolable. Electrical excitation of it can be performed with facility; a weak tetanising current applied to its central end produced the same variable movements as did the stretching of the muscle itself, but apparently less readily.

The inferior oblique muscle was employed for these observations because it can be freely isolated with little injury and displacement of other structures, and because of the length of the nerve branch supplying it. I should have preferred, otherwise, to use the externus rectus, because of the simplicity of its antagonistic coupling with the internal rectus. But the external rectus it is not easy without disturbance of other parts to isolate sufficiently to feel certain that tension put upon it remains confined to it alone. I adopted, therefore, for examining the antagonism of the external and internal recti the method of paralysing one and then examining the activities of the other. When examining in the monkey the movements of the digits obtainable by cortical excitation, if movement—*e.g.*, flexion— of the hallux or pollex is elicited, and the nerve to the flexors of the digit be then severed, renewed cortical excitation at the same spot still produces a movement;[1] this movement is generally in direction the reverse of that previously obtained; this " *reversal* " is, however, not invariably obtained; occasionally there results a feeble movement in the same direction as the movement previously obtained. In three experiments this movement has been so decided as to lead one to re-examine carefully the site of division of the peripheral nerve in order to assure oneself that it had been really severed completely. The persistence of movement in the same direction as before the flexor nerves are severed must indicate that the stimulation applied to the cortex produces at each repetition an inhibition of the tonus of the muscles antagonistic to the flexors—that is to say, of the extensor muscles. My experience of this inhibition is that it cannot, even when it occurs, be demonstrated many times in succession. The phenomenon of *reversal* is, on the other hand, obtained repeatedly with facility.

A power to inhibit the activity of striated muscle has, therefore, to be included among the attributes of the " motor " cortex of the hemisphere. In the co-ordination of the movements of the eyeballs it appears to play an important and easily demonstrable part. Ferrier[2] discovered that excitation of a particular portion of this cortex produces a conjugate movement of both eyeballs in a direction away from the hemisphere in which the stimulation is employed. If the appropriate area of the cortex of the left hemisphere be excited the movement is of both eyeballs to the right. My enquiry regarding the correlation of action of the antagonistic internal and external recti in this movement may be stated as three questions. Is the movement carried out:

(*a*) By contraction of the left internal rectus and the right external rectus, their antagonist muscles undergoing the while simply passive traction;

(*b*) By contraction of the above two muscles combined with slighter contraction (steadying) of their antagonistic muscles (left external rectus and right internal rectus); or

(*c*) By contraction of the left internal and right external rectus associated with inhibition of the tonus of their antagonistic muscles (left external rectus and right internal rectus) ?

[1] Sherrington, *J. Physiol.*, 1892, **13**, 621.   [2] Ferrier, *Functions of the Brain*, London, 1876.

The plan of experiment adopted has been as follows: The appropriate portion of the left cortex having been ascertained by excitation, and having assured myself that the desired conjugate deviation is regularly obtained, I at once sever the 3rd and 4th cranial nerves of the left side between their origin and the point of their entrance into the cavernous sinus. The position of the left eyeball in rest is, immediately after performance of that section, scarcely perceptibly different from what it has been before, nor is usually the pupil dilated immediately, although it soon becomes so. Excitation of the cortex as before is at once proceeded with. The movement obtained is still conjugate deviation of both eyeballs to the right. The right globus appears to move exactly as before; the left globus, on close examination, although it moves, clearly does not move as it did before. Its movement starts usually just perceptibly later than the movement of the right eyeball; the movement, when started, is somewhat slower than that of the right eye, and it travels only some two-thirds as far; on discontinuing the excitation both eyeballs return together.[1] Sometimes the movement of the left eye, instead of starting later than that of the right, starts simultaneously with it; sometimes it starts distinctly earlier, and this especially when the external squint that soon appears has become well developed. But the movement is never seen quite so rapid or so ample as that of the right eye. On excitation of the corresponding part of the right cortex the movement of the left eye outwards may be very slight, especially if there be marked outward strabismus; in two experiments there frequently occurred on excitation of the right cortex together with the usual movement of the right eye to the left a movement of the left eye to the right and sometimes, apparently, to beyond the primary position. A few times a double movement occurred, the left globus at first moving to the left conjugately with the right, and then suddenly reversing its movement and turning inwards to the right. At each discontinuance of the excitation of the right cortex, when the eyeballs have reacted by conjugate movement to the left, the left does not return so quickly as the right; indeed, it may be many seconds in returning.

These experiments succeed uniformly, so far as I have seen, with both *Macacus rhesus* and with *sinicus*, even when very young specimens are used. Ferrier and Munk have shown that conjugate movements of the eyes are obtainable from the cortical surface posterior to the " motor " region, and Schäfer, by demonstrating *inter alia* the great difference in the reaction time for the movements in the two cases, has provided an index for the profound distinction that must be drawn between them. I find that from this posterior region, as well as from Ferrier's " motor " region, can the tonus of the external rectus be inhibited in the orbit of the same side as the hemisphere stimulated after the 3rd cranial nerve of that side has been cut through.

---

[1] For myograph tracings of this inhibition of the extra-ocular muscles, and also limb muscles, on stimulation of the cerebral cortex, see " On the Spinal Animal," *Med.-Chir. Trans.*, 1899, **82,** 449, Plate XVI.—Ed.

An extremely interesting observation has recently been made by Mott and Schäfer.[1] Experimenting together, they have seen that by simultaneous excitation of the frontal cortex of both right and left hemispheres the two eyeballs can be set approximately in the primary position, sometimes with a slight degree of convergence. I have, in two Bonnet monkeys, repeated this experiment after having previously performed section of both right and left 3rd nerves and both right and left 4th nerves at their origin from the brain. After the section there was considerable double divergent squint, and in one of the experiments the strabismus of the left eye was distinctly the greater in degree. The effect of simultaneous bilateral excitation, approximately balanced, of the frontal cortex was to cause both eyes to be rotated inwards up to, and certainly in some trials beyond, the primary position. The double divergent squint was converted into a slight degree of convergence. Here, where the external recti were the only ocular muscles still connected with the central nervous system, convergence must have been due to simultaneous bilateral inhibition of the tonus of the right and left external recti. It is difficult to find any other interpretation for these results than that the excitation of the cerebral cortex, just as it occasionally inhibits the tonus of the muscles of the thumb or hallux, also possesses the power of inhibiting the tonus of ocular muscles, at least of the external straight muscle. Further, it would seem that this inhibitory activity of the cortex is more constantly elicitable experimentally in the case of the muscles of the eyeball than in the case of those of the hand and foot. That the cerebrum nominally exerts a more or less tonic inhibitory influence over the lower local centres subserving muscular tonicity and local muscular reflex action is a widely accepted doctrine. The above observations accord with and, as I think, extend the data for such a belief.

The above experimental results may, it seems to me, be all of them explained on an hypothesis that the cerebral cortex can inhibit muscular tonus and reduce it even to paralysation limit; but it does not seem necessary to suppose that the cortex, although it can thus inhibit tonus in striped muscle, can also inhibit the active contraction of it. This second assumption seems necessary, however, to explain the following result: If, after section of both right and left 3rd and right and left 4th nerves the left frontal cortex be excited and both eyes made to deviate to the right, excitation of the right cortex (the experiment has not succeeded unless this stimulation be somewhat strong) will not unfrequently cause the right eye to move inwards and sometimes fully up to the primary position. The active contraction of the external rectus appears to be cut short and even converted into a condition of relaxation more complete than when no cortical excitation at all is being employed.

I have watched with interest in Macacus the voluntary movements of the eyes after section of the 3rd and 4th nerves. In the early hours after the section, if, for instance, these nerves have been cut on the left side only,

[1] *Brain*, 1890, **13**, 165.

the gaze is readily directed to the left but not so readily to the right. There arises, of course, considerable external squint of the left eye. Neither when the right is directed toward the right nor when it is converged upon a light or other object just in front of the face is there more than a mere trace of movement of the left eye. Twenty-four or forty-eight hours later, when the right eye is turned to right, the left eye does perform the conjugate movement, but imperfectly, and more imperfectly and also more variably than under experimental excitation of the frontal cortex.

Another instance in which antagonistic correlation may be examined is that of the muscles which close and open the palpebral aperture. These are at least potentially antagonistic. I find that in the monkey excitation of the 3rd nerve in the cranium slightly depresses the lower eyelid at the same time that it freely raises the upper. This slight depression, often very slight indeed, is abolished by section of the branch of the 3rd to the inferior rectus muscle. The 3rd nerve (leaving out of consideration the cervical sympathetic, the action of which in opening the eye, as regards speed, direction of movement, and other characters, is different from the opening obtainable from the cortex) may be termed the nerve which opens the palpebral aperture. The 7th is the only nerve which closes it by active muscular contraction.

This latter statement applies to the monkey, not to the cat, because in the cat, after section of the 7th nerve at the stylo-mastoid foramen, I find that, although the upper and lower lids remain permanently rather widely apart, the third eyelid (membrana nictitans) shuts at short intervals with an extremely rapid sweep completely over the exposed part of the globus; and when after section of the 7th the animal sleeps the nictitating membrane is partially extended over the front of the ball. The third eyelid is therefore not innervated like the upper and lower from the 7th. Langley and Anderson[1] record that it is not innervated from the 4th, probably not from the 3rd, but that excitation of the 6th causes " great protrusion of it."

If, after section of the 3rd, the appropriate part of the frontal cortex be excited either on the same side as the nerve cut or on the opposite side, I find no movement at all result in the lids on the side corresponding to the nerve section, although the opening of the eye the other side is each time quick and wide. That is to say, there is in this instance no evidence of concomitant activity of the antagonistic muscle, either in the sense of contraction or of relaxation. But on shifting the electrodes to the suitable point of the cortex the eyes of both sides reply to the excitation by a sharp closure just as usual.

The well-known dilatation of the pupil elicitable from this region of the cortex might, in view of the above-described examples of inhibition from the cortex, perhaps, be supposed to be related rather to an inhibition of the constrictor action of the 3rd nerve than to cortical augmentation of the influence kept up via the cervical sympathetic. The dilatation of the pupil under excitation of the frontal cortex certainly is much later in onset than

[1] *J. Physiol.*, 1892, **13**, 461.

are the movements of the extrinsic ocular muscles, but that difference might be based on the difference in time of response of the two kinds of muscular fibres involved. This supposition is, however, negatived by the fact that division of the cervical sympathetic cut out dilatation that was being regularly elicited from the cortex, the 3rd nerve being undivided, in two experiments I made to test the point. In these instances, therefore, although an extreme dilatation was obtained with, for the cortex, quite weak currents, the cortex reacted by discharge directed through the sympathetic system.

Addition (April 20, 1893)

I would add to the above the following remarkable passage, which I find in *The Anatomy and Physiology of the Human Body*, by Charles and John Bell (London, 1826, vol. iii). In describing the action of the muscles of the eye, the author, after adverting to some experiments made by himself on the functions of the 4th cranial nerve, says:

" We have seen that the effect of dividing the superior oblique was to cause the eye to roll more forcibly upwards; and if we suppose that the influence of the 4th nerve is, on certain occasions, to cause a relaxation of the muscle to which it goes, the eyeball must be then rolled upwards.

" The nerves have been considered so generally as instruments for stimulating the muscles, without thought of their acting in the opposite capacity, that some additional illustration may be necessary here. Through the nerves is established the connection between the muscles, not only that connection by which muscles combine to one effort, but also that relation between the classes of muscles by which the one relaxes and the other contracts. I appended a weight to a tendon of an extensor muscle, which gently stretchted it and drew out the muscle; and I found that the contraction of the opponent flexor was attended with a descent of the weight, which indicated the relaxation of the extensor. To establish this connection between two classes of muscles, whether they be grouped near together as in the limbs, or scattered widely as the muscles of respiration, there must be particular and appropriate nerves to form this double bond, to cause them to conspire in relaxation as well as to combine in contraction. If such a relationship be established, through the distribution of the nerves, between the muscles of the eyelids and the superior oblique muscles of the eyeball, the one will relax while the other contracts."

My experiments described above show the correctness of Bell's supposition, at least as regards the external straight muscles, and that the phenomenon of inhibition of activity under volition and under appropriate cortical faradisation is not confined among the ocular group of muscles to the recti externi, the observations made seem to prove. For instance, I have divided the 6th cranial nerve of the left side at its origin from the brain, and then examined the behaviour of the eyeballs under suitable experimental conditions. The position immediately assumed by the eyeballs was that of slight convergence even when under anæsthesia (not very deep). Subsequently the internal strabismus increased somewhat, to disappear, or almost disappear, when the gaze was voluntarily turned to the right, but to be greatly increased—i.e., the angle at which the optic axes crossed becoming great—when the gaze was directed to the left. The left eye under volitional movement frequently rotated from the inner canthus outward conjugately with the right, but never passed beyond the primary (median, straight-forward) position. On the gaze being directed from the median primary position toward the right, the left eye rotated conjugately with the right eye, usually with an apparently perfect symmetry of motion, but not infrequently with a movement slower and less ample than the right. On the gaze being directed from the median primary position toward the left, the left eye did not move at all, while the right eye moved, of course, normally. It was frequently seen that the eyes remained turned to the right, apparently resting in that direction; it was so generally when the animal was sleepy or dozing. When the gaze was directed from that position over to the left, the move-ment of the left eye was not unfrequently, so far as could be seen, perfectly conjugated and symmetrical with that of the right eye as far as up to the middle line of the palpebral fissure; there it stopped short, while the right eye went a variable distance further.

On excitation of the appropriate part of the frontal cortex of the right side, both eyes being in the primary position or with a slight degree of convergence at the commencement of the excitation, the right eye swept sharply to the left, and the left either did not move or merely shifted sluggishly up to the full primary position. On excitation of the frontal area of the cortex of the left hemisphere both eyes were directed to the right, the left eye sometimes moving sluggishly as compared with the right; after cessation of the excitation, the right eye would frequently return at once to approximately the primary median position, while the left eye did not return for a considerable time, and did so in a slow unequal manner; frequently, however, both eyes remained for a long time steadily directly toward the right, and under anæsthesia that seemed to be almost as frequent a position for them to assume as was one approximating to the median primary. When the right frontal cortex was faradised, the eyes resting at the commencement of the excitation in a direction towards the right, the right eye swept over sharply to the left, sometimes with an upward inclina-tion also, more rarely with a downward; movement of the left eye invariably accompanied this movement of the right, and with a corresponding inclina-tion, but the movement of the left eye often started late, and was almost invariably slow and feeble as compared with that of the right, and it was also the more variable. When both eyes had been directed to the right by excitation of the left frontal cortex, and directly after the left side excitation had ceased, the right frontal cortex was excited, both eyes turned toward the left, but the left eye never overshot the primary median plane. When the two eyes had been directed to the right by moderate faradisation of the left frontal cortex, a somewhat strong faradisation of the right frontal cortex, the moderate faradisation of the left side being still continued, caused the left globus, and the right, to be turned toward the left, but the right eye generally started earlier and moved more quickly than the left, and the left, although sometimes brought up to the primary position, was sometimes only slightly turned towards it.[1] When a moderate excitation of the right frontal cortex had turned the right eye to the left and brought the left to the full median position, moderate faradisation of the left frontal cortex (the excitation of the right side still continuing) turned the left eye to the right so as to produce convergent squint; stronger faradisation of the left cortex successive to and concurrently with moderate faradisation of the right directed both eyes to the right. In two instances moderate excitation of the right cortex alone, near the angle of the precentral sulcus, caused the right eye to be turned to the left, and the left eye to be turned to the right, so that strong convergence resulted.

Faradisation of the left occipital cortex directed both eyes to the right with a slight downward or slight upward inclination or without any inclination, according to the area excited (Schäfer, Munk). Faradisation of the right occipital cortex, if both eyes were approximately in the primary position, caused the right eye to be slowly and steadily turned to the left, and the left eye to be steadily brought fully up to the medium primary position if it were not already in it; if already fully in the primary position, the left eyeball did not move at all. If the left eye moved at all, it very generally started its movement distinctly before the right eye and appeared to rotate less slowly than did the right. This difference was best seen if the eyes were previous to the excitation resting in a direction to the right. On then faradising with weak or moderate currents the left occipital cortex, the steady slow rotation of the left eye commenced so much before that of the right that sometimes the left had travelled half-way to the primary position before the right eye had well started. Under excitation of the right occipital cortex the movement of the left eye toward the left seemed so clearly stronger, sharper in starting, and even quicker and steadier than under excitation of the right frontal cortex, that I attempted to balance it against the movement to the right produced from the left frontal cortex. On each occasion, when tested, I found that, the two eyes being kept directed to the right by moderate excitation of the left frontal cortex, they could be sent over to the left again by moderate or strong excitation of the right occipital cortex, and in each instance the left or paralysed eye was again the first to start travelling. Three similar experiments gave results quite similar to the above in the points mentioned here.

In two experiments, one on a small *Rhesus* and one on a large *Sinicus*,

---

[1] A notable dilatation of both pupils sometimes occurred in this combination experiment. Neither the left nor the right faradisation produced by itself any dilatation of either pupil, but on the second electrodes being applied considerable dilatation of both pupils followed. There was no epilepsy.

I have combined with section of the left 6th nerve section of the left 4th nerve at its exit from the brain. The results obtained agreed in many respects with those obtained when the 6th nerve alone was severed. Points of difference were the following: In the median position of rest the left eye was turned slightly upward as well as inward. On excitation of the right frontal cortex, the eyes starting in the primary position, the right eye was turned to the left side and the left eye was turned upward more or less amply, rarely not at all; the left eye was never observed to rotate to the left beyond the primary median position. When particular points in the right frontal cortex had been found which directed the eyes not merely to the left, but upwards also, on stimulation being applied the left eye was turned upward to a greater degree than was the right. When places were found in the right frontal cortex which directed the right eyeball downward as well as to the left, occasionally the left eye moved a little downwards; more usually it moved distinctly upwards, so that there was strong divergence of the optic axes in the vertical plane, with the right pupil depressed, the left pupil elevated sometimes considerably. The same held true in the results of excitation of the occipital regions of the cortex, and the left eye generally commenced movement under excitation of the right occipital cortex distinctly earlier than did the right eye, just as when the 6th nerve alone had been divided; so that under excitation of the right occipital cortex there was usually at one phase of the movement, instead of any convergence of the optic axes, a strong divergence of them.

It was noticeable that after division of the 6th nerve, either alone or in conjunction with the 4th, also in one experiment in conjunction with the 5th, the pupil of the eye on the same side as the nerve section was slightly but distinctly larger than in the opposite eye. This observation led me to stimulate the 6th root in the monkey, but, although the eye was in result moved outwards, I could not satisfy myself that any constriction of pupil at all occurred, although the pupil was well dilated at the time. In the case of the internal straight muscle, I believed it would be less easy to sever its antagonist's nerve than in the case of the antagonist of the external rectus. I therefore made several earlier experiments, employing section of the external rectus and its nerve inside the orbit. The above description is, however, not based on the results of those earlier experiments in which the orbit was opened, because (1) it was found then impossible to be quite certain that some remnant of movement or drag in the muscle could not affect the globus sufficiently to simulate the movement that might result from a relaxation of the antagonistic muscle; (2) because when once the orbit has been opened, or its contents dissected, the movements of the globus are deranged sufficiently to beset with doubt any interpretation that can be put upon them; (3) finally, because destruction of the muscles or their nerves in the orbit or cavernous sinus involves destruction also of concomitant sensory fibres from the 5th nerve which may exert a considerable influence on the antagonistic muscle, the subject of observation. I would add, however, that the results obtained in my earlier experiments did, though open to these objections, seem to accord with those I have obtained after sections at the base of the brain; it may be that the harmony between the two sets is superficial rather than real. The experiments from which the results related here are quoted are only those in which neither the orbit nor the cavernous sinus was opened at all.

It appears, therefore, that the activity of the internal straight muscle can be directly inhibited by appropriate excitation of certain parts of the frontal cortex, still better of the occipital cortex, of the hemisphere of the side opposite to the muscle; and the inhibition is very similar to that exerted over the activity of the external straight muscle by similar regions of the cortex of the *same* side as the muscle. A point of difference—and it is a suggestive one— between the two cases appears to be that under inhibitory relaxation of the *rectus externus* from cortical excitation the globus may rotate beyond the middle line of the palpebral fissure, whereas under cortical relaxation of the *rectus internus* the eyeball may travel up to that middle line, but very rarely, if ever, trespasses beyond it.

It thus seems clear that by experiment abundant support can be obtained for the supposition put forward by Charles Bell.

3. RECIPROCAL RELAXATION A COMMON REFLEX EFFECT[1]

[*After section of the brain-stem above the level of the pons a condition of rigidity of the extensor muscles of the limbs develops (later called " decerebrate rigidity "). This rigidity relaxes when the flexion reflex is evoked, and this relaxation is a further example of the automatic behaviour of antagonists in which the one will relax as the other contracts (" reciprocal innervation ").*]

In the preceding papers attention was drawn to a particular form of correlation existing between the activity of antagonistic muscles. In it one muscle of an antagonistic couple is, it was shown, relaxed in accompaniment with active contraction of its mechanical opponent. The instance then cited was afforded by certain of the extrinsic muscles of the eyeball, but I had previously noted indications of a like arrangement in studying the reflex actions affecting the muscles at the ankle joint of the frog,[2] and it seemed probable that the kind of co-operative co-ordination demonstrated for the ocular muscles might be of extended application and occurrent in various motile regions of the body. The observations to be mentioned below do actually extend this kind of reciprocal innervation[3] to the muscles of antagonistic position acting about certain joints of the limbs.

If transection of the neural axis be carried out at the level of the crura

---

[1] Published as " On Reciprocal Innervation of Antagonistic Muscles, Third Note," *Proc. roy. Soc.*, 1896-7, **60**, 414-417.　　　　　　　[2] *J. Physiol.*, 1892, **13**, 621.
[3] The term " reciprocal innervation," which appears here for the first time (January, 1897), was defined earlier in the larger paper in *Philos. Trans.*, **190B** (here in extract on p. 153, Chapter IV), completed in 1896, read on the same day as the above, and not published until 1898.—ED.

cerebri in, *e.g.*, the cat, there usually ensues after a somewhat variable interval of time a tonic rigidity in certain groups of skeletal muscles, especially in those of the dorsal aspect of the neck and tail and of the extensor surfaces of the limbs. The details of this condition, although of some interest, it is unnecessary to describe here and now, except in so far as the extensors of the elbow and the knee are concerned. These latter affect the present subject. The extensors of the elbow and the knee are generally in strong contraction, but altogether without tremor and with no marked relaxations or exacerbations. On taking hold of the limbs and attempting to forcibly flex the elbow or knee a very considerable degree indeed of resistance is experienced; the triceps brachii and quadriceps extensor cruris become, under the stretch which the more or less effectual flexion puts upon them, still tenser than before, and on releasing the limb the joints spring back forthwith to their previous attitude of full extension. Despite, however, this powerful extensor rigidity, flexion of the elbow may be at once obtained with perfect facility by simply stimulating the toes or pad of the fore-foot. When this is done the triceps enters into relaxation and the biceps passes into contraction. If, when the reflex is evolved, the condition of the triceps muscle is carefully examined, its contraction is found to undergo inhibition, and its tenseness to be broken down synchronously with, and indeed very often accurately at, the very moment of onset of reflex contraction in the opponent prebrachial muscles. The guidance of the flexion movement of the forearm may therefore be likened to that used in driving a pair of horses under harness. The reaction can be initiated in more ways than one—electrical excitation of a digital nerve or mechanical excitation of the sensory root of any of the upper cervical nerves may be employed; I have seen on one occasion a rubbing of the skin of the cheek of the same side effective.

Similarly in the case of the hind-limb. The extensor muscles of the knee exhibit strong steady non-tremulant contraction under the appropriate conditions of experiment. Passive flexion of the knee can only be performed with use of very considerable force, the quadriceps becoming tight as a stretched string. The application of hot water to the hind-foot then elicits, nevertheless, an immediate flexion at knee and hip, during which not only are the flexors of those joints thrown into contraction, but the extensors of the knee joint are simultaneously relaxed. Electric excitation of a digital nerve or of the internal saphenous nerve anywhere along its course will also initiate the reflex.

The same relaxation of existing contraction in the extensors can be obtained by electrical excitation of the tract in the crura cerebri, when, as sometimes happens, that excitation evokes flexion at elbow or at knee. This and the previous fact which evidences that the result is obtainable after complete removal of the whole cerebrum bear out the view arrived at in my former paper that for this reciprocal and, as I believe, elementary co-ordination it is not essential that " high level " centres (Hughlings Jack-

son) be employed. I incline to think, however, that this kind of co-ordination at elbow and knee is probably largely made use of in movements
initiated via the cerebral hemispheres as well as in the lower reflexes, on the
observation of which the present note is based. This conclusion is indicated
by its occurring in response to excitation of the pyramidal fibres in the crura.
In the case of the reciprocal innervation of antagonistic ocular muscles I
was able to prove that it took place even in " willed movements." It seems,
in view of what has been shown above, legitimate to extend that result to
the additional examples afforded by elbow joint and knee.

Regarding the innervation of the *triceps brachii* and *quadriceps extensor
cruris*, it is interesting to note that these muscles, which are of all among
the limb muscles particularly difficult to provoke to action by local spinal
reflexes, are the very ones which, when the level of the transection is pontial
or prepontial, exhibit tonic contraction the most markedly. The well-known
and oft-corroborated Sanders-Ezn phenomenon of inaccessibility of the
extensors of the knee to spinal reflex action[1] has, as I have recently shown,
certain limitations, but at the same time, so long as the transection is spinal—
even when carried out so as to isolate not merely a portion of, but the whole,
spinal cord entire from bulb to filum terminale—does apply very strictly
to excitations arising in its own local region proper. And the spinal reflex
relationships of the triceps brachii in this respect, as pointed out elsewhere,
somewhat resemble those of the distal portion of the quadriceps extensor
of the leg. Alteration of the site of transection from infrabulbar to suprabulbar levels works a curious change in this. The Sanders-Ezn phenomenon[1]
then becomes subject to striking contravention. I have, after the higher
transection, several times seen excitation of the hind-foot itself provoke
unilateral ipsilateral extension of knee, a result incompatible with the
Sanders-Ezn rule[1] even under the limitations of ipsilaterality, etc., which I
consider must be attached to it. And similarly with the triceps at the
elbow.

The difference between the accessibility of the quadriceps to reflex
action after infrabulbar and after suprabulbar transection may, however,
be less abrupt than it appears at first sight, and a superficial rather than a
fundamental distinction. When *extensor rigidity* has ensued at elbow and
knee after suprabulbar transection, the reflex excitability of triceps brachii
and quadriceps cruris seems in a manner as difficult as in the presence of
exclusively spinal mechanisms. The reflex inhibitions the subject of this
note show, however, that the accessibility is not really greatly or even at
all altered; the nexus is maintained, but the conduction across it is signalised
by a different sign—*minus* instead of *plus*. The former, to find expression,
must predicate an already existent quantity of contraction—*tonus*, to take
effect upon. It seems likely enough that even when the transection is infrabulbar and merely spinal mechanisms remain in force, the same nexus
obtains, but that then that background of tonic contraction is lacking, and

---

[1] The supposed restriction of spinal reflexes to flexor muscles, see p. 142, Chapter IV.—ED.

that lacking the play of inhibitions remains invisible, never coming within the field of any ordinary method of observation.

Under the conditions adopted in my experiments, various other reflex actions, that seem probably examples of this same kind of co-ordination, can be studied—for instance, a sudden depression and curving downward of the stiffly elevated and tonically up-curved tail which can be elicited by a touch upon the perineum. But with these and also with other details regarding the reflexes at elbow and knee I hope to deal more fully in a paper to which the experiments recorded here are contributory.

Reciprocal Innervation also holds for Movements initiated by Stimulation of the Motor Cerebral Cortex or the Internal Capsule[1]

The object of the present communication is to report to the Society further on the occurrence in so-called " voluntary " muscles of *inhibition* as well as of *contraction*, as result of excitation of the *cortex cerebri*. We have obtained by excitation of the cerebral cortex some remarkable instances of what one of us has described under the name of " *reciprocal innervation* "— that is, a species of co-ordinate innervation in which the relaxation of one set of co-ordinated complexus of muscle groups occurs as accompaniment of the active contraction of another set.

The experiments, the subject of the present communication, have been carried out in the monkey (*Macacus cynocephalus*) and the cat. The appropriate region of the cortex cerebri has been freely exposed after removal of part of the cranium and subsequent slitting and turning aside of the dura mater. The cortex has then been stimulated by rapidly repeated induction shocks obtained by the Du Bois inductorium. The Helmholtz equaliser has always been employed. The intensity of the faradic currents used has been usually such as to be barely perceptible when the platinum electrodes were applied to the tongue-tip. The anæsthetics used have been either ether alone or ether mixed with chloroform in equal volumes. The degree of narcotisation forms an important condition for the prosecution of the observations. When the narcosis is too profound the results to be recorded are much less obvious than when the narcosis is less deep. It is best, starting with the animal in a condition of deep etherisation, to allow that condition gradually to diminish. As this is done it almost constantly happens that at a certain stage of anæsthesia the limbs, instead of hanging slack and flaccid, assume and maintain a position of flexion at certain joints, notably at elbow and hip. This condition of tonic contraction having been assumed, the narcosis is, as far as possible, kept at that particular grade of intensity. The area of *cortex cerebri* previously ascertained to produce under faradisation extension of the elbow joint or hip joint is then excited.

[1] Published with E. H. Hering as " Antagonistic Muscles and Reciprocal Innervation, Fourth Note," *Proc. roy. Soc.*, 1897-8, **62**, 183-187.

For clearness of description we will suppose that the left hemisphere is excited, and that, therefore, the limb affected is the right. The result of excitation of the appropriate focus in the cortex—*e.g.*, that presiding over extension of the elbow—is an immediate relaxation of the biceps, with active contraction of the triceps. As regards the condition of the biceps, the relaxation is usually so striking that merely to place the finger on it is enough to convince the observer that the muscle relaxes. The following is, however, a good mode of studying the phenomenon: In a monkey with strongly developed musculature the forearm, maintained by the above-mentioned steady tonic flexion at an angle of somewhat less than 90° with the upper arm, is lightly supported by the one hand of the observer, while with the finger and thumb of the other the belly of the contracted biceps is felt through the thin skin of the upper arm. On exciting the cortex the contracted mass becomes suddenly soft—as it were, melting under the observer's touch. At the same time the observer's hand supporting the animal's forearm tends to be pushed down with a force unmistakably greater than that which the mere weight of the limb would exert. If the triceps itself be felt at this time it is easy to perceive that it enters contraction, becoming increasingly hard and tense, even when its points of attachment are allowed to approximate, and the passive tensile strain in it should diminish. If the limb be left unsupported the movement is one of simple extension at the elbow joint. On discontinuing the excitation of the cortex the forearm usually immediately, or almost immediately, returns to its previous posture of flexion, which is again, as before, steadily maintained.

Conversely, when, as not unfrequently occurs in conditions of narcosis resembling that above referred to, the arm has assumed a posture of extension, and this is tonic and maintained, the opportunity is taken to excite the appropriate focus in the cortex, previously ascertained, for flexion of forearm or upper arm. Triceps is then found to relax, and the biceps at the same time enters into active contraction. If the biceps be hindered from actually moving the arm, the prominence at the back of the upper arm due to the contracted triceps is seen simply to sink down and become flattened. When examined by palpation the muscle is felt to become more or less suddenly soft, and the biceps at the same time to become tenser than before. The movement of the limb, when allowed to proceed unhindered, is flexion with some supination. It is noteworthy that in this experiment not every part of the large triceps mass becomes relaxed; a part of the muscle which extends from humerus to the scapula does not in this experiment relax with the rest of the muscle. This part, if the scapula be fixed, acts as a retractor of the upper arm, and is not necessarily an antagonist of the flexors of the elbow. This part of the triceps we observed sometimes enter active contraction at the same time as the flexors of the elbow. It should be remarked that under use of currents of moderate intensity we find that not from one and the same spot in the cortex can relaxation and contraction of a given muscle be evoked at different times, but that the two effects are to be found at different, sometimes widely separate, points of the cortex, and are there found regularly.

We have obtained analogous results in the muscles acting at the hip joint. When in the narcotised animal the hip joint is being maintained in flexion, the thighs being drawn up on the trunk, excitation of the region of the cortex, previously ascertained when the limbs hang slack to evoke extension of the hip, produces relaxation of the flexors of the hip and at the same time active contraction of the extensors of the thigh. We examined particularly the psoas iliacus and the tensor fasciæ femoris, also the short and long adductor muscles. Each of these was found to relax under appropriate cortical excitation. If the knee were held by the observer, it was found at the time of relaxation of the flexors of the hip to be forced downward by active extension of the hip.

Similarly with other groups of antagonistic muscles, both those of the small apical joints of the limb (e.g., flexors and extensors of the digits) and those of the large proximal joints (e.g., adductors and abductors of the shoulder). At these also instances of reciprocal innervation were obtained.

That a part of the triceps brachii (that retracting the upper arm) should actively contract exactly when another part (that extending the elbow) becomes relaxed is exactly comparable with a phenomenon which has been described by one of us in treating of spinal reflexes, both in the triceps itself and in the quadriceps femoris. And we have similarly seen in the quadriceps femoris, on exciting the cortical region yielding extension of the hip, a relaxation of a part of the quadriceps (a part which flexes the hip) with contraction of another part (which extends the knee).

We hope, in a longer communication, in which the literature can be dealt with, to give a more detailed account of other instances of co-ordination, in which inhibition of the contraction of the so-called voluntary muscles makes its appearance in result of excitation of the cortex cerebri. The examples cited in the present note are evidently intimately related to those to which attention has been already called in second and third notes on the co-ordination of antagonistic muscles already presented to the Society.

Addendum

Since the above was written, one of us (C.S.S.) has had opportunity to perform further experiments both on the monkey and the cat, and has carried out excitation of the fibres of the internal capsule, as well as excitation of the cortex cerebri. Knowledge is at present completely vague as to which of the many elements in the cortex constitutes the locus of genesis of the reaction obtained by electrical stimuli applied from the cerebral surface. It is therefore conceivable that the elements of the pyramidal tract are only mediately excited by moderate faradisation of the cortex. If so, inhibitory effects produced by excitation of the cortex might likely enough *not* occur under direct excitation of the cut fibres of the capsula interna.

As a matter of fact, however, the results obtained from the internal capsule have been as striking as those obtained from the cortex itself. From separate points of the cross-section of the capsula, relaxation of various muscles has been evoked.

Among the muscles, inhibition of which has been directly observed, are supinator longus and biceps brachii, the triceps, the deltoid, the extensor cruris, the hamstring group, the flexor muscles of the ankle joint, and the sterno-mastoid.

The spots in the cross-section of the capsula which have yielded the inhibitions are constant—that is, the position of each when observed has remained constant throughout the experiment. The area of the capsular cross-section at which the inhibition of the activity of, *e.g.*, the triceps muscle can be evoked is separate from (that is to say, not the same as) that area whence excitation evokes contraction of the triceps (or of that part of the triceps, inhibition of which is now referred to). On the other hand, the area of the section of the internal capsule, whence inhibition of the muscle is elicited, corresponds with the area whence contraction of its antagonistic muscles can be evoked. Yet synchronous contraction of such pairs of muscles as gastrocnemius and peroneus longus is obtainable from the cortex.

The observations make it clear that " *reciprocal innervation* " in antagonistic muscles is obtainable by excitation of the fibres of the internal capsule. It is probable, therefore, that the inhibition elicitable from the cortex cerebri is not due to an interaction of cortical neurones one with another. The variety of nervous reaction in which I have been able to establish existence of the reciprocal form of muscular co-ordination is now pretty extensive. In some the condition described in the previous (third) note (the state shown to ensue upon removal of the cerebrum, and in that note spoken of as " decerebrate rigidity ") was conducive to the result; in others the cerebrum was of course not removed. The reactions examined for the phenomenon with positive result include those initiated by excitation of—

(1) The skin and skin nerves (with " decerebrate rigidity ").
(2) The muscles and afferent nerves of muscle (with " decerebrate rigidity ").
(3) The dorsal (posterior) columns of the cord (with " decerebrate rigidity ").
(4) Of the cerebellum (with " decerebrate rigidity ").
(5) Of the crusta cerebri (with " decerebrate rigidity ").
(6) Of the internal capsule.
(7) Of the optic radiations.
(8) Of the Rolandic cortex.
(9) Of the occipital (visual) cortex.

Reciprocal Innervation holds for the Movement of Blinking. The Operative Procedure required Section of the 8th Nerve as well as the 7th, and the Symptoms of Section of the 8th Nerve are described[1]

In a previous communication upon this subject I gave[2] the results obtained in an experimental examination of the antagonistic correlation which at least potentially exists in the muscular action of the opening of the palpebral aperture. The *orbicularis palpebrarum* and the *levator palpebræ superioris* are to a certain extent an antagonistic couple. During the course of last year I took opportunity to examine the co-ordination of the same antagonistic muscles in the movement, not of the opening of the palpebral fissure, but of its closure. The observations having been unavoidably interrupted by removal to a new laboratory, it is only recently I have been able to confirm the preliminary observations on a sufficiently extended scale.

The monkey and the cat have been the animals employed. Under deep chloroform narcosis intracranial section of the 8th cranial nerve was performed at the point where the nerve plunges into the petrosal portion of the temporal bone. In three instances the *nervus octavus* and the *pars intermedia* were also severed with the *facialis*. In every case the side selected for operation was the left. The facial palsy caused was not detectable so long as the narcosis was maintained. As that was gradually recovered from, asymmetry of expression, etc., became marked. In those instances in which both the facialis and octavus had been severed, there appeared among the symptoms the following: Rotatory nystagmus of the left eyeball, some inequality of the pupils (the left being the smaller), some degree of impotence of the eyeballs to move so far to the right as to the left, or, expressed more objectively, the eyeballs were never observed to move freely to the right of the primary visual position, although they frequently moved well to the left; they certainly never moved far to the right; the animals rolled over about the long axis of the body, as mentioned in Magendie's original description of the effect of unilateral section of the pons. The direction of rotation, if traced from the supine position as starting-point, was towards the animal's right side, so that that side next after the back lay undermost. The monkey clutched hold of things within reach, with the apparent intention of preventing itself from rolling. If it failed to obtain some support the rolling would continue through a series of complete turns. This was the condition immediately after complete recovery from the narcosis, and at that time the left knee jerk was less brisk than the right; on the latter side it appeared to be abnormally brisk, but it is difficult to fix a normal. The actual existence of section, and whether it had included both nerves or only one, was always determined by subsequent *post-mortem* dissection.

[1] " On the Reciprocal Innervation of Antagonistic Muscles, Fifth Note," *Proc. roy. Soc.*, 1898, **64**, 179-81.

[2] *J. Physiol.*, 1894, **17**, 27.

As to the eye closure, while the animal was exhausted or sleepy, or only partially recovered from the chloroform narcosis, there was no obvious difference between the appearance of the eyelids on the two sides, as they rested half open over the globes. When the animal blinked, however, under these conditions, the palpebral opening of the right eye closed, but not that of the left—at least not to any easily perceptible extent. When on the contrary the animal was fully awake and active, with both eyes well opened, it was seen that as the right eye blinked the left eye also did so. By blinking I understand the rapidly executed movement of closure which occurs so repeatedly without attention being directed to it, although it can be voluntarily restrained—the quick movement which may be regarded as an irregularly recurring reflex that doubtless has among its objects the renewal of moisture on the corneal surface, which otherwise would become dry. This natural blinking movement seems in the monkey not to employ the orbital portion of the *orbicularis palpebrarum*, but only the palpebral. It occurs habitually as a bilateral and symmetrical movement. It is far less extensive in action than the closure of the palpebral opening, which ensues when the monkey grimaces on being threatened with a blow. That in the blinking the contraction of the palpebral part of the orbicularis is not, however, the whole of the muscular mechanism at play, is clear from the fact that in the awake and active animal with fully opened eyes the blinking still remains bilateral, subsequent to section of the facialis nerves of one side. The blinking by the right eye was of course normal in character. As the right eye blinked, the upper lid of the left eye quickly dropped three to four millimetres over the globus of that side, and was then synchronously with the lifting of the right upper lid lifted again. The left lower lid was not on any occasion detected to move at all. The quick fall of the upper lid of the left eye must have been due under these circumstances to inhibition of the tonus of the left levator palpebræ superioris muscle. This brings the co-ordination of the reaction into line with that which I have described for other movements under the term reciprocal innervation.

It is interesting that Panas, Sappey, Fuchs, Wilmart and others, who have carefully and particularly studied the mechanism of the closure of the eye, have not attributed any share to an inhibition of the levator palpebræ; one physician, however, Dr. Lor, of Brussels, has argued that in the closure of the human eye such an inhibition does under certain circumstances occur.

4. INHIBITION RESULTING FROM RECIPROCAL INNERVATION CAN BE GRADED IN INTENSITY[1]

[*The amount of relaxation in a muscle depends on the relative intensities of the excitatory and inhibitory effects. Similar antagonism occurs in visceral reflexes. Inhibition therefore does not necessarily cause complete relaxation.*]

In further prosecution of observations made in Ludwig's laboratory by Schmiedeberg[2] and by Bowditch,[3] N. Baxt[4] in 1875 carried out in that laboratory a prolonged enquiry into the effect produced on the heart's frequency by combined stimulation of the inhibitory (*vagus*) and accelerator (*accelerans*) nerves going to that organ. His observations were made on large dogs; the two nerves were faradised simultaneously. In most of his experiments stimulation of *accelerans* preceded that of *vagus* by a few seconds, to allow for the well-known longer latency of the former's reaction; the precurrent stimulation of *accelerans* alone was immediately followed by stimulation of both nerves simultaneously. Baxt found the rate of heart-beat under the combined stimulation slowed as though the vagus only and no accelerator was in operation; but, immediately following on cessation of the combined stimulation, a full accelerator effect appeared, as though no stimulation of the vagus had taken place. Baxt employed usually minimal stimulation of *vagus* and maximal of *accelerans*, for he found minimal excitation of *vagus* suffice to set aside completely, for the time being, maximal excitation of *accelerans*. In his hands the result of the combined stimulation was vagus action, even when weakest, completely obscuring accelerans action even at strongest; but, although the accelerans action showed no trace of its existence during the vagus stimulation, it appeared in full force after the vagus action had passed off. The vagus action therefore did not destroy it, but merely postponed its appearing. Baxt drew the conclusion that the inhibitory nerve and the excitatory nerve must act on separate points in the heart's mechanism and are not true antagonists. This view has since been endorsed by many,[5] but is not that of v. Cyon, the discoverer of the *accelerator*.

Another field for examination of the same problem was chosen by v. Frey.[6] He investigated the effect on the venous flow from the sub-maxillary gland of simultaneous stimulation of the vaso-constrictor (*cervical sympathetic*) and the vaso-dilatator (*chorda tympani*) nerves. The dilatating influence of the *chorda* proved to be completely overpowered by the constricting effect of the sympathetic during combined stimulation of the two.

---

[1] Extract from *Proc. roy. Soc.*, 1908, **80B**, 565, published under the title " Reciprocal Innervation of Antagonistic Muscles, Thirteenth Note. On the Antagonism between Reflex Inhibition and Reflex Excitation."

[2] *Arbeiten a. d. physiol. Anstalt z. Leipzig*, 1871.   [3] *Ibid.*, 1873.   [4] *Ibid.*, 1875.

[5] *E.g.*, Tigerstedt, *Physiologie d. Kreislaufs*, Leipzig, 1894; for a contrary view see S. J. Meltzer, *Arch. Anat. Physiol. Lpz.*, Physiol. Abt., 1892, p. 376, and v. Cyon, *Nerven d. Herzen*, Berlin, 1907.

[6] *Arbeiten a. d. physiol. Anstalt z. Leipzig*, 1876.

But on discontinuing the combined stimulation there ensued from the vein a markedly excessive blood-flow—*i.e.*, a marked chorda action ensued as an after-effect. The action of the sympathetic had therefore not destroyed the action of the concurrently excited chorda, it had only postponed its appearing. v. Frey, with his customary clearness, wrote:[1] " The antagonism between constrictor and dilatator has not as its basis a simple summing of two forces which act in opposite direction at the same point of application." The sympathetic prevails entirely for the time being as regards the surface effect, but the chorda nevertheless develops with regular course the change characteristic of its action, and does so " in some part of the excitable apparatus protected from the attack of the sympathetic: only in some other place do the actions of the two collide."[2]

Some years later Heidenhain,[3] discussing the acceleration of pulse-rate, which in the frog follows discontinuance of a stimulation of the vagus-trunk, attributed it to accelerans fibres commingled with the inhibitory in the vagus-trunk, and with them excited by the stimulus applied. He then went on to suggest that inhibitory actions fall into two classes which should be clearly distinguished one from the other. He argued that in one class the inhibitory process antagonises the excitatory process by decreasing or suppressing its actual occurrence, whereas in a second class the inhibitory process, without actually lessening, or indeed altering, the excitatory process, simply prevents the latter from, for the time being, getting access to and affecting the organ of its destination, the organ which, but for the inhibition, it would reach and affect. To this second class of inhibitions he relegated the vagus action on the heart and its interference with the accelerator on that organ. As another example of this second class, he cited similarly the opposition between sympathetic and chorda on the vessels of the submaxillary gland.

This explanation of inhibition brought forward by Heidenhain as satisfying the cases which he terms inhibitions " of the second class " resembles the hypothesis earlier offered by Rosenthal.[4] Rosenthal, after making his discovery that stimulation of the afferent *laryngeus superior* brings the diaphragm to rest in the relaxed condition, offered the following explanation of this inhibition. The rhythmic action of the respiratory centre results, he argued, from the excitation which arises in that centre not having access to the motor channels directly, but having to pass a resistance. Through this resistance the continuous excitation is transformed into an intermitting and rhythmic discharge. This resistance he supposed to be increased by stimulation of the superior laryngeal nerve; whence the inhibitory action of the nerve.

It is interesting to find Heidenhain adopting this explanation, first advanced for a central reflex inhibition, as applicable to peripheral in-

---

[1] *Arbeiten a. d. physiol. Anstalt z. Leipzig*, 1876.   [2] *Ibid.*
[3] *Pflüg. Arch. ges. Physiol.*, 1882, **27**, 283.
[4] *Die Athembewegungen u. ihre Beziehungen z. N. Vagus*, Berlin, 1862.

hibitions (therefore of his second class), but on the other hand discarding it as little applicable to central reflex inhibitions. These latter he considered as for the most part belonging to his first class. He gives no specific instance, but he is evidently expressing the impression he has derived from his work with Bubnoff,[1] published the previous year, " On Excitation and Inhibition in Motor Cerebral Centres." In " a great number of the facts known as voluntary and reflex inhibition " it is " a matter of the weakening or suppression of central excitatory processes by willed or peripheral sensory influence."[2] And ten years later Meltzer,[3] from observations " on the mutual relation of the nerve-fibres in the vagus which inhibit and excite respiration," distinctly concludes that under maximal stimuli the action of one of the opposed nerves regularly hides that of the other (just as does the vagus the accelerator's action and the sympathetic the chorda dilating action), but that with submaximal stimuli " giebt es kein Ueberwiegen, sondern ein Verschmeltzen zu einer Resultante."[4]

Reid Hunt[5] showed that, as indeed some of Baxt's own records reveal (cf. Meltzer), accelerans stimulation does express itself on beat-rate even during vagus excitation. O. Frank[6] obtained a similar result; he, however, upholds Baxt's conclusion as legitimate, stressing the fact that while accelerans quickens both systole and diastole, vagus slows diastole alone. Recently Bessmertny,[7] from experiments under Asher, also infers that these antagonists act at separate places in the cardiac mechanism. Cyon, however, has always pressed an exactly opposite view.[8] By Asher[9] the question has been tested in another case by pitting depressor stimulation against asphyxial stimulation of the vasomotor centre: there also the results he concludes confirm those already given by the experiments on vagus-accelerator and on constrictor-dilatator antagonism.

Similar questions arise in regard to the reflex inhibitions expressed by skeletal muscles. Here the seat of the inhibition is central. The skeletal muscle attached by means of its motor nerve to the centre expresses by contraction the excitation of the motoneurones of that centre and by relaxation or by restraint from contraction the inhibition of those motoneurones. In the following experiments I have chosen as field for collision of the opposed influences, excitatory and inhibitory, the motoneurones of the vasto-crureus muscle. Of the various afferent arcs acting on this field I have selected two whose reflex influences are of diametrically opposed direction. Of these, one causes flexion of the knee, the other extension. The former was excited by faradisation of the central stump of the ipsilateral peroneal nerve severed at the knee, the latter by similar faradisation of the contralateral popliteal nerve likewise severed at the knee. The vasto-crureus, with its nerve and blood supply and attachments intact, was

[1] Pflüg. Arch. ges. Physiol., 1881, **26**, 137.
[2] Ibid., 1882, **27**, 283.
[3] Arch. Anat. Physiol. Lpz. Physiol. Abt., 1892, p. 341.
[4] Ibid., p. 383.
[5] Amer. J. Physiol., 1894, **2**, 396.
[6] Sitzungsb. d. Ges. f. Morph. u. Physiol. in München, 1897.
[7] Z. Biol., 1905, **47**, 400.
[8] Nerfs d. Cœur, Paris, 1905; Nerven d. Herzen, Berlin, 1907.
[9] Z. Biol., 1905, **47**, 87.

isolated as described in previous papers.[1]   The femur was fixed by a strong clamp close above its condyles.   All nerves of the opposite leg were severed to exclude reflex movement there which might confuse the result.   The animals (cat) were decerebrate, decerebration being performed under deep chloroform-ether narcosis.   For faradisation two Berne coils with secondary values graduated in Kronecker units were employed.   In the secondary circuit containing the electrodes there was intercalated in all cases a resistance of 100,000 ohms in order to steady the stimulation values for the nerve-trunk.

In one respect the mutual antagonism of these reflex influences acting on this preparation differs from that described as obtaining in the antagonisms mentioned previously.   The difference is as follows: When both the afferent nerves are stimulated fairly strongly the ipsilateral exerts preponderant influence over the contralateral.[2]   This preponderance is evidenced in two ways: (a) The muscle, while contracting under the excitatory influence of the contralateral reflex, on fairly strong stimulation being applied to the ipsilateral afferent nerve forthwith relaxes completely so as to show no obvious contraction (see figures in previous papers).[3]   (b) The muscle, while lying relaxed under the inhibitory influence of the ipsilateral reflex already in operation, on fairly strong stimulation being then applied to the contralateral afferent nerve still remains, in spite of that stimulus, relaxed and to all appearance devoid of any contraction (see figures in previous papers).[4]

The ipsilateral afferent arc is therefore the prepotent one: its action overpowers that of the contralateral arc.   But, as has been shown elsewhere,[5] this prepotence is not inevitable.   The influence of the contralateral afferent nerve finds clear expression if its stimulation be strong at a time when that of the ipsilateral is quite weak.[6]   Whether the one influence or the other is preponderant depends, therefore, in the case of this preparation, on the relative intensity of the stimuli applied to the two antagonistic nerves respectively.   This reversibility of the sense of the reaction seemed to me to indicate the preparation as a favourable one on which to test the nature of the antagonism—the more so as in it both the excitatory reflex and the inhibitory reflex are capable of being graded in intensity with much fineness by simply grading the intensity of stimulus applied to their respective afferent nerves.

From the observations[7] it seems clear that the reflex effect of concurrent stimulation of excitatory afferent nerve with inhibitory afferent nerve on

[1] Sherrington, J. Physiol., 1907, **36**, 185.
[2] Sherrington, Integrative Action of the Nervous System, 1906, p. 224.
[3] Proc. roy. Soc., 1905, **76**, 277.   [4] E.g., Rep. Brit. Ass., 1904, p. 736.
[5] Sherrington, Integrative Action of the Nervous System, 1906, p. 225.
[6] Figured in the original paper, see fig. 42, p. 289 this volume.
[7] Loc. cit., p. 578. The details of the experimental results are here omitted, for they are summarised in the next reprint, pp. 287-291.—ED.

the vasto-crureus reflex nerve-muscle preparation is an algebraic summation of the effects obtainable from the two nerves singly, as v. Cyon has maintained for the heart. The individual effects of the two nerves " fuse to a resultant," to use the words applied by Meltzer to his results on the respiratory centre. One inference allowable from this is that in the case before us the two afferent arcs employed act in opposite direction at one and the same point of application in the excitable apparatus. They are in this sense true antagonists. The inhibition exercised by the inhibitory member of the pair comes, therefore, under Heidenhain's Class I. of inhibitory reactions. As to the common locus of operation, the point of collision of the antagonistic influences, it seems permissible to suppose either that it lies at the synapse, in which case the opposed influences may be thought of as altering oppositely the permeability of the synaptic membrane, or that it lies in the substance of the " central " portion of a neurone, probably of the motoneurone itself, meaning by " central " that part of the neurone which lies in the reflex centre. In either case the condition of the material of the common locus seems altered in two diametrically opposite ways by the two antagonistic afferent arcs.

5. REFLEX INHIBITION AS A FACTOR IN THE CO-ORDINATION OF MOVEMENTS AND POSTURES[1]

[*Reciprocal innervation requires the mechanism for an active relaxation. This mechanism is the reflex process of inhibition. It is not simple cessation of nervous discharge, but is an active nervous function which is graduated in quantity. It is regulated in amount inversely to that of the excitation of antagonists. Lack of any such reflexly-graded function results in inco-ordination.*]

Desistence from action may be as truly active as is the taking of action. In the animal organism, side by side with excitations to action run restraints from action. Only recently has account been taken of the frequency of occurrence of this restraint, and of the fact that restraint by inhibition is as fully a reaction to a stimulus as is excitatory response itself.

The nervous system, driven chiefly, though perhaps not wholly, by the external world, drives and controls in its turn the greater part of the bodily machinery, especially the motor part, and always in the interest of co-ordination. Its inner workings take expression in that way. They find material expression in no other way. Such expression, so far as physiology goes, constitutes the whole practical purpose or end of the nervous system. The powers of the environment to incite through the nervous system the activity of this or that bodily organ have long been studied; less so its powers through the nervous system to check and restrain the bodily activities.

---

[1] Published under the above title in *Quart. J. exp. Physiol.*, 1913, **6**, 251-310. Pages 285-296, with accompanying illustrations dealing with further details of action of antagonists in rhythmical reflexes, have been omitted.

Inhibition in Relation to Autonomic and to Skeletal Muscle Respectively

Nerve makes its first appearance phylogenetically in association with muscle.[1] Of all tissues muscle is the closest and most delicate exponent of nerve-action. Yet not all muscle is equally intimately tied to nervous centres. The beat of the heart, freely separable from central nervous action, proceeds unimpaired after the heart's removal from the body. Similarly the intestinal and other visceral muscles—*e.g.*, bladder[2]—continue their rhythmic contractions after rupture of all extrinsic nervous ties. Almost as full is the muscular independence of the bloodvessels. Their tonus is in many cases impaired by severance of their connections with the neuraxis,[3] yet the impairment is but transient.[4] Thus the contractile activity of these visceral and vascular muscles is fundamentally independent of central nervous influence. Yet to all these visceral and vascular muscles, including the heart itself, nerves are distributed from the central nervous system, and through these nerves that system does on occasion influence visceral and vascular activity. The nature of the influence thus exerted is in all these cases twofold. Two influences opposite in kind and direction can be exerted, and sometimes one is employed, sometimes the other. The one augments the contractile activity of the muscle, the other diminishes it: the former is termed *excitatory*, the latter *inhibitory*; and the nerve-fibres which unfold these two influences respectively are distinct from one another.

In striking contrast with this large measure of independence from the central nervous system shown by the visceral and vascular muscles stands the complete dependence on that system of the *skeletal* muscles. The contraction of a skeletal muscle is always the expression of a mandate sent to it from the neuraxis. Even with the peripheral nerve-muscle preparation a stimulus to the nerve throws the muscle into contraction more readily than a stimulus applied directly to itself. After the severance of its nerve a skeletal muscle never, except under artificial stimulation, contracts again. Hence, when removed from the body, a skeletal muscle, unlike the heart, intestine, stomach, bladder, etc., never of itself contracts again. Mere section of its nerve, even when the muscle remains *in situ*, causes it to lapse into a paralytic quietude so profound that its very structure becomes in a short time hardly recognisable as muscle. Its contractive function and its very nutrition are indissolubly dependent on the neuraxial centre which innervates it.

That stimulation of the nerve of a skeletal muscle readily and regularly

---

[1] Parker, G. H., *J. exper. Zool.*, 1910, **8**, 1.   [2] Sherrington, *J. Physiol.*, 1892, **13**, 676.

[3] By the neuraxis is meant the whole central nervous system; it is convenient to follow the practice, especially common with French and Italian neurologists, of adopting this one term for embracing the whole central nervous organ.

[4] Goltz and Freusberg, *Pflüg. Arch. ges. Physiol.*, 1874, **8**, 482.

elicits contraction of the muscle was known early. The discovery later of nerves augmenting and accelerating the contractions of the visceral and circulatory muscles fell into line with that previous knowledge, and seemed natural enough. But the discovery by the Webers[1] in 1846 that a nerve passing to the heart can stop or inhibit that muscle's contraction seemed so surprising that at first it was by many not accepted. When assured as a fact, it was, however, recognised as a phenomenon of high significance, unlikely to stand alone. Search for inhibitory nerves to other muscles was begun. The muscle of the intestine wall was shown to have an inhibitory nerve (*n. splanchnicus*, Pflüger,[2] 1857). The ring-musculature of the submaxillary artery and its branches was shown to receive an inhibitory nerve (*chorda tympani*, Bernard,[3] 1858). Meanwhile, there was always expectation of discovery of inhibitory nerves to skeletal muscle. In 1885, Pavlov[4] discovered inhibitory nerves for the adductor muscles of the bivalve mollusc Anodon; and similarly Biederman, in 1886,[5] inhibitory nerves for the claw muscles of the arthropod Astacus. For the skeletal muscles of vertebrates, however, no such inhibitory nerves have come to light.

Yet it were strange did the abundant machinery of the vertebrate nervous system provide no means for checking or curbing the contraction of the muscles of its great skeletal muscular congeries. That congeries, with its manifold individual pieces, some diametrically opposed to others, is so complex, and the confusion and waste of effort consequent were its opponent parts to obstruct each other's action, would seem so foreign to Nature's usual harmonious economy, that inhibitory as well as excitatory control appears *a priori* almost a necessity. The negative result of the search for skeletal inhibitories did not quell the expectation that they would ultimately be found; the search was often renewed. It was, however, always a search for direct efferent inhibitory nerves passing to the muscle from the central nervous system on the plan already discovered for visceral and circulatory muscles. Yet when the broad facts are kept in view, that plan does not appear as necessarily the one most likely to exist. With the skeletal muscle contraction has become so wholly dependent on the central nervous system that it contracts only when the immediate spinal or cranial motor centre summons it to do so. With a muscle which contracts solely at behest of its motor nerve-centre, a simple plan to control the muscle is to control the centre. And, in fact, it is now found that the inhibitory control over skeletal muscle is obtained by *centripetal* inhibitory nerves acting on the muscles' motor centres; the control is not by centrifugal nerves directly inhibiting the muscles themselves. Hence, unlike the autonomous muscles, visceral and circulatory, which receive two kinds of centrifugal nerves, excitatory and inhibitory, the skeletal

[1] Weber, E. H. and Edw., *Omodei annali Univers. di Med.*, 1846, **116**, 225.
[2] Pflüger, E., *U. d. Hemmungs-Nervensystem f. d. peristaltischen Bewegungen d. Gedärme*, Berlin, 1857.
[3] *Leçons sur la physiologie et la pathologie du système nerveux*, Paris, 1858, **2**, 144.
[4] *Pflüg. Arch. ges. Physiol.*, 1885, **37**, 6.   [5] *SitzBer. Akad. Wiss. Wien.*, 1887, **95**, 3 Abth., 8.

muscle receives but one nerve—namely, an excitatory or motor nerve. No inhibitory nerve is supplied to it. But its motor centre receives two kinds of centripetal nerves, excitatory and inhibitory.

The state of the skeletal muscle reflects faithfully the state of its motor centre. Its motor centre is the only source whence impulses can reach it. Upon that motor centre many nerve-paths converge, transmitting to it nervous impulses from various receptive points and from centres elsewhere. Of these nerve-paths some excite, others inhibit. The latter, by quelling or moderating the discharge from the motor centre, quell or moderate the contraction of the muscle. The inhibition of the skeletal muscle is therefore always reflex; and the study of skeletal inhibition falls wholly under the head of reflex action. The motor centre is a convergence point for various reflex influences competing, so to say, for dominance over the muscle. The motor centre lies as an instrument passive in the hands of opposing forces of excitation and inhibition, exerted by nerve channels which impinge upon it. Sometimes the one influence and sometimes the other influence prevails; often the two are simultaneously in action, and then these opponents partially cancel, either spatially in proportion to the relative intensity of their respective stimulations, or temporally by alternating with each other rhythmically in their dominance over the motor centre, thus producing rhythmic reflexes.

Nature of Reflex Inhibition

Knowledge of reflex inhibition equally with that of reflex excitation is essential for the study of nervous co-ordination. But as to the intimate nature of the inhibitory process thus reflexly elicited, at present little is known. That its seat is central is clear. Its field of operation lies in the grey matter. Whether its locus is in the perikarya, or in the dendrites, or in the synapses still waits decision. Since it occurs in reactions whose first step is the excitation of an afferent nerve, and arises from the same stimulus which in other parts of the central field provokes excitation, it is clear that at some point in the nervous arc the excitatory process must be transmuted to an inhibitory one. This inhibitory process does not amount merely to the subsidence of an excited state in its own nerve; it is more than that, for it is able to suppress excitatory processes started from other sources. A natural surmise seems that it may be of the nature of interference, somewhat as waves of sound or light by interference mutually extinguish or reduce each other. This surmise accrues from the knowledge that the nervous impulse, the excited state, is oscillatory or undulatory. Each wave of excitement is accompanied by a refractory state during which a further stimulus fails to evoke further excitement. This may be an outcome of the " all or nothing law " believed by many to hold for the nervous conductor as it does for the heart. The refractory phase, inasmuch as it precludes or lessens response to a stimulus delivered during its persistence, resembles a state of inhibition. Experiments on peripheral nerve-muscle preparations (Keith Lucas[1]) indicate that with certain frequencies of repetition of stimuli the impulses generated and transmitted along the nerve-fibre are too weak to be conducted across places of higher resistance in the line of conduction. The synapses of the nervous arc may be such points of higher resistance. Possibly in such phenomena we have the beginning of an explanation of the nature of reflex inhibition. It certainly seems likely that inhibition is not a conducted state, but one that at some restricted locus breaks or bars the transmitting power of the conductor. It may be that the points where this occurs are those where synaptic conduction occurs. J. S. Macdonald,[2] however, insists on the significance of a difference revealed by microchemistry between axones and nerve-fibres on the one hand, and perikarya and dendrites on the other. The latter have, in addition to the material possessed by the former, a material seen in " fixed " preparations as the well-known Nissl-bodies. Interaction between these two materials might modify conduction in the dendrites and perikarya in ways impossible in the axone, where they do not coexist. Inhibition might be an expression of this interaction. But whatever inhibition is, it can occur in the peripheral nervous system as well as in the central.

A fact to be reckoned with is that the excitatory effect of one afferent and the inhibitory effect of another can be so pitted against one another as to neutralise in their final result. There naturally suggests itself the idea of two delicately gradable antithetic processes or states which can balance in a resultant.[3] Assimilation and dissimilation,[4] alkalinity and acidity, electropositivity and electronegativity, precipitation and resolution[5]— paired opposites like these, as attributes of a reversible reaction, rise to mind and have been suggested.

But while much is still obscure in regard to nervous inhibition, certain types of its action have gradually become familiar in physiology, and help the physiologist to decipher certain of the biological purposes which inhibition serves. A summary of these in the case of reflex inhibition is the main object of the present paper.

REFLEX INHIBITION AS A FEATURE OF SIMULTANEOUS CO-ORDINATION—THAT IS, AS A FACTOR IN THE REFLEX FIGURE

In any systematic study of co-ordination a useful arrangement of its phenomena is into those concerning muscular events which proceed contemporaneously, and those concerning muscular events which follow in

---

[1] *J. Physiol.*, 1911, **43**, 88.   [2] *Quart. J. exp. Physiol.*, 1909, **2**, 65.

[3] A summary of work relating to intermediate grades of antagonism between excitatory and inhibitory effects on the heart, and comparison with reflex effects in voluntary muscle, will be found in Sherrington, *Proc. roy. Soc.*, 1908, **80B**, 565, reprinted here p. 265.—ED.

[4] Gaskell, *J. Physiol.*, 1887, **8**, 404, and Hering, E., *Z. Theorie d. Vorgänge i. d. lebend. Substanz*, Prague, 1888.

[5] Macdonald, *Proc. roy. Soc.*, 1905, **76**, 343, and 1907, **79**, 17. See also discussion in *Integrative Action*, 1906, p. 196.

successive order. Also it is helpful to keep separate the two main forms in which muscular contraction occurs—namely, to distinguish the phasic contractions which execute movements from the tonic contractions which maintain postures. The first step attempted may be to trace the occurrence and significance of inhibition as a factor in the co-ordination of the action of muscles simultaneously involved in the execution of a movement, and for the sake of simplicity the movement chosen may be one of purely reflex kind.

A.—In the Execution of Movements

(i) *Reciprocal Innervation of Anatagonistic Muscles ; Identical Innervation of Synergic Muscles*

Reflex inhibition in the interest of co-ordination intervenes in the taxis of antagonistic muscles. In the anatomical arrangements of the muscula-ture individual muscles are frequently so placed as to exert their pull in diametrically opposed directions. Striking examples of this occur at hinge joints, such as the elbow and the knee, where extensor and flexor muscles act on the same bony lever in exactly opposite senses. Experiment shows that in reflex flexion of the joint the afferent nerve evokes at one and the same time a reflex contraction of the flexor muscle and a reflex relaxation of the extensor (Fig. 37). Conversely, a simple reflex contraction of the extensor is accompanied by a reflex relaxation of the flexor (Fig. 38, and *cf.* Fig. 9A and Fig. 10, *Proc. roy. Soc.*, 1909, **81B**, 260, 262). It is useful to avoid periphrasis by terming that muscle which contracts the protagonist and that which relaxes the antagonist.

In this co-ordination, as in all here discussed, the inhibition is not peripheral but central—that is, it has its seat, not in the muscle nor in the peripheral nerve, but in the nervous centre, probably about the starting-point of the " final common path."[1] The muscle relaxes because the motor discharge from that centre is abated.

This reflex concurrence of excitation with inhibition which the paired centres of an antagonistic muscle-couple exhibit stands in strong contrast with the reflex concurrence of excitation with excitation which the centres of synergic muscles exhibit. As examples of synergic muscles two common types are the following:

(1) Muscles which act mechanically in the same direction at the same joint, such are *semitendinosus* (Fig. 40, A, т) and *biceps femoris posterior* (Fig. 40, A, в) (cat); both are flexors of knee, the one on the outer aspect, the other on the medial of the joint. The reflexes of the limb deal with them identically.[2]

(2) Muscles which act similarly at two neighbouring joints which commonly flex or extend together—for instance, hip and knee. Such muscles are *psoas* (Fig. 40, A, 1) and *semitendinosus*, one flexing hip,

[1] *Brit. Ass. Rpt.*, 1904, p. 730, see this vol., p. 441, and *Integrative Action*, 1906.
[2] *J. Physiol.*, 1910, **40**, 28, and this vol., p. 170.

the other knee. The reflexes of the limb deal with these apparently identically.

In short, muscles which are synergic at the same joint or at neighbouring joints are found to behave identically in the reflex execution of movements; they contract together and relax together. If the reflex flexes the

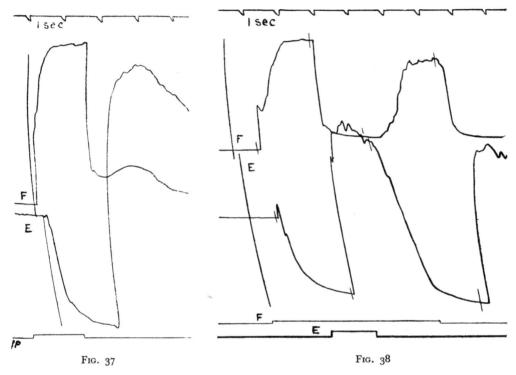

FIG. 37   FIG. 38

FIG. 37.—RECIPROCAL REFLEX OF ANTAGONISTIC MUSCLES OF KNEE

F, *semitendinosus*, a knee-flexor; E, *vasto-crureus*, a knee-extensor. IP, ipsilateral popliteal nerve. The inhibition of the extensor is followed by marked rebound contraction, which is accompanied by a simultaneous relaxation of the flexor muscle. Decerebrate cat. Time marked above in seconds. The signal line signals upward. The myograph writer for extensor muscle is set a little to right of that for flexor muscle, in order that the two may clear each other: the ascent of F and the descent of E are therefore, in fact, practically synchronous

FIG. 38.—RECRIPROCAL REFLEX OF ANTAGONISTIC MUSCLES OF KNEE

F, flexor of knee, *semitendinosus*; E, extensor of knee, *vasto-crureus*. Of the signal lines, the upper marked F marks, by its rise, the period of stimulation of the ipsilateral peroneal nerve; the lower marks similarly the stimulation of the contralateral peroneal nerve. Decerebrate cat. Time above in seconds

limb, all the true flexor muscles contract (Fig. 40, A) and all the true extensors relax concurrently, strongly if the stimulus be strong, weakly if weak. Conversely, if the reflex extends the limb, all the synergic flexors are inhibited and all the synergic extensors (Fig. 40, B) are thrown into contraction. On synergic muscles, therefore, the reflexes operate by identical innervation (as outlined above, pp. 169-172), on antagonist muscles by reciprocal innervation.

Instances of reciprocal innervation of antagonistic muscles are easily obtained for study in the laboratory. Thus in an appropriate reflex preparation it is easily seen at knee or elbow during the flexion-reflex of the limb. While the flexor muscle contracts, the extensor muscle relaxes, and

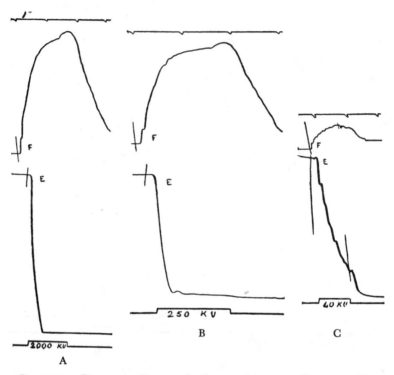

Fig. 39.—Reciprocal Reflex of Flexor, F, Semitendinosus, of Knee, and Extensor, E, Vasto-crureus, of Knee, excited by Stimulation of Afferent End of Ipsilateral Popliteal Nerve

In A the stimulus is moderately strong; in B it is weaker, and in C weakest. The numbers indicate the intensities in Kronecker units of the Berne inductorium. Decerebrate cat. Time above in seconds. The hesitant, slightly tremulant character of weak inhibition is seen in tracing C

the relaxation of the one runs *pari passu* with, and proportionately to, the contraction of the other (Fig. 39, A, B, C).

While thus laying stress on the reflex co-ordination of antagonistic muscles by reciprocal innervation, it must be remembered that not all muscles and pairs having antagonistic mechanical effects are dealt with in this way. The mechanical antagonism of muscles exhibits two main types. Muscles, according as they act directly on one joint or on more than one, are distinguishable into a single-joint class and a double-joint class, and so on. Single-joint muscles exert their pull from origin to insertion across one joint only; they *directly* affect that one joint alone. The most direct and simplest case of antagonism is that between a single-joint flexor and a single-joint extensor acting on one and the same hinge, such as *brachialis* flexing elbow, and humeral head of triceps extending elbow, the lateral and medial muscles of the eyeball rotating the ball in opposite directions about the same vertical axis, or *tibialus anticus* (Fig. 40, A, A) and *soleus* (Fig. 40, B, 8) acting upon the ankle. In all cases of this direct an-

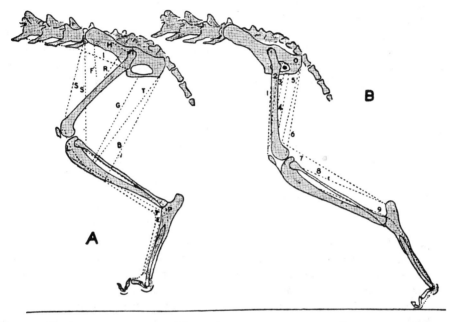

Fig. 40.—Figure illustrating the Muscles actually observed by Experimental Analysis to be engaged in Contracting in the Flexion-phase A and in the Extension-phase B of the Reflex Step of the Cat

Those which contract in the flexion-phase are relaxed by inhibition in the extension-phase, and conversely

A.—A, tibialis anticus; B, biceps femoris posterior; E, extensor brevis digitorum; F, tensor fasciæ femoris; G, gracilis; I, psoas; L, extensor longus digitorum; M, gluteus minimus; P, peroneus longus; R, rectus femoris; S, sartorius lateralis; S', sartorius medialis; T, semitendinosus

B.—o, quadratus femoris; 1, crureus; 2, vasti; 3, adductor minor; 4, adductor major (a part); 5, semimembranosus; 6, biceps femoris anterior; 7, gastrocnemius; 8, soleus; 9, flexor longus digitorum

tagonism the co-ordination of the antagonistic muscle pair is by *reciprocal innervation.*

A less simple kind of antagonism occurs where double-joint muscles are involved—muscles which act directly on two joints. At the knee the *vasto-crureus* (Fig. 40, B 1 and 2) muscle, which passes across that joint only, is the great extensor of the joint, while a double-joint muscle, *semitendinosus* (Fig. 40, A, T) is the main flexor of the joint; but this latter, besides flexing the knee, extends the hip. If the hip be prevented from extending, and, still more, if it be actually flexed, the action of *semitendi-*

nosus as a knee-flexor is enhanced. Experimental examination of the reflex act of flexion of the knee shows[1] that when *semitendinosus* contracts to produce flexion, its antagonist at knee is relaxed by inhibition; but at the hip, where *semitendinosus* is an extensor, it and the hip-flexors are contracted together. The analysis of the reflex shows that *semitendinosus*, although potentially from its position an extensor of hip as well as a flexor of knee, is employed in fact by the nerve centres as a knee-flexor and not as a hip-extensor; nor is there evidence that it is ever used in any other than the former way. In using it the nervous system favours its effect at knee by simultaneously inhibiting its direct antagonist there; but it throws into contraction its antagonists at hip, thus immobilising the point from which the muscle as a knee-flexor takes its pull. A muscle which by fixing a joint enhances the effect of another muscle crossing that joint to act on a more distant one is termed the pseud-antagonist of the latter. *Pseud-antagonists*, unlike true antagonists, are dealt with[1] by " identical innervation "—that is, they contract together and relax together. Thus, in reflex flexion at the hip, when the hip-flexors contract, *semitendinosus*, although a potential extensor of hip, contracts. It is used as a knee-flexor, and knee-flexion often accompanies hip-flexion. But *semimembranosus* (Fig. 40, B, 5), which lies alongside of *semitendinosus*, never contracts with the hip-flexion; it relaxes; it is a hip-extensor and a true antagonist of the hip-flexors, and is always used as such; it is used as if it had no influence at knee. Pseud-antagonists are a numerous class; they fix a joint in order that double-joint muscles crossing it may act better at another joint. True antagonism is dealt with by " reciprocal innervation "; pseud-antagonism, which is really a form of synergism, is, like other synergism, dealt with by " identical innervation."[1]

Reflexes in which " identical " and " reciprocal " innervation are perhaps most easily observable are those where the movement provoked, although maintainable (subject to fatigue) in an enduring fashion, is nevertheless simply single in the meaning that it occurs in one direction only. Such instances are well afforded by the nociceptive flexion-reflex of the limb, where in result of a harmful stimulus the stimulated limb is drawn up and folded as it were out of harm's way; or where, as under cortical stimulation, the eyeballs are turned laterally, directing the gaze sideways.

The question remains whether reciprocal innervation holds good also in rhythmic and alternating reflexes with their more or less rapid reversals of phase and direction—for instance, in the stepping-reflex, the scratch-reflex of the hind-limb, and in consensual nystagmus of the eyeball. In the stepping reflex, with its relatively slow alternation of phase, it is not difficult by myographic analysis to show, with the muscles suitably isolated, that reciprocal innervation of the antagonists does in fact obtain just as in the flexion-reflex itself.[2,3] The limb-muscles employed in the execution of

[1] *J. Physiol.*, 1910, **40**, 28; extracts in this volume, pp. 163-172.
[2] *Ibid.*; here extracts on pp. 185-188.
[3] Graham Brown, T., *Proc. roy. Soc.*, 1913, **86B**, 140.

the flexion phase of the stepping-reflex are found[1] to be those same ones which are employed in the flexion-reflex. And they behave as in the flexion-reflex, and exhibit reciprocal innervation and identical innervation just as in that reflex.[1] That is, the true antagonists are reciprocally innervated; the synergic muscles, those whose contractions mechanically harmonise, including the pseud-antagonists, are identically innervated. And in the extension phase of the reflex, where the extensors instead of the flexors are the protagonists, reciprocal and identical innervation also appear, exemplifying the same rules of distribution to protagonists and antagonists and synergic muscles as in the flexion phase. In fact, the extension phase of the stepping-reflex proves under analysis to be an abbreviated and rhythmically recurrent replica of the extension-reflex just as the flexion phase is of the flexion-reflex.[1]

The scratch-reflex is, like the stepping-reflex, rhythmic—that is, the reflex response is one of rhythmic alternation, although the eliciting stimulus is continuous[2, 1]—e.g., faradic excitation, heat, mechanical friction, etc. But its rhythm is twice as fast as that of the stepping-reflex. The limb-muscles engaged in it are the same as in the stepping-reflex.[3] As regards those of hip, knee, and ankle, they are simultaneously grouped on the same plan as in the step-reflex, although the contraction phase is briefer, if we leave out of account the element of tonic flexion, which the present question does not involve. The higher rate of alternation of the reflex makes it more difficult than in the case of the stepping-reflex to be sure that the phases of contraction of protagonists synchronise with those of relaxation of antagonists. But tracings obtained with the double myograph by T. Graham Brown,[4] using tibialis anticus and gastrocnemius soleus, demonstrate that this is actually the case. In this rhythmic reflex also, therefore, as in the stepping-reflex, reciprocal innervation holds good for the individual phases of the rhythm.

The rhythmic reflex of lateral nystagmus of the eyeball has been examined by Bartels[5] in the rabbit, with analysis of the behaviour of the antagonist muscles, internal and external rectus. The animal was placed on a turntable and the reflex elicited by a turn of the table. A turn to the right causes the eyes to be sharply turned to the right, and this deviation relatively slowly passes off and is then sharply repeated, and so on with rhythmic recurrence. There the double movement consists of quick phases alternating with slow. In each of these phases active relaxation of antagonist synchronises perfectly with active contraction of protagonist (Bartels, Fig. 5, *op. cit.*). So also in the after-nystagmus which ensues in the opposite direction after cessation of the turntable's rotation. Reciprocal innervation holds also, therefore, in this rhythmic movement of the eyeball,

[1] *J. Physiol.*, 1910, **40**, 28.
[2] Sherrington, *J. Physiol.*, 1904, **31**, 18, and 1906, **34**, 1.
[3] *Idem, Quart. J. exp. Physiol.*, 1910, **3**, 213.   [4] *Quart. J. exp. Physiol.*, 1911, **4**, 150.
[5] *Von Graefes Arch. Ophthal.*, 1911, **78**, 129.

just as in its movement of gaze, volitional[1] and under experimental stimulation of the cortex.[2]

(ii) *Biological Meaning of and Peripheral Examples of Reciprocal Innervation*

If we attempt to decipher the biological meaning of reciprocal innervation, such examples as have been given seem to say plainly that it arises when the functional problem to be solved is mechanical antagonism. Where there are two muscles of opposed effect, reciprocal innervation is the principle by which the centres contracting the opponent muscles are dealt with. Also, where there is but one muscle, governed, however, by two nerves influencing it oppositely, one contracting it, the other relaxing it, reciprocal innervation is again the principle by which the two opponent centres are co-ordinated.

In the examples so far cited the reciprocal innervation is always reflex. It may be asked whether reciprocal innervation is entirely limited to reflex and to higher nervous reactions, or whether its distribution in the nervous system is not wider than that, descending, so to say, into simpler and more primitive mechanisms, as might be expected were its significance fundamental.

The musculature of the intestine, with its lowly organised local nervous system of molluscan nerve-net type, has to meet, simple though it be, certain problems of mechanical antagonism. The purpose of its peristaltic movements is evidently propulsion of the intestinal contents down the visceral tube. The ring-muscle below a bolus has to be regarded as in a sense antagonistic to the ring-muscle above the bolus, for its tonus tends to obstruct the passage of the bolus downward under the propulsive contraction of the ring-muscle above. Experiment shows (Bayliss and Starling[3]) that in fact stimulation of the intestinal wall by a bolus excites contraction of the tube above the bolus and relaxation of the tube below the bolus. The relaxation is inhibitory; inhibition of the ring-muscle below accompanies, therefore, contraction of it above. The inhibition obviates the antagonism in a way fundamentally analogous to that by which at a hinge joint inhibition of an extensor muscle obviates mechanical obstruction to the work of a contracting flexor. The neuro-muscular mechanism operative in peristaltic movement, however, need not, and often does not, involve any reactions of the central nervous system. It must be ascribed to the lowly organised local nervous system, the Auerbach plexus, of the intestinal wall. The reciprocal reaction is therefore not reflex in the ordinarily accepted sense of the term. A further problem of mechanical antagonism is presented in the intestine by the axes of contraction of its ring-muscle and its longitudinal muscle being at right angles to each other. It may be that where the ring-muscle contracts, the longitudinal relaxes by inhibition, and conversely. Concerning this we have at present no sufficient data for analysis.

---

[1] Sherrington, *J. Physiol.*, 1894, **17**, 211, and A. Topolanski, *v. Graefes Arch. Ophthal.*, **46**, 452.
[2] P. 249, this volume. [3] *J. Physiol.*, 1899, **24**, 99.

Two other cases of reciprocal innervation which are peripheral may also be cited. One of these is the well-known antagonism of the muscles of the arthropod claw. Stimulation of the cut nerve of the claw distal to its section causes contraction of the one muscle and inhibitory relaxation of its opponent.[1] A point of further interest is that change in the intensity of the stimulus changes the direction of the reciprocal effect. Weak stimulation contracts the abductor and relaxes the adductor; strong stimulation contracts adductor and relaxes abductor. The innervation is a reciprocal one, and its direction changes with change in intensity of stimulus, as does that of the reflex reciprocal innervation of the antagonistic knee muscles evoked from the afferent peroneal nerve,[2, 3] and much as does that of the antagonist muscles at the ankle evoked by stimulation of the afferent nerve, saphenus internus (T. Graham Brown).[4]

The second case is that of the cervical sympathetic and the iris muscle. Langley and Anderson[5] showed that in the mammalian iris there exist in addition to its well-known sphincter muscle some radially arranged contractile elements upon whose contraction dilatation of the pupil in large measure depends. Waymouth Reid,[6] following on the lines of Gaskell's experiment,[7] which demonstrated a positive variation of the demarcation current in the auricle accompanying vagus inhibition of that muscle, examined the effect of stimulation of the cervical sympathetic on the demarcation current of the iris. He used two positions for the galvanometer electrodes applied to the iris—a radial position for tapping the demarcation current of the dilatator muscle, a concentric position for that of the sphincter muscle. He obtained a negative variation in the concentric position of the electrodes when the pupil constricts, in the radial position when it dilates; and a positive variation in the radial position when the pupil constricts, in the concentric when it dilates. He concludes that in the dilatation of the pupil the tone of the sphincter of the iris is inhibited simultaneously with contraction of the dilatator; and that in constriction of the pupil the tone of the dilatator is inhibited simultaneously with contraction of the sphincter. In this peripheral neuro-muscular act reciprocal innervation is the principle on which the antagonist muscles are dealt with, just as in that of the muscles of the arthropod claw.

(iii) *Reciprocal Innervation and Symmetrical Muscles*

In all the above instances the problem solved by reciprocal innervation, whether central or peripheral in seat, is that offered by direct mechanical antagonism of two muscular structures. The distribution of reciprocal innervation extends, however, beyond cases of pure mechanical antagonism. The reflex relation obtaining between the two knee-extensors right and

[1] Biedermann, *S.B. Akad. Wiss. Wien*, 1887, **95**, 3 Abth., 8.
[2] Sherrington and Sowton, *Proc. roy. Soc.*, 1911, **83B**, 435, and **84B**, 201.
[3] Sherrington, *Ibid.*, 1913, **86B**, 219.   [4] *Quart. J. exp. Physiol.*, 1912, **5**, 296.
[5] *J. Physiol.*, 1892, **13**, 554.   [6] *Ibid.*, 1895, **17**, 433.   [7] *Festschrift f. Ludwig*, 1886.

left is, on the whole, reciprocal[1, 2]—that is, the same stimulus which excites reflex contraction of the one evokes reflex inhibition of the other. Here the two muscles are not antagonistic in the ordinary sense; they do not operate on the same lever, nor even on the same limb; one is on one side of the body, the other on the other. And a similar reflex relation holds between many other pairs of symmetrical muscles, not only extensors, but flexors such as the right and left *semitendinosus* muscles and right and left *tensores fasciæ femoris*,[1] also presumably between such a pair as the sterno-mastoidei. It is noteworthy that here the bifurcation of the afferent path which leads to the reciprocal effect sits astride the median longitudinal plane of the body. Also that between the reciprocal innervation of symmetrical extensors and that of symmetrical flexors there is the difference, that in the former the inhibition is in the muscle ipsilateral with the stimulus, and the reflex contraction is contralateral, whereas in the latter the reciprocal signs are converse.[1]

Analogous further is the reciprocal influence exerted by a stimulation of a suitable cortical point in regard to the right and left rectus externus muscles of the eyeballs; and again on the right and left rectus internus muscles. In these cases the same cortical point influences the right and left muscles reciprocally.[3]

But the reflex reciprocity of these muscle-pairs, both of limbs and eyes, presents a difference from that obtaining between the two muscles of an antagonistic couple acting on one and the same joint. In the latter it appears doubtful whether they are ever normally actuated otherwise than reciprocally. In the former the muscle-pair, though perhaps more usually actuated reciprocally, is certainly not rarely actuated identically. Thus the extensors of the two knees, though reacting reciprocally in the walk and trot, react fairly identically in the gallop and in standing. The afferent nerve *genito-cruralis* exerts commonly an excitatory influence concurrently on both vasto-crurei. Again, with the internal recti of the eyeballs, the direction of the gaze laterally is executed by reciprocal innervation, but convergence always involves identical innervation of them, and stimulation of certain brain-points exhibits that kind of innervation in execution of the artificially excited convergence.

It is evident, then, that reciprocal innervation is a mode of taxis not restricted in its application to cases of inevitable mechanical antagonism merely. One field of its application is that of the symmetrical right and left side muscles of the limbs and some other parts. With them, however, reciprocal innervation, although a usual, is not the invariable form which the neural handling of them takes, for sometimes they are dealt with by identical innervation (*v. infra*, Reversal, etc., p. 304).

---

[1] Sherrington, *Proc. roy. Soc.*, 1913, **86B**, 219.   [2] *J. Physiol.*, 1910, **40**, 28.
[3] See also the study of deglutition, and its reciprocal relationship with respiration, by Miller and Sherrington, *Quart. J. exp. Physiol.*, 1915, **9**, 147.—ED.

B.—In the Assumption and Maintenance of Postures

Turning from the execution of movements to that other form of muscular action which evidences itself as the maintenance of posture, a question is whether identical and reciprocal innervation, as disclosed in the taxis of movements, hold also when the muscular function is tonus—that is, posture. As regards muscles forming true antagonistic pairs and their co-ordinatives when engaged in posture, A. Forbes[1] gives arguments for the existence of inhibitory tonus as well as excitatory tonus. Direct experimental evidence on the point is not very easily obtainable. The tonus of skeletal muscle is a reflex state readily upset by operative interference, and liable to vanish under the very procedure required for its analysis. Moreover, true antagonists in most cases consist of a flexor and an extensor muscle, and tonus is particularly difficult and uncertain of production in flexor muscles; so that the criteria for judgment are not regularly open to access in their case.

That reciprocal innervation with its inhibitory factor does hold good for tonus and posture as well as for execution of ordinary movements can be shown, however, by appeal to symmetrical muscles, choice being made of a pair each member of which exhibits demonstrable tonus. Right and left vasto-crurei, extensors of knee, form a suitable symmetrical pair.[2] As shown above, their innervation in ordinary movements is reciprocal. When observed in regard to changes of their tonus in the tonic (decerebrate) preparation, the tonic shortness of the one muscle is seen to decrease as that of the other increases (Fig. 41), in result of, for instance, a few repetitions of stimulation of an appropriate afferent nerve such as peroneal. The innervation of these symmetrical muscles is reciprocal, therefore, also in respect to tonus.

As to reciprocal innervation in respect to tonus of true antagonists acting on one joint, a clear answer is furnished by experiments on the motor cortex.[3] In some grades of narcosis tonic contraction of the flexor muscles becomes marked. It often happens that a muscular contraction evoked from the cerebral cortex under this condition of narcosis subsides only partly after withdrawal of the electrical stimulus. A tonic after-action persists, and on restimulating the cortical point a few seconds later the renewed contraction starts from a higher level again, to lapse only partially on cessation of the stimulus and leave behind a tonus increment—that is, an accentuation of posture—additional to that previously induced. In this way, besides the actual movement induced by each stimulation, there is built up, as in the experiments just mentioned with symmetrical extensors, under successive stimulations, a more or less lasting tonic posture of the reacting muscle. Observation with separated antagonistic muscles shows that *pari passu* with this increase of postural contraction of the protagonist

---

[1] *Quart. J. exp. Physiol.*, 1912, **5,** 149.   [2] *Proc. roy. Soc.*, 1913, **86B,** 219.
[3] Graham Brown and Sherrington, *Proc. rov. Soc.*, 1912, **85B,** 250.

muscle goes decreased postural contraction—*i.e.*, increased postural relaxation of its antagonist—just as with the above-cited symmetrical extensors. Reciprocal innervation holds good for the co-ordination of antagonists in their postural tonus, just as it does for that of symmetrical muscles in their postural tonus, and as it does for both in the execution of ordinary reflex movements.

Also in the innervation of the musculature of the arteries, Bayliss[1] finds

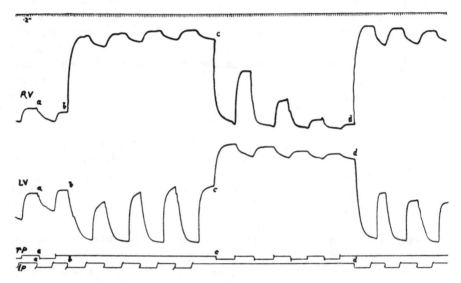

FIG. 41.—RECIPROCAL REFLEXES OF POSTURE, AT THE KNEE-JOINTS RIGHT AND LEFT, GIVING PROPRIOCEPTIVE " SHORTENING " AND " LENGTHENING " REACTIONS

RV, vasto-crureus, the single-joint extensor, of right knee; LV, vasto-crureus of left knee. At *a a* the right peroneal nerve, *rp*, and the left peroneal nerve, *lp*, are faradised concurrently, causing inhibitory relaxation of both the muscles, followed on withdrawal of the stimuli by some post-inhibitory rebound in both muscles. At *b* the left nerve alone is faradised, causing contraction of right muscle and relaxation of left muscle. This stimulation is repeated for three more brief periods in succession; the right muscle retains a postural condition of marked contraction, broken only by small relaxations between the periods of stimulation; the left muscle's postural condition of relaxation is broken by rebound contractions in the intervals between stimulation. At *c* the right nerve alone is faradised; the right muscle then drops into a posture of relaxation, and the left enters into contraction; the stimulus is repeated for three more brief periods, and the right muscle retains its relaxed posture, broken only by rebound contractions between the stimulations; conversely, the left muscle retains its posture of contraction. At *d* stimulation of the left nerve only is reverted to, and the reciprocal posture of the two muscles previously assumed at *b* is again reverted to. Decerebrate cat. Time above in fifths of seconds

that reflexes unfold simultaneous excitatory and inhibitory influences reciprocally. From the central nervous system two sets of efferent nerves pass to the arterial ring-musculature—vaso-dilatators and vaso-constrictors. Some arterial regions receive both these supplies, others the vaso-dilatator only. The musculature is, unlike the heart which is engaged pre-eminently in executing movements, engaged in contraction eminently postural. It

[1] *Proc. roy. Soc.*, 1908, **80B**, 339.

maintains a certain posture of the artery wall in regard to the contained blood, a postural contraction technically known as tonus. Alterations of this posture occur in two directions: the postural tonus is either lessened so that the artery sets in a more open condition, or is increased, the artery maintaining a posture of greater narrowing. The postural tonus of the arterial muscle expresses the tonus of the nerve-centres governing it. In these nervous centres, however, their tonus, unlike that of the centres governing the postural tonus of skeletal muscles, is maintained, not reflexly, but appears to be autochthonous, arising in the nerve-centres themselves. But it can be reflexly influenced. The question investigated by Bayliss is the following: When excitation of an afferent nerve causes a reflex fall of arterial pressure, does it do so by inhibiting the tonus of the vaso-constrictor centres, or by increasing the tonus of the vaso-dilatator centres, or by a combination of both of these? He shows that the possibility last mentioned is what actually occurs. Stimulation of the depressor nerve produces simultaneously with lowering of the action of the vaso-constrictor centres on, for instance, the splanchnic arteries a heightened action of the vaso-dilatator centres on the arteries of, for instance, the submaxillary gland and the limbs. Conversely, when the arterial pressure rises on stimulation of the central end of an ordinary afferent nerve, such as the median nerve of the fore-limb, the reflex reaction includes, along with heightened action of the vaso-constrictor centres, an inhibitory depression of the tonic action of the vaso-dilatator centres. In these general vaso-motor reflexes, therefore, the centripetal impulses act reciprocally on the nerve-centres of antagonistic influence; in raising the arterial pressure the reflex excites the vaso-constrictor centres and inhibits the vaso-dilatator; in lowering it the reflex excites the vaso-dilatator centres and inhibits the vaso-constrictor.

When the afferent nerve from any particular organ is excited, it produces along with the usual rise of general blood-pressure a vaso-dilatation in the organ itself. This latter local part of the reflex is called a Lovén reflex, after Lovén,[1] who first described it, in the ear and in the hind-limb (rabbit). Bayliss[2] has examined also the Lovén reflexes in respect of their exhibiting reciprocal innervation. He finds that the local dilatation is brought about by the reflex causing inhibition of the local vaso-constrictor centres simultaneously with excitation of the vaso-dilatation. The local vaso-motor reflexes, therefore, like the general vaso-motor reflexes, exhibit reciprocal innervation.

DOUBLE RECIPROCAL INNERVATION

The simple reciprocal innervation described above must be regarded as probably a relatively artificial reaction, because the experimental conditions under which it is produced are not merely more crudely produced, but much less complex than are natural happenings. The isolated stimulation of just

---

[1] *Ber. sächs. Ges. Wiss., Mat.-phys. Cl.*, 1866, p. 92. [2] *Loc. cit. sup.*

one whole afferent nerve, the rest of the nervous system lying plunged at the time in approximately complete quietude, is a state of things little resembling the ordinary occurrences of waking life. Usually in the latter the reactions of the nervous system result from the combination of a number of stimuli playing concurrently on its afferent channels, and some impelling to one action and some to another. Any particular motor centre, whether for flexion or extension, lies then under at least a twofold influence, tending on the one hand toward excitation and on the other toward inhibition. Such twofold influence can be imitated and its reflex results studied, in an elementary way at least, by taking a pair of antagonistic muscles and two afferent nerves, the one nerve exerting an opposite reflex effect to the other upon the muscle-pair in question.

If we voluntarily hold the arm semiflexed, nothing is easier than to make both flexor and extensor contract together; by simply feeling the hardness of the muscles through the skin we can assure ourselves of that fact. This concurrent contraction of both antagonists scarcely ever results under normal circumstances from simple reflex stimulation of any single point or any single nerve. But it can be obtained in pure reflex-flexion of the joint produced in another way. If two afferents, one producing flexion of the joint, the other extension, be stimulated simultaneously, it is not difficult to find a grade of conjoint stimulation producing some flexion of the joint. In this flexion there is, if suitable strengths of stimuli are chosen, some contraction of the extensor muscle as well as of the flexor muscle; yet the contraction of the flexor may predominate, and hence the joint is flexed.[1] What happens is instructively studied by the myograph. If the reaction of the muscles in response to either of the single stimuli is compared with their reaction under the double stimulus, the motor centre for the flexor is shown in the latter case to be under a twofold influence; similarly the extensor centre is also under a twofold influence.[1] Of the two afferents concurrently stimulated, that one which when stimulated alone causes *flexion* of the joint *excites* the flexor half-centre and *inhibits* the extensor half-centre; and the other afferent, which when stimulated alone causes *extension* of the joint, *excites* the extensor half-centre and *inhibits* that of the flexor. When both afferents are stimulated simultaneously with appropriate intensity, the discharge from the flexor half-centre represents the algebraic sum[2] of the opposed excitation and inhibition which the two afferents individually exert on it, and the discharge from the extensor half-centre similarly represents the algebraic sum of its opposed excitation and inhibition (Fig. 42). If the intensity of the stimuli be suitably chosen, both flexor and extensor motor centres discharge, but the discharge of neither is as great as it would be were the antagonistic influences not present.[1]

Certain reflex actions in their natural occurrence similarly exhibit in some cases a contemporaneous contraction of antagonists. Thus, stepping

---

[1] Sherrington, *Proc. roy. Soc.*, 1909, **81B,** 249. See especially Figs. 9 and 10, pp. 260, 262, in this connection.   [2] *Idem, ibid.*, 1908, **80B,** 565.

consists essentially of alternate extensions and flexions of the limb, and its reflex execution appears due to the interaction of two sets of stimuli, one set causing extension of the limb and the other flexion of the limb. Two antagonistic influences compete at the extensor and flexor half-centres, and predominate alternately. When the step is full and free one influence for a moment practically completely suppresses the other. Full rest and unimpeded discharge thus alternate in each half-centre in turn.[1] But in some forms[2] of stepping, as when the step is not free but crouched, one of the two influences never wholly suppresses the other. Each half-centre then predominates in turn, but in one of them at least—e.g., in the flexion half-centre—the discharge is at no time wholly quelled. That half-centre, therefore, never obtains complete rest. It is probable that faulty habits of walking, running, etc., frequently have this latter character. The gracefully balanced stepping which proper systems of drill and exercise cultivate owe their excellence to physiological avoidance of this imbalance. The proper execution of the act ensures a moment of complete rest to each of the opposed motor centres engaged. Fatigue is in this way minimised.

It is sometimes assumed that under reciprocal innervation two antagonist muscles necessarily can never be in contraction at the same time, and that the antagonistic half-centres never exhibit discharge of motor impulses concurrently. That this need not be the case is clear from the above examples. Not unfrequently the antagonists are concurrently in contraction, and their centres concurrently discharging. What reciprocal innervation does provide is that, in the execution of a muscular act by antagonists, augmentation of contraction or motor discharge shall not occur concurrently in protagonist and antagonist, nor conversely decrease of contraction or discharge occur concurrently in the two. These latter appear only possible when, breaking in on a condition of rest of both half-centres or opponent muscles, there ensues one of those instances of double reciprocal innervation in which the balance between inhibition and excitation is such as to allow both half-centres to discharge, although unequally; or when to such a state of double reciprocal innervation there succeeds a reversion of both half-centres into rest, the stimuli which evoked the double reciprocal innervation subsiding together. Except under these circumstances, reciprocal innervation secures that any increase in the contraction or discharge of the protagonist shall be accompanied by corresponding diminution of the contraction or discharge of its antagonist, even to complete suppression of the latter.

GRADING OF MUSCULAR CONTRACTION BY REFLEX INHIBITION

Study of double reciprocal innervation therefore incidentally reveals a further important office served by inhibition in the interest of co-ordination. It reveals inhibition as not only a suppressor of reflexes but as a delicate

[1] Sherrington, *Science Progress Twent. Cent.*, 1911, p. 584, and *Brain*, 1910, **33**, 1.
[2] See pp. 185 and 371, this volume.

adjuster of the intensity of reflex contraction (Fig. 42). This it effects by grading the intensity of the nerve-centre's centrifugal discharge. In a reflex preparation the grading of the intensity of the contraction can be arrived at in either of two ways: (*a*) by grading the intensity of the stimulus applied to the excitatory afferent nerve; (*b*) by combining with the stimulation of the excitatory afferent the stimulation of an inhibitory afferent; in this latter case, the opposed influences sum algebraically, and can be adjusted to produce any desired grade of contraction. This latter method is important, because it probably represents a mode of gradation which occurs very commonly under natural circumstances. The grading which simply follows different intensities of stimulation of an excitatory nerve contributes, of course, importantly toward securing that the degree of muscular action shall be suited to the circumstance evoking it. It is an obviously useful factor in the co-ordination of motor reactions. The grading of the reflex intensity conformably with grading of the exciting stimulus follows with great fidelity when studied in the laboratory under conditions which, so far as possible, exclude all but the one stimulus, and ensure as far as possible absence of activity from the whole nervous system except its one reacting arc.

But under natural circumstances it is usual not for one stimulus nor even one group of stimuli, but many groups to be playing on the organism concurrently through many and varied afferent paths (*Integrative Action*, p. 182). Double reciprocal innervation shows that a weak discharge of impulses from a motor centre does not invariably mean weak stimulation of the excitatory afferents of that centre. The motor discharge may be weak, although the excitatory afferents are excited strongly, because the influence of these latter on the centre are being counteracted by concurrent operation of inhibitory afferents. The opposed influences collide. Representing the influence of the pressor afferent by + and that of the inhibitory by −, the contraction resulting from concurrent stimulation of the two afferents appears as the algebraic sum of + and − quantities. The muscle excited through a purely pressor afferent exhibits for each intensity of stimulus theoretically but one particular grade of intensity of contraction. But under the less simple though more natural condition, where several afferent channels of opposed effect are concurrently at work on the centre, any particular grade of contraction may represent any one of many different combinations of intensity of opposed stimuli. Even where only two different channels are competing, it is impossible to know what state of interaction the state of the muscle represents except by quantitative observation of one at least of the stimuli.

Observation shows that if the one influence is very much stronger than the other total suppression of the weaker takes place; the issue then is as though the weaker opponent were for the time being wholly ineffective. But this is not what happens when the two influences are better matched in intensity.

The two processes of reflex excitation and reflex inhibition are to be regarded as coequal in their importance for co-ordination. They are

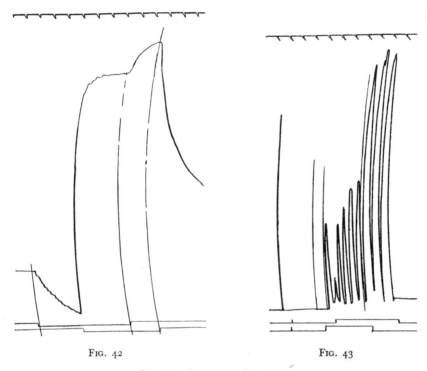

FIG. 42   FIG. 43

FIG. 42.—ALGEBRAIC SUMMATION

Reflex reaction of vasto-crureus muscle under, at first, the influence of an inhibitory afferent nerve (upper signal line); then the conjoint influence of that nerve and of an excitatory afferent (lower signal line) concurrently stimulated; and, finally, the influence of the excitatory afferent alone. The observation illustrates the algebraic summation of the two opposed influences. The excitatory afferent was contralateral popliteal nerve, the inhibitory ipsilateral popliteal. Decerebrate cat. Time above in seconds. (From *Proc. roy. Soc.*, 1908, **80B**, 572)

FIG. 43.—REFLEX STEPPING IN ISOLATED KNEE-EXTENSOR, VASTO-CRUREUS, PRODUCED BY STRONG STIMULATION OF CONTRALATERAL POPLITEAL NERVE IN SPINAL PREPARATION (DECAPITATE CAT)

The stimulation is marked by rise of the signal line. Observation opens with stimulation of ipsilateral popliteal nerve (lower signal line); this remains without obvious effect, owing to the toneless state of the extensor muscle preventing reflex inhibition from being apparent. Stimulation of the contralateral nerve (upper signal line) is then begun. Under this concurrence of the stimulation of the two antagonistic nerves the muscle begins to contract rhythmically, alternate contractions and relaxations of it ensuing rhythmically about twice a second. The stimulation of the ipsilateral nerve is then withdrawn, the contractions at once increase in size, and the rhythmic reaction ceases when the contralateral stimulus is finally withdrawn. Time above in seconds

commonly combined, in the sense that the accuracy of a muscular contraction, delicately adjusted to the extent and force of the movement which is required, is usually a result of the graded combination of both inhibitory and excitatory influences coalescing upon the motor centres involved. The depressor influence of an inhibitory afferent is just as capable of graded intensity as is the pressor influence of its excitatory antagonist. Each therefore is not only itself capable of finely graded adjustment of intensity, but each forms also a means of finely grading the intensity of the other (*cf.* Figs. 5 and 6, *Proc. roy. Soc.*, 1909, **81B**, 254, 255). Reflex inhibition with its gradation constitutes, therefore, a main means for co-ordinating to the momentary requirements of the organism the intensity of activity of its chief motor machinery, the skeletal musculature.

And there is another way in which reflex inhibition appears in the grading of muscular contraction. Postural tonus can be studied under very favourable conditions in the extensor muscles after decerebration (cat). The tonus is reflex. The afferent fibres concerned are among those distributed to the tonic muscle itself; the centres engaged seem to be twofold, one in the post-cerebral part of the brain about the pontine region, and probably another one subsidiary to that in the spinal cord in the locality of the spinal arc of the muscle. The reflex posture has a feature which has been termed its plasticity; the extensor tonus prevents the joint, for instance knee, yielding under the weight of the body, but when the joint is forcibly flexed, as it may be by the observer forcibly bending it, the tonus yields, and on release of the joint retains the joint-posture thus passively imposed on it. For example, suppose the initial attitude of the knee to be full extension, and the observer then, while holding the thigh, to proceed to forcibly flex the joint against the tonus of the extensor muscle, he feels the muscle when a certain degree of pressure is put upon it yield suddenly and allow itself to be carried into a new posture—for instance, semiflexion. On then ceasing to apply the strain further, it is found that the tonus of the extensor now retains its new tonic length (*cf.* Fig. 58, this volume, p. 353), holds the joint in its new attitude, and does not tend, or tends only in the course of minutes, to reassume its previous posture and initial tonic length. And the *tension* of the muscle in its new tonic length is the same, or very nearly the same, as it had in its initial tonic length. The length of the muscle has been changed greatly by an adjustment-reaction, while its tension has remained unchanged. The reaction has been termed the "lengthening reaction." It is a nervous reaction. It requires the afferent nerves from the muscle and their nerve-centres. The relaxation produced by the forcible stretch of muscle seems to be a *proprioceptive* reflex of inhibitory character. There is, conversely, a "shortening reaction" of excitatory character, but that does not concern us here. These two imbue the tonus of the muscle with plasticity. The plasticity appears to meet the requirement that, for instance, in "standing" the posture of the limb may vary, provided always that each joint maintains a resistance sufficient to counteract the superimposed weight of the body. Standing postures, especially in the quadruped, include variable degrees of flexion at hip and knee. One hind-foot may rest close beside or in advance of or behind the other. Yet in all cases, though the tonic length of the muscle varies much, its tonic tension varies little and does not fall below that required to bear the superincumbent load. In this postural reflex the extensor or anti-gravity muscles are in v. Uexküll's[1] terminology acting as " Sperr-muskellen." Just as the sea-urchin rests supported on its spines by the " Sperr-reflex " of the tonic muscles of the spines, so the decerebrate cat and dog stand in virtue of the " Sperr-reflex " stiffening the jointed framework of the animal by means of the tonus of the anti-gravity muscles. In the adjustments and gradings of the length of the muscle in this postural tonus, inhibition exhibited by a proprioceptive reflex appears to play an important rôle.

Reflex inhibition is also able to grade the amplitude of rhythmic reflexes, such as stepping. Fig. 43 shows the decrement of the stepping reflex exercised by faradisation of the ipsilateral peroneal nerve as afferent upon the reflex stepping excited by faradisation of the contralateral peroneal. On removing the former stimulus the stepping is much ampler. Since the rhythmic step itself consists of an equipoise between inhibition and excitation (*vide infra*), the reflex inhibition by peroneal must arrive at this issue in a complicated manner.

REFLEX INHIBITION AS A FACTOR IN SUCCESSIVE CO-ORDINATION— THAT IS, IN REFLEX SEQUENCE

So far it has been inhibition as a factor in the co-ordination of muscles reacting simultaneously that has been followed. We have now to turn to the rôle played by inhibition in the co-ordinate sequence of reflexes.

A.—*Reflex Inhibition and the Transition from One Muscular Act to Another*

One muscular act follows another, and the same musculature is commonly employed for different effects in succession. Not only in the co-operation of muscles at one and the same moment does inhibition play a part, but also in the co-ordination of successive steps in a reflex series. The execution of the change from the old muscular act to the new is ushered in by an inhibitory suppression of the discharge of motor centres prevailing previously (*cf.* Figs. 37 and 38, p. 275), as well as by discharge of motor centres previously at rest. Take the case where a reflex (decerebrate) preparation is exhibiting the steady postural reflex of standing, and then draws up one foot on that foot being pinched. As the animal stands the extensors of the leg are in contraction; if then one foot be squeezed, the foot is lifted and drawn up out of harm's way. In this action not only are the flexors of knee, hip, and ankle thrown into contraction by the new reflex, but the extensors of knee, and hip, and ankle, which were engaged in contraction by the previous reflex of standing, are thrown out of action and their motor centres brought to rest by inhibition. In the transition from one reflex to another,

[1] *Z. Biol.*, 1899, **37**, 381.

a muscle's activity is inhibited if it would offer obstruction to the new reflex. Inhibition ushers in the new reflex by wiping out any antagonistic persistence of the old. In default of this inhibition one of two things must happen: either the stimulus which is exciting the old reflex must cease exactly as the stimulus exciting the new one begins—a state of things of obviously exceptional occurrence under natural conditions—or there will persist during the new reflex activities belonging to the old with, in result, confusion of the two. Rarely, indeed, can it happen normally that the reflex machinery in executing a train of different reflexes is actuated by a train of different stimuli, each one of which abruptly ceases just as the next one begins. The reflex machinery is constantly exposed to whole constellations of stimuli, and the different items of the constellations overlap each other widely in time. Yet one act succeeds another without confusion. The items composing the array of environmental and internal agents acting concurrently on the animal exhibit correlative change in regard to it, so that one or other group becomes —generally by increase in intensity—temporarily prepotent. Thus there dominates now this group, now that, in turn. And the inhibitions of the dominant group prevail over the excitations of the subsidiary, just as the excitations of the dominant over the inhibitions of the subsidiary.

Further, a feature of the reflex discharge of centres is that on withdrawal of the stimulus exciting it the discharge does not cease and subside immediately. With strong stimuli the discharge of a spinal centre may dribble on with somewhat irregular decline for several seconds,[1] giving a slow tremulous waning of the muscular contraction. This after-discharge is suppressed strikingly easily and completely by reflex inhibition. The tremulously persistent remainder of excitement in the centre is suppressed by the inhibition and the centre steadied to its new state of rest. Reflex inhibition thus cures the disability which would result from the natural tendency of the discharge of a motor centre to outlast considerably the duration of the stimulus provoking it. It renders the action of the reflex arcs, despite their inherent inertia and momentum, practically dead-beat. Its utility in this respect somewhat resembles that of simultaneous contrast in vision which, as Hering has pointed out, corrects the spatial blurring due to irradiation of the image by giving it a sharper psycho-physiological boundary.

For orderly and unconfused sequence of reflex acts—also of willed acts —central inhibition is a necessary element of co-ordination in the transition from one muscular act to another.

Further, the increased tendency of a motor centre after inhibition to discharge impulses forms obviously a factor making for co-ordination in reflex sequences where alternate phases of inhibitory restraint from discharge and excitatory production of discharge are required from one and the same centre in succession. The rôle of reflex inhibition here is exactly the converse of reflex fatigue. Reflex fatigue favours the influence of inhibition upon the centre;[2] a centre the reflex excitation of which is even slightly fatigued

[1] *Integrative Action*, 1906.   [2] *Cf. Proc. roy. Soc.*, 1911, **84B**, 208, Fig. 7.

is more readily amenable to reflex inhibition. In a centre which is to be alternately driven by excitation and reduced to quietude by inhibition, reflex fatigue favours the transition from the phase of excitatory discharge to that of inhibitional restraint from discharge, and conversely, post-inhibitory exaltation favours the transition from the phase of inhibitional quietude to that of excitatory discharge.

Again, just as reflex inhibition corrects the inertia of the reflex excitatory mechanism and the momentum of the excitatory process seen, for instance, in the after-discharge of an excited centre, so does reflex excitation obviate the inertia and momentum of the reflex inhibitory mechanism and its process. The effect of strong reflex inhibition can be observed to consider-ably outlive the cessation of its evoking stimulus. To this post-stimulatory persistence of inhibition seems due the long latency of the post-inhibitory rebound contraction.[1] A tendency to regard inhibition as a mere negation of action may make it appear strange that inertia and momentum should attach to it. But reflex inhibition, although antithetic to excitation in its purpose, has to be regarded as, like it, an active process. This emerges perhaps particularly clearly in cases where an afferent nerve inhibits an inhibitory centre. Such an instance is furnished by the vasomotor reflexes analysed by Bayliss.[2] A vaso-dilatator centre is, in view of its end-effect —i.e., relaxation of the ring-musculature of the artery—an inhibitory centre: yet its effect can be reflexly inhibited, as in the usual pressor reflex obtain-able from ordinary afferent nerves.

Processes at work in the transition from one reflex to another are pre-sented relatively simply in the turning-points of reflexes of rhythmic alternating direction. Thus in stepping, with its alternate phases of limb flexion and limb extension. To say that a refractory period rhythmically oscillates across the two half-centres flexor and extensor is even descriptively unsatisfying. One question is, How far is such oscillation intrinsically produced in the centre itself? T. Graham Brown has obtained evidence indicating that it is indeed essentially intrinsic in origin. In experiments with the isolated and de-afferented knee extensor I frequently found it " step." The further question rises, How far do proprioceptive reflexes originating in the muscles, etc., of the moving limb react on, accentuate, and modify in detail, and especially in " tempo," the intrinsic oscillations of the centres? The mere gentle passive arrest of the moving limb often leads to subsidence almost immediately of the rhythmic reflex either of step or scratch,[3] the reflex being found to be no longer in operation on release of the limb after a brief arrest. And the passive arrest of the stepping movement in one limb often immediately arrests it in the other fellow-limb, although that remains free from all restraint.

One factor assisting the transition seems certainly to be inhibition in virtue of its appended post-inhibitory rebound. In the stepping of the

[1] Sherrington, *Proc. roy. Soc.*, 1905, **76B**, 160; 1906, **77B**, 478; and 1907, **79B**, 337.
[2] *Proc. roy. Soc.*, 1908, **80B**, 339.   [3] Sherrington, *J. Physiol.*, 1904, **31**, 18.

decerebrate cat this influence is particularly clear in the transition from flexion phase to extension phase. A series of complete active diphasic steps can be excited and maintained at any desired " tempo " by suitably repeated flexor-stimuli alone (Fig. 44). Post-inhibitory exaltation helps the transition from the one phase to the next. If rebound contraction be included as part and parcel of the reflex response (*cf.* Fig. 37, *supra*), the whole reflex effect of a single stimulus is one of successive double sign. Thus, with knee-extensor when reflexly excited by an ipsilateral nerve, if by − we denote inhibition and by + excitation, the reflex result runs − + —*i.e.*, as regards that muscle one complete cycle of the reflex step. The rebound contraction which ensues in the previously inhibited half-centre is accompanied in the antagonist half-centre by its reciprocal excitation. If both opponent muscles be viewed together—*e.g.*, flexor and extensor of knee —the formula for the response to a single stimulus runs thus:

$$\frac{F \;\; + \;\; -}{E \;\; - \;\; +}.$$

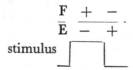

stimulus

B.—*Post-Inhibitory Exaltation*

After subjection to reflex inhibition the activity of the motor centre of a skeletal muscle tends for a time to show exaltation; the muscle often contracts seemingly spontaneously (*cf.* Fig. 37, *supra*). Hence the application of a stimulus which excites flexion of the limb, and consequently inhibition of the extension half-centre, is followed in cessation of that stimulus by an active extension of the limb. The inhibition of the extensor half-centres during the flexion phase of the step favours and predisposes them for their activity in the following extension phase of the step.

To such an extent is this the case sometimes that the extension or second phase seems self-induced by the inhibition. The central discharge ensuing on withdrawl of an inhibitory stimulus has been termed rebound discharge, and the contraction by which the muscles evidence it rebound contraction. How potent it is in reflex stepping is shown by the fact that a stimulus which excites the muscle group figured in A of the diagram, Fig. 40, is followed on its cessation by a rebound contraction of all the muscles figured in B. So that the flexion phase of the step evoked by the stimulus is succeeded by a complete extension phase without further stimulus at all. This extension phase is at once cut short by inhibition on reapplying the stimulus appropriate for flexion. A series of the complete diphasic acts of stepping can thus be produced by simple repetition of a single stimulus (Fig. 44). The same phenomenon is observable in the rhythmic alternating reflex of respiratory movement of the chest (H. Head).[1]

[1] *J. Physiol.*, 1889, **10**, 279.

A condition favouring reflex rebound—at least in the case of the extensor phase of the step—is the co-operation of the afferent nerves of those muscles which exhibit the rebound contraction. If these nerves are severed the rebound is much less easy to evoke, less regular, and less pronounced.[1] These same nerves are responsible for the reflex tonus of their muscles; this tonus, which forms so marked a feature of the postural tonus in the decerebrate animal, is lost on severance of these nerves.

But the proprioceptive nerve of the muscle is not essential for the rebound, since the muscle may be de-afferented and still exhibit rebound,[1]

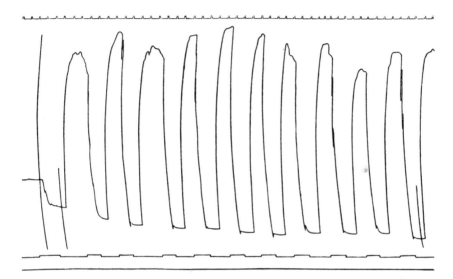

FIG. 44.—KNEE-EXTENSIONS BY REBOUND: ISOLATED EXTENSOR MUSCLE

On applying the electrical stimulation (first rise of the signal line) to the foot-nerve, the myogram line falls and remains down during the stimulation, showing the reflex inhibition of the tonus. After three seconds the stimulus is discontinued (fall of the signal line); a post-inhibitory rebound contraction ensues during this discontinuance of the stimulation. This contraction is then cut down by reapplication of the stimulus (second rise of signal line), the muscle being again relaxed by inhibition. On withdrawal of this stimulation a rebound contraction re-ensues. This is repeated eleven times, each lapse of the stimulus giving an active extension of the knee. Decerebrate cat. Time marked above in seconds. Observation by S. C. M. Sowton and C. S. Sherrington

though in my own experience with vasto-crureus, an extensor muscle, not readily. T. Graham Brown,[2] however, using tibialis anticus, a flexor muscle, found rebound occur even more markedly after the muscle was de-afferented than before.

The rebound contraction usually lasts but a few seconds—apart from semblance of longer persistence due to an appended " shortening reaction." The latency of the rebound contraction is long; as counted between the moment of cessation of the inhibitory stimulus and the first onset of the ensuent contraction it may amount to a second or even more. The

[1] See p. 348 this volume.   [2] *Quart. J. exp. Physiol.*, 1911, **4**, 369.

elicitation of the rebound is closely dependent on intensity and duration of the precurrent inhibitory stimulation. That stimulus must not be of very prolonged duration; moderate intensity and brevity seem favourable. To elicit the rebound it is not necessary that the inhibited muscle should actually lengthen at all. The process determining the rebound is not anything happening in the muscle; it is evidently of central locus.[1]

Besides ordinary rebound there is another form of post-inhibitory exaltation which is considered by Forbes[2] to differ fundamentally from the rebound just described. This second form is termed by him " subsequent augmentation." In Forbes' experiments subsequent augmentation is studied as follows: The reflex inhibition of a muscle is maintained for a considerable period—e.g., thirty seconds or more; on then, after withdrawal of the reflex inhibition, applying a reflex excitation of known effect, the response of the motor centre as indicated by the muscle contraction is greater than before the inhibition. A similar phenomenon is probably the augmentation of the extension-reflex of the knee observable when the reflex is elicited just after a strong flexion-reflex of knee which has been maintained for half a minute or more.

That a state of superactivity or superexcitability often obtains in the nerve-centre after it has been inhibited is evident from post-inhibitory rebound contraction and the phenomenon allied to that, which I classed with it, but by Forbes separated from it, and called " subsequent augmentation." I included both under the term successive induction, to distinguish them from immediate or spatial induction. The chief outward difference between post-inhibitory rebound and subsequent augmentation is that the former may occur very quickly, in less than a second, whereas the latter manifests itself over much longer times.

It is a question how to explain the superactivity commonly supervening in a centre after release from inhibition. Is it a result of the precurrent inhibition? It is one of the phenomena which Graham Brown[3] designates " terminal," because ensuing on termination of the applied stimulus. A first inquiry is, " Is rebound contraction always preceded by inhibition ?" in other words, is there evidence that the stimulus on cessation of which the rebound occurs is in all cases inhibitory during its application? Usually the evidence is quite clear that the stimulus has actually been producing inhibition. And among this class of cases must be included those instances where a weak stimulus while in progress causes, as in certain conditions it does,[4] an initial contraction which partially subsides and is followed on its withdrawal by a terminal increase of contraction. In such cases it has been shown that the decline of the contraction is due to an inhibitory influence possessed by a mixed afferent nerve, the inhibitory

[1] Proc. roy. Soc., 1905, **76B**, 160; 1906, **77B**, 478; 1907, **79B**, 337; and J. Physiol., 1907, **36**, 185.
[2] Quart. J. exp. Physiol., 1912, **5**, 149. [3] Ibid., 1911, **4**, 331.
[4] Sherrington and Sowton, Proc. roy. Soc., 1911, **83B**, 435, and 1911, **84B**, 201. Also Fröhlich, Z. allg. Physiol., 1904, **4**, 468.

effect gradually dominating an excitatory influence also possessed by the nerve. The case offers, therefore, no difficulty for the view that the terminal rebound contraction is then post-inhibitory.

But there are cases of terminal access of contraction where the stimulus throughout its duration has been producing a considerable maintained contraction (*cf.* Fig. 45, *infra*). Graham Brown[1] has described such instances and has discussed their significance. In them the rebound contraction is preceded either during or immediately after the stimulus by some evident relaxation which may well be inhibitory since, as he points out, it is accompanied by contraction of the antagonist muscle. He concludes " that rebound contraction is a post-inhibitory phenomenon, and where it appears after the contraction of a muscle it may still be due to the cessation of an inhibitory factor " which has been concealed in the contraction.

In yet other cases it would seem that terminal access of contraction occurs without any good evidence of an inhibitory factor in the precurrent reflex behaviour of the muscle.[2] And it has to be remembered that reflex excitation of a centre does often, if not carried to excess, leave the centre in a temporary condition of facilitation (bahnung) which must itself be taken as a sign of exalted activity. Thus, when the condition of a reflex centre is tested at four-second intervals by single break-shocks, and is giving in response a series of equal reflex " twitches," the interpolation of a moderate reflex tetanus for even so short a period as three seconds is often followed by marked augmentation of the height of the reflex twitches immediately following the tetanus.

There is next the question whether inhibition is *always* followed by superactivity as a terminal phenomenon. If the inhibition be quite weak and brief sometimes no ensuent superactivity is demonstrable, but over a wide range of period and intensity of inhibition the terminal rebound contraction increases with increase of the precurrent inhibition. If, however, the inhibitory stimulus be increased or prolonged beyond certain limits, the terminal rebound contraction does not occur. And Forbes[3] has shown that similarly, using reflex response to a definite excitatory stimulus as a test for post-inhibitory exaltation, inhibition of more than a certain " critical " intensity leaves behind it not an exaltation, but a depression of the centre's reflex response to excitation.

Further, Graham Brown[4] has recently pointed out that in many cases the terminal relaxation following an excitatory reflex may be regarded as of the nature of an inhibitory rebound, and that occasionally a form of terminal relaxation presenting the appearance of inhibitory rebound ensues after an inhibitory reflex.[5] In this last case the observations were made on an extensor muscle, gastrocnemius-soleus, in the decerebrate preparation.

[1] *Quart. J. exp. Physiol.*, 1911, **4**, 331.   [2] See Figs. 6 and 10, *Integrative Action*, 1906.
[3] *Quart. J. exp. Physiol.*, 1912, **5**, 149; and *Proc. roy. Soc.*, 1912, **85B**, 289.
[4] *Loc. cit. sup.*   [5] *Quart. J. exp. Physiol.*, 1912, **5**, 233.

It is possible, of course, to suppose here that there was an excitatory component in the precurrent reflex masked by concomitant inhibition, but there was no evidence that such was the case.

The above somewhat complex evidence does not preclude our asking how it comes about that a precurrent reflex inhibition of a centre should, as is so often observable, be followed by superactivity of the centre. Forbes[1] brings cogent evidence against supposing that the inhibition effects this by, so to say, damming up the effect of a concurrent autochthonous or reflex excitation which, when the inhibition is withdrawn, bursts forth with accumulated power. He shows that concurrent excitation along with the inhibition lessens instead of increasing the subsequent augmentation. He suggests that post-inhibitory superactivity may be due to fatigue of an inhibitory tonus which, constantly operative through the inhibitory afferents, drops to a lower intensity after prolonged electric stimulation of those nerves owing to their temporary fatigue.

It must be borne in mind that many of the afferent nerves possess individually two influences, excitatory and inhibitory, on the same centre. As Forbes points out, it may be that when such an afferent is stimulated the excitatory component in its effect, though masked and overcome by the inhibitory during the electric stimulation, on withdrawal of that stimulus outlasts the inhibitory effect. A somewhat similar effect is seen on the heart when its acceleration and inhibitory nerves are stimulated concurrently.[2]

Forbes,[3] who has systematically studied subsequent augmentation, considers it essentially different from rebound. He finds, however, that, like rebound, subsequent augmentation has as a factor in its production the intensity of the inhibitory stimulus. He shows that if the intensity of the inhibitory stimulus is above a certain " critical value," the subsequent effect is depression of excitatory response instead of exaltation. The degree of intensity which the inhibition must overstep in order to leave behind it this depression of the motor centre varies in different preparations. An interesting result established by Forbes is that the critical value of this inhibition is reached with lower intensities if inhibitory stimulation runs concurrently with reflex excitation of the centre applied from some other source. In other words, a state of subsequent depression of the centre is more easily brought about by combined excitation and inhibition than by inhibition alone.

The reflex provoked by a stimulus on cessation of that stimulus very frequently exhibits not a mere waning of the motor discharge from the excited half-centre, but phenomena of which one salient type is the rebound motor discharge from the inhibited half-centre. Graham Brown[4] has recently described very fully the several forms which these " terminal phenomena " assume in various circumstances. The aspect of them of concern

[1] *Loc. cit.*

[2] Baxt, N., *Arbeiten a. d. Physiol. Anstalt z. Leipzig*, 1875; see discussion, p. 265 this volume.

[3] *Loc. cit.*   [4] *Quart. J. exp. Physiol.*, 1911, **4**, 331.

here is whether or no they respect and exhibit " reciprocal innervation." Examination has shown that the post-inhibitory rebound contraction so commonly met in the decerebrate extensor muscle is usually accompanied by reciprocal relaxation of the contracted flexor (*cf.* Fig. 37). Also the post-stimulatory increase of contraction, not shown rarely by the knee-flexor in the flexion-reflex, is usually accompanied clearly by synchronous augmentation of relaxation of the knee-extensor (Fig. 45). Again, post-inhibitory rebound contraction of the ankle-flexor is shown by Graham Brown[1] to be accompanied by a synchronous relaxation of the ankle - extensor. Graham Brown has also met and described " rhythmic rebounds "; in these " the process of contraction in one muscle is slightly preceded and is thereafter accompanied by an act of relaxation in the other. Shortly after the first muscle begins again to relax the second begins to contract; and the contraction coincides in time with the relaxation of the first."

It is clear that " reciprocal innervation " holds for reflex-rebounds. Indeed, the various " terminal phenomena " furnish striking examples of it, if we except the rare form " rebound relaxation after inhibition "

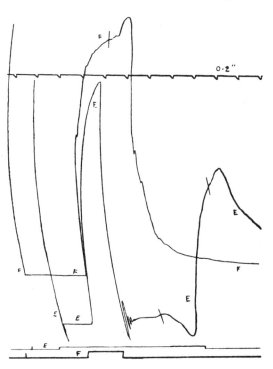

FIG. 45.—RECIPROCAL INNERVATION OF ANTAGONISTIC MUSCLES

F, knee-flexor, *semitendinosus*; E, knee-extensor, *vasto-crureus*. The observation begins with faradisation of the contralateral popliteal nerve (E signal line); this causes contraction of the extensor muscle, but has no apparent effect on the already relaxed flexor. Then follows faradisation of the ipsilateral popliteal (F signal line); the flexor muscle immediately contracts, and the extensor is inhibited. On cessation of this stimulus there follows a terminal contraction of flexor along with a reciprocal terminal increase of inhibition of the extensor; this latter is later followed by a return of contraction in the extensor under the influence of the still continued faradisation of the contralateral nerve, E. Decerebrate cat. Time marked above in fifths of seconds. The recording writing-points, in order to clear each other, are not in the same vertical, the extensor muscle's writer lying well to the right of the flexor's, as is marked at the beginning

(Graham Brown[2]), where flexor still shows subsidence of contraction although extensor is relaxing.

Turning from the antagonistic muscle-pair to the *symmetrical* muscle-

[1] *Quart. J. exp. Physiol.*, 1911, **4**, 331.   [2] *Ibid.*, 1912, **5**, 233.

pair, and taking as a type of this latter the extensor muscle, vastro-crureus, of right and left knee, it is common enough in these to see as a terminal effect following a reciprocal reflex a rebound contraction ensue in the inhibited muscle synchronously with relaxation of the contracted muscle. But it is also quite common in my experience with these muscles to see terminal rebound contraction ensue in only one of the muscles, although both have simultaneously suffered inhibition. Also, with synchronous stimulation by closely equal strong stimuli, post-stimulatory rebound contraction usually occurs symmetrically in both muscles (*cf.* Fig. 41, *a*, *supra*; and Fig. 3, *Proc. roy. Soc.*, 1913, **86B,** 223). It is evident, therefore, that in the case of the centres of these muscles the rebound is a reaction which can be confined to one of the symmetrical centres without obvious concomitant either reciprocal or identical in the other centre.

An interesting feature of post-inhibitory rebound contraction is that of all forms of contraction it is the one most easily inhibited. It provides, therefore, the most delicate of all test-objects for the detection of inhibitory power in an afferent nerve. An inhibitory quality which remains latent under all other tests may often be readily demonstrated if a background of rebound contraction can be obtained against which to test it.

C.—*Reflex After-discharge and Inhibition*

It is characteristic of reflexes that they tend to outlast the duration of the stimulus which provokes them. A very common form which this persistence takes where the muscle is, for instance, a flexor of hip or knee is a slow waning of the contraction, outlasting the end of the stimulus sometimes by many seconds. This may be taken to mean that the excitement in and discharge of impulses from the excited centre subsides relatively slowly. We have here to inquire whether similarly the state of inhibition in the antagonistic half-centre likewise subsides thus slowly. In other words, does the inhibitory mechanism exhibit similarly to the excitatory a momentum and an inertia in its reaction? If so, it forms a feature of likeness in the two antithetic processes. The answer is that when the behaviour of the two opponent muscles is examined, the post-stimulatory persistence of contraction in the one is accompanied by post-stimulatory delay of recovery from inhibitory relaxation in the other (Fig. 45). The post-stimulatory continuance of excitation in the one half-centre is accompanied by post-stimulatory continuance of inhibition in the other. This suggests that the post-stimulatory persistence of reflex action is not due to momentum in the motoneurones and *final common paths* of the centres, but to continuance of activity of some elements in the reflex arc upstream above the motoneurones. The motoneurones and final common paths have *per se* no power, so far as we know, to inhibit skeletal muscle, though they have power to excite it. The post-stimulatory persistence of inhibitory relaxation of the antagonistic argues a relatively slow subsidence of the inhibitory process playing on its motoneurones from some point above them.

D.—*Reflex Inhibition and the Production of Rhythmic Reflexes*

It has been shown above that inhibition as an element in reciprocal innervation takes its share in the execution of rhythmic reflexes, such as stepping, scratching, and eyeball nystagmus. It contributes also to the production of nervous rhythms, even where generated itself by a continuous stimulus. It proceeds to, as it were, cut up a continuous steady contraction into rhythmic pieces (Fig. 46). This it does by alternately breaking through and then reyielding to the effect of the similarly continuous

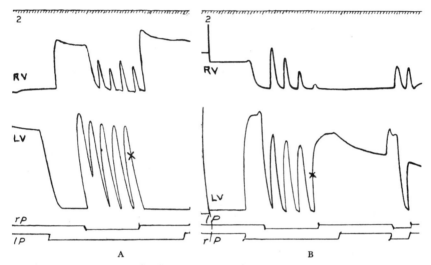

A   B

FIG. 46.—SYMMETRICAL EXTENSOR MUSCLES

RV, vasto-crureus, of right knee, LV, of left knee. Rhythmic reciprocal stepping under concurrent
    stimulation of the antagonistic afferent nerves, *rp*, right peroneal, *lp*, left peroneal. The
    reflex effect of either of these nerves alone is steady reciprocal excitation and inhibition in the
    two muscles respectively, as shown in the figure; but so soon as the stimuli are concurrent
    the reflex becomes rhythmical in both muscles, though still maintaining its reciprocal effect in the
    two. In Fig. A the observation begins with faradisation of the left afferent, and that of the
    right is intercalated; in Fig. B the arrangement is reversed. The reversed results are shown
    by the muscles. Decerebrate cat. Time marked above in fifths of seconds. Crosses mark
    point of withdrawal of intercurrent stimulus. (Further examples given in the original paper)

excitatory stimulus opposed to itself. In this way it is that double reciprocal innervation, brought into play by symmetrical afferents, establishes, under certain conditions, as its outcome on symmetrical muscles—*e.g.*, extensors of right and left knees—*reflex stepping*,[1] the rhythmic steps taken by the two isolated muscles being alternate and reciprocal in phase in the two limbs r. and l. (Fig. 46, A and B). Here the two antagonistic influences—namely, excitation and inhibition—exerted together on each of the two motor centres results in a see-saw of excitatory and inhibitory effect.

Reflex inhibition of a centre tends to superinduce in it a state of super-

[1] *Proc. roy. Soc.*, 1913, **86B**, 233.

activity, just as conversely, as has long been known, the reflex excitation of a centre tends to superinduce in it a state of depressed activity, fatigue. It is therefore not surprising that when the two antagonistic influences are concurrently at work on a centre, and are nearly balanced, there should result a rhythmic oscillation of the two; and presumably the rate of their alternation will depend largely on the nicety of balance, and on the intensity with which the processes are acting. The rhythmic stepping of the hind-limbs which can be evoked by unipolar faradisation of the cross-section of the cervical spinal cord (decapitate cat) is slow when the stimulus is weak, and fast when the stimulus is strong.

The genesis of rhythmic reflexes by inhibition appears in yet another light from the following considerations. Muscles, broadly taken, fulfil two more or less separable mechanical functions: they execute movements and they maintain postures. A muscle may be employed at one time in main-taining a posture (postural tonus), and at another in executing a movement. Very often while one set of muscles is maintaining a posture, others are engaged in executing movements. For instance, in walking,[1] while the tonus of many groups is maintaining the erect posture of trunk, neck, and head, the extensor and flexor muscles of the lower limbs are executing the alternating phasic contractions of the step. But very often also one and the same muscle is at one and the same time occupied both in executing movement by phasic contraction, and in maintaining posture by steady contraction. A good simple reflex example of this is furnished by the scratch-reflex.[2] The hind-limb is brought forward to a flexed posture at hip, and is somewhat extended at knee, so that the hind-foot may reach the shoulder; and at the same time it performs on the top of, and in addition to, the steady postural contraction those rhythmic alternating five per second movements so characteristic of the scratch. If a hip flexor, such as sartorius, be isolated, and its behaviour examined with the myograph, the form of its contraction reveals two elements: a maintained postural, and a phasic beat executive of movement.[2] To such cases Graham Brown[3] applies, on the basis of further experiment, an explanation which invokes inhibition for the mechanism of production of the rhythmic movement. In substance he considers that the rhythmic movement is obtained by a rhythmic set of inhibitory discharges, puffs of inhibition, so to say, which notch more or less deeply the maintained postural contraction.

In the rhythmic stepping produced by two concurrent excitatory and inhibitory stimuli it is of interest to note what happens after withdrawal of the stimuli. The stepping always ceases, but the exact manner of its cessation differs according to the particular phase of the step reached at the moment of time at which the stimulus is withdrawn (Fig. 46).

It is to be remembered, of course, that faradisation of single afferent nerves can produce reflex stepping[4] and other rhythmic reflexes—for instance,

---

[1] *Brain*, 1910, **33**, 1.   [2] *Quart. J. exp. Physiol.*, 1910, **3**, 213.
[3] *Ibid.*, 1911, **4**, 19.   [4] *Cf. Integrative Action*, 1906, p. 91, Fig. 32.

the scratch-reflex, swallowing, etc. The exercise of double reciprocal innervation in the way indicated in this section is therefore not the only experimental procedure for obtaining the reflex.

De-afferentation of the Muscle and Reflex Inhibition

The ataxic condition of a muscle after destruction of its afferent nerve fibres shows itself in various ways. Its invalidation for steady postural tonus, as shown by its exclusion from the stato-tonus after decerebration, is one of these. Another evidence of the upset of balance which its nervous centre undergoes in consequence of de-afferentation is the increased susceptibility of its reflex contractions to inhibition. A stimulus which on the normal fellow-muscle produces a reflex contraction not easily quelled by a given inhibitory stimulus causes in the de-afferented muscle a contraction which, though it may appear on the myograph not unlike the normal, is found to yield much more easily and also irregularly to a reflex inhibition. The activity of the reflex centre of the de-afferented muscle appears depressible by inhibition more readily than normally.

Fatigue of Reflex Inhibition

Reflex inhibition undergoes fatigue. Its fatiguing is well shown in experiments by Forbes.[1] An inhibitory afferent, yielding an ascertained degree of effect when opposed against a certain reflexly-excited contraction, was tested for its effect on the specified degree of contraction immediately before and after being strongly employed for thirty seconds or more. Its inhibitory effect was found to be lessened. To avoid confusion with mere " local polarisation " or " local nerve-trunk fatigue " at the seat of the electrodes, two pairs of electrodes were applied to the afferent nerve and the test stimulations made through the proximal, the prolonged intercurrent stimulation through the distal. The impairment of subsequent inhibition was often as marked when two pairs of electrodes were used as when one. The fatigue of inhibition is clearly central. Recovery from the fatigue is rapid, and may be complete in twenty to thirty seconds from cessation of the prolonged inhibition. Forbes also shows that fatiguing the inhibitory effect of one afferent nerve on a given motor centre does not fatigue the inhibitory effect of another afferent nerve on that centre. The central fatigue of the inhibitory arc is therefore " not a true fatigue of the inhibitory mechanism as a whole, but only of the particular arc employed." It may be a fatiguing of the excitatory process in the earlier upstream part of the arc.

It might be thought that the fatigue of reflex excitation of a motor centre would be prevented or delayed by a concurrent reflex inhibition of the centre sufficient to suppress any apparent effect of the centre's excita-

[1] *Quart. J. exp. Physiol.*, 1912, **5,** 149; and *Amer. J. Physiol.*, 1912, **31,** 102.

tion. Forbes shows that this is not in fact the case. The inhibition, although it suppresses the excitation effect on the centre, hastens rather than delays the fatiguing of the excitation.

In regard to the place of incidence of reflex fatigue, Forbes finds that both in the case of fatigue of inhibition and fatigue of excitation, the fatigue, though central, does not involve the reflex centre " as a whole, but merely the particular channel of approach employed." We may suppose that the popliteal and peroneal nerves are connected with the motoneurones through two independent sets of synapses, and that fatigue in one set does not affect the other. It is interesting in this connection to recall the experiments of Camis,[1] showing that maximal stimulation of one afferent nerve does not evoke all the reflex excitation of which the centre is capable.

REVERSAL OF REFLEX INHIBITION

A phenomenon not remote from processes of transition from one reflex to another is reflex reversal (*umkehr*). It is not all kinds of reversal which are germane here, but rather that one kind which Magnus[2] terms " shunting," elucidated especially by himself and v. Uexküll and Matula.[3] In it initial posture acts as a determinant of the sense or even of the existence of a reflex. As instance may be cited a mammalian example discovered by Magnus.[4] The pendent tail of the spinal cat is moved laterally in response to a skin stimulus. The direction of the reflex movement is determined by the inclination of the tail to the long axis of the body. If the tail in its initial posture hangs to the left the reflex response is movement to the right, and *vice versa*. Again, the stimulus which causes the spinal dog's hind-limb to be flexed if the initial posture of the limb is extension causes it to be extended if the initial posture is flexion. Again, the stimulus which excites scratching of the left leg if the dog lie on its right side excites scratching of the right leg if the dog lie on its left. These postures are passive. Magnus shows that in several such types of reversal the shunting influence is traceable to the deep afferents, the proprioceptive, and that the influence is a tonic one.

Besides reversals due to passive postures there are others due to active postures. Graham Brown[5] has well stressed this point and gives examples of it. If the decerebrate guinea-pig is held up the hind-limbs usually assume a state of maintained extension; pinching the femoral fold then excites a reflex movement of extension of the limb. But if the initial active posture of the limb be flexion, the pinching evokes flexion of the limb.

What concerns us here is that in some cases the reflex influence modifying the sense or distribution of the reflex evidently includes inhibition. The points at which excitation previously was operative become places where inhibition is operative, and *vice versa*.

[1] *J. Physiol.*, 1909, **39**, 228.   [2] *Pflüg. Arch. ges. Physiol.*, 1909, **130**, 219.
[3] *Ibid.*, 1911, **138**, 388.   [4] *Ibid.*, 1910, **134**, 545.   [5] *Quart. J. exp. Physiol.*, 1911, **4**, 273.

Certain drugs facilitate reflex inhibition—that is to say, favour it rather than reflex excitation. Chloroform and ether are such agents. Occasionally at a certain stage of narcosis by chloroform an excitatory reflex may be reversed to an inhibitory one. Bayliss has noted this for vasomotor reflexes, and Sowton and myself for the limb-reflexes of skeletal muscle.

On the other hand, strychnine in certain doses changes the inhibition of the ordinary limb-reflexes into excitatory effect.[1]

Allied to functional normal reversals is the case of the change from reflex-extension of the limb to reflex-flexion, which occurs when a nociceptive stimulus applied to the foot or afferent nerve of one limb is accompanied by a similar stimulus to foot or nerve of the other limb. The reflex figure, which under the unilateral stimulus is ipsilateral flexion and contralateral extension, is changed under the bilateral stimulus to bilateral flexion.[2] The explanation of this is that on experimental analysis of the ipsilateral and contralateral effects on isolated extensor and flexor muscles[3] it is found that, with moderate and strong stimuli (and nociceptive stimuli are never weak), the intensity of the ipsilateral excitation is greater in the flexor muscle than is the intensity of the contralateral inhibition, and conversely with the extensor muscles. Under the combined right and left stimuli the algebraic summation of the inhibitory and excitatory effects leads to contraction of flexors and inhibitory relaxation of extensors.

Departures from Reciprocal Innervation

Is reciprocal innervation an invariable rule of reflex behaviour in antagonist muscles? The question may perhaps be put better thus: When afferent impulses play on the twin half-centres representing a pair of antagonistic muscles, do they always, while exerting excitatory influence on the one half-centre, exert inhibitory influence on the other? In lieu of examining directly the twin half-centres themselves, the procedure available is to examine two muscles representing the half-centres, and from their behaviour to infer the inhibition and excitation of the half-centres themselves.

There is a source of confusion for this question in the circumstance that it is not always easy by mere inspection to know which muscles are antagonistic to each other. In the first place, many double-joint muscles act in opposite ways on the two joints they cross.[4] Thus gastrocnemius (Fig. 40, B, 7) is an extensor of ankle and also potentially a flexor of knee, semitendinosus (Fig. 40, A, т) is a flexor of knee and also potentially an extensor of hip, tibialis anticus (cat, dog) is a flexor of ankle and also potentially an extensor of knee, scapular head of triceps is an extensor of elbow and also potentially a flexor of shoulder; and so on. But analysis of the part taken by the several muscles of the limb in the various specific limb-

---

[1] *J. Physiol.*, 1907, **36**, 185.
[2] Schäfer's *Textbook of Physiology*, 1901, **2**, 842; and *Integrative Action*, 1906.
[3] *Proc. roy. Soc.*, 1913, **86B**, 219.   [4] *J. Physiol.*, 1910, **40**, 28.

reflexes (flexion-reflex, crossed extension-reflex, stepping-reflex, scratch-reflex) shows that one and the same muscle is used in all these reflexes either always as a flexor or always as an extensor. The reflex taxis does not employ such a muscle sometimes as a flexor and sometimes as an extensor. Once a flexor always a flexor, once an extensor always an extensor. Hence semitendinosus was spoken of above as a *potential* extensor (of hip), because it is always employed as a flexor (of knee), and its ability from its mechanical position to extend hip is not given the opportunity for fulfilment, although at the same time taken advantage of to the full as a means of enhancing its action as a flexor (at knee). The reflexes always throw it into contraction along with the other great flexors of the limb, and inhibit it along with the inhibition of the other great flexors. Used in this way its relatively feeble power to extend the hip is completely overriden by the contraction of the great flexors of that joint. But the circumstance that it passes across the extensor aspect of the hip enables the flexors of the hip to act as flexors of knee by means of semitendinosus, and thus they enhance the action of this latter as a knee-flexor. If the observer, desirous of studying reciprocal innervation, so isolates the semitendinosus that he artificially renders it powerless at knee, and wishing to examine with it the flexors of the hip, detaches them so that they can no longer operate there, he finds that a muscle which appears to him an extensor of hip contracts reflexly simultaneously with, and conversely undergoes inhibitory relaxation simultaneously with, the flexors of that joint. What he is really examining is, however, a flexor of knee along with a flexor of hip. The identical innervation of synergics is in this way liable to appear as though antagonists were identically innervated.

Another pitfall exists in the circumstance that some muscles named by the anatomist on the tacit assumption that they are functionally homogeneous are in fact compounded of functional antagonists. As examples may be cited biceps femoris, triceps brachii, and quadriceps extensor femoris. Biceps femoris (Fig. 40), although to inspection a homogeneous muscular mass, especially where as in many animals it has only one head, proves on physiological analysis to be compounded of two antagonistic portions. One of these is a powerful extensor of hip, the other a powerful flexor of knee, and potentially a weak extensor of hip. The former is treated by the limb-reflexes as an extensor, is excited to contract when the other limb-extensors contract, and inhibited when they are inhibited. The latter is dealt with by the same reflexes as a flexor, contracts with the rest of the flexor muscles, and is inhibited when they are inhibited. The distinction between the two seems to have escaped notice; an observer, unaware of it, might fail to observe the reciprocal innervation really obtaining between one part and the other. In reality the muscle in itself forms a suitable preparation for study of reciprocal innervation.

Similarly, triceps brachii is functionally compounded of antagonistic muscles. That part of it which is humeral in origin is extensor; that part of it which is scapular in origin is flexor. So likewise with quadriceps extensor femoris; that part of it which may be called vasto-crureus is an extensor muscle, but the rest of it—namely, rectus femoris—is flexor. And the reflex taxis deals with the two as antagonists, and innervates them reciprocally; the distinction between them finds expression also in the fact that vasto-crureus yields a tendon-reaction—the knee jerk—like other extensor muscles, while rectus femoris is in no wise implicated in the knee-jerk reaction.

A circumstance altogether different in source from the above, yet like them tending to conceal reciprocal innervation of antagonists, is the following. If when a pair of antagonists have been isolated for the examination of reciprocal innervation, the condition of the preparation is such that both the twin half-centres lie at rest, the reflex when it breaks on the half-centres, although it exerts a reciprocal influence on them, will only reveal its effect on one half-centre—namely, on that half-centre where its influence is excitatory. The inhibitory influence playing on the twin half-centre will not show itself in the myogram, because the centre lying at rest, the muscle, is already relaxed and can relax no further. The reciprocal innervation is then not apparent.

Another way, somewhat related to the preceding, in which seeming departures from the rule of reciprocal innervation of antagonists may come about is the following. Suppose twin half-centres E and F to be in repose, and suppose a reciprocal reflex influence A breaks on them with $+$ influence on E, and $-$ influence on F, and also a reciprocal influence B converse in direction to A. Suppose influence A have a value 10, its excitatory influence being $+10$, its inhibitory -10; and suppose influence B have a value 5, its excitatory being $+5$, its inhibitory -5. The point from which these values are measured is, that condition of the centre which corresponds with a medium state of the muscle midway between full excitation and full inhibition—that is, midway between full contraction and full relaxation. Then, as was shown above in the experiments on double reciprocal innervation, the muscle of E under the algebraic sum of the two influences A and B exhibits a degree of contraction greater than the medium contraction by $10-5=5$, and the muscle of F conversely a state of contraction less than the medium contraction by $5-10=-5$. That is, the one muscle shows a contraction of numerical value 5 above medium contraction, the other a contraction of numerical value 5 below medium contraction. If both muscles are in a condition of medium contraction when the compounded reflex sets in, reciprocal innervation is clear, because one contracts further and the other relaxes. But if the reflex sets in when both twin half-centres are at rest, and their muscles therefore fully relaxed, both muscles are seen to contract, although that of E's muscle is much greater than that of F's muscle. In experiments where two separate suitable afferent nerves are concurrently stimulated, this concurrent contraction of both antagonists has been shown, as above mentioned under double reciprocal innervation.

It has to be remembered that there is a good deal of evidence that in some afferent nerves there appears to be a mixture of afferent fibres, some with excitatory and some with inhibitory influence on the same muscles. In such cases double reciprocal innervation may accrue from stimulation of a single afferent nerve. Some of the cases where both antagonists, or both of two symmetrical muscles, are thrown into contraction together by stimulation of one single afferent nerve (Fig. 47) may have their origin in this way, and be seeming rather than real exceptions to reciprocal innervation. Conversely, in such cases both the opponent muscles may relax concurrently when the stimulation ceases. Further, cortical stimulation must often be equivalent to concurrent stimulation of two or more afferents of diverse effect, and to the seemingly anomalous results of cortical excita-

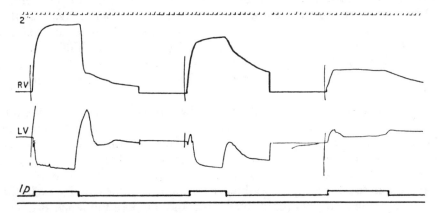

FIG. 47.—REFLEX OF SYMMETRICAL EXTENSOR MUSCLES OF KNEES, RIGHT, RV, AND LEFT, LV,
EVOKED BY FARADISATIONS OF LEFT PERONEAL NERVE, *lp*

The rise of the signal line marks commencement of the stimulation. The reflex is " reciprocal " in the two muscles when the stimulation is strong—*i.e.*, the first of the three faradisations—and is then followed by terminal rebounds. The reflex is " identical " in sense in the two muscles, and without rebound when the stimulation is quite weak—*i.e.*, the last faradisation of the three. With faradisation of intermediate strength the reflex is " identical " in sense at outset and soon becomes reciprocal. Time above in fifths of seconds. Decerebrate cat

tion on antagonists the above line of argument can be justifiably applied. It would seem from the observations on rhythmic reflex of stepping that stimulation of a point in the white column of the cord may be equivalent to combined stimulations of excitatory and inhibitory nerves acting on the same centre.

But there is a class of cases, and it is a large class, in which the mode of innervation of two muscles is reciprocal, although the muscles do not stand to each other in the relation of mechanical antagonists in the usual meaning of the word. In this class of case it seems clear from experiment that though some nerves exert reciprocal influence on the muscle-pair, others exert identical influence (*vide supra*), and that reciprocal innervation is not the only mode of innervation obtaining in regard to the muscles, even when the afferent nerve employed is the same throughout the observations. An instance of this is given by the right and left knee-extensors, vasto-crurei, the afferent nerve being peroneal. With moderate and strong stimulation, the result on the two muscles is always reciprocal, ipsilateral muscle being inhibited, contralateral excited; with quite weak stimulation the result is that both muscles contract, the innervation being, so far as I have seen, truly identical. The contraction though not strong is quite clear (Fig. 47). With stimuli of intensities intermediate between fairly weak and liminal, the effect on the two muscles opens by being contractive in both, and then during the continuance of the stimulation quickly changes to reciprocal by reason of contraction of the ipsilateral muscle passing over into inhibitory relaxation of that muscle. If a surmise as to the significance of the two modes of reaction may be hazarded, it would be that to the very weak stimulation the reflex response is the reflex act of standing, involving mild steady extension of both knees, whereas to the stronger stimulation the response is the nociceptive withdrawal of the ipsilateral limb by knee-flexion, and the stepping-reflex of " running " away with the contralateral limb. Conformably with this, the contraction of the contralateral extensor is often distinctly rhythmic.

Occasionally, but in my experience very rarely, the reflex effect of an afferent limb nerve upon the contralateral extensor (of knee), instead of being pure contraction as usually, opens with distinct though short-lasting inhibition (Fig. 48), which changes over into contraction while the stimulus is still running, even in the course of a second. This is, of course, the exact converse of

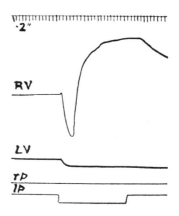

FIG. 48.—SYMMETRICAL EXTENSORS
RIGHT AND LEFT

RV, vasto-crureus of right knee; LV, vasto-crureus of left knee. When the left peroneal nerve, *lp*, is fara-dised (lower signal line), the ipsi-lateral extensor, LV, shows the usual inhibitory relaxation; the contralateral RV exhibits an initial relaxation soon followed by con-traction. The reaction of the muscles as a pair begins, there-fore, by being " identical " in sense, and then quickly passes over into the usual " reciprocal " form. Decerebrate cat. Time above in fifths of seconds

what is not uncommon with the reflex reaction of ipsilateral extensor (of knee)—namely, the commencement of the reaction with con-traction which passes over rapidly into the usual inhibition. In those rare cases where the contralateral reflex on the extensor opens with inhibi-tion, there is, for the brief time during which the inhibition lasts, a bilateral relaxation of both extensors (Fig. 48). Thus, instead of a reciprocal reac-tion, an identical reaction is obtained, but only for the opening second, then reciprocal action re-establishes itself.

The Motor Cortex Cerebri and Inhibition

Of the effects observable in skeletal muscles on stimulation of the motor region of the cerebral cortex, inhibitory relaxation is one of the most common. When the effect of stimulation of a cortical motor point upon antagonistic muscles is examined by the myograph, reciprocal innervation of the muscle-pair is often exhibited with great clearness. Protagonist contracts, antagonist relaxes.

Often, however, results evidently of considerable complexity are seen, and among these appears relaxation or contraction in one member of the muscle-pair without or with only a trace of the converse effect in the other. Often, too, the one effect may appear in the myogram much later than the other, instead of both processes starting together or nearly so, as in simple reflex reactions. These seeming anomalies are referable in part at least to the different degrees of tonus obtaining from time to time in the opponent muscles. Variations in the degree of narcosis seem answerable for much of the variability of the tonus. If the tonus of both of the muscles —and the tonus of the muscles merely mirrors the tonus of their motor centres—is low, as may easily be the case when the narcosis is profound, contraction clearly shows, but inhibitory relaxation is difficult of exhibition because there is no background of tonus upon which it can evidence itself. Contraction of the one muscle then appears without obvious inhibitory relaxation of the other.

The narcosis of chloroform and ether is one of the necessary difficulties attaching to such experimental study of cortical reactions involving the sketetal musculature. A certain grade of the narcosis is often accompanied by marked tonic states, flexor or extensor. Very profound narcosis annihilates the tonus of the skeletal muscles altogether. More embarrassing still, the chemical narcosis seems to depress the tonus and reactions of the respective muscle-centres variably and unequally. Thus the eyeballs exhibit a variety of malpostures under such narcosis. When the narcosis is profound the eyes are sensibly parallel, the tonus of all their muscles being annulled. But in the approach towards and in the recovering from such profound narcosis the eyeballs pass through a variety of deviations from parallelism, showing the relative inequality of action of the narcotic on the several centres of the different muscles. Similarly with the centres of extensor and flexor muscles, the narcosis from period to period influences unequally flexor and extensor respectively. Hence it is perhaps not surprising that the cortical stimulation which inhibits the one muscle of the pair not rarely fails to produce contraction of the opponent. It has to be remembered also in this regard that chloroform and ether tend to favour inhibition and to depress reflex excitation, and tend to suppress the latter more than the former.

Instances occur, whatever their explanation, which show a cortical effect on antagonist muscles in which inhibitory relaxation of one member of the antagonist pair is sundered, as far at least as the myograph evidence goes, from all contraction of the other.[1] And this result is not uncommon with the cortex under experimental conditions. Nor is narcosis probably the only influence accounting for it. Another cause seems traceable in instances such as the following.[1] A cortical point E, which usually gave contraction of the extensor and inhibitory relaxation of the flexor, was stimulated immediately after stimulation of an antagonistic point F, a point which evoked contraction of flexor and inhibition of extensor. The point E then gave inhibitory relaxation of flexor, though not so markedly as before, but it gave no obvious contraction at all of extensor. The antagonistic influence of point F on point E seemed to be still persisting as regards the extensor muscle, although it had largely passed away as regards the flexor muscle.

Reactions of cortical points on antagonistic muscles are prone to " reversal "—that is, the direction of the reciprocal effect which the point exerts on the muscle-pair may under various circumstances be diametrically reversed.[1] When such reversal occurs, it is not very uncommon for the excitatory effect to be reversed, inhibition replacing contraction in regard to one of the muscles, and yet for no contraction to appear in the opponent muscle.

Concluding Remarks

There are close correspondences in many points between reflex inhibition and reflex excitation, although the process of E and that of I may be viewed as polar opposites, and though the one is able to neutralise the other. Both undergo fatigue; the fatigue of the one favours the supervention of the other; both outlive and outrun their stimulation periods for a little time, and in proportion as their evocation has been intense; the latent period of both appears about the same; many of the time relations of the one closely resemble those of the other. While two reflex arcs make use of the same " final common path," the same degree of independence and of dependence appears in the two arcs when tested by inhibitory reactions on extensors as when by excitatory on flexors.[2] An inference from such correspondences may well be that the two processes consist essentially of one reaction which is reversible in direction, so that when proceeding in one direction its outcome is excitation, and when in the other inhibition.

It has, however, to be remembered that the process of reflex excitation as studied in reflex reactions is always commenced by excitation—that is, opens with excitation of some afferent nerve-trunk. It is somewhere in the further course of the reaction and further downstream in the reflex arc that the process inhibition begins. The above-mentioned features of resemblance between the inhibitory and the excitatory reflexes may be, in part at least, due to the earlier parts of the reflexes in both cases being concerned with the same process—namely, excitation.

[1] Graham Brown and Sherrington, *Proc. roy. Soc.*, 1912, **85B**, 250.
[2] Forbes, *Amer. J. Physiol.*, 1912, **31**, 102.

The power of the environment operating through the nervous system to incite this or that animal activity has long been known and studied; knowledge of its converse power to stem and to call halt to such activity has been elaborated only more recently.   Reflex inhibition is the expression of this latter power.   The skeletal musculature offers a field especially favourable for its examination.   The intimate nature of the reflex inhibitory process remains still obscure.   Started by nervous excitation though it is, it yet seems detail by detail to present an exact antithetic counterpart to nervous excitation.   Often the two processes meet and neutralise each other according to dosage, in appearance much as do acidity and alkalinity.

Whatever the intimate nature of its process, certain rules regarding the times and places and circumstances of occurrence of reflex inhibition, and the purposes which it serves, are becoming more clear.   It takes regularly a part in the correlation of action of antagonistic centres, and therefore of their muscles, both when such muscles are executing movements either steady or rhythmic, and also when they are in so-called " tonus " maintaining attitudes and postures.   Waste of nervous and muscular energy in the correlation of antagonists is thus avoided.

It is a great factor in the due grading of muscular contraction.   It grades the degree of contraction of muscles in their execution of a particular act under particular combinations of circumstances.

It plays a part in the production of rhythmic reflexes, tending to generate them when balancing the opponent excitatory process, and regulating their rate of alternation of phase by intensity, degree of equipoise, and via proprioceptive channels (breathing, stepping).

In the sequence of reflexes of opposed and partially opposed effect, it secures co-ordination by suppressing a pre-existent reflex to make room for a new one which employs the muscles differently.   It tends to cure the momentum of the reflex discharge of centres and makes their reactions more dead-beat.   By inducing excitatory discharge as an after-effect sequent to itself, it interconnects the phases of alternating reflexes and facilitates transitions between reflexes of opposite effect by post-inhibitory rebound.

In all these uses of inhibition we see it as an associate of, and a counterpart or counterpoise to, excitation.   Whether we study it in the more primitive nervous reactions which simply interconnect antagonistic muscles, or in the latest acquired reactions of the highly integrated organism, inhibition does not stand alone but runs always alongside of excitation. In the simple correlation uniting antagonistic muscle-pairs, inhibition of antagonist accompanies excitation of progatonist.   In higher integrations where, for instance, a visual signal comes by training to be associated to salivary flow, the key of the acquiring of the reflex and of its maintenance is attention.   And that part of attention which psychologists term negative, the counterpart and constant accompaniment to positive attention, seems as surely a sign of nervous inhibition as is the relaxation of an antagonist muscle the concomitant of the contraction of the protagonist. In the latter case the co-ordination concerns but a small part of the mechanism of the individual and is spinal and unconscious. In the former case it deals with practically the whole organism, is cortical and conscious. In all cases inhibition is an integrative element in the consolidation of the animal mechanism to a unity. It and excitation together compose a chord in the harmony of the healthy working of the organism.

VIII

ON POSTURAL REFLEXES

[The investigation of tonic contraction in mammalian voluntary muscle was enormously facilitated by the discovery of decerebrate rigidity in 1896. This condition was shown to be modifiable by the limb reflexes, and to be a reflex itself. The afferents for the reflex, lying in the nerves side by side with afferents inhibitory for the reflex, were difficult to stimulate artificially. Nevertheless, the presence of a self-contracting reflex from muscle was established, and the reactions concerned systematised in their relation to attitude and posture (the " proprioceptive system," 1906). The difficult proof that the plasticity of tonic muscle was also reflex was accomplished in 1909. In 1915 " tonic " muscular reactions in general, including both visceral and skeletal muscular tone, and the modifications of the latter by the neck reflexes and labyrinth, were brought within the one clarifying conception of postural adaptations.

*Just as the discovery of reciprocal innervation, by giving precise meaning to inhibition, enabled its closer analysis, so the conception of postural reflexes immediately gave impetus to investigation of all the problems related to sustained contraction in voluntary muscle. The difficulty in measuring the contraction in a muscle while it was being stretched or released was eventually overcome by the isometric method of recording, and in 1924 the fundamental postural reflex, " the stretch reflex," was demonstrated, and its adequate stimulus fully defined.—*Ed.]

1. DECEREBRATE RIGIDITY, ITS NATURE, AND RELATIONSHIP WITH OTHER LIMB REFLEXES[1]

IN a communication to the Royal Society in 1896[2] I described under the name *decerebrate rigidity* a condition of long-maintained muscular contraction supervening on removal of the cerebral hemispheres. The condition is one possessing considerable physiological interest, but I have not succeeded in finding any description of it prior to the above mentioned. Although continued experimentation still leaves me in doubt concerning the actual focus of origin of the rigidity, it will be useful to give here a further account of the phenomenon and of some points connected with it.

When in the monkey after ligation of the carotid arteries and under

---

[1] Published under the title " Decerebrate Rigidity, and Reflex Co-ordination of Movements," *J. Physiol.*, 1898, **22**, 319-32.

[2] " Cataleptoid Reflexes in the Monkey," describing the long after-discharge in reflex reactions in the decerebrate animal, *Proc. roy. Soc.*, 1896-7, **60**, 411 (see also p. 414), and defined as " decerebrate rigidity " in *Philos. Trans.*, 1898, **190B**, 178, and also mentioned on pp. 159, 161 and 174. The latter paper was communicated in 1896.—Ed.

deep chloroformisation the cerebral hemispheres are removed, and little hæmorrhage has occurred, the respiratory movements proceed, after a slight temporary check, regularly as before, and the chloroform narcosis can be somewhat relaxed because profound unconsciousness has resulted from the ablation itself. Then ensues, often almost at once—*i.e.*, in a few minutes—sometimes, however, only after an interval of an hour or more, a status characterised by a peculiar rigidity of certain joints. The elbow-joints do not allow then of the usually easily made passive flexion, the knee-joints similarly are stiffly extended. The tail is stiff and straight instead of flexible and drooping. The neck is rigidly extended, the head retracted, and the chin thrown upward.

In my observations I have been accustomed to support the animal freely above the table. In that way opportunity is afforded for separate inspection and investigation of the individual parts of the trunk and limbs. The joints are then free to move with little hindrance. Moreover, the existence of and even the degree of paralysis of different regions is indicated very valuably by the extent to which the attitude is determined by mere gravitation. If in a monkey or cat transection below or in the lower half of the bulb has been performed, the animal, artificial respiration when necessary being kept up, hangs from the suspension points with deeply drooped neck, deeply drooped tail, and its pendent limbs flaccid and slightly flexed. The fore-limb is slightly flexed at shoulder, at elbow, and, very slightly, at wrist. The hind-limb is slightly flexed at hip, at knee, and at ankle. On giving the hand or foot a push forward and then releasing it the limb swings back into and somewhat beyond the position of its equilibrium under gravity; and it oscillates a few times backward and forward before finally settling down to its original position.

To this condition of flaccid paralysis supervening upon transection in the lower half of the bulb the condition ensuing on removal of the cerebral hemispheres offers a great contrast. In the latter case the animal, on being suspended just in the same manner as after the former operation, hangs with its fore-limbs thrust backward, with retraction at shoulder-joint, straightened elbow, and some flexion at wrist. The hand of the monkey is turned with its palmar face somewhat inward. The hind-limbs are similarly kept straightened and thrust backward; the hip is extended, the knee very stiffly extended, and the ankle somewhat extended. The tail, in spite of its own weight—and it is quite heavy in some species of monkey—is kept either straight and horizontal or often stiffly curved upward. There is a little opisthotonus of the lumbo-sacral vertebral region. The head is kept lifted against gravity, and the chin is tilted upward under the retraction and backward rotation of the skull. The differences in general attitude assumed after transection in the lower half of the bulb and after ablation of the cerebral hemispheres respectively is indicated in the diagrams (Fig. 49, *a* and *b*). When the limbs or tail are pushed from the pose they have assumed considerable resistance to the movement is felt, and, unlike the condition after bulbar section, on being released they spring back at once to their former position and remain there for a time more stiffly than even before.

The phenomenon of this decerebrate rigidity occurs with little variation in the monkey, dog, cat, rabbit, and guinea-pig. In all these species the effect upon the fore-limb seems more intense than on the hind-limb. In the hind-limb the knee is the principal joint affected. In the rabbit the phenomenon in the hind-limb has so far as my observations go been particularly well seen. It is noteworthy that the wrist and ankle are comparatively slightly implicated in the rigidity, the ankle more than wrist. I have never in any instance been able to satisfy myself that the digits are implicated at all.

The rigidity is immediately due to prolonged spasm of certain groups of voluntary muscles. The chief of these are the retractor muscles of the head and neck, the elevators and dorsal flexors of the tail, and the extensor muscles of the elbow and knee, and shoulder and hip. This prolonged spasm I have seen maintained in young cats, with some intermissions, for a period of four days. It is increased, and even when absent or very slight may be soon developed, by passive movements of the part. For example, passive flexion and extension of the elbow will suffice to " develop " in a few seconds a high " extensor rigidity " of that joint. This will, after continuing a short time, then tend to slowly relax again, and then again it can be recalled by repetition of the passive movements. There is no obvious tremor in the spasm in the earlier hours of its continuance; later it does sometimes become tremulant.

Administration of chloroform and ether, if carried far, quite abolishes the rigidity. On interrupting the administration the rigidity again rapidly returns.

Section of the dorsal columns of the spinal cord does not abolish the rigidity. Section of one lateral column of the cord in the upper lumbar region abolishes the rigidity in the hind-limb of the same side as the section. Section of one ventro-lateral column of the cord in the cervical region destroys the rigidity in the fore- and hind-limbs of the same side.

It would be possible to ascribe these results to interruption of the pyramidal tract. The following, however, cannot be explained by appeal to the pyramidal section. Section of one lateral half of the bulb in the lower half of the floor of the fourth ventricle and quite above the level of the decussation of the pyramidal tracts abolishes the rigidity in the limbs *on the same side as the section*. And, further, transverse severance of the lateral region only of this part of the bulb without interference to either pyramidal tract produces similar abolition of the rigidity of the homonymous limbs. Finally, excitation of this lateral region with rapidly alternating series of induction shocks reinforces the rigidity in the homonymous side.

If instead of both cerebral hemispheres one only—say, the right—be ablated, the decerebrate rigidity appears, though not with the same certainty as after double ablation, chiefly on the *same* side as the hemisphere removed. The monkey when slung after ablation of one—*e.g.*, the right—hemisphere exhibits generally the following attitude. The right limbs are extended in the pose above described as characteristic for decerebrate rigidity, the tail is strongly incurvated toward the right—that is, its concavity is toward the right and its tip is also toward the right. It resists passive movement to the left, and if displaced thither immediately on being released flies back. The head also is pulled toward the right and retracted. The left fore-limb —and the point will be returned to—is sometimes distinctly more flexed than would be expected in the paralysed condition of the animal: the left knee likewise. The same results are seen in the cat. The contrast between the attitude of the crossed and homonymous sides is very striking. They

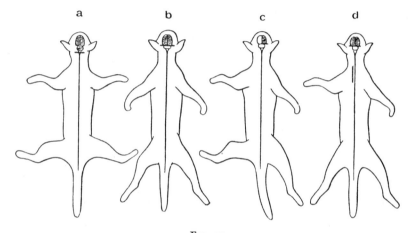

FIG. 49

a. Position of animal after transection at calamus scriptorius
b. Position of animal after ablation of cerebral hemispheres when decerebrate rigidity has developed
c. Position of animal after ablation of one cerebral hemisphere when decerebrate rigidy has developed
d. Effect on decerebrate rigidity of severance of afferent spinal roots of left fore-limb

are indicated by the diagrams (Fig. 49, *b* and *c*). The retraction and bending of the head cannot, however, be well shown in a diagram taking the dorsal view.

Homonymous extensor rigidity consequent on ablation of one hemisphere is, however, neither so constant of production nor so persistent when it has appeared as the rigidity following bilateral ablation. After coming on it may totally subside and again reappear, and so on several times over. There would seem under these circumstances a struggle between two conflicting influences, as though a tonic influence from the still intact crossed hemisphere at times overcame and at times was overcome by another opposed influence from a lower centre. Some amount of extensor rigidity on the side opposite to the lesion is not uncommon.

Afferent Nerve-roots and Decerebrate Rigidity

If after ablation of both cerebral hemispheres, even when the rigidity is being maintained at its extreme height, the afferent roots, which have been previously laid bare and prepared, are carefully severed, the limb at once falls into flaccidity. From the stiffly extended position it drops into the slightly flexed position it assumes when flaccid under gravity. The result is quite local, as indicated in Fig. 49, *d*.

A question arises: Is this setting aside of the rigidity by severance of afferent spinal roots a result of their paralysis or of their irritation? Is it due to pure interruption of the afferent path leading from the periphery to the spino-cranial centres, or is it due to mere irritation of the afferent fibres by the mechanical process of severing them and the irritation of the injury set up in them? The former seems the explanation on the following grounds. Firstly, the abolition of the rigidity is long-lasting—*i.e.*, persists for several hours—however the mechanical stimulation be minimised, the roots being cut through with as little disturbance as possible at the single closure of a sharp pair of scissors. Secondly, the rigidity develops either very imperfectly or not at all when the afferent roots have been severed some time—*i.e.*, a number of days prior to carrying out the operation which produces the rigidity. Of this the following are examples:

Cat.—The dorsal (afferent) roots of the 5th, 6th, 7th, and 8th right cervical and of the right 1st thoracic nerves were severed in the vertebral canal. Marked ataxy of the right fore-limb ensued with obvious weakness of the right fore-paw (ankle). Ten days later under deep anæsthesia the cerebral hemispheres were removed. In the course of half an hour *decerebrate rigidity* fixed both knees and the left elbow in the extended position. The right elbow remained flaccid, although perhaps not quite so flaccid as is usual after transection at the stimulus. After the animal had been subsequently killed, the onset of rigor mortis was much delayed in the extensors of the right elbow as compared with those of the left.

Cat.—The dorsal (afferent) roots of the 6th, 7th, and 8th right cervical of the right 1st thoracic nerve were severed in the vertebral canal. There resulted distinctly less ataxy in movements employing the paw than in the above example; there appeared also less weakness at the wrist, but in the erect position the animal stood with its wrist less dorsal-flexed than its right. In jumping the animal appeared always to alight on the left fore-foot a little before the descent of the right. In walking each step forward with the right fore-limb brought the foot far round, sometimes even to the left of, the left foot. Twelve days later the cerebral hemispheres were removed under deep anæsthesia. *Decerebrate rigidity* rapidly ensued, fixing in the extended position both the two knee-joints and the left elbow; but the right elbow remained flaccid. After killing the animal rigor mortis set in much later in the right than in the left triceps. Histological examination of the spinal cord revealed degeneration in the dorsal column of the right side but no further lesion. The ventral (motor) roots were quite intact.

Monkey (Macacus rhesus).—The afferent (dorsal) roots of the 5th, 6th, 7th, and 8th left cervical nerves and of the left 1st thoracic nerve were severed in the vertebral canal. Marked ataxy of the left arm ensued. The movement of " grasp " by the left hand was lost. Twenty-one days later the cerebral hemispheres were removed under deep anæsthesia. *Decerebrate rigidity* rapidly supervened in both knees and in the right elbow, also to some extent in the ankles and in the right wrist. There was for some time no rigidity at all in the left elbow, which remained flaccid. In the course of three hours the rigidity increased considerably, and there were dubious traces of rigidity in the left elbow, although certainly there was no rigidity in the left wrist. After the killing of the animal subsequently the onset of rigor mortis was much later in the extensors of the left elbow than in those of the right. Histological examination showed the lesion to be confined to the afferent roots mentioned above, and the degeneration to their continuations in the dorsal column of the cord.

Monkey (Macacus sinicus).—The dorsal (afferent) roots of the 5th, 6th, 7th, and 8th left post-thoracic spinal nerves severed in the vertebral canal. There ensued the usual symptoms of ataxy and enfeebled grasp-movement noted by Mott and myself. The left knee jerk was abolished. As the animal ran about it kept its left limb flexed at hip and knee. There was no actual " contracture " in the limb. Five weeks after the initial operation the cerebral hemispheres were removed under profound anæsthesia. *Decerebrate rigidity* soon developed in high degree. Both elbows became fixed in the extended position, as also the right knee. At first there was no rigidity in the left knee, and later even when the rigidity elsewhere was extreme it was doubtful whether at the left knee any developed; but I do not think the knee was so flaccid as it would have been after transection at the calamus. Subsequently after killing the animal rigor mortis set in much later in the left knee than in the right. Histological examination showed the lesion to implicate only the afferent roots above mentioned.

The decerebrate rigidity seems therefore in some way dependent on integrity of the afferent paths of the limbs. This dependence points to centripetal impulses from peripheral sense-organs of the limb as important for the production and maintenance of decerebrate rigidity in the muscles of the limb in question. Normal tonus of limb-muscles has been shown (Brondgeest, v. Anrep, etc.) to be similarly dependent on centripetal impulses from the limb; and in the case of tonus the afferent paths from the skin have been found less important (Mommsen[1]) than those from deep structures, and especially from the muscles themselves.[2] I find that similarly the afferent nerves from muscles can exercise a great local influence on decerebrate rigidity. Electrical excitation of the central end of a nerve-trunk distributed purely to muscles—*e.g.*, the hamstring nerve of the cat—produces immediate relaxation of the rigid extensors of the knee. On discontinuing the excitation the extensor rigidity of the knee returns. A ligature drawn tightly round this nerve keeps the knee of the homonymous side relaxed, presumably by acting as a continual slight stimulus. The extensor rigidity of the knee of the crossed side seems, on the other hand, somewhat increased. Mere section of the hamstring-nerve did not, however, in three experiments made with a view to determining the point, prevent the development of the rigidity of the knee.

It is noteworthy that in the second example given above the sensory spinal roots severed in the brachial plexus were exactly those in which exist the afferent nerve-fibres coming up from the triceps (extensor of the elbow) muscle itself—namely, from the muscle especially affected by the decerebrate rigidity. Also it should be stated that in all of the experiments

[1] *Virchows Arch.*, 1885, **101,** 22. [2] Sherrington, *Proc. roy. Soc.*, 1893, **53,** 407 (here p. 244).

performed the afferent roots cut were roots in which the extensor muscles—
the seat of the rigidity—are represented.

These results are strikingly in accord with views that Mott and myself[1]
have put forward, and especially with an argument advanced by Bastian[2]
in discussing the condition of the limb in our experiments on the effect
of severance of the sensory spinal roots upon the movements executed by
the limb.

J. R. Ewald[3] has pointed out that destruction of the otic labyrinth
reduces the tonus of the skeletal musculature of the homonymous half of
the body. He also found[4] the onset of rigor mortis delayed in the muscles
of the homonymous side. Similarly also I found[5] section of the afferent
nerve-roots of a limb delay considerably the onset of rigor mortis in it.
Decerebrate rigidity undoubtedly hastens the onset of rigor mortis in the
muscles it involves. It seemed, therefore, desirable to enquire whether
section of the nervus octavus would affect the development of decerebrate
rigidity. In a monkey the 8th cranial nerve of the left side was accordingly
cut intracranially between its surface origin and the internal auditory
meatus. Nystagmus, lateral rolling movement, and other effects more or
less striking ensued. Five hours later the cerebral hemispheres were removed
under profound anæsthesia. Decerebrate rigidity then quickly set in and
developed with about equal rapidity and in about equal degree on the left
as on the right side.

Forms of Extensor Rigidity allied to Decerebrate Rigidity

While attempting, however, to obtain as above some nearer view of the
causation of decerebrate rigidity it must be added that other mutilations
than ablation of the cerebral hemispheres induce phenomena of extensor
rigidity bearing at least superficially much resemblance to that produced
by removal of the cerebrum.

After median section of or ablation of the cerebellum a rigidity often,
but not always, sets in somewhat similar to that ensuing on removal of the
cerebral hemispheres. That the two conditions are identical I am not
convinced. The uncrossed nature of the decerebrate rigidity suggests a
causal connection between the cerebellum and the rigidity, perhaps through
the nucleus of Deiters, which, as first shown by Ferrier and Turner, possesses
large efferent connections from the side of the cerebellum. On the other
hand the crossed cerebello-cerebral and crossed cerebro-cerebellar paths,
in the anterior and middle peduncles on which Mingazzini's histological
work has recently thrown more light, may form a circuit whose function
is upset in much the same way whether cerebellar or cerebral ablation be
performed. This might explain the supervention of a similar condition
after either one of these injuries. Median section of the cerebellum also

[1] *Proc. roy. Soc.*, 1895, **57**, 481.   [2] *Ibid.*, 1895, **58**, 96.
[3] *Nervus Octavus*, Wiesbaden, 1892.   [4] *Pflüg. Arch. ges. Physiol.*, 1894.
[5] *Proc. roy. Soc.*, 1893, **53**, 407.

causes some extensor rigidity of the limbs. It will be remembered in this connection that the paths ascending by the inferior peduncle and reaching the superior vermis largely decussate there across the median line (Mott, Thomas, etc.).

It is significant that decerebrate rigidity sometimes persists after removal of the cerebellum, if the latter ablation be performed without any serious amount of hæmorrhage.

These allied forms of extensor rigidity further resemble decerebrate rigidity in similarly being readily broken down by appropriate central and peripheral excitations, among the former of which are to be included excitations applied to the Rolandic area of the cortex cerebri.

Decerebrate Rigidity inhibited by Central Stimuli

One of the chief interests of decerebrate rigidity attaches to it as a field for examination of the play of inhibition. For this it gives a wider scope than can be usually obtained, and it has revealed to me an almost unexpectedly significant number of examples of depressor effect generally, perhaps always, in combination with pressor effects—that is to say, in the form of *reciprocal innervations*.

Electrical excitation of the *dorsal spinal columns* in the cervical region provokes such inhibitions. Similarly, as mentioned in my first paper, electrical excitation of the *crusta cerebri* sometimes inhibits the rigidity, evoking reciprocal innervation of antagonistic muscles at elbow, knee, etc. So also excitation of the *pyramidal tract*. In the monkey similar inhibition of the decerebrate rigidity can be produced by excitation of the anterior (cerebral) surface of the *cerebellum*,[1] as mentioned in my previous paper. Faradisation of points in a large area extending from near the middle line far out toward the lateral border of the cerebellar surface causes relaxation of the rigid neck and tail muscles, and relaxation of the rigid limbs, especially of the uncrossed side.

But the homonymous extensor rigidity which frequently ensues, as above mentioned, on ablation of one cerebral hemisphere presents an opportunity for examining the effect of excitation of the cerebral cortex itself (of the remaining hemispheres) upon the activity of the extensor muscles of the crossed elbow and knee. I find in the Rolandic region of the monkey a cortical area which gives, markedly and forthwith, inhibition of the contraction of the extensor of the elbow; and another cortical area which similarly when excited inhibits the contraction of the extensors of the knee. This is in accord with the results obtained under different conditions by H. E. Hering and myself.[2] Also, as Hering and myself in those other experiments noted, the areas of cortex whence inhibition of the active

[1] *Philos. Trans.*, 1898, **190B**, 174 (p. 150, this volume), reported in 1896, read January, 1897; see *Proc. roy. Soc.*, 1897, **60**, 408. In the following month its occurrence in the dog and cat was reported, somewhat contentiously, by Loewenthal and Horsley, *Proc. roy. Soc.*, 1897, **61**, 20.

[2] See p. 259.

extensors is elicited are not the same areas as those whence contraction of the extensors is elicited, but on the other hand coincide with the areas whence contraction of the flexors can be excited.

Decerebrate Rigidity inhibited by Peripheral Stimuli

Besides the inhibitions from the central nervous system inhibition of decerebrate extensor rigidity can be evoked by excitations applied to the periphery.

Thus on excitation of the central end of the 2nd cervical nerve, or of a branch, even a small twig of that nerve, the high-held retracted head drops almost as if knocked down by a blow from above. The muscles causing the contraction can be seen and felt to relax at once under the excitation; the completeness and suddenness of the relaxation is surprising.

Similarly, after removal of the cerebral hemispheres, when it is easy to apply electrodes to the divisions of the trigeminus on the floor of the middle fossa of the cranium, a touch with the electrodes is enough to cause the relaxation of the rigid neck muscles: and the stimulation need not be strong in order to similarly evoke relaxation in the fore-limb, the hind-limb, and in the tail. Indeed, the erected tail drops almost as easily and suddenly as the retracted neck. Excitation of even small twigs of distribution of the 5th effects the same; even the faradisation of certain spots of the dura mater suffices. Stimulation of a digital nerve or of the radial trunk causes relaxation of a similar kind, but commencing in the limb. Stimulation of the saphenous nerve as mentioned in my previous paper[1] similarly causes relaxation commencing in the hind-limb and tail.

Electric stimulation of the optic nerve is less effectual.

Excitation of the skin itself produces similar results, and here it is easier to obtain more restricted play of the inhibitions, and therefore results more instructive in regard to the mutual distribution and co-operation of depressor and pressor reactions.

On excitation of the pinna of the ear—e.g., the left, whence the afferent paths are 5th cranial and 2nd cervical (in dog, cat and rabbit 1st cervical also) admixed—a complex reflex reaction to the following effect occurs:

The head, high-held and retracted, is somewhat dropped and turned away toward the right, the stiffly extended left fore-limb is flexed at elbow, extended at wrist, and brought forward. The left hind-limb is thrust backward, its existing extension at hip and knee being increased. The right fore-limb is thrust backward, its existing extension at elbow and shoulder being increased. The right hind-limb is flexed at hip and knee and ankle. The erected tail is dropped. (Fig. 50, compare b and c.)

In this reaction there occurs (1) inhibition of the rigid left triceps, with contraction of the antagonistic prebrachial muscles, (2) further increase of the maintained spasm of the extensors of the left knee and hip, (3) further

[1] *Proc. roy. Soc.*, 1897, **60**, 411.

increase of the maintained spasm of the right triceps brachii with relaxation of the antagonistic prebrachial muscles, (4) inhibition of the rigidly maintained spasm in the extensors of the right knee and hip with contraction of the hamstring and tibialis anticus muscles of the right hind-limb.

In this reflex the turning of the head away from the stimulus forcibly gives the impression of an attempt to escape from the irritation; and the concomitant raising and moving forward of the left fore-paw forcibly gives the impression of an attempt to remove the source of irritation.

If instead of the left pinna the skin of the left hand (or in cat the pad of the fore-foot) be the site of stimulation, reaction occurs to the following effect (Fig. 51, *b*):

The high-held retracted head is let fall somewhat and turned *toward* the side stimulated. The stiffly extended left fore-limb is flexed at elbow, extended at wrist, and brought forward. The left hind-limb already extended is extended even further, especially at the hip. The right fore-limb is thrust backward and its already existing extension at elbow and shoulder is increased. The right hind-limb is flexed at hip and knee and ankle, its pre-existing extensor rigidity being broken down. The erected tail is dropped.

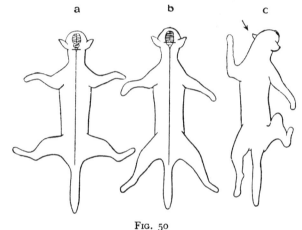

FIG. 50

a. Position of animal after transection at calamus scriptorius
b. Position under decerebrate rigidity
c. Change of attitude from *b* evoked by stimulation of left pinna

Between this reaction and the foregoing the chief difference is in regard to the movement of the head. In the foregoing the movement resembles one employing the left sternomastoid—but inspection proves that at least other muscles besides the sternomastoids are involved in it. In the latter the movement seems due to lateral flexors of the neck in combination with relaxation of some of the retractors of the head.

If the cutaneous point excited instead of being in the hand be in the left foot (*i.e.*, be in cat the left hind-pad) the reaction which occurs is to the following effect: The extensor spasm in left hind-limb at knee and hip is broken down, and flexion at hip, knee, and ankle occurs. The tail is drooped from the stiff erect position. The left fore-limb has its extensor rigidity not diminished but increased. The right hind-limb also undergoes not a relaxation of its extensor spasm but an increase. In the right fore-limb the extensor spasm is broken down, and the limb is advanced with flexion at elbow, extension at wrist, and advancement at shoulder. The head is somewhat drooped. These results as illustrated in the cat are indicated in Fig. 51, *c*. Here again the movement is forcibly suggestive of a *purpose*—namely, the withdrawal of the limb from the place of an irritation.

In this reaction the relaxation of the extensors of the left knee and hip is accompanied by active contraction of the hamstring muscles, of the part of the quadriceps cruris which flexes the hip, and of the tibialis anticus and pretibial flexors, also in some cases of the peroneus longus. The relaxation of the right triceps brachii is accompanied by active contraction of the prebrachial flexor.

Further examples of local restriction of the inhibitory effect are those which I gave in my first communication: a touch on the skin of the perineum producing inhibition often confined to relaxation of the spasm of the extensors of the stiffly elevated and tonically upcurved tail; rubbing of the cheek producing inhibition of the spasm of the muscles retracting the neck and head.

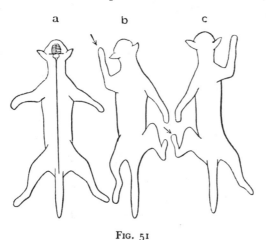

FIG. 51

a. Position under decerebrate rigidity
b. Change of attitude from *a* evoked by stimulation of left fore-foot
c. Change of attitude from *a* evoked by stimulation of left hind-foot

Regarding the inhibition of triceps brachii and quadriceps cruris, and to a less extent of the gastrocnemius, it is interesting to note that these muscles, which among the limb muscles are particularly difficult to provoke to action by local spinal reflexes, are seen in these experiments to be easily accessible when inhibition and not merely augmentation is taken into account. The well-known observation that the extensors of the knee are very inaccessible to spinal reflex action has, as I have recently shown, certain important limitations. But at the same time so long as the transection is spinal—even when carried out so as to isolate not merely a portion of the spinal cord, but the whole cord entire from bulb to filum terminale—does apply really very strictly to excitations arising in its own local region proper. And the spinal reflex relations of triceps brachii in this respect, and also of gastrocnemius, somewhat resemble, as I have elsewhere pointed out, those of the distal portion of the quadriceps extensor of the leg. The difference between the accessibility of the quadriceps and triceps to reflex action after infrabulbar and after suprabulbar transection it seems to me is a matter of superficial rather than fundamental distinction. The *manner* of reply of triceps brachii and quadriceps cruris seems not different in the two conditions. When the conduction across a nexus is signalised by a minus sign instead of a plus, the former, to find expression, must predicate an already existent quantity of contraction—tonus or spasm—to take effect upon. Against a background of maintained contraction effects otherwise invisible, because in the nature of inhibition and therefore finding expression as relaxation, become visible. It seems likely enough that even when transection in infrabulbar, and therefore when merely spinal mechanisms remain in force, the same nexus obtains, but that then, since that background of maintained contraction is lacking, the play of inhibitions remains invisible, never coming within the field of ordinary methods of observation.

When the rigidity is developed after ablation of one cerebral hemisphere only, besides the extensor spasm on the uncrossed side there is usually some flexion on the crossed side, and this especially, I think, when the cortex is inexcitable, owing to anæmia, etc. In connection with this I would add that, in conformity with results in the dog recently reported by Wertheimer and Lepage, I have in examining in repeated experiments the movements obtainable from the *homonymous* limbs by excitation of the cerebral cortex never seen flexion of the limbs but always extension, whereas from the crossed limbs it is easy, as is well known, to obtain both flexion and extension separately.

The results arrived at in the above communication can be shortly summarised thus:

" Decerebrate rigidity " is but a type of extensor spasm of which allied examples follow various other lesions of the cerebello-cerebral region.

The development of " decerebrate rigidity " in a limb is largely determined by centripetal impulses coming from the limb in question.

The contraction of the muscles active in " decerebrate rigidity " can be readily inhibited by stimulation of various regions of the central nervous system, and, among others, of the sensori-motor region of the cerebral cortex.

The activity of the rigid muscles can be readily inhibited by stimulation of various peripheral nerves, and, among others, of the afferent nerve-fibres proceeding from skeletal muscles.

Reflexes obtained from the decerebrate animal exhibit contraction in one muscle-group accompanied by relaxation, inhibition, in the antagonistic muscle group (" reciprocal innervation "), and this in such distribution and sequence as to couple diagonal limbs in harmonious movements of similar direction.

2. THE PROPRIOCEPTIVE SYSTEM[1]

[Discussion of the function of the proprioceptors. They may be regarded as a functional system concerned in the maintenance of attitude.]

It is often asked, What may be the utility of the tonus of skeletal muscles? A suggestion may be hazarded which is germane to the present argument. One function this tonus may serve is that of an adjuvant to so-called muscular sense. The steady, mild tension which the muscles exert in virtue of their reflex tonus may, by acting on joint surfaces, tendons, and muscles, etc., assist the functioning of the sense organs belonging to those structures, much as the reflex tonus of the constrictor pupillæ is adjuvant to the visual receptive surface, and affords the eyeball a favourable condition for its function. But the reflex tonus of skeletal muscle still persists, after destruction of the higher centres to which we have to relegate the operations of sense, and *inter alia* those of the so-called " muscular sense." And it is clear that the receptors of muscles, joints, etc., are concerned with much outside the production of sensations. The reflex tonus of skeletal muscles must therefore have, it would seem, a purpose outside that of directly subserving muscular sense. I would suggest that this reflex tonus is the expression of a *neural discharge concerned with the maintenance of attitude.* Though of many reflex reactions the outcome is movement and the muscles reacting are thus used as organs of motion, much of the reflex reaction expressed by the skeletal musculature is not motile, but postural, and has as its result not a movement, but the steady maintenance of an attitude. The bony and other levers of the body are thus held in certain positions, both in relation to the horizon and to one another. The frog, after removal of its cerebral hemispheres, rests squatting in its tank preserving an attitude very different from that which gravitation would give it were its musculature not in action. Evidently a great part of its skeletal musculature is steadily active all the while, antagonising gravity in maintaining the trunk semi-erect, the fore-limbs semi-extended, and the hind-limbs tautly flexed. Innervation and co-ordination are as fully demanded for the maintenance of a posture as for the execution of a movement.

A posture of the animal as a whole, a *total* posture, is a complex built up of postures of portions of the animal, segmental postures, just as movement executed by the animal as a whole, *total* movement—*e.g.*, locomotion—is compounded of segmental movements. With only the hinder portion of its spinal cord intact, the hind-limbs of the frog still maintain a posture. Owing to spinal reflex action, the hind-limbs are then kept flexed at hip, knee, and ankle. When displaced from that posture they return to it. The deep receptors of the limbs, the proprioceptors, give to their segments —namely, those of the hind-limbs—by local spinal reflex action a definite *attitude.*

[1] Extract from " On the Proprioceptive System," *Brain*, 1906, 474. See also *Integrative Action*, 1906, p. 129, and *Ergebn. Physiol.*, 1905.

The vertebrate animal, as regards the scheme of arrangement of its spinal and cranial reflex arcs and the musculature which they innervate, may be regarded as a fore-and-aft series of segments. In each segment there tend to recur reflex arcs of similar functional kind to those occurring in the other segments. For instance, to each segment there belong reflex arcs arising at the skin surface (exteroceptive) and arcs arising in joints, muscles, tendons, etc. (proprioceptive). The arcs of analogous function belonging to successive segments unite to a homogeneous reflex system extending more or less continuously through the length of the animal. Thus it is that the proprioceptors and their reflex arcs have, in their sum total, to be treated as a *proprioceptive system*.

As the segments—*e.g.*, of a vertebrate—are followed towards the head end of the animal—that is, towards the end which leads in habitual loco-motion—the receptor organs are found to exhibit in the head or leading segments a greater development and general importance than in the other segments. This is strikingly obvious in the receptors of the external surface. It is at the leading end of the animal that the great exteroceptors consti-tuting the eye and the organs of hearing and of smell are met. This leading end it is which, when the creature moves in the direction of its habitual locomotion, explores that portion of the environment into which the body is about to pass. And when the creature is not itself in active locomotion, but, as often happens, allows a moving environment—*e.g.*, a stream of water or a current of air—to drift by, the posture assumed by it is usually such as makes the moving environment impinge upon the head segments first. It is not surprising, therefore, that the reflex arcs are centres of the head or leading segments are found to dominate the arcs of analogous function in all the segments behind their own. A segmental series of reflex arcs of analogous function in its integration to a unified system tends to exhibit a functional hierarchy, in which the reflex arcs belonging to the head are supreme. As regards the system of the proprioceptive arcs, it remains to inquire whether there also the head segments are of higher general im-portance than the rest and exert a special predominance in their system.

Taking the case of the vertebrate, in it there lies in one of the leading segments (head segments) a receptor organ, the *labyrinth*, recessed off from the surface as a sort of cyst. This receptive organ is adapted to mechanical stimuli. It consists of two parts, both endowed with low receptive threshold and with refined selective ability to differentiate stimuli. One part, the otolith organ, is adapted to react to changes in the incidence and degree of pressure exerted on its nerve-endings by contents of higher specific gravity than the fluid otherwise filling the organ. The second part, the semicircular canals, appear to react to minute mass movements of fluid contained within it. These two parts may be taken as typically constituting the labyrinth. The incidence and degree of pressure of the otoliths upon their receptive bed alter with changes in the position of the segment in which the labyrinth lies, relatively to the horizon line. Similarly, movements of the segment stimulate the labyrinthine receptors through the inertia of the labyrinthine fluid as well as of the otoliths. There are some obvious resemblances between these labyrinthine functions and the functioning of the proprioceptors, *e.g.*, of a limb. In the stimulation of the labyrinth the active agent which directly excites the receptor is a portion of the organism itself, and is not an item of the environment. Moreover, the stimulation is provoked commonly by a reactive movement of the organism itself, and that reactive movement is commonly in its turn a response to an environmental stimulus acting on some receptor of the exteroceptive surface. Both these are points of resemblance to the conditions above shown to obtain in regard to the stimulation of the proprioceptors, *e.g.*, of a limb. The segment to which the labyrinth belongs is commonly rigidly conjoined with the other segments composing the head. Postures and movements of the head are thus the immediate causes which stimulate the labyrinth. Thus the labyrinthine receptors, like the proprioceptors in other segments, are stimulated by the animal itself as agent, though secondarily to action of the environment at work upon the animal.

There is another functional likeness between the labyrinth and proprioceptors elsewhere. The latter, as was mentioned, are the source of a reflex tonus in the skeletal muscles. J. R. Ewald and others have shown that to the labyrinth is traceable a share of the neural tonus of many muscles. Ewald concludes his work on the labyrinth by designating it the tonus labyrinth. And these tonic actions of the proprioceptors and of the labyrinth appear to reinforce mutually. Thus the tonus of the extensor muscle of the knee, in the cat and dog, appears to have, under many circumstances, a combined source in the proprioceptors of the limb and in the receptors of the labyrinth.

A further functional resemblance between the labyrinth and other proprioceptive organs lies in both of them initiating compensatory reflexes. It was mentioned that to the proprioceptors of the hind-limb seems traceable in the spinal animal the active reflex resumption of a posture temporarily disturbed by an intercurrent movement. The limb is returned to its original attitude by help of a movement which is reflex and traceable to afferent nerves from the articulo-muscular mechanisms of the disturbed part. Similarly, the reflex posture and the compensatory reflexes of the head are largely traceable to the receptors of the labyrinth. From the labyrinth are excited reflexes which adjust its segment—and with that segment the others of the head are rigidly conjoined—to the horizon line. That the adjustment is to the horizon line seems particularly shown by the eyeballs. The retinæ, those refined photo-receptive patches of the head surface, conduct reflexes delicately differential in regard to space. The due reaction of the animal to stimuli, active above or below, or to right or to left, in the photo-receptive patches, depends on a fairly constant relation being kept between the normals of the patches and true horizontality. This is the meaning of the laws of Donders and Listing regulating eyeball movements. The photo-receptive patches are set movably in the head. By the action of muscles they can retain their bearing to the horizon, although the head itself shifts its bearing to the horizon. The reflex control of these muscles lies largely in the power of impulses from the labyrinth. When temporary causes disturb the usual relation of the normal of the head to the normals of the retinæ, compensatory reflexes bring back the parts to their previous habitual relation both to each other and to the horizon line. These compensatory reflexes, as well as the habitual maintenance of that primary harmonious attitude, are largely traceable to the operation of the reflex arcs which arise in the receptors of the labyrinth. Thus, *as the proprioceptors of a limb are in large measure responsible for the reflex posture and the compensatory reflexes of the limb, so the labyrinthine proprioceptors are largely responsible for the reflex posture and the compensatory reflexes of the head.*

3. ON THE PLASTICITY OF REFLEX POSTURE[1]

[*The reflex nature of the plasticity of tonic muscles. The capacity of a muscle to adapt its length to postures passively applied to it, or actively adopted by it, can be analysed in terms of the " lengthening " and " shortening " reactions. Both of these are proprioceptive reflexes.*]

PROPRIOCEPTIVE REFLEXES OF THE HIND-LIMB IN THE SPINAL ANIMAL

(a) The " Shortening Reaction "

Subsequent to spinal transection, either thoracic or cervical, and after the period of spinal shock has passed, there are obtainable from the extensor muscle of the dog's knee some reactions, unmentioned in the literature, which appear significant for reflex co-ordination. Of these reactions one can be elicited and observed as follows: The animal is held supported under the shoulders with the hind-feet hanging free. Suppose the right limb to be examined: the observer lifts the knee of that pendent limb by simply supporting it from beneath under the tibial component of the joint. In this way the knee is raised with the knee-joint itself extended, but with the hip flexed. It is then found that the extensor muscle of the knee exhibits a considerable tonic contraction; if the supporting hand be shifted upward so as no longer to support the tibial part of the joint, the knee still remains extended, its extended posture being maintained by the tonic contraction of the extensor muscle. This much is obvious to inspection, but can be appreciated better if the observer attempt to forcibly flex the knee. The extensor muscle then opposes the forced flexion, and a considerable resistance to the flexion is experienced.

Modifying in various ways the procedure for this reaction, one is led to the conclusion that the condition essential for thus eliciting the extensor's

---

[1] " On Plastic Tonus and Proprioceptive Reflexes," *Quart. J. exp. Physiol.*, 1909, **2**, 109-56.

contraction is approximation of the end-points of the muscle. The bringing nearer together its insertion and origin appears to induce in the muscle a heightened tonus. This reaction may be termed, for brevity, the " shortening reaction " (Fig. 52, *Sr*).

(b) The " Lengthening Reaction "

A reaction, in several respects the converse of the above " shortening reaction," can then be proceeded to. Suppose the " shortening reaction " to have been evoked and the extended posture of the knee due to tonic

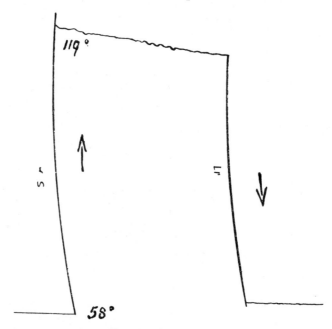

FIG. 52.—SPINAL DOG

" Shortening reaction " *Sr*, " lengthening reaction " *Lr*. The figure 58° signifies the angle of flexure of the knee when the myograph marked the base line; 119° signifies the angle of the knee when marking the top line[1]

contraction of the extensor to be going on. If the observer then, with one hand still supporting the lower end of the thigh, take with his other the leg near the ankle, and bend the knee against the knee-extensor's contraction, he feels the opposition offered by the extensor give way almost abruptly at a certain pressure; the knee can then be flexed without opposition. On then releasing the ankle, the knee is seen to remain flexed (Fig. 52, *Lr*) approximately in that degree of flexion to which it had been carried by the manipulation. The tonic contraction previously exhibited by the extensor has disappeared. Various modifications of the procedure

[1] All the figures read from left to right; the time line where given is near the top of the figure and marks one-second intervals.

producing this result indicate that the factor essential to it is forced stretch of the extensor muscle. The forced stretch causes a relaxation of the tonic extensor, and this condition of relaxed tonus persists after the forced stretch itself has ceased. This reaction may, for brevity, be termed the " lengthening reaction."

The shortest interval after spinal transection at which I have found these reactions present is sixteen days, but on that occasion they disappeared, again to return more permanently about a month after the transection. In the early days following thoracic spinal transection the hind-limbs, on the animal being held in the way above mentioned, hang almost flaccid and with both knees equally flexed under the action of gravity. Later— e.g., four weeks—on the animal being held up in this way, the hind-limbs droop differently; it can be seen that the posture of the two knees is asymmetrical, one being less flexed than the other. On examining the less flexed knee, evident tonic contraction of the vastocrureus is found. It is with this asymmetry of posture of the two knees that the " shortening reaction " becomes obtainable. Concurrent with the appearance of asymmetrical posture in the spinal limbs and of elicitability of the " shortening " and " lengthening reactions," there appear the first walking movements; this co-appearance of the three phenomena is significant of their association in the co-ordinative processes underlying normal stepping. Later still, it is not uncommon to find at times both legs concurrently exhibiting extensor tonus. The reflex posture then assumed is that of standing.

In the spinal dog it is not uncommon for the " knee jerk " to evoke not merely a twitch, but a long-lasting tonic contraction. What then occurs seems as follows: The " knee jerk " elicits a twitch; the shortening of the muscle by the twitch elicits a " shortening reaction." The result is a tonic extension instead of the transient jerk.

(c) Crossed Reflexes

The " shortening reaction " is frequently accompanied by a crossed reaction at the opposite knee. At this opposite knee the tonus of the extensor is relaxed and the knee undergoes flexion. A good way of eliciting this crossed reflex is the following: One thigh (e.g., right) is lightly supported from underneath so that the hip is semi-flexed and the knee, owing to the shortening reaction, is tonically extended; the other knee (e.g., left), which is hanging flaccid in the flexed posture owing to the weight of the leg below the knee, is gently but quickly extended by a passive movement raising the leg. This, especially if the hip be somewhat flexed, also induces the shortening reaction in the left knee extensor. There follows at the opposite (right) knee a subsidence of the tonic extension, so that the right leg below the knee drops down into flexion under its own weight. The latency of this crossed effect is relatively long. Accompanying the crossed effect, there is often a contraction of the quadriceps extensor of the limb in which the passive knee-extension was performed, so that extension of knee occurs in it together with some flexion at hip, just as if this leg were engaged in the forward phase of the step, while the opposite leg engaged in the backward phase. As to whether or no in this crossed flexion of knee a contraction of the flexors occurs, it is difficult to satisfy oneself; my impression is that it does. As to the relaxation of the crossed extensor there is not any doubt. But this crossed flexion of knee is not a regular accompaniment of the " shortening reaction "; sometimes no crossed reflex accompanies it, and sometimes I have seen it accompanied by a crossed extension of knee instead of crossed flexion. That is, a reflex of standing or galloping is produced instead of reflex trotting.

The " lengthening reaction " is, on the other hand, regularly accompanied by a crossed reflex at the opposite knee, the movement being always extension of the crossed knee. This crossed reflex accompanying the " lengthening reaction " appears to me to be undoubtedly a reflex already described by Philippson,[1] and designated by him " crossed reflex III." Speaking of his spinal dogs he writes, " Forced flexion of the leg upon the thigh provokes in the opposite limb extension of the leg and foot, the thigh remaining flexed." It may be remembered that stimulation, either mechanical or electric, of the central stump of the cut nerve of vastocrureus excites reflex contraction of the fellow-muscle of the opposite limb, as was pointed out by myself in a former paper.[2]

M. Philippson cites[3] Freusberg's name in connection with this crossed reflex, but I find in Freusberg's excellent papers[4] no explicit mention of it. I do not know any published reference to the reflex prior to that of M. Philippson. A good way of observing Philippson's reflex is, in my experience, the following: The animal, reclining on the lap of an assistant, is so placed that its back is turned from the observer, the hind-quarters resting but little lower than the fore-quarters. In this supine posture both hips are passively flexed under the weight of their limbs. One knee—e.g., left—is then supported so as to be somewhat extended; to let the knee rest on a finger placed under it affords it usually quite sufficient support. The " shortening reaction " then sets in in the extensor muscle of this knee (left). The knee of the opposite limb (right) now lies passively flexed, as also is the hip of that limb. The observer then, lightly holding with his free hand the left leg near the ankle, forces into flexion this tonically extended left knee. Extension of the right knee immediately results. The force required to flex the left knee is usually slight, but varies with the degree of tonic contraction of the left knee-extensor.

In my experience it is necessary for the occurrence of this crossed reflex that the forced flexion should be executed *against resistance from contraction of the knee-extensor*, though the amount of that resistance may be small. In other words, it seems essential for eliciting the crossed reflex that the forced stretch of the knee-extensor should be made when that muscle is exhibiting tonic contraction. Also in my experience it is favourable for the reaction that in the extensor muscles of the crossed knee (right) there should, at the time when the other knee (left) is flexed, be no active contraction.

[1] *Trav. d. Lab. de Physiologie, Instituts Solvay*, publiés par P. Heger, 1905, **7**, 2, 31, Bruxelles.
[2] *Proc. roy. Soc.*, 1906, **70**, 490.　　　　　　　　　　　[3] *Loc. cit.*
[4] *Pflüg. Arch. ges. Physiol.*, 1874, **9**, 358; 1875, **10**, 174; *Arch. expt. Path. Pharmak.*, 1875, **3**, 204.

Exhibited, therefore, by the extensor muscle of the knee are four re-actions, two ipsilateral and two crossed; and these are so coupled that the crossed *flexion* of knee when it occurs is a concomitant of the ipsilateral *shortening* reaction, and the ipsilateral *lengthening* reaction is regularly accompanied by crossed *extension* of knee.

Another reflex of the same kind remains to be mentioned. When the spinal dog is held up in the manner mentioned, stepping movements set in as noted by Goltz and Freusberg[1]—their " marking time " reflex. In these movements there occurs alternate flexion of the two legs, the hip and knee of one limb flexing as those of the fellow-limb extend. If, while these cyclic movements are in progress, the thigh of one side be gently supported in the flexed posture by a finger or pencil, etc., placed beneath it, the walking movement at once ceases in both limbs.[2] So long as the support is continued the cyclic reflex remains absent. When the support is with-drawn and the thigh drops, the hip of that side undergoes a passive extension. Even before this passive extension reaches its full, there sets in at the oppo-site hip a movement of flexion. Passive extension of one hip excites a crossed reflex of flexion of the opposite hip. The same reflex can also be excited by taking one leg below the knee and gently performing a forced extension of the hip of that limb; this causes a marked flexion of the opposite hip. But in my experience this latter method of producing the crossed hip-flexion is not so reliable. More often this forced extension of one hip excites rhythmic stepping of the opposite limb. I have seen it do so when, owing to spinal depression, the limbs, although pendent in the proper pose for exhibiting the reflex stepping, are hanging motionless. A slight passive extension of one hip will then excite stepping in the opposite limb; but this stepping in the opposite limb opens with flexion at hip. The stimulus occasioned by the extension of the hip is due, at least in part, to stretch of ilio-psoas and tensor fasciæ femoris muscles; the stimulus, in part at least, is a proprioceptive one. In the decerebrate animal passive extension of hip after severance of all the skin nerves of the limb and groin and lower part of abdominal wall, and after severance of all the muscular nerves except those of ilio-psoas and tensor fasciæ femoris, and after free resection of the glutei and all the muscles inserted into the trochanters and inter-trochanteric line, still causes reflex contraction of the vastocrureus of the opposite knee. A proprioceptive reflex therefore is originated by stretching these flexors of the hip, and has the effect of producing extension of the opposite knee. It might be expected from this that passive relaxation of the hip flexors would conversely produce a reflex flexion of the crossed knee, especially if with the flexion of hip an extension of the same side knee were induced. This can be tested by inducing the " shortening reaction " by lifting one thigh in the manner above described, and then, when the tonic extension of knee has set in, passively flexing the other hip and inducing in that limb the shortening reaction. The passive flexion of hip and active

---

[1] *Pflüg. Arch. ges. Physiol.*, 1874, **9**, 358. [2] Sherrington, *Proc. roy. Soc.*, 1906, **77B**, 479, Fig. 1.

extension of knee induced in the second limb is seen to be followed almost at once by a dropping of the other tonically extended knee into flexion. Obviously a reflex inhibition of the crossed vastocrureus has taken place. Sometimes this crossed inhibition of extensor of knee is excited by passive flexion of hip alone.

(d) Reflexes in Decapitated Mammal

From frequent experience of the above-described reactions I was led to suspect them to be proprioceptive. Skin nerves seemed inessential to them. They sometimes occurred when the area of skin handled or stretched had had its afferent nerves paralysed by cocaine or by actual severance.

A difficulty in the way of their analysis lies in the long time and considerable cost required in preparing the material. Traces of the reactions can, it is true, be met in the spinal mammal immediately after transection of the cord. I have found them best with the decapitated cat. From the cat, during some eight hours or more after decapitation, many spinal reflexes can be excellently obtained—e.g., flexion reflex of limb, crossed extension reflex, scratch reflex. Artificial respiration is of course employed and the animal prevented from cooling by supplying the air warm and heating the table on which the animal lies. The knee jerk is brisk and strong, and I have seen it remain so even twelve hours after the decapitation. There is, however, little tonus in the extensor muscles, except during the first half-hour or so following the decapitation. During that period there is commonly both in fore-limb and hind-limb some approach to the extensor rigidity which follows transection through midbrain and destruction of forebrain (decerebrate rigidity). In this first half-hour the lengthening reaction and the shortening reaction can be got from the quadriceps extensor cruris, gastrocnemius-soleus, triceps brachii, and supraspinatus, etc., although not to any great perfection. But the reactions wane quickly and the tonus decreases, until in a short time all practically disappear. The preparation does not, therefore, lend itself well to analysis of the reactions.

I turned, therefore, to the decerebrated in place of the decapitated cat, in belief that they might there be more accessible for analysis. The event showed that isolated preparation of the vastocrureus in the decerebrate cat offers good opportunity for their study, especially when made doubly—i.e., of both right and left vastocrurei in the same experiment.

PROPRIOCEPTIVE REFLEXES IN DECEREBRATE CAT

(a) Method

The suitable preparation in the decerebrate cat can be obtained as follows:

The animal being deeply narcotised with chloroform and ether, the cranium is exposed by partial eversion of one temporalis from its origin; a trephine hole is made and enlarged with the bone forceps. The animal is then placed supine, the skin reflected in a semicircular flap from the groin—*e.g.*, left—n. cutaneus femoris anterior externus[1] (external cutaneus) severed just above the inguinal fold, the m. ilio-psoas completely severed well above its insertion, and the n. saphenus and sartorius branches of the n. femoralis (anterior crural) severed at their origins from that nerve-trunk. In cutting through the ilio-psoas muscle the lumbo-sacral cord and the next following two roots of origin of the sciatic may be met with and severed. The pectineus muscle is then cut completely through, and at its edge, somewhat deep, the n. obturatorius is found emerging from the obturator foramen, and its divisions, both superficial and deep, are severed; n. lumbo-inguinalis (genito-crural) lying close by, alongside the external iliac artery, is also cut through. An incision is then made midway between great trochanter and tuber ischii, and through it the sciatic nerve (peroneal, popliteal, hamstring, and cutaneus branch of n. ischiadicus lying close together) is severed. Enlarging the incision upwards, the n. cutaneus femoris posterior (small sciatic), n. cutaneus clunium inferior and n. pudendus internus above and to the median side of the tuber ischii are found and cut through, as also is the little tenuissimus muscle. Gluteus maximus (both parts) and tensor fasciæ femoris are resected completely up from their insertions and the great trochanter thus exposed. Then all the muscles inserted into the trochanter are freely dissected from it and from the capsule of the hip-joint, and in doing this it does not matter if the joint cavity be opened and exposed. Quadratus femoris and gemelli are dissected off from the femur, in doing which it is helpful for the limb to be rotated somewhat inwards. A free incision near the mid-ventral line along the lateral face of the pubes frees the mechanical connection of the adductor group of muscles (left) from the adductor group of the opposite limb. Finally, a loop of thread is placed round each carotid artery in the neck and a cannula is inserted in the trachea. The animal is then placed in the prone position again, and while the threads on the carotids are drawn so as to temporarily occlude those arteries, a blunt knife is inserted through an opening in the dura mater and, with the edge of the bony tentorium as a guide, the midbrain is transected at its junction with the hindbrain or through the level of the posterior colliculi. The brain in front of this is broken up or removed through the opened cranial vault. This transaction does not usually endanger the respiratory movements; if it does temporarily do so, artificial respiration is employed through the tracheal cannula. The carotid arteries can usually be freed without danger of hæmorrhage in less than five minutes after the decerebration. After decerebration has been performed the chloroform and ether narcosis can be relaxed. Decerebrate rigidity then develops.[2]

[1] In mentioning the nerves, the names here used are those employed by Ellenberger and Baum in the *Anatomie d. Hundes*: the nomenclature of the muscles is that given by Mivart in the cat, and by Jayne in his *Mammalian Anatomy*. The names introduced in parenthesis are those of the structures in human anatomy with which the parts appear to correspond.

[2] The description given is that of the standard method of decerebration (often called the " trephine " method to distinguish it from the " guillotine " method) used for investigation in the cat, dog, and monkey. In the Oxford laboratory the procedure was amended a little as follows: Under anæsthesia the preparation of the muscles was made, laminectomy performed if nerve-roots were to be examined, the trachea intubated, both carotids then *tied*, then the incision made in the scalp, the temporal muscle reflected, the trephine opening made and enlarged, the dura incised widely. At this point the anæsthesia was deepened and the assistant grasped the neck behind the atlas firmly to occlude the vertebral arteries temporarily. With a blunt spatula the operator pulled the occipital lobe forward exposing the tentorium and the colliculi, and made the section at the desired level. The remainder of the brain was rapidly scooped out and wool applied to the level of section. The vertebral arteries were then released. Artificial respiration was usually unnecessary owing to the rapidity of the procedure. Anæsthesia is abolished immediately the section is made.

For student work in the mammalian physiology class the " guillotine " method was used on account of the rapidity of its performance. It also has advantages for the observation of pharyngeal reflexes, for which it was first devised. Detailed description of this method will be found in the paper by Miller and Sherrington, *Quart. J. exp. Physiol.*, 1915, **9**, 147; Sherrington, *J. Physiol.*, 1915, **49**, *Proc. Physiol. Soc.*, **52**; and in Liddell and Sherrington, *Mammalian Physiology*, 2nd ed., 1929.

The level of section of the brain stem commonly used was that termed " intercollicular," and

Before examining the reflex, I reflect the denervated skin from the thigh and expose the sartorius, and then take off the whole of that muscle, itself already denervated, right up to its origin, either leaving it reflected or removing it altogether. This allows the rectus femoris portion of quadriceps extensor cruris to be completely seen. The whole pelvic attachment of the rectus femoris is then carefully and fully resected, and a free transverse incision across it below where it merges in the rest of the quadriceps is found not to impair the reactions from this latter, while still further ensuring the exclusion of the rectus femoris itself. In this way a preparation is obtained in which the sole muscle and nerve in the whole limb remaining connected with the spinal cord is the m. vastocrureus and its nerve branch from m. femoralis (anterior crural). Vastocrureus is a single joint muscle. Its blood-supply and mechanical attachments, except for that small part of its upper end which unites with rectus femoris, remain untouched. If care be taken to preserve its exposed surface from cooling and drying, it yields the reactions to be described for several hours after the decerebration. The tonic rigidity characteristic of decerebrate rigidity is not interfered with by any part of the above procedure except that the operation limits the rigidity of course entirely to vastocrureus muscle, and thus in effect wholly to the knee.

The preparation thus obtained is a unilateral one, in the sense that the vastocrureus of one limb only is isolated. For many observations it is preferable to have the vasto-crureus isolated in both limbs. I therefore usually make the preparation a double one by carrying out the above-described procedure on both limbs instead of on one only.

The ipsilateral reactions can be observed as soon as decerebrate rigidity sets in. For the crossed reactions it is better, in my experience, to allow an hour or so to elapse after the decerebration and the ending of the deep narcosis.

(b) *Plasticity of the Extensor Muscle in Decerebrate Rigidity*

In a first paper[1] on decerebrate rigidity attention was drawn to a peculiar plasticity of the musculature as characteristic of that condition. In decerebrate rigidity a limb passively moved from one posture to another retains the new posture thus given it. In this respect the decerebrate condition offers some resemblance to a cataleptic state. After describing instances of this behaviour, I related it to the long-drawn form possessed by reflex movements evoked after decerebration, a sluggishness not of commencement but of subsidence—that is, of subsidence unless effected by inhibition. To this plasticity I recall attention here, for in it seem comprised the phenomena which now concern us.

Forced flexion of knee in the decerebrate vastocrureus preparation provokes in the muscle a marked lasting change. Starting with the knee

---

passed obliquely forwards from between the anterior and posterior corpora quadrigemina to emerge two to three millimetres forward of the emergence of the third nerves from the midbrain. This level of section gave the optimum rigidity. For some purposes a " precollicular " section was made (Liddell and Sherrington, *Proc. roy. Soc.*, 1925, **97B**, 267) then passing from above the anterior colliculus to emerge in the region of the corpora mammilaria or infundibulum (" midbrain animal " of Magnus). With the trephine method the level of section could be chosen as desired, and for some purposes the basal ganglia were left attached to the brain stem to make a " thalamic preparation."

No detailed study of the histology of the structures involved by these sections was published except that of Bazett and Penfield, *Brain*, 1922, **44**, 185. This subject has, however, been exhaustively studied since that time in other laboratories (Magnus, Rademaker, Lorente de Nó).—Ed.

[1] *Proc. roy. Soc.*, 1896-7, **60**, 411.

in a posture of extension, due to its extensor's rigidity, the observer forces it into flexion. On cessation of the flexing force the knee is found to remain approximately in the new posture. If the degree of flexion to which it has been subjected be but partial, the knee remains flexed partially. If then forced to fuller flexion, it remains flexed more fully (Fig. 53, *l*). Conversely, if from one of these flexed postures the observer moves it back to an extended one, the knee is found on its release to remain extended; it remains extended not quite to the full to which the manipulator moved it, but yet extended far more than it had been in the flexed posture it was moved from. The decerebrate vastocrureus therefore exhibits under forced movements of the knee two converse reactions. When subjected to a stretch it remains, after the application of the stretching force has ceased,

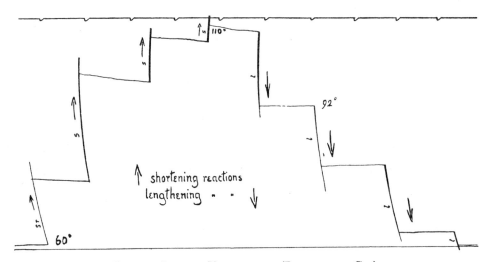

FIG. 53.—ISOLATED VASTOCRUREUS (DECEREBRATE CAT)

s, s, s, s, " shortening reactions "; *l, l, l, l*, " lengthening reactions "; 60° and 110° mark the angle of the knee in the respective postures. Time marker 1 second intervals

at a new and increased tonic length. This reaction appears to be the same as that which in the spinal dog was referred to above the as " lengthening reaction."

Conversely, when the points of origin and insertion of the muscle are passively approximated, the decerebrate muscle remains, subsequent to the execution of the passive movement, at a new and shortened tonic length (Fig. 53, *s*). This reaction is that which in the spinal dog was called above the " shortening reaction." The two reactions together confer on the preparation a tonic plasticity which is characteristic.

This property is exhibited under decerebrate rigidity not by vasto-crureus only, but by many other muscles; thus, gastrocnemius and soleus, and supraspinatus at shoulder, and triceps at elbow. It is noteworthy that all these are extensor muscles.

There is, however, a difference between the "lengthening" and "shortening" reactions as observable in the decerebrate and in the spinal animal respectively. In the latter it is less easy to grade the extent of these reactions. For instance, although it is easy, by a forced stretch of the knee extensor, to change the posture of the knee from one of tonic extension to one of flexion, it cannot so easily in spinal animals be made to retain intermediate postures.

The "lengthening reaction" of vastocrureus can be elicited in the decerebrate preparation by simply faradising the distal end of the cut nerve of the flexors of the knee. The contraction of the flexor then overpowers the tonic contraction of vastocrureus, stretching the latter and bringing the knee into flexion. On discontinuing the faradisation, the flexors of course cease to contract, but if the animal be supine, so as to allow gravity to reveal the condition of the knee, the flexed knee still remains flexed; the forced stretch of vastocrureus due to the contraction of the flexor has caused the former to assume a new and increased tonic length.

Conversely, on approximating the ends of the muscle by active contraction of the muscle itself, there ensues the "shortening reaction," just as after passive approximation by manipulation. This can be seen when the isolated vastocrureus is thrown into contraction reflexly. Suppose the animal supine and the nerve stimulated to be the central stump of the cut peroneal nerve of the crossed side, the stimulation exciting the reflex may be with advantage brief, such as weak faradisation for one second, or the quick tightening of a ligature. The extension of knee caused by this stimulus does not pass away forthwith; the knee remains extended, and continues so even for several minutes. The reflex bears the appearance of one on which has supervened and to which has affixed itself a "shortening reaction." This suggestion is strengthened by the observation that if, during the application of the exciting stimulus and for a second or so longer, the muscle, although contracting, be mechanically prevented from shortening, on then releasing the limb the reflex is found to have already subsided, while if left to its natural course its reflex contraction would have lasted far longer. The mechanical restraint from shortening has cut out the tonic after-action of the reflex.

Likewise, by flexing the knee during the after-continuance of the extension reflex, the limb is found on release not to return to extension. The passive stretch of the muscle has suppressed the remainder of the reflex. In other words, a "lengthening reaction" has been produced, so that in this respect also the condition of shortened length which in the decerebrate animal characteristically prolongs the reflex contraction of the extensor, and long outlasts the duration of the external stimulus, resembles the tonus of decerebrate rigidity; in both conditions a passive stretch of the muscle permanently removes the shortened state. In other words, in both conditions the "lengthening reaction" can be produced.

(c) *Philippson's Reflex and Crossed Reflexes of Knee in Decerebrate Cat*

In the vastocrureus preparation of the decerebrate cat I find Philippson's reflex usually obtainable with ease. Suppose the vastocrureus preparation to be of the left limb. With the animal either supine or lying on its (right) side, the knee end of the other (left) thigh is lightly supported from the sides or behind, so as to avoid touching the vastocrureus or its attachments. A movement of flexion is gently imposed on the knee by pressing back the leg at the ankle; the knee of the opposite limb is then seen to extend by reflex action. This reflex extension of the right knee is not accompanied— at least not usually—by noticeable extension at the right hip; it seems, however, usually accompanied by some extension at the right ankle. This reflex is doubtless the same as that excitable by stimulation of the central end of the cut vastocrureus nerve itself.[1]

The forced flexion of the knee excites this crossed reflex more surely and more markedly when executed rather quickly. The experiments of Goldscheider[2] upon sensations evoked by the passive movements of joints have shown that the speed of the movement of the joint influences greatly the elicitation of sensation, a quicker movement being more effective than a slow one. In the case of the reflex provoked by flexing the knee in the vastocrureus preparation the question rises—Is the reflex excited from the joint (knee-joint) or from the muscle (vastocrureus) ? The nerve of vasto- crureus is generally credited with supplying some nerve-fibres to the knee- joint.

To examine the possibility of an articular origination of the reflex I proceeded as follows : The lateral extensions of the lower attachment of the vastocrureus were cut away throughout their length down to the tibial insertion. The sides of the muscle thus freed, it was next separated along its deep surface from the whole of the lowest fourth of the femur. The knife was then carried down between the deep surface of the tendon and the whole of the joint, severing entirely all its attachments to the joint, and stopping only at the tibial tubercle. Finally, the patella, which remained with the thus freed tendon, had the whole of its deep (articular) face removed with a strong knife, and the cartilaginous face of the lower end of femur pared in the same way. When this had been done the muscle still retained its decerebrate rigidity; and flexing the knee still as before evoked the crossed reflex of extension of the opposite knee. The same was true when in the vastocrureus preparation the knee-joint cavity was injected with cocaine (0·5 per cent. solution); the extensor rigidity, the " lengthening reaction," the " shortening reaction," and the crossed reflex still persisted.

It appears, therefore, that these reactions, in so far as they are reflex, are initiated by excitation of receptive organs belonging to the vastocrureus muscle itself, apart from any belonging to the joint. After this elimination of the knee-joint, the crossed reflex and the extensor rigidity are not perhaps so marked as they were before, but the process of elimination is severe, and can hardly be carried out without inflicting some damage on the muscle itself. The observations, therefore, while they allow the supposition that

---

[1] Sherrington, *Proc. roy. Soc.*, 1906, **77B**, 490.   [2] *Arch. Anat. Physiol. Lpz.*, 1889, 369.

the crossed reflex may, when the nerves of the joint are intact, be excited partly through articular receptors, show that the chief and essential seat of initiation of the reflex lies, not in the joint, but in the vastocrureus muscle.[1]

Sometimes a slight degree of flexion will excite the reflex, but often it is necessary that the flexion be considerable.   In the latter case a source of fallacy has to be guarded against.   When the knee flexion is carried to extreme degree the heel may touch the skin of the ischial region.   From the skin of that region, if n. cutaneus femoris posterior and n. pudendus internus of the (left) limb have not been severed, a crossed reflex extending the opposite (*i.e.*, right) knee and ankle can be easily excited, sometimes even by a light touch.

When the crossed extension does not set in until the forced flexion has carried the ipsilateral knee into a fairly fully flexed posture, crossed extension *follows* the ipsilateral flexion rather than *accompanies* it.   I do not, however, regard this as the natural time-relation; it seems more likely that this tardiness of response is due merely to the severity of the conditions under which the observations are made—*e.g.*, recent decerebration and heavy narcosis.

As in the spinal dog, so also in the decerebrate cat the contraction of the crossed vastocrureus excited by forced stretch of the other vastocrureus occurs only when the stretching of the latter is carried out against resistance offered by tonic contraction of the muscle.   If there be no tonic resistance, there is, in my experience, no reflex.   Further, a favourable condition for the appearance of this crossed reflex seems to be an attitude of flexion at the crossed (*i.e.*, right) knee at the time of the forced bending of the other (*i.e.*, left) knee.   Reflex flexion of the right knee just preceding the forced flexion of the left is also favourable to the appearance of the crossed reflex of extension.   The muscle which the crossed reflex employs in extending the crossed knee is the vastocrureus of that side; this is well seen with the double preparation, the only muscles then remaining innervated in the two limbs being the vastocrurei right and left.   The reflex arc therefore begins in receptor neurones of one vastocrureus and ends in effector neurones of the fellow vastocrureus of the opposite limb.

In the spinal animal the crossed extension of knee is not usually so long maintained—that is, it does not assume the character of a lasting posture of extension.   In the decerebrate animal it is usually maintained, so as to amount to the assumption of a tonic posture of extension.

I have looked to see whether stretching the gastrocnemius and soleus will similarly provoke a crossed reflex at the opposite knee.

For this observation the above-mentioned preparation is modified.   The vastocrureus nerve, instead of remaining intact, is severed, and the nerves of gastrocnemius and soleus, instead of being severed, are untouched, all other branches of the popliteal nerve being cut through.   To leave the gastrocnemius-soleus nerves while cutting the others is not

---

[1] I am including here, under the term muscle, not only the fleshy part, but also the aponeurotic and tendinous parts.

difficult, since the nerves to the two muscles are the uppermost branches given from the popliteal trunk. With a preparation modified in this way, the decerebrate rigidity appears in the gastrocnemius-soleus and not in vastocrureus. The muscle can be easily stretched by flexing the ankle, or by amputating the heel and pulling directly on the tendo Achillis.

I obtain a crossed reflex at the opposite knee much less easily by stretching gastrocnemius-soleus than by stretching vastocrureus; it is, however, obtainable, and its effect on the crossed knee appears in the form of contraction of the vastocrureus. In this case the joints both of knee and ankle are altogether excluded from contribution to the effect, because the nerves of gastrocnemius-soleus give no articular branches whatever, and all other nerves of the limb were severed.

These observations furnish evidence that the stretching of an extensor muscle by flexing a joint over which the muscle or its tendon passes can excite a reflex after the joint itself has been desensitised; the reflex is therefore excited through the afferent apparatus of the muscle. The excitation is sufficiently easy and the mode of stimulation sufficiently natural to warrant the inference that this stretching forms an " *adequate* " stimulus for receptor endings in the muscle. We have therefore *in this crossed reflex a proprioceptive reflex excited by its adequate stimulus.*

The other crossed reflex—namely, the flexion of the opposite knee, which in the spinal animal frequently accompanies the " shortening reaction "— is met also under decerebrate rigidity. In my experience, however, with the double isolated vastocrureus preparation, it occurs far more rarely than does the converse crossed reflex just described. Its latency is also longer. The " shortening reaction " is occasionally accompanied by a crossed reflex of extension of opposite knee—in this latter case bilateral extension of the knee is the result. This variant on the more usual asymmetrical reflex falls into line with the similar variant that not unfrequently replaces the more usual asymmetrical bilateral reflex of hind-limbs in response to excitation of a fore-limb, or conversely of the fore-limbs in response to excitation of a hind-limb. It may be related to reflex standing instead of reflex stepping—that is, its appearance may indicate the substitution of reflex stepping by reflex standing or reflex galloping.

The De-afferented Knee-extensor in Regard to Proprioceptive Reactions

If the " shortening " and " lengthening " reactions are reflex, they must, since they are obtainable from the isolated vastocrureus preparation, originate from stimulation of receptive nerves which lie within the muscle itself. If reflex, these reactions should therefore disappear on severance of the afferent fibres of vastocrureus nerve. In that nerve-trunk itself the afferent fibres are inextricably commingled with motor. But the two sets of fibres separate in passing through the spinal roots. The spinal roots through which in the cat these afferent fibres pass[1] are in the prefixed form of plexus the 4th and 5th lumbar, in the postfixed the 5th and 6th lumbar; in some intermediate forms they go through the 4th, 5th, and 6th lumbar.

(a) Method

In a series of experiments the afferent roots of the 4th, 5th, and 6th lumbar nerves of one side were cut, under full asepsis and deep narcosis. Then, after an interval varying from two hours to 140 days subsequent to the root-severance, the isolated vastocrureus preparation in the decerebrate animal was made in both limbs. The reactions of the de-afferented preparation and of the other, which may here be briefly termed the " normal," preparation were then compared.

In one experiment in the series two afferent roots only—namely, 4th and 5th—were severed. This was done because it had been noted by palpation that the animal seemed to possess twelve ribs only instead of the usual thirteen. It was inferred, therefore, that the plexus would be fully prefixed. Post-mortem, it was found that there existed in fact thirteen ribs, but the thirteenth was very small; the plexus proved to be, as had been suspected, fully prefixed. The n. femoralis received fibres from the 4th and 5th lumbar roots only. The results obtained from this experiment agreed completely, in regard to vastocrureus, with those obtained from the rest of the series.

In all the experiments certain marked differences appeared between the reactions of the " normal " and of the de-afferented preparation.

(b) Difference between Reactions of De-afferented and " Normal " Vastocrureus Preparations in the Decerebrate Animal

1. The de-afferented preparation exhibited no trace of decerebrate rigidity; the " normal " preparation always did. Severance of the afferent spinal roots, confined entirely to those particular roots through which pass the afferent fibres of the vastocrureus nerve itself, suffices to prevent the occurrence of any trace of decerebrate rigidity in vastocrureus muscle, and this holds whether the roots have been severed two hours previously or 140 days previously. This, with the converse fact that decerebrate rigidity occurs with completeness after severance of every other nerve in both limbs excepting only the vastocrureus nerve itself, shows that the afferent nerve of the vastocrureus itself is the afferent, and the only afferent, in both limbs, which is essential for this reflex tonus of that muscle, and that it by itself suffices completely as afferent channel for this reflex tonus. This reflex tonus depends, therefore, on an afferent nerve of the proprioceptive class, and the particular proprioceptive nerve necessary is the afferent nerve of the muscle which itself exhibits the tonus. This reflex tonus is therefore autogenic; the one reflex arc essential for it is the muscle's own reflex arc, meaning by that the arc which, besides ending wholly in this self-same muscle, also arises wholly in it.

[1] Sherrington, J. Physiol., 1892, **13**, 621.

2. The " normal " preparation exhibited the " knee jerk " always, and always in exaggerated form, as is usual in the decerebrate condition. The de-afferented muscle never exhibited any trace of " knee jerk." Opportunity was taken to try to produce in the de-afferented preparation a " knee jerk " by throwing its muscle into reflex contraction of various grade through stimulation of various extrinsic afferent nerves. By extrinsic afferent nerves are meant nerves arising elsewhere than in that vasto-crureus muscle itself under observation. The vastocrureus, when reflexly contracting either weakly or strongly under stimulation of various extraneous afferent nerves, never exhibited any trace whatever of knee jerk. Nor was a knee jerk elicitable from it when afferent arcs were stimulated with induced currents just subliminal for evoking actual reflex contraction. Similarly, when the de-afferented muscle was contracting under strychnine I failed to elicit a knee jerk from it.

3. *The " Shortening Reaction."*—The normal preparation always yielded the " shortening reaction "; the de-afferented preparation never yielded any trace of the reaction. It did so neither when at rest—*i.e.*, not reflexly contracting—nor when rested during various grades of reflex contraction under excitation of extrinsic afferent nerves.

4. *The " Lengthening Reaction."*—The normal side in every experiment yielded this reaction. On the de-afferented side there was no tonic rigidity to serve as basis on which to try the reaction. But since the de-afferented muscle readily contracts reflexly on stimulation of appropriate afferent nerves—*e.g.*, of the crossed hind-limb—it was attempted to obtain the " lengthening reaction " from the de-afferented preparation when its muscle was moderately contracting reflexly under excitation of an extraneous afferent nerve. This the normal preparation will do. It yields the " lengthening reaction " not only when in tonus, but also when in moderate reflex contraction under actual stimulation of an extrinsic afferent nerve. On trying the de-afferented muscle I inclined at first to think that it did sometimes[1] under this condition exhibit the lengthening reaction, though in incomplete form. Further examination of this semblance of the reaction brought forward, however, a different explanation of the result. The reflex contraction of the de-afferented muscle is apt, especially under weak stimulation of the afferent nerve exciting the reflex, to wane quickly and almost abruptly. When passively stretched during the reflex contraction, the muscle on being released from the forced stretch springs back to its shorter (reflexly contracted) length; but if the reflex contraction has already waned during the short time which the passive stretch occupied, the return of the muscle is not to its previous height of contraction, but merely to that grade of contraction to which the reflex has declined during the interval. In this

---

[1] Figured in the original paper. The degree of lasting impairment of the contraction is slight, and the reassumption of this new level takes two seconds. This degree of impairment is now recognised as an effect which can be produced when the muscle of a simple nerve-muscle preparation is forcibly stretched during a tetanic stimulation (*cf.* Gasser and Hill, *Proc. roy. Soc.*, 1924, **96B**, 398). It is therefore not reflex.—ED.

way semblances of incomplete lengthening reaction are sometimes produced. The ordinary result of trying to obtain a lengthening reaction in the de-afferented preparation is entire failure to produce it. Fig. 54 shows a moderately weak reflex contraction of the de-afferented muscle produced by stimulation of the central stump of the contralateral popliteal nerve. During this reflex three forced stretches of the muscle made in fairly rapid succession failed, as the graphic record shows, to evoke any trace of "length-

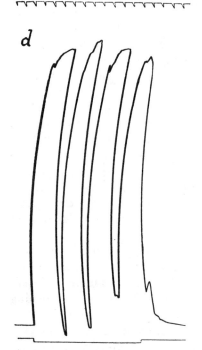

ening reaction," and this is the usual result.

5. Since, therefore, the de-afferented preparation exhibits neither "shortening reaction" nor "lengthening reaction," it shows none of that *plasticity* which characterises the tonic condition of the extensor muscles both in decerebrate rigidity and to a lesser degree in the spinal condition after subsidence of spinal shock.

6. The various afferent nerves which reflexly influence the vastocrureus preparation may, for clearness of description, be separated into *intrinsic* and *extrinsic*. By the intrinsic afferent is understood the afferent of the muscle itself; the extrinsic afferents comprise all other afferent nerves which influence the muscles, whether from skin or from deep structures such as muscles other than vastocrureus itself, including among the extrinsic nerves that of the fellow vasto-

Fig. 54.—Isolated Vastocrureus (Cat)

De-afferented; three forced stretches of the muscle while it is contracting under faradisation of the opposite peroneal nerve: the stretches fail to produce any trace of "lengthening reaction"

crureus of the other thigh. Among the extrinsic afferent nerves which I have used for exciting the vastocrureus reflexly in the isolated decerebrate preparation have been (contralateral) internal saphenous, which is purely cutaneous, the (contralateral) vastocrureus nerve, which is purely proprioceptive, and (contralateral) peroneal and popliteal, which are mixed. Their normal effect on the vastocrureus preparation is to cause reflex contraction, and this they continue to do when the muscle has been reduced to the de-afferented state.

The instance of the crossed vastocrureus nerve may be taken first. Faradisation of the central stump of this nerve excites reflex contraction of the fellow muscle of the opposite limb. But the afferents of this nerve can, as shown above (Philippson's reflex), be stimulated by passively bending the knee (*e.g.*, right) when that joint is in a tonically extended posture under decerebrate rigidity. The reflex contraction thus excited in the (left) vastocrureus when that muscle has its own afferents intact is not usually of great amplitude, but is of considerable duration; the contraction rises deliberately to a maximum, which is maintained for some seconds and then slowly declines, so that the extended posture the knee attained persists with little diminution for a minute or more. But in the de-afferented preparation the course of the reflex contraction runs otherwise. It is often of very ample excursion, rushes to its maximum, and then as quickly or almost as quickly subsides, presenting hardly a trace of the prolonged

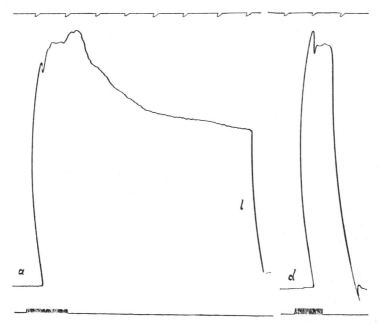

FIG. 55.—ISOLATED VASTOCRUREUS (CAT)

Crossed extension reflex excited by faradisation of the opposite popliteal nerve *a* expressed by the muscle with normal afferent nerve-fibres, *d* by the muscle with its afferent nerve-fibres destroyed 100 days previously: at *l* a lengthening reaction was induced to cut short reflex *a*

maintenance and slow decline characteristic of it in the decerebrate muscle still possessing afferents.

This difference between the reflex reaction of the normal and the de-afferented extensor muscle comes out even more strikingly where the stimulus used for the afferent nerve—*e.g.*, contralateral popliteal—is electric (Fig. 55). The cessation of the stimulus is then doubtless more abrupt than in the previous instance, and with the cessation of the stimulus there ceases at once the reflex contraction of the de-afferented vastocrureus (Fig. 55, *d*); in the " normal " preparation the reflex contraction continues long after the actual external stimulus is at an end; finally, I cut it short by inducing a lengthening reaction (Fig. 55 at *l*). So sharp and abrupt is the disappearance of the contraction in the de-afferented muscle that the extended leg, on falling back to the flexed posture, gives at the end of its fall a vibratory shake (Fig. 55, *d*), its slackening is so sudden and complete. There is a tendency, too, for the onset of the reflex contraction to be more abrupt in the de-afferented than in the normal muscle (Fig. 55), and for the movement of extension to be of ampler excursion, as though its momentum were less controlled than on the " normal " side.

These differences are well illustrated when the reflex stimulus consists of relatively slowly repeated single stimuli. I have shown elsewhere that the flexion reflex of the limb can be easily excited by a single induction shock of even weak intensity.[1] I find the same holds true for the crossed reflex of extension. In the decerebrate animal a series of weak break shocks applied to the central stump of the severed popliteal nerve at the rate of 2·5 per second excites a reflex contraction of the crossed vastocrureus of sustained character. A similar series of break shocks similarly applied excites in the de-afferented vastocrureus a reflex contraction far more clonic in character. Similar differences are observable when, instead of electric stimuli to naked nerve-trunk, there are employed mechanical stimuli to the skin—*e.g.*, touches on the ischial or the perineal region. A touch on that region normally excites a bilateral reflex extending both knees. The reflex contraction in the bilateral isolated vastocrureus preparation is in the " normal " vastocrureus long maintained; in the de-afferented fellow muscle, though perhaps more ample in excursion, it subsides almost at once; it is a mere flash, instead of a maintained effect. One outcome of this is that a series of touches produces on the " normal " side a tonic summed effect (Fig. 56, *a*), but on the de-afferented side a coarsely clonic effect (Fig. 56, *d*). The same result is seen with electric stimuli (break induction shocks), even as slowly repeated as in Fig. 57—*i.e.*, fourteen per 10 seconds. The contraction of the de-afferented muscle is more ample, less steady, and subsides abruptly on cessation of the stimulus, instead of persisting further for a time.

The prolongation of reflex contraction which occurs on the " normal " side cannot be obtained on the de-afferented by any increase of mere intensity of stimulation. It is absent alike when the stimuli and resulting contractions are strong and when they are weak.

An obvious inference from these comparisons is that when, under decerebrate rigidity, the " normal " extensor muscle—*i.e.*, with its intrinsic afferents intact—is thrown into reflex contraction by stimulation of other afferent nerves than its own extrinsic afferents, the contraction thus excited in it induces a " shortening reaction," and that the maintenance of the contraction after the application of extrinsic stimulus has ceased is referable to the " shortening reaction " for which the intrinsic afferents of the muscle itself are responsible. In other words, *in the muscle with its afferent nerve*

---

[1] *Proc. roy. Soc.*, 1905, **76**, 160.

intact a proprioceptive autogenous reflex adds itself to reflexes caused by extrinsic afferents. In the de-afferented muscle the proprioceptive autogenous reflex is impossible, because the intrinsic afferents have been severed; hence the want of maintenance of the reflex effect, and the want of fusion of the reflex effects of serial stimuli repeated at slow intervals (Figs. 56, 57).

The autogenous proprioceptive reaction (" shortening reaction ") seems to graft itself upon a reflex contraction more perfectly than upon a shortening produced passively, and to be itself more perfect when elicited by active contraction than by mere passive extension of the knee under ex-

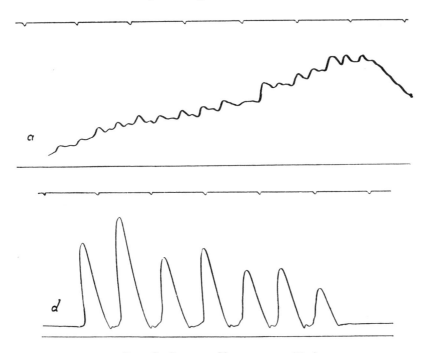

FIG. 56.—ISOLATED VASTOCRUREUS (CAT)

Perineal reflex excited by a series of touches on the skin, *a* expressed by the " normal " muscle, *d* by the de-afferented muscle. Time tracing in Figs. 54-59 in seconds

ternal mechanical manipulation. Fig. 55 shows crossed reflexes obtained by faradisation of the central end of the popliteal nerve; *d* is the reflex responses of the de-afferented muscle, *a* of the normal muscle. These show how completely the contraction initiated by the extrinsic afferent (contralateral popliteal) is supplemented and maintained by the autogenic proprioceptive reaction. Often no feature in the curve betrays the actual point of union of the two; the reinforcement is effected smoothly and without hitch.[1]

In these reflex contractions of de-afferented vastocrureus the myograph

_____
[1] Illustrated in the original paper.

lever falls so immediately on cessation of the exciting stimulus that there
seems practically no after-discharge from the excited arc.   My observations
include experiments in which the interval between severance of the afferent
roots of vastocrureus nerve and final examination after decerebration was
at shortest two hours, and at longest 140 days.   Fig. 55 instances 100 days.
All these experiments agree in yielding from the de-afferented muscle reflex
contractions whose duration of contraction practically does not outlive
the actual duration of the external stimulus.   In some, however, of the
experiments of shorter interval—*e.g.*, two hours, eighteen hours, three days,

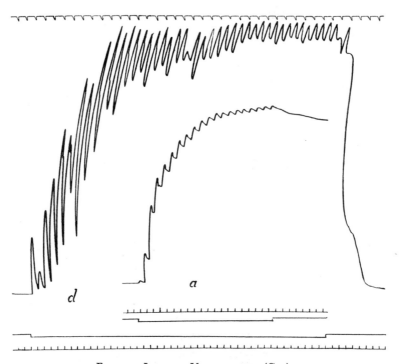

FIG. 57.—ISOLATED VASTOCRUREUS (CAT)

Crossed extension reflex excited by break shocks (lowest signal) at slow repetition delivered to
     popliteal nerve (of opposite limb) during period marked by lowest signal but one.   *a* the reflex
     in the muscle with afferents normal, *d* in the de-afferented muscle

five days, and twenty-six days—the reflex contractions of the de-afferented
preparation, although not showing any maintained after-effect nearly
approaching that of the " normal " side, and although exhibiting not only
premature but abrupt subsidence unlike that of the normal side, do yet
outlive the withdrawal of the exciting stimulus for a period which, while
brief—*e.g.*, five seconds—is nevertheless clearly longer than in observations
in the general run of the experiments.   That is to say, from the preparations de-afferented for a shorter period, a distinct though quite brief after-
discharge does present itself in some of the reflexes.   The duration of this

brief after-discharge is less brief with more intense stimulation than with weaker—in other words, more intense reflexes have more after-discharge than have less intense. This after-discharge, in my experience, rapidly wears off under a few quickly following repetitions of the reflex, and may recur again with the first fresh reflex after a long pause. In the reflex contractions yielded by the vastocrurcus preparations that have been de-afferented for longer periods, even this brief after-continuance of the contraction beyond the actual application of the external stimulus has very rarely, in my experience, occurred.

The course run by the reflex contractions of the de-afferented preparation seems to provide data for analysis of the after-action seen in the reflexes of the fellow extensor muscle still possessed of its afferent nerve. The after-action of this latter would seem to be built up of two factors: (*a*) an " after-discharge " greater with stronger stimuli than with weaker, and referable directly to the externally stimulated extrinsic reflex arc; and (*b*) a " shortening reaction " grafted on the extrinsic reaction, and indirectly occasioned by it, but directly due to the extensor muscle's own intrinsic proprioceptive arc. This double source of the after-action explains naturally an observation mentioned above—namely, that if during the application of an exciting reflex stimulus, and for a second or so longer, the muscle, although contracting, be mechanically prevented from shortening, on then releasing the limb the reflex is found to have already subsided, whereas if left to its natural unimpeded course the extension of the knee by the reflex would have endured for much longer. The mechanical restraint from shortening has cut out the tonic after-action of the reflex— *i.e.*, has suppressed the " shortening reaction " which would have grafted itself upon the extrinsic reflex.

7. As to the threshold value of stimulus for reflex contraction in the de-afferented as compared with the " normal " preparation, it has sometimes, so far as I could judge, been the same for both. Sometimes, however, it has seemed distinctly different on the two sides, but the difference has not always been in the same direction. On the other hand, my experience has been repeatedly that the de-afferented extensor replies more easily than does the normal to forced flexion of the crossed knee (Philippson's reflex). The reflex excitability of the de-afferented muscle does often appear to be abnormally great.

8. The de-afferented muscle is certainly capable of giving graded responses conformably with grading in intensity of the external stimulus applied to the extrinsic afferent source. How far this grading compares in fineness[1] with that of the " normal " preparation, the observations have not as yet determined.

9. The reflex contractions of the de-afferented muscle can certainly be readily inhibited by stimulation of appropriate extrinsic afferent nerves which normally cause reflex inhibition of the reflex contractions of the

[1] Sherrington, *Quart. J. exp. Physiol.*, 1908, **1**, 67.

muscle. But I have not yet made any careful comparison in this respect between the de-afferented and the normal sides.

10. It was pointed out in a previous paper that reflex inhibition of the vastocrureus and other extensor muscles in decerebrate rigidity is followed regularly, under certain circumstances, on withdrawal of the inhibitory stimulus, by a rebound contraction (successive spinal induction).[1] Examining the de-afferented preparation for this effect, I have found it present, and in one experiment in fairly marked degree; but the rebound contractions, even though moderately ample in height, have not been of prolonged duration, as they often are in extensor preparations with the intrinsic afferents intact.

11. *Fatigue.*—The reflex contractions of the de-afferented preparation appear to tire more quickly than do those of the preparation whose muscle still possesses its afferent nerve. This waning of reflex contraction occurs earlier with reflexes excited by weak stimuli than in those excited by strong stimuli, just as was noted with the scratch reflex in the spinal dog.[2] This premature fatigue is one of the difficulties met with in looking for the " lengthening reaction " in de-afferented preparations. The waning of the reflex of the de-afferented preparation is apt, after it has set in, to progress rapidly, and abruptly to complete disappearance of the reflex contraction. Under strong reflex stimuli the reflex contraction of the de-afferented muscle, the muscle being lightly loaded, may maintain its full amplitude for a minute or a minute and a half; then, in my experience, it begins to fail, and its failure tends rapidly—*i.e.*, in a few seconds—to become complete, just as with weak stimuli. Polarisation at the seat of stimulation in the afferent nerve has to be remembered in such an experiment, and I am not prepared to discount such a complication in the observations made. The observation is mentioned here merely to contrast with it the results observable under similar circumstances in the fellow preparation, in which the afferent nerve of the muscle has remained intact. In this " normal " preparation, instead of the contraction disappearing after a minute or a minute and a half, it can be maintained for five or ten minutes with very little decline of amplitude. Moreover, in this latter case the decline, when it comes, is very gradual, without any of that abruptness of subsidence shown by the de-afferented preparation.

12. The contraction of the contralateral vastocrureus which occurs when the tonic vastocrureus of one limb is stretched, also the relaxation of the contralateral vastocrureus which ensues when the vastocrureus of one limb is relaxed by extending the knee of that limb, are not obtainable when the latter muscle has been de-afferented.

---

[1] *Proc. roy. Soc.*, 1905, **76**, 160; 1906, **77**, 478; 1908, **80**, 55; *Quart, J. exp. Physiol.*, 1908, **1**, 67.
[2] *J. Physiol.*, 1906, **34**, 42, and *Integrative Action*, 1906, p. 219.

REFLEX NATURE OF THE PROPRIOCEPTIVE "REACTIONS"

(a) *Relation of these "Reactions" to the Reflex Arc of the Muscle*

From the foregoing it is clear that both "lengthening reaction" and "shortening reaction" of vastocrureus are indissolubly connected with afferent nerve-fibres distributed in that muscle itself. The functioning of the intrinsic proprioceptive arc—*i.e.*, the proprioceptive arc of vastocrureus itself—is essential to these reactions, and no other arc is essential. So much seems proved. Yet, to connect these reactions with the functioning of the intrinsic proprioceptive arc, and to show, as above, that that arc is indispensable to them, and uniquely indispensable, does not prove that the reactions themselves are strictly reflex. It is conceivable that the functioning of that arc confers upon the muscle-fibres a state—*e.g.*, *tonus*—with properties which render the muscle-fibres plastic in the above-mentioned sense, so that when subjected to mechanical changes such as shortening and stretching, they retain the shortening and lengthening impressed upon them.

That this latter view of the relation of "lengthening reaction" and "shortening reaction" to the reflex arc of the muscle is a possible alternative to a pure reflex view is evident from the analogy of another reaction obtainable from this same muscle and preparation. In the "knee jerk" we have a phenomenon which is thought to bear just such a relation as this to the intrinsic proprioceptive arc of the muscle. The functioning of that arc seems absolutely and uniquely essential for the phenomenon; yet the phenomenon, there seems good reason to think,[1] is not truly reflex, but a peripheral (muscular) event. A state or condition necessary for the phenomenon is conferred upon the muscle by the functioning of the intrinsic proprioceptive arc. A like relation to the reflex arc possibly exists also in the case of the "lengthening reaction" and "shortening reaction."

(b) *The "Lengthening Reaction" as compared with Reflexes* sensu strictiore

To discuss this some further details must be given concerning tonic "plasticity," and that aspect of it presented by the lengthening reaction. When the forced flexion is begun resistance, even considerable, is felt opposing it. Under continuance of the strain this resistance almost suddenly subsides; the tonic contraction of the muscle abruptly gives way; the resistance from that moment onward is less; the flexing of the knee and the forced stretching of the muscle meet with little further opposition. On discontinuing the force the joint is found to remain almost, though not fully, at the new angle imposed on it—in other words, the muscle has adapted its tonus nearly, though not quite, to the increased length to which the manipulation has extended it. Thus the knee, if flexed from an initial angle

[1] In 1909 the latent period was still thought by many to be too short to be that of a reflex. See *Integrative Action*, p. 87.—ED.

of about 120 degrees to an angle of about 60 degrees, remains on release at an angle of about 65 degrees. This change wrought in the tonic length is a relatively enduring one. Although induced in a couple of seconds (Fig. 58), it persists for several minutes. Indeed, the period of execution of the forced flexion which produces it does not sometimes exceed half a second. If, however, the rigidity be great, and the angle through which the forced movement is carried be wide, the new posture is better retained when passively continued for a few seconds. This indicates that the passive posture itself is in some way acting on the reflex process of the rigidity. The muscle exhibits, if the rigidity be marked, a gradual return in the direction of its former shorter length. This is well shown by the posture of the knee. The knee shows a slow recovery from flexion towards extension, frequently as a series of minute step-like increments of the angle of its flexion. Minutes usually elapse before much recovery has been made towards the attitude of extension which the knee possessed before. But the actual time consumed in appropriately regaining the original degree of extension varies with the extent of departure which the flexion had enforced, and with the intensity of the decerebrate rigidity.

The "lengthening reaction" exhibits various grades of completeness, meaning, by completeness, the degree to which the muscle after passive stretch—e.g., by flexing the knee—preserves when released from manipulation, that length to which it has been stretched by the manipulation. The "lengthening reaction" tends to be incomplete (Fig. 58) when the decerebrate tonus is unusually intense. But at a time when a forced flexion of the knee if brief fails to produce the reaction with completeness, a flexion longer maintained may produce it with completeness. A more prolonged passive stretch produces, as a rule, a more complete "lengthening reaction" than does a briefer though otherwise similar passive stretch. At times when the decerebrate tonus becomes very great, the passive stretch may fail altogether to induce the reaction; a plastic tonus has been replaced by an elastic tonus. My experience is that the "lengthening reaction" is not obtainable from the vastocrureus preparation during the rigidity caused by strychnine. I have failed to obtain either "lengthening reaction" or "shortening reaction" when the muscle is steadily contracting under faradisation of the distal stump of the nerve. In various grades of steady contraction thus produced, repeated trials to obtain either reaction have been unsuccessful. On the other hand, when in the decerebrate animal a mild degree of reflex contraction is being evoked by faradisation of an afferent nerve—e.g., of the opposite limb—I find both the "lengthening reaction" and the "shortening reaction" obtainable during the actual continuance of the external stimulation. If, however, the reflex contraction is made intense by stronger faradisation of the afferent nerve, the "lengthening reaction" becomes unobtainable; an elastic contraction has then replaced a plastic contraction. There is then also no opportunity for determining the presence of a "shortening reaction" either.

The " lengthening reaction " is obtainable from the animal either supine or on its side; in the latter case I sling the limb horizontally from a ceiling 6 metres above the table. The strain of the weight of the limb on the extensor muscle then alters little in the various postures of the knee. The retention by the muscle of its greater length after the forced flexion can then hardly be due to its being more heavily loaded in the flexed than in the extended posture of the knee. The load on the vastocrureus, the

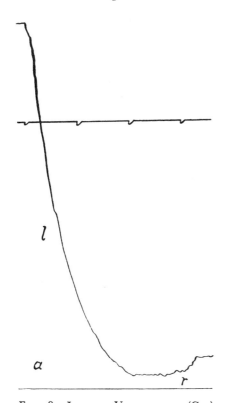

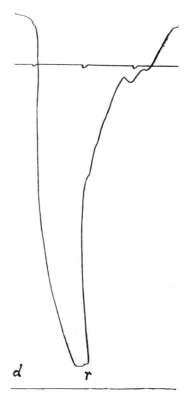

FIG. 58.—ISOLATED VASTOCRUREUS (CAT)

" Lengthening reaction " to show the time relations. The muscle was forcibly stretched during the descent *l*, and the stretch maintained until *r*, when the muscle was released. Time tracing notched at 1 second intervals

FIG. 59.—ISOLATED VASTOCRUREUS (CAT)

Attempt to produce a " lengthening reaction " in a de-afferented preparation: shows the release at *r* and the time relations of the elastic rebound. Compare with Fig. 58

femur and pelvis being fixed, is composed chiefly of the weight of the leg below the knee and the weight and tension of the hamstring muscles. The latter are paralysed by nerve section in the preparation above described, but they can further be severed close to their insertion or cut away altogether without interference with the phenomena of tonic plasticity. As regards the weight of the leg and its alteration as a load on the vastocrureus in various postures of the knee, I have minimised that further by immersing the limb in warm saline at the same time as having it slung from the ceiling above. The "lengthening" and "shortening" reactions succeed under these conditions. I have also amputated the limb close below the insertion of the extensor tendon, but observations on the tonus then become difficult, owing to difficulty in following the changes in the angle of the knee. In obtaining graphic records, the reactions have been taken when a long, weak spring is further stretched by extension of the knee, and less stretched by flexion of the knee. The "lengthening reaction" then somewhat relaxes the spring, the "shortening reaction" somewhat stretches it. I do not think, therefore, that the load on the muscle was greater in its lengthened state than in its shortened state.

To form some estimate of the relative intensity of the tonus when it keeps the muscle in the shortened state (knee extended) and in the lengthened state (knee-flexion) respectively, I have looked for the difference between weights which the tonus just supports in the two postures respectively.

The limb being horizontal and the animal on its side, the femur was secured by transfixion through the lower part of the shaft. The weight of the leg below the knee was supported at the ankle by a thread from the ceiling 6 metres above. A weight carried by a thread passing over a very freely running pulley was attached to the tibia 11 centimetres from the axis of rotation of the knee. The pull of this weight through its thread was in a plane parallel to the plane of rotation of the knee-joint and at right angles to the long axis of the tibia, and in a direction such as to flex the joint. It was noted, using successive increments of load, what weight just sufficed to begin flexing the knee against the tonic rigidity of the isolated vastocrureus, (a) when the posture kept up by the rigidity was fairly full extension of knee, (b) when the posture was fairly full flexion. The pull of the thread was arranged in each case to be at right angles to the tibia.

Such differences as detected were very small. Thus, 46·5 grammes with the knee at 105 degrees and 47 grammes with the knee at 65 degrees; or, 43 grammes with the knee at 102 degrees, and the same with the knee at 70 degrees; or again, 42 grammes with knee at 110 degrees, and 42·5 grammes with knee at 50 degrees. The lapse of time between the observations of the weight borne in the shortened and in the lengthened state of the muscle respectively would not be more than two minutes in these cases. It is, however, difficult to decide at what exact weight the tonic muscle begins just to yield, for where the weight and the tonus nearly balance the yield is slow, and occurs in little steps. It seems evident, however, that *in this tonic condition the muscle may maintain very different lengths under loads which differ from one another very little.*

In this respect the tonic preparation of this extensor muscle resembles in its reactions the retractor preparation of Sipunculus,[1] and preparations of Ophioghypha[2] and Edimus[3] described by v. Uexküll. A. Mosso and Pellacani[4] early demonstrated that the urinary bladder may with the same

[1] *Z. Biol.*, 1903, **44**, 269.   [2] *Ibid.*, 1904, **42**, 1.
[3] *Ibid.*, 1900, **39**, 73.   [4] *Arch. ital. biol.*, 1882, **1**, 97, 291.

internal pressure contain greatly different quantities of fluid. P. Schultz[1] found for the muscle of the frog's stomach a great divergence between isometric and isotonic contractions; and v. Uexküll[2] says of the retractor of Sipunculus, " The tensions and the shortenings by no means go hand in hand, but exhibit great independence one of another." Grutzner,[3] reviewing this whole question in a luminous essay, *Die glatten Muskeln*, adds, " I believe even striped muscle exhibits in this respect a certain analogy with unstriped." The tonic preparation of an extensor muscle (cat, dog) in decerebrate rigidity certainly does so. And in Sipunculus, if I follow v. Uexküll aright, the tonic basis for the reaction is not peripheral but central. Magnus[4] has shown it is set aside by an early stage of cocaine poisoning.

v. Uexküll[5] writes: " When an unstriped muscle is stretched it readily follows the stretch. If the stretch is removed the muscle does not then quickly return, but remains elongate and returns quite gradually to its former length. It finds itself, therefore, after the discontinuance of the stretch, in a condition of excitation different from before the stretch. For although it is again loaded only with its own weight, it is nevertheless longer than before." These words I find quite applicable to the tonic preparation of the vastocrureus muscle of cat and dog. They practically describe the " lengthening reaction " of that preparation.

As to the differences in the length of the muscle which a " lengthening " or a " shortening reaction " may bring about, the following supply a rough estimate. With a well completed " lengthening reaction," the tonic posture of the knee may be altered from an angle of 115 degrees to an angle of 60 degrees. The length of the fleshy part of the muscle, as measured on its anterior surface, was then found to increase from 82 mm. to 96 mm. The full extension which can be caused by contraction of the vastocrureus opens the cat's knee to an angle of about 160 degrees, the angle of the knee in full flexion being reduced to about 50 degrees. The length of the fleshy part of vastocrureus in this latter posture of knee being 96 mm., its length under full contraction from stimulation of its motor nerve fell to 72 mm.

(c) Data for Reflex View of " Lengthening Reaction "

The tonic contraction of vastocrureus in decerebrate rigidity is reflex in origin. The change which forced flexion of the knee induces in the decerebrate vastocrureus may therefore be a change in the muscle's reflex condition. The enduring elongated state produced in the tonic muscle by the forced stretch may be due to reflex inhibition of the tonus of the motoneurones supplying the muscle; the process of stretching the muscle may act as a mechanical stimulus to receptors in or adjunct to the muscle itself.

[1] *Arch. Anat. Physiol. Lpz., Physiol. Abtg.*, 1897, 322.   [2] *Loc. cit.*, **44,** 285.
[3] *Ergebn. Physiol.*, iii. Jahrg., Abt. 2, p. 80, 1904.   [4] *Arch. exp. Path. Pharmak.*, 1903, **1,** 86.
[5] *Ergebn. Physiol.*, iii. Jahrg., Abt. 2, p. 7, 1904.

In considering this possibility the following points have weight:

1. The " lengthening reaction " disappears under chloroform and ether narcosis with the disappearance of other reactions which are indubitably reflex.

2. Afferent nerve-fibres proceeding from the vastocrureus and contained in the nerve-trunk belonging to that muscle produce, when stimulated mechanically or electrically, a reflex relaxation of the muscle.[1] When the central end of any severed subdivision of the vastocrureus nerve is stimulated directly by either of the above-mentioned means, the invariable result, in my experience, is that in all that part of the muscle supplied by the uncut remainder of the nerve there ensues reflex relaxation. There must, therefore, exist in the nerve-trunk of the muscle a number of afferent fibres which can produce reflex lengthening of the tonically contracted muscle.

3. The sudden yielding of the tonically contracted muscle when the knee is forced into flexion is, to palpation, indistinguishable from the yielding of the muscle which occurs in known instances of its reflex inhibition.

4. Philippson's reflex—*i.e.*, the reflex extension of one knee produced by bending the other—occurs together with, or very slightly later than, the onset of the yield in the tonic ipsilateral vastocrureus subjected to the stretch. The crossed reflex being one of extension of the knee, a reflex having as its effect flexion is just the kind of reflex which, from analogy with other cases, would be expected in the ipsilateral knee; the " lengthening reaction," if reflex, is in fact a flexion reflex of the knee. Both the ipsilateral and the crossed reactions possess in common the feature of being protracted in their subsidence. That the crossed reaction does not usually appear regularly at each repetition of the elicitation of the ipsilateral is in accord with the general fact that crossed reflexes are not so readily evoked as are ipsilateral, and fail more readily. Now, the occurrence of a crossed reflex *without* an ipsilateral to pair with it is very exceptional. In regard to Philippson's reflex and the " lengthening reaction," my experience is that the former is never obtained without the latter. If, then, the " lengthening reaction " is not the ipsilateral reflex accompaniment of this crossed (Philippson's) reflex, where is that accompaniment ? Philippson's reflex is never obtained by stretching a vastocrureus the afferent nerve-fibres of which have been severed.

5. A difficulty for the reflex explanation of the " lengthening reaction " arises in that the relaxation of the muscle might be expected if reflex to relax the muscle not merely to that particular length which the forced stretch attained, but completely. But observation shows that the degree of relaxation induced by the lengthening reaction in instance after instance conforms nearly with the lengthening actually produced by the forced stretch. Now it has been found (Chapter VII, p. 276) that reflex inhibitions of vastocrureus follow with fine gradation the grades of intensity

---

[1] Sherrington, *Proc. roy. Soc.*, 1906, **77B**, 490; 1907, **79B**, 339.

of their exciting stimuli. The degree of inhibitory lengthening follows step by step the degree of intensity of the inhibitory stimulus, even when that stimulus is wholly artificial, and is applied not to receptive organs but to the raw nerve-trunk. If stretching the muscle constitutes a stimulus, and if a greater stretching constitutes a stronger stimulus, then more ample reflex relaxation will certainly result from greater stretching than from less. Moreover, the stretching of the muscle probably constitutes not merely a stimulus, but verily the *adequate* stimulus. The relation between the amplitude of the forced bending of the knee and the amplitude of the resulting inhibitory relaxation of vastocrureus would then be expected to be finely graded. The " lengthening reaction," if reflex, would be expected to follow closely the amplitude of the forced stretch, just as in fact it is found to do.

It has been shown that with weak stimuli the inhibitory relaxation of vastocrureus in ordinary reflexes increases *pari passu* with prolongation of the operation of the stimulus. A slowly executed forced flexion would, therefore, be competent to relax the muscle to the same extent as a more violent one acting for a shorter time; with this the actually observed results agree.

6. For the " lengthening reaction " to be reflex in nature need not imply that the inhibitory stimulus outlasts the actual brief period of forced stretch. It is not suggested that the muscle continues at its increased length in virtue of the continued action of some inhibitory stimulation persisting after the actual execution of the forced flexion of the knee has ceased. Three facts indicate that if the execution of the forced movement really produces an inhibitory stimulation, it is in operation as an inhibitory stimulus only during the actual execution of the movement, or but little longer: (1) After cessation of the forced movement the muscle often, although remaining nearly at the increased length reached under the movement, begins, if the rigidity is fair, on its release from manipulation, to shorten again, though but slowly and slightly. If the inhibitory stimulus were still in progress the muscle would, instead of shortening, relax further, at least in all those cases in which the " lengthening reaction " did not elongate it to the full limit to which reflex inhibition can carry it. (2) That the muscle remains in its new elongated state for a period long outlasting the duration of the inhibitory stimulus given by a transient stretch agrees fully with the actual course observed in inhibitory reflexes of vastocrureus due to transient inhibitory stimuli in decerebrate rigidity. Thus the lengthened state following relaxation evoked through a skin-nerve very usually endures several minutes after the brief stimulus has ceased, especially if the stimulus be weak and the degree of rigidity prevailing at the time be not extreme. It is when the degree of rigidity is not extreme, and when rebounds (successive induction) are not prominent, that the " lengthening reaction " and plasticity are best seen. (3) If the elongated condition assumed by the tonic muscle after a passive stretch were to signify a con-

tinued state of inhibition, the threshold of reflex excitation might be expected to be higher than it was previously—*i.e.*, before the forced stretch which induced the elongated state. If, on the other hand, it was a tonic state merely following on a transient inhibited state, the threshold of reflex excitation might be expected to be lowered.

To test this point the crossed reflex exciting the vastocrureus—*e.g.*, from an afferent nerve of the other (*e.g.*, left) limb—has been in several experiments examined for its threshold value of stimulus immediately before and immediately after a " lengthening reaction " was induced. The observations[1] fail to detect any clear difference in the threshold of reflex reaction, either for excitatory or inhibitory effect when the tonic length of the muscle has been increased by the " lengthening reaction " or shortened by the " shortening reaction." The observations, therefore, do not support the supposition that the " lengthening reaction " and the " shortening reaction," after their respective occurrence, leave the reflex arc in a perceptibly altered condition of excitability. It is difficult, therefore, to regard the " lengthening reaction " as leaving the muscle in an elongated condition by leaving the reflex arc in a state of inhibition. It must be remembered, however, that in these experiments it is the threshold of reaction, not of the proprioceptive arc of the muscle itself, but of extrinsic reflex arcs which is tested; the test nerve for the excitatory reflex was the crossed peroneal, for the inhibitory reflex the ipsilateral peroneal.

7. In decerebrate rigidity, manipulations such as kneading, pulling, etc., applied direct to the fleshy portion of the exposed vastocrureus *in situ* in the thigh can be seen to produce sudden partial elongations of the muscle. When the limb is suitably held, each such interference causes some dropping of the knee toward flexion. Running the end of a blunt seeker along the lines of attachment of the muscle at the sides of the lower part of the shaft of the femur causes similar smart partial elongations of the muscle. These reactions are obviously reflex inhibitions. They seem referable to mechanical excitation of inhibitory afferents belonging to the muscle and distributed within it.

8. Occasionally, when the reflex excitability of the preparation is high, the relaxation of vastocrureus caused by stretching it in forced knee-flexion is quickly followed by a rebound to a degree of tonic contraction greater even than before. This rebound resembles to all appearance the rebound seen to follow reflex inhibition under conditions favouring successive induction.

9. Strychnine diminishes or completely sets aside the property of the decerebrate muscle to assume increased tonic length in consequence of a forced stretch; it upsets the " lengthening reaction." It has been shown that strychnine also upsets reflex inhibition. The influence of strychnine upon the " lengthening reaction " conforms, therefore, with the view that that reaction is itself of the nature of an inhibitory reflex.

[1] Details of an experiment are given in original paper.—Ed.

Several facts, therefore, support the supposition that forced stretch of the extensor muscle in decerebrate rigidity gives a new tonic length to the muscle by an inhibitory reflex—in other words, that the " lengthening reaction " is reflex.

(d) Data for Reflex View of " Shortening Reaction "

As to the " shortening reaction," there are somewhat similar grounds for regarding it as reflex. That the nerve of vastocrureus contains afferent fibres arising in the muscle, and that these can promote a tonic reflex contraction of that muscle itself, seems clear from several facts:[1] among others, this, that severance of the afferent spinal roots belonging to that nerve precludes and abolishes the tonic contraction of the muscle characteristic of decerebrate rigidity. The " shortening reaction," if reflex, is a tonic reflex, for its result on the muscle is an increased tonic shortening. There are two ways in which such a reflex might be brought about: (1) The passive relaxation of the muscle when the knee is extended by external manipulation might cut short a stimulus which was keeping the muscle elongated by reflex inhibition. But, as pointed out above, there seems no firm ground for assuming that persistent inhibitory stimulus is then at work. (2) The passive relaxation of the muscle might itself act as a stimulus to intramuscular receptors, productive of reflex tonic excitation of the muscle. The latter view postulates the possession by the muscle of afferent nerve-fibres which can excite it to reflex contraction. Now the conditions essential for decerebrate rigidity seem to prove that such afferent fibres are possessed by the muscle. A difficulty regarding them is that they are not revealed by direct stimulation, either mechanical or electrical, of the vastocrureus nerve itself, although it is in that nerve that they must lie. Similarly, their presence in the afferent spinal roots is not demonstrable, in my experience, by direct stimulation, either mechanical or electrical, of those roots. The explanation of this may be that they are there commingled with afferents of opposite effect, and their reflex influence is thereby masked or prevented when the whole afferent nerve or root is artificially excited. Regarding their mode of excitation, the alteration of the muscle in shape and tension when passively relaxed by manipulative extension of the knee must, it would seem, if it act as a stimulus to the receptors of these fibres, be a stimulus of mechanical kind. It may excite them selectively—that is, it may selectively excite one certain class of intramuscular receptors—namely, those which cause reflex tonic contraction. In considering such an explanation, it must be remembered, however, that a frequent feature of the " shortening reaction " is that the leg, on release from the passive extension at knee, drops a little from the full posture given it. It drops till the tightening of vastocrureus checks its further fall. It is then caught, as by a ratchet, and prevented from dropping further. A difficulty arises as to by which of two ways the tonic contraction of vastocrureus which thus

[1] Sherrington, *Proc. roy. Soc.*, 1906, **77B**, 478.

checks the fall at the knee has been produced. The tonic length of the muscle, when it thus checks the fall of the leg, is obviously much shorter than it had been a second before, when the passive extension of the knee was begun. The speed and extent with which the approximation of the attached ends of the muscle is carried out may exceed the rate at which the tonic shortening of the muscle can proceed. In that case, on releasing the leg from the manipulation, the knee cannot be supported at the point to which the manipulation has carried the leg, but drops till it finds support from vastocrureus at that grade of tonic shortening which the muscle has then had time to acquire. In this case the new tonic length of the muscle is merely revealed by the check in the fall of the limb.

But there is another possibility—namely, that the drop of the limb released by the manipulator actually excites, by the slight stretch it gives to vastocrureus, a tonic reflex in that muscle, and that the check in the fall of the leg is due to a tonic contraction not previously present, but now excited from the muscle by the stretching action of the fall itself. Remembering that certain skeletal muscles are directly excitable by mechanical strain (tortoise, frog), it at one time seemed to me that, as the leg dropped, the stretch so caused in the vastocrureus excited in that muscle a contraction, which itself then checked the further fall of the leg. More extended experience of the phenomenon has brought out two facts against that view: (1) In the " lengthening reaction " we have passive stretch of the tonic muscle, causing a reflex elongation of it, and not a reflex contraction. (2) The " shortening reaction " not unfrequently occurs without any dropping back of the knee toward flexion; a dropping of the knee cannot in those cases be the excitant of the reaction. This absence of any dropping back of the knee is rare when the " shortening reaction " is brought about by passively extending the knee (Figs. 52, 53), but is fairly common when the approximation of the ends of the muscle is effected by moderate reflex contraction of the muscle itself (Fig. 55). The reflex contraction requisite for this may be excited from any of various appropriate afferent nerves, either ipsilateral or contralateral. This extension of the knee called forth by extraneously initiated reflex contraction is seen to merge on cessation of the extrinsic stimulus in an autogenous " shortening reaction " without any lapse toward flexion intervening between the two. The support of the extraneous reflex by the autogenous reaction tends to be more complete with reflexes of moderate or weak intensity than with strong, perhaps because the weaker reflex contraction occurs rather more slowly, and the development of the " shortening reaction " can better keep pace with it. With strong reflexes, especially when also brief, the amount of tonic shortening developed by the " shortening reaction " seems to lag behind the degree of shortening actually reached by the active contraction itself, so that at the end of this latter the muscle drops back to the grade of shortness given it by the more sluggishly developed " shortening reaction." The occurrence with moderate reflexes, even brief, of an unbroken transition from shortened state due to the extrinsic reflex, to an after-following shortened state due to concomitant " shortening reaction "—the transition being so smooth that no feature of the myogram indicates where one ends and the other begins—shows that the " shortening reaction " can take place perfectly without any precurrent partial elongation of the muscle. Its excitation, therefore, is neither in strong reflexes nor in passive manipulations due to the " drop " of the knee.

We are driven back to the supposition that the excitant for the " shortening reaction " is actually the approximation of the ends of the tonic muscle, and that this evokes the reaction both when brought about passively by external means and when brought about actively by contraction of the muscle itself—e.g., when it contracts in reflex response to stimulation of any of various afferent nerves in its own or in the fellow limb. The " shortening reaction " of the muscle seems more perfectly evoked when the approximation of its ends is performed by the muscle's own contraction than when it is passively executed under external manipulation.

On this view—namely, that approximation of the ends of the muscle evokes the " shortening reaction "—the knee jerk, although a peripheral phenomenon, should be competent to evoke it. I find this actually the case frequently in the spinal dog; it proves also to be so under the more strictly analysed conditions of the isolated vastocrureus preparation in the decerebrate cat. The knee jerk in these cases often takes the form, not of a twitch, but of a lasting tonic extension of the knee.

But if the " shortening reaction " is evoked by approximation of the ends of its muscle, how is it capable of gradation in amplitude ? The muscle's degree of tonic shortness under the reaction remains set at any desired grade—e.g., the knee keeping at 80, 90, 100 degrees, or any other angle between flexion and full extension. If the muscle as it shortens under an extrinsic reflex keeps inducing an intrinsic " shortening reaction " as it proceeds, the twofold process might be expected to form a self-maintaining cycle of activity which would cease only when the muscle was shortened to the full extent of which it is ultimately capable. In other words, a reflex extension of the knee, once started, would proceed to maximal extension, and not stop at any intermediate stage. And similarly with the " lengthening reaction "; if more stretching of the tonic muscle evokes the " lengthening reaction " pari passu as it proceeds, one would expect that, once started, the double process could not stop short until the maximal elongation of the muscle had been reached—i.e., until in the isolated vastocrureus preparation the knee had fallen into full flexion. But, as a fact, the knee can be set by the " lengthening reaction " at any degree of flexion greater than that from which the passive stretch began. The answer may lie in the fact, for which a good deal of evidence has been given, that the " shortening reaction " and the " lengthening reaction," as regards their effect on the muscle's length, often exhibit a lag behind the primary change in muscle length which excites them: this seems to be the reason why slowly induced " lengthening reactions " tend to be more complete than very quickly induced ones, just as more slowly induced " shortening reactions " tend to be more perfect than very quickly induced. The change which constitutes each of these reactions seems itself to be a secondary change which follows but hardly runs abreast of, certainly never gets ahead of, the primary change—namely, either forced stretch or passive or active approximation of muscle ends, as the case may be—which is its forerunner and provokes its appearance. If this is so, the brevity of latent period which is the chief reason for regarding the knee jerk as not a true reflex is not a feature of the " lengthening reaction " or the " shortening reaction." There seems, therefore, no valid ground for not regarding these reactions as reflex. And as reflexes, they belong to the proprioceptive class.

Summary of Conclusions

1. Certain reactions (the " *lengthening reaction* " and the " *shortening reaction* ") which confer upon the extensor muscle of the knee a quality of plasticity both in the spinal and especially in the decerebrate animal are dependent on the proprioceptive arc of the muscle itself, and all other spinal afferents than those of that arc are inessential to them.

2. The " *lengthening reaction* " is as follows: When the tonic muscle is stretched it assumes, by virtue of its proprioceptive arc, a new tonic length, which is approximately that to which it has been stretched. In this reaction the behaviour of the muscle bears resemblance to the behaviour of preparations of unstriped muscle as noted by v. Uexküll (Sipunculus retractor preparations), Grutzner, Magnus, and others.

3. Conversely, when in the tonic preparation of the knee extensor the muscle is shortened, either passively or by active contraction of the muscle itself, the muscle retains approximately the shortened length thus given it. This is the " *shortening reaction*."

4. The vastocrureus muscle, when de-afferented by severance of the particular afferent spinal roots through which its afferent fibres reach the spinal cord, reacts in the decerebrate animal differently from the muscle with afferent nerve intact. It shows from the earliest period examined after section of its afferents—namely, two hours—up to the latest period examined—namely, 140 days—certain defects. Among these defects are the following: The de-afferented muscle is toneless, and yields no trace either of " shortening reaction " or of " lengthening reaction." Manipulation of it fails to evoke either contraction or inhibition of the fellow muscle of the opposite limb. Under decerebrate rigidity, its reflex contraction, excited from whatever source, instead of being prolonged beyond the duration of the external stimulus, ceases immediately on withdrawal of that stimulus, the muscle then lapsing at once into full relaxation. In response to slowly repeated reflex stimuli, the de-afferented muscle exhibits a coarsely clonic instead of a steady tetanus. Its failure in duration of contraction is due to

absence of any " *shortening reaction* " coming to reinforce and maintain the reflex excited through the extrinsic afferent arc. This defect in the reflexes of the de-afferented muscle bears out what has been previously[1] indicated, that *proprioceptive reflexes normally fuse with other reflexes as adjuvant to them.*

Further, in the de-afferented muscle a reflex contraction excited from an extrinsic arc cannot be cut short by a forced stretch of the contracting muscle, as is the case with extensor muscles still possessed of their normal afferent nerve-fibres. This indicates, as has been pointed out previously,[2] that a *function of proprioceptive reflexes is to produce a compensatory reaction cutting short a reflex, and restoring the* status quo ante *existing before that reflex set in.*

The de-afferented muscle presents no tonic reflexes, and this is in accord with what has been previously pointed out—namely, that proprioceptive reflexes tend especially to be tonic in character.[3]

The reflex contractions of the de-afferented extensor muscle appear to suffer fatigue sooner than those of the muscle with afferent nerve intact. Its contractions wane under prolonged stimulation earlier and more abruptly than is the case with muscle still possessed of afferents.

5. The proprioceptive apparatus of the vastocrureus and other extensor muscles seems *specially adapted to stimuli of mechanical quality;*[4] the apparatus reacts both to stretch of the muscle and to the converse of that, and its response is different in the two cases.

6. The proprioceptive reflex apparatus of the vastocrureus muscle yields four reactions, two reacting on the muscle itself and two on its fellow muscle of the opposite limb. These reactions are coupled in pairs which are not interchangeable. For one pair of these reflexes the *adequate stimulus is shortening,* it matters not whether passive or active, of the muscle; this stimulus induces shortening of the tonic length of the muscle itself, and the reflex relaxation (more rarely reflex contraction) of the fellow muscle of the opposite limb. For the other pair of reflexes the *adequate stimulus is stretch of the tonic muscle*: this stimulus causes reflex lengthening of the muscle itself, and reflex contraction of the fellow muscle of the opposite limb.

Of these four reactions, those with contralateral effect are indubitably reflex; the present investigation has found no valid reason against supposing that those with ipsilateral effect are truly reflex also: one relation in which they stand to the reflex nervous system emerges with clearness—namely, that the integrity of the intrinsic reflex arc of their own muscle is absolutely essential to their production.

7. The plastic tonus of the extensor muscles is *autogenous,* being in each muscle dependent on afferent nerve-fibres from that muscle itself.

[1] Sherrington, *Integrative Action,* 1906, p. 139.   [2] *Ibid.,* p. 341.
[3] *Ibid.,* p. 338.   [4] *Ibid.,* p. 336.

4. REFLEX STANDING[1]

1. *Spinal.*—The execution of stepping movements by the limbs does not of course in itself amount to walking. For this latter act the reflex stepping of the limbs has to be combined with reflex maintenance of the erect posture of the body. In regard to this the question rises, Can the spinal preparation stand ? In my experience the decapitate preparation (cat) certainly cannot stand. Placed in the erect posture it immediately sinks; limbs, neck, and tail drop; they are without power to antagonise gravity. The stepping movements of the limbs so readily excited in this preparation are ineffective for locomotion; the extension phase of the step is usually unable to straighten the limbs effectively under the superincumbent weight of the body.

But a different condition is observable after a period has elapsed following the spinal transection—*e.g.*, at 10th thoracic level. In the course of some months or weeks the hind-limbs become able to stand (dog).[2] If placed symmetrically in the standing posture with the hind-feet together and the fore-limbs supported by an assistant, the hind-limbs are found capable of maintaining the extended posture and supporting the weight of the hind-quarters, even for minutes at a time. In some experiments, as was described earlier, the standing can be executed by one hind-limb without help from the other, so that the animal stands on three legs, but such standing lasts in my experience only for a short time, rarely a full minute. Spinal standing is subject to sudden lapses. At times by no device can the spinal limbs be made to stand. And there is little latitude in the exact pose of the limbs compatible with the standing. In my experience the limbs need to be symmetrically placed, and there must be no wide departure from the vertical. In short, there is in the tonic reflex which maintains standing in the purely spinal condition little of that plasticity which the natural act exhibits.

2. *Decerebrate.*—If, however, we turn to the decerebrate preparation the condition is different. The state of that preparation is, as regards the innervation of its skeletal musculature, more constant and homogeneous than that of the decapitate or spinal. The decerebrate preparation is exhibiting a steady reflex in continuous operation. It is in a state of reflex equilibrium such as the purely spinal preparation rarely approaches. In the decerebrate preparation there obtains a characteristic rigidity. The limb muscles are stiffened by tonic reflex action to the extent that they successfully counteract the weight of the body. In short, in the limbs a static reflex is in progress. A tonic reflex keeps the limbs extended, the neck and tail lifted, the back and head horizontal, and the lower jaw closed against the upper. This reflex rigidity maintains the preparation in a definite posture. The tonic contraction which thus maintains a reflex

[1] Extract from *J. Physiol.*, 1910, **40**, 103-13.

[2] *Cf.* Philippson, *International Congress of Physiologists, Heidelberg*, 1907, p. 130, and p. 132 this volume.

attitude does not involve all muscles in the limb and other regions; it is confined to certain muscles and is absent from the antagonists of these. It is present in the extensors of the limb, the retractors of the head, and the elevators of neck and tail and lower jaw. The tonic reflex contraction is therefore confined to those muscles which counteract gravity in the usual erect posture of the animal. And the grade of contraction of these muscles in the decerebrate state commonly just suffices to support the creature in the erect attitude when passively set upright. This static reflex, though its effect covers a wide field of musculature, is nevertheless a homogeneous entity. The tonic excitation produced by it is distributed to muscles which form one functional system compassing one common result—namely, the counteracting of gravity in those parts whose weight has to be duly supported for the maintenance of the erect posture of the animal. The source whence proceed the centripetal impulses maintaining this reflex has been traced to be in those muscles which themselves exhibit the tonic reflex contraction. The reflex arises therefore from a source which is itself of unitary functional character—namely, that system of muscles which in the erect posture of the animal antagonises the displacements which gravity would produce. This reflex employs a prespinal centre situate between anterior colliculus and hind-edge of pons. It ceases when that region is removed. Originated via one particular set of proprioceptive afferents and subserving one unitary purpose, the reaction constitutes a single though composite proprioceptive reflex.

In it, as in the kinetic reflexes (flexion-reflex, crossed extension-reflex) analysed above, reciprocal innervation of antagonistic muscles seems to obtain. The tonic excitation is supplied only to one member, the extensor, of antagonistic muscle pairs. There is evidence that the flexors are under a mild tonic inhibition, the counterpart of the tonic excitation of extensor motoneurones.

(1) The reflex contractions of the flexors in decerebrate rigidity show less prolonged after-discharge than they show in the purely spinal condition. (2) The threshold stimulus for reflex contraction of the flexors of the limb is often seen to be slightly lower in the decapitated preparation than in the decerebrate. (3) Alternating reflexes are facile in the decapitate preparation but are much less so in the decerebrate. The latter is occupied by the tonic extensor reflex, the former not. In the decerebrate preparation occasionally the tonic extensor reflex (rigidity) does not develop or lapses; when this happens the alternating reflexes are more facile than usual in the decerebrate preparation. Reflex flexion is involved in the alternating reflexes and some of them—e.g., scratch reflex—open with flexion. (4) In spinal preparations myographic work with the flexors is commonly disturbed by reflex twitchings of the muscles. This is especially the case when afferent nerves of the limb have been prepared for stimulation, etc. The twitches can be temporarily subdued by reflex inhibition. Work with the decerebrate preparation is not disturbed in this way. The twitching of the flexors seems suppressed. In decerebrate rigidity a stimulus A which reflexly excites the flexor muscles produces marked relaxation of the extensors of that limb. Conversely, a stimulus B which excites the extensor muscles inhibits the flexor muscles, as can be shown by its suppressing a contraction just previously produced in them. Yet in decerebrate rigidity stimulus B produces in the flexors no further elongation (relaxation) than they already show. The inference is that the flexors are already completely relaxed.

These points indicate that in the decerebrate preparation the postural reflex which keeps the extensors in tonic contraction is keeping the flexors relaxed by tonic inhibition. This static reflex which the decerebrate preparation so constantly exhibits is the attitude of " standing " reflexly executed. It seems unnatural that experimental search should find, so far as " acute " preparations go, reflex *stepping* obtainable as a purely spinal reflex, but for reflex *standing* have to resort to a preparation retaining hind-brain and part of mid-brain as well as cord. An explanation lies, I imagine, in the circumstance that the latter, the postural reflex (standing), is an extensor reflex, whereas the former is a flexor as well as an extensor reflex. Extensor reactions usually suffer more than flexor from loss of subcortical prespinal centres. After the " shock " has passed as pointed out above a modicum of standing remains even in the spinal preparation.

And to ascribe to " standing " such widespread muscular action as is seen in decerebrate rigidity may seem somewhat opposed to views in general acceptance which tend to attribute it mainly to ligaments, joints, and organs of purely static function. But R. du Bois Reymond, our best authority on such matters, writes:[1] " In the study of joints the idea of the bones and ligaments acting as stops, which was at first alone visualised, has with time become ever more restricted. In its stead the doctrine of the checking of the joint movements by muscles has arrived."

" Standing " appears to be the functional meaning of decerebrate rigidity. The preparation " stands " and maintains its " standing " as a continuous reflex even for hours at a time. The transection through mid-brain seems to set into action or to free from higher control a reflex " standing " which unfettered persists whatever the passive position of the animal as a whole. The tonic postural reflex still goes on when the preparation is laid upon its side. That the animal still stands when laid upon its side may seem an extravagant statement. It merely implies that in the decerebrate preparation the standing posture is largely beyond control by the otic labyrinths. Similarly in the dog with spinal hind-limbs the hind-limbs often execute for long periods the stepping reflex when lying in the stall sidewise and on the flank. The reflex standing of the decerebrate preparation is not broken down even by complete inversion of the animal. And that the reflex is in large measure independent of the otic labyrinth and nervi octavi is indicated by its not being annulled nor sometimes obviously impaired by removal of both labyrinths (cat) or severance of both nervi octavi (cat, monkey) subsequent to onset of the rigidity. Nor has it been by destruction of both labyrinths four days prior to decerebration. The longest period over which the observations on this point range has been in an experiment in which one labyrinth was removed eight days and the other three days before decerebration. In this and other experiments on this point I had the advantage of the able co-operation of Dr. S. Sewell. After decerebration the tonic postural reflex appeared as usual and without

[1] *Arch. Anat. Physiol. Lpz., Physiol. Abt.*, 1902, p. 37.

obvious difference in the right and left sides. Nervus octavus can, it is true, regulate, adjust, and modify the reflex standing of the decerebrate preparation. But the reflex posture of standing can be maintained even in complete absence of both otic labyrinths and after severance of both nervi octavi. These receptors and receptive nerves are therefore not essential to the fundamental execution of the standing posture. And this agrees with the fact that the spinal hind-limbs of the dog after spinal shock has passed are able to stand, although less perfectly than is the decerebrate preparation.

Although the tonic postural reflex persists even when the animal is completely inverted, its intensity is favoured by placing the animal upright on its feet. It is markedly increased by lifting the preparation from shoulders and loins and setting it briskly on its feet a few times in succession. With each setting down the extensor attitude of the limbs stiffens and the head and tail, which before the manœuvre may be drooping, rise with the increasing tonus of the neck and tail muscles. Centripetal impulses from the soles of the feet contribute, as with reflex stepping (see Chapter V, p. 181), little toward the reflex. The afferent nerves of the feet may be severed without clear lessening of the reflex, just as similar severance does not obviously impair the execution of the standing posture when assumed naturally (horse,[1] pigeon,[2] cat[3]). The afferents from practically the whole of the skin of the limb may be severed without obviously lessening the reflex. The skin may be removed from the whole preparation and the reflex " standing " of the preparation still continue. The reflex is clearly proprioceptive. In other words, the stimuli exciting and maintaining it come not from the environment but from the body itself acting as stimulating agent to its own afferent nerves.

The reflex tonus which thus executes the posture of standing in the decerebrate preparation has " plasticity "—*i.e.*, capacity for local modification in regard to the length of this or that particular muscle or muscle-group without disturbance of the tonic tension of the muscle. Each such local modification is given by an intrinsic proprioceptive reflex. This plasticity appears to meet the requirement that in " standing " the posture of the limb may with advantage vary a good deal provided always that each joint maintain a resistance sufficient to counteract the tendency to double up under the weight it bears. Ordinary standing postures (*usustatus*[4]) include various degrees of flexion at hip and knee and extension is usually less at the former. One hind-foot may rest close beside the other or much in advance of or behind it. Yet the plastic tonus allows the tonic length of the muscle to vary without its tonic tension falling too low to bear the superincumbent load. In v. Uexküll's[5] terminology the extensors in this postural reflex of standing are acting as " sperr-muskeln." They secure

[1] Chauveau, *Brain*, 1891, **14**, 153.   [2] *Ibid.*   [3] *V. supra*, Chapter V, p. 181.
[4] Schaefer, K., *Pflüg. Arch. ges. Physiol.*, 1887, **41**, 582.
[5] *Ergebn. Physiol.*, 1904, **3**, Abt. 2, 7, and *Umwelt u. Innenwelt für Thieren*, 1909.

that in the various positions of the joints in standing the tonic tension of the muscles shall still continue adjusted to the support the limb requires under the standing animal. Reflex " standing " is a " sperr-reflex."

The reflex standing of the decerebrate preparation differs from that exhibited by the spinal preparation in its equable, steady, long-persisting character, in its immunity from sudden lapses, in its reliability of occurrence, and in its plasticity allowing latitude to the exact form of standing posture assumed.

In the hind-limb (cat, dog) the muscles observed to be contracting in this tonic postural reflex of standing in the decerebrate preparation are as follows (Fig. 60):

Biceps femoris anterior.	Crureus.
Semimembranosus.	Adductor minor.
Quadratus femoris.	Adductor major (in part).
Vastus lateralis.	Gastrocnemius.
Vastus medialis.	Soleus.

Other muscles as well—particularly I would suspect flex. long. digitorum —may be contracting, but only those in which observation by the isolation method has ascertained their contraction without any doubt are included in the above list. Similarly the following are muscles in which absence of contraction in this reflex has been ascertained clearly:

Psoas magnus.	Gracilis.
Tensor fasciæ femoris.	Tibialis anticus.
Sartorius.	Peroneus longus.
Semitendinosus.	Extensor digitorum longus.
Biceps femoris posterior.	Tenuissimus.

These lists make clear that the same principles of co-ordination are adhered to in the execution of this static reflex as in that of the kinetic reflexes above analysed. Hence the term protagonists seems preferable to that of prime movers for the main muscles executive of the reflexes. For the latter term is inapplicable to the static reflexes, since in them posture but not movement results. Contracting muscles used at one joint as direct execu- tants of the posture serve also as fixators for the direct executants of the posture at another joint. Contraction is arranged to reinforce passive mechanical effects due to contraction elsewhere. Rotation of the limb at certain joints is avoided by balanced action of partially antagonistic muscles. All those items of taxis traced in the kinetic reflexes are observable also in this postural static one.

3. *The Initiation of Reflex Stepping during Reflex Standing.*—Between decere- brate rigidity signifying the reflex attitude of standing and the flexion- reflex or extension-reflex of the limb signifying the execution of a step the nexus is natural and close. When in the decerebrate preparation a stimulus is applied such as by quality and locus would in the decapitate preparation excite reflex stepping, the kinetic reflex of a step-phase breaks in on the

static reflex of " standing." Suppose the stimulus one which gives flexion as the opening phase of the step, and the limb in which the reflex is initiated to be the right hind. The extensors of the limb are in reflex plastic tonus when the kinetic reflex opens. The kinetic reflex at once inhibits the tonic standing contraction of quadratus femoris, semimembranosus, and biceps femoris anterior, extensors of hip, of vasti and crureus, extensors of knee, of gastrocnemius and soleus extensors of ankle, and also of adductor minor and part of adductor major of thigh. While inhibiting the motoneurones of these muscles it excites the motoneurones of psoas magnus, sartorius, rectus femoris, tensor fasciæ femoris brevis, flexors at hip; gluteus minimus, a flexor and abductor of hip; semitendinosus, biceps femoris posterior, gracilis, sartorius and tenuissimus, flexors at knee; tibialis anticus, a flexor at ankle; extensor longus digitorum, a flexor at ankle and extensor of toes; extensor brevis digitorum, an extensor of toes; peroneus longus, an abductor of foot; and a part of the adductor of the thigh. These muscles the reflex found at its outset in a state probably of slight tonic inhibition. By these inhibitions and excitations the reflex flexes the limb, lifts it slightly from the ground and swings it forward.

This reflex effect on right limb is accompanied by a converse action on the left limb. There the muscles which are in tonic contraction under the postural reflex of standing are reinforced in their contraction by the kinetic reflex. This is proved for semimembranosus and biceps femoris anterior, extensors of hip; adductor minor and part of adductor major, adductors and extensors of hip; vastus lateralis, vastus medialis and crureus, extensors of knee;

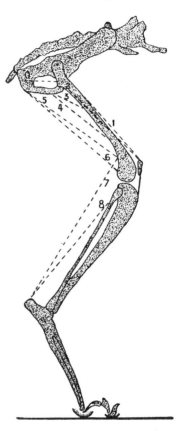

Fig. 60.—Muscles observed by Direct Analysis to be engaged in the Reflex Tonic Contraction of the Standing Posture [Decerebrate Preparation (Cat, Dog)]

1. Crureus and vastus medialis
2. Vastus lateralis
3. Adductor minor
4. Adductor major (a part)
5. Semimembranosus
6. Biceps femoris anterior
7. Gastrocnemius
8. Soleus (absent from dog)
9. Quadratus femoris

gastrocnemius and soleus, extensors of ankle. It is so sometimes with quadratus femoris, but reflex stepping in the decapitated preparation only occasionally actuates this muscle. Late in its course the kinetic reflex causes contraction of flexor longus digitorum, but that this muscle is engaged in the tonic reflex of standing I have not been able actually to see. And in this left limb also the kinetic reflex exerts inhibitory besides excitatory influence. The inhibition is distributed to semitendinosus, biceps femoris posterior, sartorius, and tibialis anticus, and almost certainly to other flexors as well, but with these others my observations have not actually dealt in this respect. To detect the inhibition in this case meets with the difficulty, as already mentioned, that the muscles on which it is exerted are much relaxed at the time when the inhibitory influence is exerted. The combined effect of these inhibitions and excitations by the kinetic reflex in the left limb is an accentuation of the extensor position previously maintained in it by the " standing " reflex. The foot is pushed backward against the ground and the body forward and somewhat upward as the limb extends.

Thus the kinetic reflex of the step so grafts itself on the tonic postural reflex of standing that its flexion phase is an interruption of the static reflex, its extension phase is an accentuation of the static reflex. One of the features of the tonic postural reflex is that although systemic and unified in its effect it is of multiple origin. Its source, although homogeneous in character, is multiple in seat, arising in the afferents of the widely spread groups of muscles which it causes to contract. In each region it is originated by centripetal impulses from the muscles of that region. Thus that part of the reflex which keeps the neck supported against gravity arises through the deep afferents of the neck; that part which supports the fore-limb under the weight of the fore-quarters arises through the afferents of supraspinatus, humeral triceps, and other extensors of the fore-limb; that which keeps the hind-limb extended under the weight of the hind-quarters arises from the afferents of the hind-limb extensors, and so on. The reflex posture in each body-region is not, of course, *wholly* independent of afferents in other regions. Thus passive flexion of elbow and shoulder often provokes in the decerebrate preparation heightening of the tonic extension of ipsilateral knee and ankle, and lowering of it in crossed knee and ankle. Again, active or passive rotation of neck on its long axis in the decerebrate preparation inhibits extensor tonus in hind-limb on the side of the lowered prima and causes active flexion of knee; and does so after severance of both cranial 5ths and both octavi. Again, in the de-afferented vastocrureus (decerebrate preparation), though the steady enduring tonus ensuing on decerebration is characteristically absent from the muscle, nevertheless from time to time for relatively short periods tonic contraction of it occurs traceable to afferent sources altogether headward of hind-limb.

But apart from these exaltations and depressions of tonus which are *regulative* of the reflex posture but not part of its essential basis, the broad fact remains that the reflex maintaining the erect posture of each region has its source in the proprioceptive afferents of that region itself. This holds even to the extent that the source of the decerebrate posture of the extensor of the knee is traceable almost entirely if not absolutely entirely to afferents of the knee-extensor itself. A result of this is that although the individual components traceable from these several sources all involve a central mechanism between anterior colliculus and hinder edge of pons, and combine to one united static reflex of " standing," the resultant systemic reflex can be modified piecemeal. Hence a kinetic reflex such as the flexion phase of a step upsets the systemic postural reflex of standing only in its own limb and leaves it unbroken elsewhere.

Reflex walking therefore consists in an alterative innervation locally disturbing in due sequence parts of a general tonic reflex. A rhythmic series of kinetic reflexes breaks a systemic static reflex in each limb in turn, but leaves it in force elsewhere. In regions other than the limbs the erect posture continues maintained by the systemic tonic reflex during walking and running even as during standing. And the erect posture is as necessarily contributive to them as to standing itself. This does not, of course, mean that outside the limbs the static postural reflex necessarily remains everywhere wholly unmodified during the kinetic reflexes of progression. The tail exhibits rhythmic lateral movement during the spinal stepping of the hind-limb, and the same stimulus which excites the flexion phase of the step excites a lateral motion of the tail to the ipsilateral side; the same is true of the neck in relation to the flexion-reflex of the fore-limb. Yet apart from these details the broad fact is that the general postural reflex which maintains the erect posture is modified only piecemeal by the kinetic reflexes which execute the step. The successive and simultaneous interruptions and reinforcements of the static reflex in its various parts by the kinetic reflexes grafted upon it in the several regions permute the general static reflex into the composite acts of walking and running. The fundamental relation of these reflex acts to the reflex posture of standing becomes clearer when this interweaving of the kinetic and static reflexes is recognised.

5. REFLEX WALKING[1]

Reflex stepping movements of the hind-limb (cat, dog) are less easy to evoke in the decerebrate preparation than in the decapitate. They are of a more effective character when evoked in the latter. Reflex stepping movements of the limbs even when including all four limbs timed in appropriate sequence yet of themselves alone do not constitute a complete reflex act of walking or running. For this they must be duly combined with the general static reflex maintaining erect posture of head, neck, trunk, and tail. A greater efficiency of the reflex stepping when evoked in the decerebrate preparation as compared with the decapitate seems traceable to two factors:

(1) The extensor phases of the stepping movement are more vigorous. In other words, that prespinal mechanism which importantly contributes to standing contributes also to the extensor phase of the movement of the

[1] From *J. Physiol.*, 1910, **40**, 115-16.

step. It reinforces by its adjuvant action each extension phase whether primary or due to rebound. This adjuvant action is therefore added to the factors of the reflex step in the more complete form in which the step occurs in the decerebrate preparation.

(2) The stepping movements of the limbs are combined with the tonic reflex which maintains the erect position of the animal as a whole.

In virtue of these two factors the performance of mere stepping movements as exhibited by the decapitate preparation is amplified in the decerebrate preparation into the performance of actual walking and running— imperfect, it is true, especially in regard to equilibrium, the regulation of which is almost entirely wanting, but nevertheless amounting to a certain measure of effective locomotion.

As to what nervous mechanism it is which, present in the decerebrate preparation and absent from the spinal, contributes so importantly to reflex standing and to the extensor phase of the step, and tends to convert alternating reflexes into tonic postures by suppressing refractory phase, a main portion of it clearly lies between the levels of anterior colliculis and hinder edge of pons. It can hardly be the otic labyrinths, for their bilateral destruction leaves these reactions still elicitable. The paracerebellar nuclei[1] are within the confines of the region to which the reaction is traced. Whatever the morphological field of the mechanism it is clear that its removal exerts at first a depression amounting to annihilation of reflex standing and to great weakening of the step, especially of the step's extensor phase. Gradually in the course of weeks and months both reflexes recover partly. The recovery, however, never in my experience amounts to full qualitative restitution of the original reactions in which the prespinal mechanism participates.

6. PARAPLEGIA IN FLEXION[2]

[*In the spinal monkey the lower limbs often come to assume a flexed posture (paraplegia in flexion). This appears to be the result of an unequal recovery of reflexes, the extensor reflexes usually remaining in abeyance in this animal. When posture is long-continued structural shortening of the muscles (contracture) occurs.*]

The cord having been transected in the lower thoracic region, the monkey frequently develops, in the course of some weeks, marked rigidity of the lower limbs. Certain muscles become spastic and rigid, and gradually cease to be ever fully relaxed, and structural rigidity may in time supervene. The hypertonic and rigid muscles are especially the flexors of the hips and of the knees. In five months' time the position permanently assumed by the limbs is as follows: they are drawn up and somewhat crossed. The flexion of hips and knees may be extreme, the adduction of the thighs is less. I cannot myself escape the conviction that the position assumed

---

[1] Thiele, *J. Physiol.*, 1905, **32**, 358; Horsley, *Brain*, 1906, **29**, 455.
[2] Extract from *Philos. Trans.*, 1898, **190B**, 158.

by the limb, and the late rigidity itself and its distribution in the musculature, is the natural outcome of the fact that after the cord had been
sundered from the brain the inequality of incidence of the local stream of
centripetal impulses, and the fact that at its *embouchement* it selects, employs,
and discharges motoneurones for flexion of hip and knee, and neglects
the antergic extensors, leads, in due course, to a permanent upset of balance
between the two, in which relative over-action is continuous in the one,
and atrophy, yielding, and under-action existent in the other.   In one
monkey the amount of rigid flexion of the hips and knees was unequal
on the two sides, the left hip and knee being kept more flexed than the
right: in this animal reflexes were more easily elicited from the skin of the
left limb than of the right, but owing to the more rigid condition of the left
limb, the movement obtained was generally less in the left than right limb.
It was, in fact, easier to obtain movement of the right hip and knee from
many parts of the skin of the left limb than from the skin of right itself.
From the front of the left thigh, flexion of the left hip and adduction of the
right thigh, with slight extension of the right knee, could be regularly
evoked.   The greater rigidity was, therefore, present in that limb which
possessed the greater sensitiveness.   This supports, therefore, the view of
the spinal reflex origin of the late rigidity which I here put forward.   The
same explanation, with little modification, may apply to the later rigidities
occurring in limbs, subsequent to lesions of the limb areas of the cortex
cerebri.   After reading the recent admirable account, by Hermann Munk,[1]
of rigidities after cerebral ablations in the monkey, I should quite agree
with him that in the constant assumption of the sitting pose in cramped
cages, an important adjuvant condition in the production of late rigidity
in the monkey has been discovered by him.   At the same time, in the
occurrence of late rigidity of the lower limbs after spinal section, I look
upon a natural inequality of reflex spinal play in, or employment of, individual spinal mechanisms (*e.g.*, reflex spinal flexion of knee, and reflex
spinal extension of knee respectively), and the gradual, almost inevitably
resulting loss of functional balance between antergic sets of spino-muscular
apparatus, as the prime factor.   For instance, flexors of the knee become
contracted when the cord is transected, because extensors, practically
inaccessible to spinal reflexes of short path and of ordinary stimulus-intensity,
never exert that normal maximal stretching which, even if artificially given
from time to time, successfully defers their surrender to contracture.   My
view is that the contracture is the expression and result of the over-balance
of the spinal tonus of the extensors of hip and knee by that of the flexors.   I
look upon its origin as of reflex nature, and this is borne out by the fact that
in my monkeys it could, in its earlier stages—*i.e.*, before structural changes in
the muscles set in—be set aside by chemical anæsthesia, and by applying an
Esmarch bandage to the limbs.

[1] *SitzBer. preuss. Akad. Wiss.*, 1895.

7. TONE CONSIDERED AS A POSTURAL REACTION

[Discussion of the meaning of muscular " tone." Its relation to posture. Postural reactions as a general property of muscle both voluntary and involuntary. The postural reflexes of striped muscle are a function of the proprioceptive system.]

[1]A fairly literal meaning attaching to the term " tonus " is, of course, " mechanical tension." In this sense it fits well the slight, steady, enduring tension so characteristic of muscles in their state of reflex tonicity. This meaning of the term is evident in the definition quoted from Hughes Bennett. But in its early use, by J. Müller and writers of that period, the term carried also or soon came to carry the implication of " automatism."[2]

One meets the term in Humboldt's[3] *Researches on Muscle and Nerve* of 1907; there it is applied to nerve, and though used only occasionally, evidently refers to some then current view which postulates an intrinsic activity of the nerves and nervous system generally. That meaning out-lived considerably the discovery that the tonus of which Müller[4] spoke was reflex and not the outcome of automatism of nerve-centres. The connotation of the term has drifted in various directions from the literal meaning of mechanical tension. It is applied to the activity of nerve-centres, thus: " tonic nerve-centres," " tonic discharge of nerve-cells," and the " bio-tonus " of living matter. In these departures there is always more or less prevalent the signification " lasting " and " enduring " muscular or nervous action as contrasted with evanescent or passing. Today we commonly speak of the action of a muscle or nerve as tonic when we wish to indicate that it is relatively long-lasting. The term has become somewhat vague by reason of the multiplicity of meanings attached to it. But one service expected of a technical term is that it should be precise and unequivocal.

And the conception itself, as well as the term, labours in one important respect under vagueness. Physiology pursues analysis of the reactions of the body considered as physical and chemical events; but, further, it aims at giving reasoned accounts of the acts of an organism in respect of their purpose and use to the organism *qua* organism. This may be called a teleological aim, yet belongs to a teleology not foreign to the scope of natural science. In animal behaviour the more complex the act the less equivocal usually its biological meaning. The physiologist in analysing animal reactions seeks, as a rule, components more elementary than those toward which the " behaviourist " directs his work. Thus the " behaviourist " examines a train of acts characterising some instinct; he seeks to describe the sequence of events from their outset in initiatory stimuli onward to

---

[1] Extract from " Postural Activity in Muscle and Nerve," *Brain*, 1915, **38**, 192.

[2] See also the " Note on the History of the Word ' Tonus ' as a Physiological Term," Sherrington, contribution to *Medical and Biological Research dedicated to Sir William Osler*, 1919, **1**, 261.

[3] v. Humboldt, A., *Versuche ii. Muskeln. u. Nerven*, Fraser, 1797.

[4] Müller, J., *Handbuch d. Physiol.*, 1834.

movements and turning-points of movements often each one of high complexity and intricate co-ordination, and yet each one sufficiently unitary to serve for his present purpose as one separable piece of the train of behaviour he is fractioning. The physiologist aims at yet simpler units—for instance, at the characteristics of a synaptic function, or the dissociation of the periodicity of a nerve-centre's activity from that of a muscle's activity. He takes for his problem reflexes usually much simpler than those studied by the " behaviourist." Yet every reflex is in its own measure an integral reaction, and is purposive in that it bears some biological purport for its organism. Every reflex can therefore be regarded from the point of view of what may be called its " aim." To glimpse at the aim of a reflex is to gain hints for further experimentation on it. Such a clue to purpose is often difficult to get; and attribution of a wrong meaning may be worse than absence of all clue. But the difficulty is generally inversely as the complexity of the reflex. Thus the larger the muscular field involved in the reflex effect the plainer usually its purpose. A slight movement confined to a single limb or, in appearance, to a single muscle, a transient rise of arterial pressure—these observed alone lie open to many interpretations and admit of no security of inference. They are fractional reactions which may belong to any of many general reactions of varied aim. Thus reflexes observed in paraplegic man have been notoriously difficult to refer to their functional purpose. On the other hand, in lower animals where depression of spinal function and spinal shock are less, the ampler reflex actions, embracing by irradiation wider groups of associated muscles, often write their own meaning clear, and can indeed give a clue to the meaning of the analogous reactions less obviously decipherable in man.

When the spinal dog in response to an irritative stimulus of the scapular skin brings the hind-foot to the irritated point and scratches there, the purpose of the reaction is clear. And a reflex of simple kind may have as much purposive completeness as a complex one. Thus the reflex emptying a viscus, though it involves but a restricted field of musculature, may be as complete for its purpose as is such a reflex as walking, which involves skeletal musculature practically throughout the body.

Further, among data helpful for assigning its purpose to a reflex is the fashion of its elicitation, the nature of the adequate stimulus. That a faradic stimulus applied to the back of the tongue in a decerebrate cat interrupts the rhythm of the respiratory movements is an observation which may leave us in doubt as to the biological meaning of the result. But the same result when caused by putting a few drops of water on the back of the tongue suggests an obvious " purpose," and the interpretation is clinched by the reflex swallow which ensues.

As to muscular tonus, much of it is reflex. To know the biological purpose of such a reflex reaction is to have suggestions for lines along which to investigate it. The question arises, Does muscular tonus carry the same biological meaning in all its examples, or does it in some cases meet one

purpose, in other cases meet another? The decipherment of what biological meanings its various instances possess should help towards obtaining
a broader standpoint for evaluating the whole phenomenon itself. A
step toward this is to consider manifestations of it in particular cases. In
the first place a field of musculature may be taken which is skeletal, because
although complex its very specialisation reveals the more clearly the particular purpose it effects.

[1]The tonus of skeletal muscle can be studied favourably in the mammalian preparation. Removal of the brain from the posterior colliculi
forwards in the cat provides an excellent tonic preparation of the extensor
muscle of the knee. This tonus is still retained by the muscle to the full
after severance of all the skin nerves of both hind-limbs. Further, the
muscle still retains its full tonus after severance of *all* nerves of both limbs
excepting only the nerve of the tonic muscle itself. That nerve consists,
of course, of fibres afferent as well as efferent. The afferent fibres are
traceable partly from the muscle's tendon, but mainly from the muscle
itself. These afferent fibres reach the spinal cord via the dorsal (posterior)
roots of two spinal nerves (the 5th and 6th lumbar in the cat). If these
two afferent dorsal roots are severed, the tonus at once vanishes from the
muscle, although the corresponding ventral roots containing the motor
fibres for the muscle remain intact, and although all the other nerves of
the limbs remain intact as well. And similar experiments with other
muscles exhibiting tonus—*e.g.*, gastrocnemius, semimembranosus, triceps,
supraspinatus—meet the same result. In each case the tonus of these muscles
requires the afferent fibres of the tonic muscle itself, and in the decerebrate
cat preparation no other afferent fibres than those of the tonic muscle itself
are actually essential for the exhibition of the tonus.

The tonus of these muscles in this decerebrate preparation is not a
phenomenon requiring for its detection and demonstration any refined
apparatus, or indeed any apparatus at all. It and its features are palpable
and obvious; graphic records of it are obtainable by relatively coarse
methods. The extensor muscle of the knee, m. vastocrureus, lends itself
well to the purpose. That and the three other muscles mentioned above
are specimens of the tonic muscles in this preparation. But many other
muscles in this preparation show the tonicity as well. In the hind-limb
the distribution of the tonicity in the musculature shows the following
feature: If the reflex act of stepping is examined, as it may be both in the
spinal and in the decerebrate preparation (cat), the act is found to consist
of two phases. In one phase—the flexion phase—the foot is lifted slightly
from the ground, and the limb is swept forward by flexion of hip, accompanied by flexion at knee and ankle, so that the foot may clear the ground
in its advance. In this phase all the flexor muscles of the limb are excited

[1] Extract from *Brain*, 1915, **38,** 195.

to contract, and all its extensor muscles are inhibited by reflex inhibition. The other phase—the extension phase—is that in which the foot being in contact with the ground, the limb is straightened at knee and ankle, and kept from bending under the body's weight by the extensors of those joints; and at the hip the extensors, using the foot's *point d'appui* against the ground as a fulcrum for the leverage of the limb, push the body forward. In this phase all the extensors of the limb are in active contraction, and the flexors are reflexly inhibited. The distribution of the reflex tonus of the decerebrate preparation in the musculature of the limb is exactly to those muscles which are in active contraction in the extensor phase of the step, to those and to no others.

In the fore-limb, though this analysis of the exact distribution in the musculature of the extensor phase of the step has not been so completely made, the analysis, so far as it goes, shows again exact correspondence between the musculature exhibiting the tonus and those engaged in contracting the extensor phase of the step. The two phenomena involve, and are confined to, the same group of muscles. It is in the extensor phase of the step that the limb is supporting the weight of the body.

The distribution of the tonus in the limb musculature reveals, therefore, arrangement on a plan of strict co-ordination. It is, however, not confined to the musculature of the limbs. It is as markedly present in various other regions. In the trunk it obtains in the muscles which bend the vertebral column upwards (opisthotonos); in the neck in those muscles which lift (retract) the neck and head; in the caudal region in those which lift the tail; in the head in those which close the jaw. It is not present in those muscles which bend the spine downwards, droop the neck and tail, flex the head, depress the jaw. It seems to be present, but of this I am not entirely sure, in the ventral muscles of the abdominal wall. Evidently, therefore, the distribution of this reflex tonicity embraces just those muscles whose contraction tends in the erect position of the animal to counteract the effect of gravity on the various several regions, the muscles which prevent those parts, and the animal as a whole, from sinking to the ground. And from the muscles antagonistic to these the reflex tonicity is absent. In other words, the reflex tonus obtains in, and is confined to, those muscles which maintain the animal in an erect attitude. That this is so may be demonstrated by setting the decerebrate preparation on its feet; it is then seen that the preparation stands. Thus this reflex tonicity, which when seen in a single isolated muscle prepared for the myograph does not carry on the face of it any very obvious biological purpose, does carry a clear and unmistakable biological purpose when the phenomenon is followed in the musculature as a whole. The reflex tonus is postural contraction. Decerebrate rigidity is simply reflex standing. The reflex tonicity of the skeletal muscles of the decerebrate cat and dog is shown by its co-ordination, its effects, and its distribution in the musculature, to be a reflex which differs from the reflexes more commonly studied mainly in this, that the latter execute *movements* while this maintains *posture*. The reflex tonus is, in short, reflex posture, and in this case the posture maintained is that of *standing*. And the reflex posture is modifiable on the supervention of certain additional stimuli, and the modifications of posture thus obtained are so intelligible as forms of standing adapted to particular purposes that they carry on the face of them that significance. If the head of the reflexly standing decerebrate preparation be forcibly flexed, the postural contraction of the extensor muscles of the fore-limbs is inhibited, and the animal's fore-quarters sink, while at the same time the postural contraction of the extensors of the hind-limbs increases, raising the hind-quarters. The preparation thus assumes the attitude of a cat looking under a shelf. On the contrary, if the head of the preparation is passively tilted up and back the postural contraction of the extensor muscles of the fore-limbs increases, raising the fore-quarters, and at the same time the postural contraction of the extensors of the hind-limbs is diminished so that the hind-quarters sink. The preparation thus assumes the posture of a cat looking up to a shelf. There goes further with each main posture of the head even passively imposed upon the decerebrate preparation a corresponding reflex modification of the reflex posture of the limbs. Magnus and de Kleijn,[1] to whom is owing the elucidation of this subject, have described these fully, and shown their constancy, and shown further that the centripetal impulses causing these reflex modifications of the reflex standing are traceable for their one part to the otic labyrinth, for their other part to the deep afferent nerves (proprioceptors) of the neck itself. These experimenters have succeeded in separating the reflex results from the two sources, and have thus determined what part each source plays in the combined effects which under natural conditions are those of usual occurrence.

As mentioned above, the afferent nerves producing and maintaining this postural reflex of standing are the afferent nerves of the posturally contracting muscles themselves. The whole reflex posture of standing is thus one great compound reflex built up of a number of component reflexes. To the making of the total reflex posture there goes the postural reflex of each limb, similarly the postural reflex of the neck, of the trunk, of the tail, of the head. And the reflex posture of each component region is in large measure separable from that of the rest, and is capable, within limits, of modification, although remaining still contributory to the general posture of standing. This is in accord with the natural occurrence of, for instance, such a modification of the erect posture as " sitting " in the cat or the rabbit —a posture half-way between lying down and standing, the fore-limbs " standing " and the hind-limbs lying down.

And the local reflex posture, say, of a limb, can be modified by local influences. It is in the examination of these that we meet with exemplification of characteristics of postural contraction to which attention will be drawn in dealing with the postural contraction of muscular walls of the

---

[1] Magnus, R., and De Kleijn, *Pflüg. Arch. ges. Physiol.*, 1912, **145**, 455, and following papers.

hollow viscera and bloodvessels. In the posturally acting skeletal muscles these characters appear as what have been termed the " lengthening " and " shortening reactions." The " lengthening reaction " and the " shortening reaction " are given by the skeletal muscles of the cat in postural contraction, and they are given also by the smooth muscle of the viscera and of invertebrata. Just as the postural configuration of the knee or elbow is adjustable by these means, so likewise is that of the bladder or the stomach.

The skeletal musculature by reason of these lengthening and shortening reactions allows that latitude of pose which is so useful and familiar a feature in natural attitudes. The animal may stand with right foot in advance of left, or left in advance of right, or with the two feet abreast of each other; all these differences in detail from local posture to local posture are compatible with the general posture of standing in the animal as a whole. The postural reflex contraction is plastic in this sense, hence the term *plastic tonus*[1] has been applied to it. The skeletal muscle in this form of reflex contraction can quite readily adjust itself to different lengths while counteracting one and the same load.

The alterations in posture, to which the limb is subjected in showing its power of adjustment, may be alterations imposed by passive movement. The observer moves the limb into the new attitude which the reflex postural contraction then takes up and lightly fixes. But the reflex adaptation to the new posture occurs just as well, or better, when the changed position of the joint is brought about by active reflex movement excited, for instance, by faradising an afferent nerve-trunk. Thus in the postural reflex preparation when a reflex extension movement of the knee has been provoked, the shortening reaction appends itself to the reflex contraction, and on discontinuing the stimulus which caused the extension movement the extensor muscle still remains shortened, and the knee still continues in the extended position.

[2]The existence in various invertebrata of muscles separately differentiated for execution of movements and for maintenance of posture respectively seems without parallel in the skeletal musculature of vertebrates. In the latter, one and the same muscle is used for the two purposes, though some muscles are predominantly concerned with the one, some with the other function. Perhaps the nearest approach to muscles of purely postural function in mammals are the sphincter muscles controlling orifices. But in most of the more complex reflex acts the reflex while employing some muscles for execution of movement simultaneously employs others for maintaining posture. Thus, in the scratch-reflex, while one hind-limb is engaged in the rhythmic scratching movement the reflex employs the muscles of

[1] Sherrington, *Quart. J. exp. Physiol.*, 1909, **2,** 109, and *Proc. roy. Soc.*, 1908, **80B,** 552.
[2] From *Brain*, 1915, **38,** 205.

the other three limbs and of the neck and head for the maintenance of a characteristic posture which continues so long as the reflex scratching continues. Similarly, in a powerful nociceptive flexion-reflex, while the stimulated limb maintains the attitude of flexion the other limbs frequently perform stepping movements, just as in the intact animal that has stepped on a thorn the injured foot is held folded up and the other legs run away. And with these skeletal muscles one and the same muscle may at the same time exhibit both postural contraction and phasic or movement contractions. Thus, in the scratch-reflex, there is required in order that the hind-limb reach the neck and apply there its scratching movement a certain posturing of the limb as well as rhythmic movement of it. For this there is demanded some postural flexion of the hip. It is found that the sartorius muscle, which is a flexor of hip and knee, shows in this case a well-marked degree of steady postural contraction as well as, over and above that, the characteristic four per second rhythmic contraction of the scratching movement itself.

A question which arises is whether in all cases the reflex postural action of skeletal muscle depends normally upon the afferent nerve of the posturing muscle itself. In the reflex posture of standing exhibited by the decerebrate cat that does largely seem to be the case. Severance of the afferent spinal roots of both hind-limbs in the dog (Bickel[1]) renders standing with those limbs impossible for a considerable period; but in the course of time the animal becomes able to support itself upon them, a compensation traceable to labyrinths, cerebellum, and motor region of cerebral cortex. In the pigeon, severance of the afferent roots of both hind-limbs makes standing impossible (Trendelenburg). Severance of the afferent roots of one leg impairs also the flexion posture assumed by the hind-limb during flight. Section of the afferent roots of the wing affects little, if at all, the folded posture maintained by the wing when not in flight—e.g., during standing or walking. Nor has the source of the postural contraction of the flexors of the wing been found. Here, as in the case of the iris, the postural contraction if, as is presumable, reflex, lies in receptors not those of the contracting muscles themselves—is, in short, allogenous, not autogenous.

That receptors other than those of the contracting muscles themselves can be adjuvant to the reflex postural action maintained by these latter is evidenced in many observations. For instance, Ewald[2] has shown that the postural closure of the pigeon's beak is impaired by destruction of the labyrinth; and after splitting the lower bill into its two lateral halves he found that destruction of the right labyrinth weakened the postural contraction of the right half much more than that of the left: the movement of closure was often fully executed, but with the right half the closed posture was less powerfully maintained; this was clearly demonstrable by hanging upon each of the separate halves one of a pair of equal weights—the right

[1] Bickel, A., *Unters. ü. d. Mechanismus d. Nervösen Bewegungsreg.*, 1903.
[2] Ewald, R., *Nervus Octavus*, 1892.

half did not maintain the closed posture under so heavy a load as did the left, an observation recalling those on the pecten shell.

And Magnus and de Kleijn[1] have shown the existence of a number of important postural reflexes of labyrinthine origin affecting the extensor muscles of the limbs. To excite the labyrinth they employed modes of stimulation natural to it, " adequate " stimuli—namely, posings of the head in regard to the direction of gravitational force. The labyrinth is a receptive organ specialised for reacting to gravitation force, hence it initiates sensations reporting on the spatial relation of the head to axes running through it and the earth's centre—in short, to the vertical—and the reflexes which the labyrinth initiates consist in adjustments of the head, including eyeballs and jaw, to the vertical. The action of the muscles in the posture of standing is anti-gravitational. Hence it is not surprising that the labyrinth reactions should be related to and influence the anti-gravitational reflex of standing, though this latter has its origin in the receptive organs of the standing muscles themselves. Magnus and de Kleijn show that the labyrinthine influence on the postural contraction of the extensors of the limbs is adjuvant and symmetrical for each limb-pair—that is, right and left fore-limbs are affected similarly and together, and right and left hind-limb similarly and together. They show that the adjuvant influence is greatest when the head is inverted, least when the head is right side up, and that in lateral positions of the head the influence is of intermediate degree. In these experiments the influence of neck posture was excluded by fixating the neck in plaster of Paris or by severance of the afferent roots of the upper cervical nerves.

They examined also the influence of neck posture on the posture of the limbs in reflex standing. To do this the labyrinths were destroyed. Postures of the neck in which the head retains a symmetrical relation to the body affect the postural contraction of the right and left limbs symmetrically. Flexion of the neck, bending it ventrally, decreases the postural contraction of the extensor muscles of the fore-limbs and increases that of the extensors of the hind-limbs. Extension of neck, lifting it dorsally, increases the postural extension of the fore-limbs and decreases that of the extensors of the hind-limbs. Postures of the neck bringing the head out of symmetrical relation to the body influence the limb postures asymmetrically; the limbs of that side to which the lower jaw and snout are turned exhibit increased extensor action, the contralateral decreased extensor action.

The labyrinth affects not only the limb posture but also the neck posture. The head (labyrinth) posture which most supports the extensors of the limbs likewise most supports the postural contraction of the retraction of the neck, and conversely. Since the neck and head commonly alter their posture in combination their influences act usually in combination on the limbs. The strange postures assumed after labyrinthine extirpation and disease are largely traceable to abnormal postures thus imposed on the neck and influencing in their turn the postures of the limbs.

[1] Magnus, R., and de Kleijn, *Pflüg. Arch. ges. Physiol.*, 1912, **145,** 455, and following papers.

The modifications shown by Magnus and de Kleijn to occur in the postural reflex of decerebrate rigidity by influences coming from the labyrinths and muscular afferents of the neck are all of them confirmatory of the inference that that postural reflex is reflex standing. As mentioned above, depression of the neck such as occurs when the normal animal looks under a low shelf causes lowering of the fore-quarters and the assumption of just such a modification of standing as occurs normally in that act. The raising and retraction of the head and neck increase the extension of the fore-limbs and lower the hind-quarters just as when the normal animal looks up at a high shelf. The bending of the neck and head to the right causes increased extension and advancement of the fore-limb as normally occurs when the animal modifies its attitude for gazing round to the right. The increase of extension of the limbs when the preparation is inverted is also what happens in the normal animal when it is inverted; of course, the normal animal usually struggles against such an attitude being forced upon it, but, when that resistance is over, it, just as Verworn has shown in the guinea-pig, keeps the limbs extended strongly upwards, and may, by what is sometimes termed hypnosis, maintain that protective posture for a long time, even when left to itself and free from restraint.

That in the reflex standing of the decerebrate cat and dog the postural contraction of the anti-gravity muscles, which is its essential mechanism, is in the main a proprioceptive reaction whose afferent nerves are those of the anti-gravity muscles themselves is clear. As to the nervous centres involved, the following seem the main facts: In the dog after transection of the spinal cord in the hinder thoracic region, when in the course of some months the depression of spinal function, termed spinal shock, has subsided, the hind-limbs are not rarely able to stand. They can bear erect the superincumbent hind-quarters, so much so that the observer placing his hand under the hind-feet can find that, on lifting the hand suddenly, the erect posture of the hind-limbs is sufficiently strong to maintain itself, while the hinder portion of the animal is danced up and down by the hand so placed. And the spinal hind-limbs will maintain their standing posture for half an hour at a time. But it is subject to sudden lapses the cause of which may not be obvious, although it is often some evident stimulus to the foot or elsewhere exciting intercurrent reflex flexion of the limb. But although spinal centres isolated from prespinal are, after the period of spinal shock has passed, able *per se* to maintain the posture at least in fair degree in cat and dog, they cannot in the period immediately following the isolating transection. Normally, some prespinal centre, or probably several centres, is adjuvant either in the sense that the postural reflex besides employing the spinal centres employs prespinal as well, or in the sense that the spinal centres which the reflex employs are kept up to the mark for that reaction by influence exerted on them by prespinal. As to where these prespinal centres lie the following can be said: Unessential for crude maintenance of the act of standing in cat and dog are the whole fore-brain and mid-brain back to and inclusive of the posterior colliculi. Likewise the labyrinths are not necessary since they can be destroyed and the reflex posture persist. Further, the cerebellum can be removed without the posture being annulled. Evidently the prespinal centres necessary lie in the pontine region or bulb, or both, though mainly in the former.

But though the neural mechanism of the standing posture does not essentially demand for its crude performance those mid- and hind-brain regions, these do afford it assistance, and, as Magnus and de Kleijn's observations prove for the octavus nerves, provide for it reflex adjustment in manifold important ways. And Weed's[1] experiments indicate that the cerebellum commonly lends it a large amount of support and doubtless of refined adjustment and correlation too.

[2]Posture may be passive or active. The former—for instance, the postures of a dead body impressed on it by gravity, etc.—are of course outside this inquiry. Active posture largely compasses the counteraction of those effects which gravitation, etc., produce in the dead body. Active postures may be described as those *reactions in which the configuration of the body and of its parts is, in spite of forces tending to disturb them, preserved by the activity of contractile tissues, these tissues then functioning statically.* The rôle of muscle as an executant of movements is so striking that its office in preventing movement and displacement is somewhat overlooked. When a movement, whether active or passive, has brought about a change in the configuration of a limb —*e.g.*, by flexing one of its joints—an important function of the musculature may be to maintain the new configuration, the posture. In doing this the muscle *prevents* movement, not makes it; it then acts statically and, though in a state of contraction, does no mechanical work whether the tension it develops in thus maintaining its and the limb's new configuration be great or small. Just as the limb assumes, in result of a movement either passively imposed upon it or actively executed by it, various configurations and can maintain each of these with various degrees of tension—for instance, the arm horizontal with a 2 kg. weight in the hand for a 6 kg. weight— so the hollow muscular viscus after partial evacuation, or after introduction of more content, assumes a new configuration, conformably with the changed volume of content, and this new configuration is in both cases maintained by the activity of the muscle functioning statically. Here the assumption of a new configuration and the maintenance of it are muscular in the viscus just as in the limb, and the essential nature of the muscular reaction exhibited is in the viscus that which it is in the limb. Such reaction in the musculature of the limb is called postural; it is conducive to clearness if in the viscus also it be termed postural. Both are instances of the postural contraction of the muscle; though the relation of the central nervous system to the postural activity is very different in the two cases. But the essential

[1] Weed, L., *J. Physiol.*, 1914, **48**, 205.   [2] From *Brain*, 1915, **38**, 217.

identity of the two cases justifies, and is helpfully kept in view by using, such phrases concerning a muscular reservoir viscus as that it exhibits a quarter-pint posture, or a half-pint posture, and so on, according to the amount of its contents, and that both in the one and in the other posture it may exert one and the same pressure on its contents.

The bladder is no isolated instance of a muscular viscus exhibiting these volumetric postures.

[1]The upshot of experiments on unstriped muscle is that this type of muscle, besides producing movement contractions or beats, is able to maintain itself at various lengths, exerting under all those various lengths approximately one and the same tension. The wall of a hollow viscus is thus able to hold the fluid contents of the viscus at approximately the same pressure whether those contents are copious or not, because of the ability of its fibres to exert the same tension whatever the form, shorter or longer, within a certain wide range, which they have assumed. And their differences in length during this activity can be so great as to allow differences in the capaciousness of the organ suggestive of actual slipping of the muscle-fibres upon each other. Tonus as applied to such a condition seems an equivocal term. If the pressure of the wall on the viscus content be taken as criterion of tonus, then tonus has nothing to say about the state of shortness or of elongation of the muscle, for these are independent of the pressure. If tonus be transferred from its literal meaning to one descriptive of form, and be used to indicate the state of shortness of the muscle—thus if the bladder when maintaining a small or restricted volume be considered to have more tonus than maintaining a large and " dilated " capacity—then, since these states of size have no constant relation to states of tension, tonus appears a misnomer, since it then retains nothing at all of its original and literal meaning. Skeletal muscle exhibits exactly the same properties as these just described in unstriped muscle, and skeletal muscle exhibits them when it performs one of its chief functions—namely, the maintenance of posture. With the unstriped muscles of the viscera and bloodvessels, just as with the striped muscles of the skeletal frame, it seems therefore preferable, because more direct, to speak of this form of activity as postural.

The application of the term tonus to sphincter muscles illustrates its employment as meaning posture. A sphincter is described as exhibiting tonus when it maintains a closed posture of the orifice it guards. Tonus here means nothing but postural contraction.

[2]In a previous contribution to *Brain*[3] an outline was attempted of what was there termed the proprioceptive division of the nervous system. That

---

[1] Extract from *Brain*, 1915, **38**, 224.   [2] *Ibid.*, 1915, **38**, 233.
[3] Sherrington, *Brain*, Hughlings Jackson number, 1906, **29**, 467.

division, it was shown, has distinctive features anatomical and functional, rendering advisable its consideration as a mechanism with peculiarities sufficiently its own to warrant its being dealt with broadly as an entity by itself. The postural action of muscles and nerves, the subject of the present paper, is a main outcome of the functioning of the proprioceptive part of the nervous system—at least it is so as regards the skeletal musculature, perhaps as regards the visceral and vascular musculature also. Reflex maintenance and adjustment of posture is a chief portion of the reflex work of the proprioceptive system, just as sensation of and perception of posture is a chief portion of the psychical output of that system.

8. THE STRETCH-REFLEX AS BASIS OF POSTURE[1]

[*The postural reflex can be analysed in each muscle in terms of its reaction to stretch (the " stretch-reflex "). The proprioceptors in muscle include end-organs other than the stretch receptors, with different reflex effect.*]

The receptors played upon by the events of the external world supply their " drive " to the muscles. In reflex action they do so far more simply and for far more simple purposes than when the trains of reaction they set going have to thread the mazes of the higher brain, and, so to say, obtaining mental sanction, issue in acts remoter from the original stimulus. Yet in both cases the muscles lie at the behest of the receptors, as instruments of their hand.

We should go too far, however, did we infer that the muscles themselves are instruments entirely passive under drive of the receptors acting on them from without. That they are agents not purely passive is shown by their possession of receptors of their own. On their own behalf they send messages into the central exchanges. This must mean they have some voice in their own conditions of service, perhaps ring themselves up and ring themselves off. Let us attempt to penetrate into the significance of this their " receptivity."

It is a receptivity differing obviously from that of other receptors, rightly more commonly chosen to exemplify receptive function, such as retina, ear, tongue, tactile organs, and so on, for in the case of the receptors of muscle, instead of being stimulated directly by agents of the external world, they are stimulated by happenings in the microcosm of the body itself—namely, events in the muscles themselves. In muscular receptivity we see the body itself acting as stimulus to its own receptors. The receptors of muscle have therefore been termed " proprioceptors."

Following the functional scheme of all receptors, we may be sure that the central reactions provoked by the receptors of muscle will be divisible into, on the one hand, the purely reflex, and on the other hand, those which subserve mental experience.

[1] Extract from " Problems of Muscular Receptivity," Linacre Lecture, *Nature*, 1924, June 21 and 28.

Let us turn to the simpler of these divisions, the purely reflex. For that purpose, appeal can be had to what may with justification be regarded as a partially surviving animal—an animal which, its cerebral hemispheres having been removed, is a wholly inconscient and purely reflex automaton. From it no sight or sound evokes evidence of perception. There is total inability to evoke from it any sign of mentality, of emotion, let alone intelligence. It remains motionless hour after hour; yet if planted upon its feet in the upright position it stands, and statuelike continues to stand.

Now, standing is a postural act, and one of course of high importance. In maintaining posture the muscles, though they perform no external work, are active with an activity often technically termed "tonus," a postural contraction. In this maintenance of the erect posture by the decerebrate animal, we meet a co-ordinated posture involving many separate muscles harmoniously co-ordinated reflexly. For this reflex postural act of standing some stimulus must be at work evoking and maintaining it. We have to ask what that stimulus may be.

If the afferent nerves that pass from a limb to the spinal centres be severed, the standing posture in that limb is no longer fully executed or maintained. The stimulus exciting the posture in that limb must be something which is applied to the receptors of that limb itself. The skin surface of the limb is rich in receptors, one region especially rich being the sole of the foot. On the receptors of the skin of the sole of the foot the external world may evidently be acting as a stimulus in the form of pressure from the ground upon the skin. To test whether that is the source of the reflex posture, the skin of the foot can be deprived of all its receptors by severing their nerves. This is found to exert no obvious influence upon the posture. Nor does severance of all the receptive nerves from the skin of the whole limb, nor, indeed, from that of all the four limbs. The stimulus producing and maintaining the posture is therefore not pressure of the skin against the ground, nor indeed any cutaneous stimulus whatsoever. On the other hand, if, even without interference with the skin nerves, the receptive nerves of the limb-muscles—the motor nerves, of course, remaining intact—be severed, the reflex posture disappears at once from the limb. The stimulus which produces and maintains the posture is something which is acting on and exciting the receptive nerves of the muscles of the limb.

What are the muscles which, by their contraction, execute this postural act? The posture keeps the head and neck from sinking, the trunk straightened and the spine supported, the tail from drooping, the limbs from yielding and folding under the superincumbent weight of the body. In a word, this habitual reflex posture counteracts in the various parts of the body the effect of gravity on them in the erect attitude. Experimental analysis shows that throughout the muscular frame of the animal all those muscles, and only those, are in action, the activity of which counteracts gravity in the erect attitude—for example, in the hind-limb the muscles which extend hip, knee, and ankle. The muscles which execute the reflex we may, in short, term " antigravity " muscles. Even the jaw is included; the lower jaw, which, but for its postural tonus, would drop, is held lifted against the upper.

If in the limb the receptive nerve of one of these antigravity muscles be cut, that muscle no longer contributes to the reflex posture. On the other hand, severance of the receptive nerves of all the other muscles does not destroy the postural reflex of the muscle the receptive nerve of which remains intact. The stimulus which is the source of this reflex standing is therefore one acting on the receptors of those limb-muscles which are themselves executants of the posture.

The excitability of a receptor is selective. That is, construction fits the receptor to respond to stimuli of one particular kind only, the so-called " adequate " stimulus; thus, the retina to light, a taste papilla to " sweet," and so on. Hence Pavlov's term " analyser " for the receptors, because by them the various complex events which play upon the body and cause reactions of it through the nervous system are to some extent analysed. A wave breaking on the shore excites the retina by its reflected lights, the ear by sound vibrations, and, maybe, the skin by the spray dashed up. The wave as " object " and stimulus from the external world is thus partially analysed by the receptors.

Seeing that the receptors of muscle are an appendage of an organ mechanical in function, a near supposition is that their adequate stimulus is of mechanical kind. What is the adequate stimulus at work in these antigravity muscles in their posture of standing ?

A muscle representative of the whole antigravity group is the extensor of the knee. Suppose it isolated from the rest and its freed tendon attached to a stiff spring, and to the spring a light lever so fixed that movement of the lever-point is photographically recorded. If then, by its bony attachments, the muscle be pulled against the spring, we can passively stretch the muscle and record the tensile strain developed in it by the stretch. Let us take the case of the muscle paralysed by severance of all nerves both afferent and efferent which connect it with the nerve-centres (Fig. 61). The tension developed in the muscle as it is stretched yields a curve resembling that given by various fibrous and elastic tissues of the body, not unlike that given by a strip of indiarubber. Let us repeat the observation, but with the difference that the muscle retains unimpaired its purely efferent motor nerve. The stretching produces the same tensile curve as before, a curve practically indistinguishable from that of the wholly paralytic muscle. Then let us make the observation, with the further difference that the muscle this time retains not only its motor nerve but its receptive nerve as well. We find the muscle yields now a completely different curve of tensile strain. The tension developed by it is much greater, and its curve under equable progressive increase of the stretch runs, tensions being ordinates, convex instead of concave to the abscissa line. The muscle in response to the stretch now replies not merely by passive strain but also by active contraction of its muscle-fibres. In the muscle with its reflex arc intact, the passive pull provokes a reflex contraction of the muscle.[1] Evidently a mechanical stretching of the muscle supplies an adequate stimulus for receptors in the muscle.

The reflex is closely graded by the degree of stretch; and the degree of stretch required to excite reflex contraction is quite small. Mr. Liddell and I have seen a stretch, extending the muscle's resting length by less than 1 per cent., produce a reflex contraction registering 2,000 grammes of active tension. The reflex contraction provoked by the stretch tends to produce equilibrium between the extending force and the contractile resistance of the muscle, and thus to prevent further elongation of the

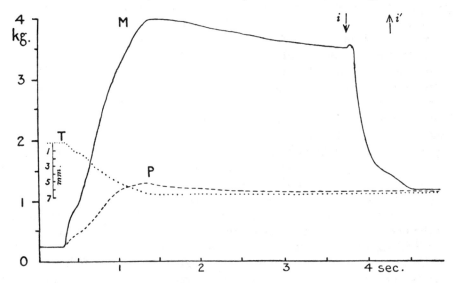

FIG. 61.—KNEE EXTENSOR MUSCLE

Effect of reflex inhibition, evoked between *i* and *i'* from afferent nerve, on the muscular reaction M to 6·5 mm. stretch T compared with reaction P of the " paralysed " muscle to similar table-stretch. Myograph multiplies tendon-movement 62 times. Time in seconds. (Liddell and Sherrington, *Proc. roy. Soc.*, 1924, **96B,** 212)

muscle. This is so whether the passive stretching is applied slowly or quickly. So soon as the stretch ceases to be increased, increase of the reflex contraction promptly ceases.

Reflex contractions produced in this muscle by other means than stretch have not such dead-beat character. Commonly, they long outlast the receptive stimulus which excites them. Stretch-reflexes, though with cessation of further increase of the stretch-stimulus further increase of the reflex contraction ceases, show persistence of the degree of contraction already reached after the progressive stretch has ceased. The question arises whether this persistence of the contraction is due, as in those other

[1] Liddell and Sherrington, *Proc. roy. Soc.*, 1924, **96B,** 212, and 1925, **97B,** 267.

cases, to continuance of central reverberation after the exciting stimulus has ceased, or whether the residual passive stretch constitutes a persisting stimulus—whether, in fact, under appropriate conditions the stretch-reflex can present itself in a purely static form. The question is not unimportant, because, if the residual stretch is a stimulus exciting and maintaining the reflex contraction, then a passive stretch-posture is exciting an active postural contraction.

This question can be examined in several ways. One is as follows: It is possible to subject the reflex arc of the muscle to inhibition—in other words, to throw it out of action temporarily. Such inhibition annuls a stretch-reflex already in progress and, if suitably timed, prevents contraction in response to a stretch however powerful. The muscle passively stretched when the inhibition is in operation exhibits the same curve of merely passive tension as does an entirely paralytic muscle. This being so, we can arrange for the inhibition to begin before and continue while the stretching movement, the " kinetic stretch," is being applied to the muscle and then, when the stretching movement is over and the residual, merely static, stretch remains, remove the inhibition. In this way the reflex arc of the muscle on which the stretch-reflex depends is, so to say, put to sleep during the kinetic stretch and until the stretching movement is finished, and then, when that is over, the reflex arc is, so to say, allowed to wake. On doing so it will find its muscle has assumed a state of stretch, of steady strain, a passively stretched posture. The result observed by this method is that the muscle on its nervous arc so waking immediately develops a reflex contraction, and then steadily maintains it (Fig. 62). The passive stretched posture acts *per se* as a stimulus. The proprioceptive nervous arc of the muscle reacts to the passive stretched posture imposed upon the muscle, and its reaction results in the production and maintenance in the muscle of an active contraction posture which opposes the passive stretch to which the muscle is subjected.

Let us revert now to the reflex " standing " exhibited by the decerebrate animal. We traced it to a postural contraction of the antigravity muscles, in each of which the contraction was due to a proprioceptive reflex excited somehow in that muscle itself. We can take as an example of the antigravity muscles the knee-extensor muscle. The tendon of that muscle bridges the extensor aspect of the knee-joint, and the superincumbent weight of the body in the erect posture tends to flex the knee. Knee-flexion stretches the extensor muscle. Gravity in the erect posture acts, therefore, on the knee-extensor as a stretching force. We have seen that such a stretch is a stimulus to certain receptors in the muscle and provokes a postural contraction which counteracts the stretching force. The reflex standing of the decerebrate animal appears, therefore, as a postural stretch-reflex.

A peculiarity which distinguishes the stretch-reflex from other reflexes is that, whereas in other reflexes the reflex contraction excited from a single source implicates whole groups of the limb-muscles, the stretch-reflex excites in its limb just the one muscle stretched. The reflex standing of the limb is an harmonious *congeries* of stretch-reflexes, each component reflex being the self-operating reaction of an individual extensor muscle. This mode of production of the reflex posture allows it latitude in detail. The standing pose is still maintained though the observer shift in detail, within limits, the position of the feet. Thus a foot may be advanced or set backward, and the shift alters the position in detail, but the reflex animal still stands. The altered incidence of gravity involved by the shift compensates itself, and greater and lesser stretch wherever they occur excite,

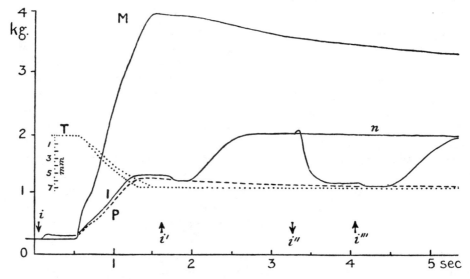

FIG. 62.—SUCCESSIVE REACTIONS M OF NORMAL, I OF REFLEXLY INHIBITED, AND P OF PARALYSED MUSCLE TO STRETCH T OF 7 MM.

The inhibition (by afferent nerve) was on first occasion from *i* to *i'*, on second occasion from *i'* to *i''* and again from *i''* to *i'''*, giving therefore on second occasion the fall from and reascent to the plateau line *n* of the first occasion. The inhibitory nerve gave slight concomitant contraction, so that full inhibitory effect is seen only close subsequent to cessation of the inhibitory stimulation. The less steep dotted line T gives the stretch for observation M; the other for observations I and P. Myograph multiplying tendon-movement 62 times. Time in seconds. (Liddell and Sherrington, *Proc. roy. Soc.*, 1924, **96B**, 212)

as we have seen, a correspondingly greater or lesser contraction which antagonises further yield and compensates the altered stretch.

The living reaction of plants and animals to gravity is called geotropism, and standing is a geotropic reaction. The stretch-reflex of the extensor muscles offers an explanation of how the limbs can antagonise gravity and stand, but that reflex provides no mechanism by which the reflex animal can, when non-erect, assume the erect posture; for that, as Magnus and de Kleijn have shown in a fascinating series of experiments, other reflexes provide, reflexes initiated by special gravity receptors in the head, the otolith organs. It is interesting to note that a group of stretch-reflexes operated by gravity should dovetail in with special gravity reflexes from the head, giving gravity still further reflex control of the whole animal's posture as regards standing. In instance of this further control there is the reflex discovered and elucidated by Magnus and de Kleijn in which, the reflex animal's initial posture being standing, a passive tilt of the head upward, thus inclining the head's gravity organs, changes the reflex posture from that of standing to that of sitting and looking up at a shelf. The hind-limbs bend and sink, the fore-limbs straighten more, bearing upward the inclined neck and head. Conversely, a passive downward tilting of the head causes, Magnus and de Kleijn have shown, the fore-limbs to crouch, bringing the fore-quarters lower than the hind-, thus modifying the standing position to that for taking food from a platter. Accepting the stretch-reflex of the limb-extensors as existent in this reflex standing, the otolith organs, reacting in postures of the head, evidently suitably control that limb-reflex, depressing or reinforcing it as circumstances dictate. The stretch-reflex of the limb-extensors is, however, a reaction essentially independent of the otolith organs, although it can be regulated by the otolith organs; it still obtains (Liddell and Sherrington) after bilateral severance of receptive nerves of the latter.[1]

Elicitation by gravity of the stretch-reflex of the limb-extensor suggests itself as a basic factor in this static geotropic reflex of standing. As such it offers an explanation of the postural contraction counteracting gravity, of the proprioceptive nature of that reaction, and of the latitude of detail allowed to the standing posture of the reflex limb. As to accepting without reserve this scope for the stretch-reflex, certain experimental facts enjoin caution. When, in obtaining the reflex preparation, the portion of brain removed encroaches backward—*i.e.*, is larger—the standing of the limb is exaggerated in degree; whereas when the decerebration is more restricted—*i.e.*, more of the brain-stem remains—the creature, though purely reflex, exhibits (Magnus and de Kleijn) a standing in which the postural contraction is practically normal in degree. In the former type, assuming for it the stretch-reflex, that reflex is giving an exaggerated caricature of standing rather than truly normal standing. This may, however, merely mean that for full normality of reflex standing several reflex factors, involving successive brain levels, co-operate, among them being the stretch-reflex of the limb-extensors, and that this reflex occurs in exaggerated form when " released " by removal of co-ordinate centres further forward. Such would have analogy with the " release " exaggeration of the reflex postural extension of the fore-limbs, which regularly ensues when the post-brachial spinal cord is severed. There the " release " seems due to severance of an inhibitory path studied in cerebellar (vermis) cortex by Banting and Miller, by Camis,

---

[1] Liddell and Sherrington (*Proc. roy. Soc.*, 1925, **97B,** 267) later reported that the stretch-reflex was obtainable after section of the 8th nerves, and after precollicular section of the brain stem as well as the more usual intercollicular level of decerebration. It is also the basis of the extensor postures of the hind-limbs of the spinal dog when these have recovered from spinal shock (Denny-Brown and Liddell, *J. Physiol.*, 1927, **63,** 144).—ED.

and by Bremer; and by Bremer traced from spino-cerebellar afferents, through cerebellum and mesencephalon, and thence back to reach spinal centres of the limb-extensors.

A more obstinate ground of difficulty appears in the experimental fact that the reflex creature, decerebrate through posterior colliculi and with otolith organs out of action by nerve-severance, retains a postural contraction of its limb-extensors when the line of gravity runs not lengthwise in the limb.

In reflex standing we met the stretch-reflex in its postural form. But, as we saw, it can also operate movements. Now locomotion, whether of walking or running, is a rhythmic movement of the limb grafted upon the erect attitude of the body. Just as the erect posture can be maintained by pure inconscient action of the nervous system, so likewise can the stepping of the limbs. In this inconscient stepping the contact of the foot with the ground might be thought to supply an important skin-stimulus reflexly evoking the step. But the receptivity of the skin seems not to actuate reflex stepping any more than it does reflex standing. Indeed, from the observations of Professor Graham Brown, an intrinsic automatic activity of the spinal centres seems the essential nervous mechanism responsible for inconscient stepping, a central activity comparable with that of the respiratory centre in the bulb, and like this latter, highly regulable by reflex action.

The motion of a limb in the step is broadly divisible into two phases—a flexion phase in which the hip, knee, and ankle are flexed, carrying the foot forward clear of the ground, and an extension phase in which the hip, knee, and ankle are extended, bringing the foot to the ground and pushing the body forward from the ground as point of support. In the flexion phase the bending of the knee by the flexor muscles stretches, of course, the extensor muscle of the knee. But, at that time, judging by analogy from the well-known " flexion-reflex," the proprioceptive arc of the extensor muscle lies under inhibition, a reciprocal inhibition, one of the main purposes of which may indeed be to preclude a potential stretch-reflex from impeding the active flexion. At completion of the flexion phase the lapse of its concomitant inhibition of the nervous arc of the extensor muscles must leave the stretch-reflex free. The step, in fact, repeats, though probably less abruptly, the experiment in which the stretch-reflex wakes to post-inhibitory freedom. The precurrent flexor phase thus, so to say, compresses the spring which, when released, does the main work of the step. The extension phase itself in its turn, during the course of its performance, by straightening the knee, effects relief of the stretch of the extensors, and so terminates itself by abrogating its own promoting stimulus.

Further contribution by the stretch-reflex to the extension phase of the step occurs also in another way. When the extensor muscle is actively contracting, a stretch applied to it enhances immediately and greatly its contraction. The myograph record (Fig. 63) exemplifies this from an experiment meeting the requisite conditions. A passive stretch, amounting

to but 2·5 per cent. of the length of the active muscle, causes the contraction-
tension of the muscle to become three times as great. Now, a part of the
knee-extensor muscle, the " double-joint " portion, bridges across the hip
as well as the knee. It lies across the flexor aspect of the former. In the
extension phase of the step the angle of the hip, like that of the knee, opens.
This opening of the angle of the hip necessarily stretches the part of the knee-
extensor bridged across it. Thus a stretch is given to this part of the extensor
not by its antagonists, but by its own ally-muscles, the extensors of the hip.
This, happening as it does during the extension phase, occurs when the

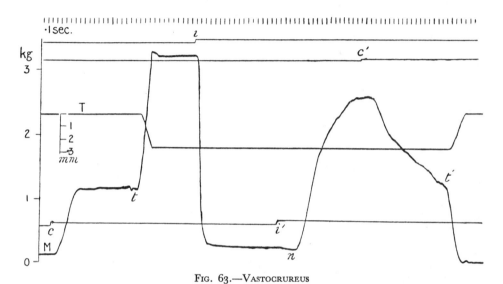

FIG. 63.—VASTOCRUREUS

From C to C′ stimulation of contralateral afferent peroneopopliteal nerve (break-shocks at 40 per
sec., coreless primary fed by 0·2 amp., secondary coil 16.3 cm. from primary) evoking reflex
contraction. At *t* a 2·5 mm. stretch; at *t′* relief of the residual stretched-posture. From *i* to
i′ stimulation of inhibitory afferent nerve; this nerve as frequently evoked, besides inhibition
of the contralateral nerve's reflex contraction, slight reflex contraction on its own part, so that
full inhibition revealing the passive tension component in the reaction to this stretch is fully
evident only at *n*, where on cessation of the ipsilateral stimulus the slight ipsilateral contraction
passed off though the inhibition temporarily remained. Myograph multiplying tendon-
movement 62 times. Time in 0·1 sec. (Liddell and Sherrington, *Proc. roy. Soc.*, 1924, **96B**
212)

extensor muscle is already in action and obviously not under inhibition.
This stretch must therefore, as our experiment shows, enhance further the
reflex contraction already in operation, and do so at the period of mid-
progress of the extension phase when the foot is in contact with the ground
and the weight of the body bears most on it, because acting approximately
vertically above. Later, with fuller straightening of the knee towards the
end of the extension phase, this stretch upon the double-joint portion of the
muscles diminishes and lapses, and with it the enhancement of contraction.
The stretch-reflex thus in two respects plays an important part in the extension phase of the action of the step.

Study of the stretch-reflex in its greater completeness and entirety has been but recent.   There can, however, be little doubt that the " knee jerk," a reaction long familiar to the physician, is a fractional manifestation of it. The " knee jerk " is a slight twitch-like contraction of the muscle of the front of the thigh.   The physician evokes it by a light tap directed close below the knee-cap.   This stretches the thigh muscle slightly, and evokes from the muscle a slight contraction lasting some tenth of a second.   The routine of the physician employs this brief reaction as a test where there is question of certain diseases of the nervous system.   Where there is, as in tabes dorsalis, degeneration of the receptive nerves of muscle, absence or impairment of the knee jerk is apt to be an early symptom.   Of common occurrence in tabes dorsalis, along with impairment of the knee jerk, are two other symptoms—namely, defect of the normal ability to walk or run, and impairment of normal ability to stand, especially with the eyes closed. The physician in testing the knee jerk is in fact testing the stretch-reflex of an antigravity muscle.   We have seen the rôle which that stretch-reflex plays in the performance of the step and in the maintenance of standing. In the light of that we can appreciate more clearly the bearing of the little evanescent twitch, the " knee jerk," on the two fundamental acts, motor and postural, of stepping and of standing.   That bearing emphasises the contribution made to the inconscient reflex performance of these acts by the receptivity of the muscles which they employ.

We have thus glimpsed something of the contribution made to bodily posturing and movement by reflex action arising in the muscular receptors. These same receptors connect also with the mental region of the brain. What kind of mental experience do they enable ?   I do but mention this in order that, regarding muscular receptivity, there shall not escape us the similarity which exists between its reflex and its sensual scope.   This latter concerns the perception of our postures and our movements, their intensity, their direction, speed, and extent.   In their sensual aspect the muscular receptors serve as means whence mental experience can work toward attainment of yet finer delicacy and precision for the muscular acts of the body, and arrive even at trains and combinations of them that, in so far, are acquisitions altogether new.   The two reactional aspects, the sensual and the purely reflex, of muscular receptivity reveal therefore as two sides of, broadly taken, one singly-purposed function addressed to a single problem, in brief, the taxis of execution, the management—from rough adjustment onward into minutely refined *finesse*—of the acts of our skeletal muscles, which is to say, in the language of the older physiologists, the movements and postures of our life of external relation.

Though the general problem is thus broadly definable, its content of unanswered questions is legion.   Passive stretch applied to the extensor muscle provokes reflex contraction in it.   The stretch stimulates receptors which through the receptive nerve of the muscle provoke contraction. The nerve of the muscle consists of several branches.   Take one of these branches, cut it across, and stimulate its central end, the end connected with the nerve-centres. The receptive nerve is thus stimulated not, it is true, through the medium of stretch applied to its receptors, but directly. Yet no contraction of the muscle results. We should not, of course, expect contraction in that part of the muscle the nerve-branch of which has been cut, because from that part we have, by cutting the branch, withdrawn the motor nerve-supply. But from the rest of the muscle with motor supply intact, we might expect reflex contraction. Not only is there none, but further, the muscle, if reflexly contracting at the time, is thrown out of contraction. Instead of reflex contraction, there is therefore reflex inhibition. Evidently the muscle is provided with more than one kind of receptor; it possesses certainly two kinds with diametrically opposed functional effect. Like the heart, it has two opposed nerves, one of augmentor function, one of inhibitory function—only in the case of our skeletal muscle these two opposed nerves are afferent and not efferent.

The significance of this is at present obscure. The " lengthening reaction," it is true, may involve a reflex inhibition and is certainly proprioceptive. We must also not forget that muscles can give rise to pain. Cramp, rheumatism, muscular fibrositis, and neuritis evidence this only too commonly. Even a small partial rupture of a muscle makes it a seat of pain when it contracts. In all such cases the treatment that the physician's experience enjoins is rest—that is, the treatment that Nature herself seems to aim at, for she enforces it, in the last resort prescribing pain, if rest be departed from. Existence of these inhibitory afferents from muscle suggests she enjoins involuntary desistence from contraction by reflex inhibition. Some involuntary, as well as voluntary, restraint from use of his lumbar muscles restricts the lumbago patient in rising from his chair. But the problem of the proprioceptive nerve, which inhibits its own muscles, certainly cannot be satisfied wholly in this way. Among such proprioceptives are some which, while reflexly inhibiting their own muscle, excite contraction of the antagonist, thus causing for their own muscles a stretch scarcely likely to be soothing to inflammation. Moreover, there are muscles which seem not to possess proprioceptors inhibitory of themselves.

The microscope likewise separates the receptors of muscle into species of more than one kind, well-differentiated forms, muscle-spindles, Golgi tendon-organs, basket-endings, tendril-terminals, Pacinian corpuscles, and so on. It is unlikely that for all these the adequate stimulus can be the same, or the functions identical. In perception of postures and movements there seem traceable, as underlying data, degrees of muscle-length on one hand and, on the other, degrees of muscle-tension. Some muscle-receptors may be length-recorders, others tension-recorders; one would suppose the Golgi tendon-organs among these latter. As to the " muscle-spindles," the muscle-fibres they enfold, though differing within the spindle from those outside, yet receive motor terminals; one would suppose active contraction to supply their stimulus. Through them and through other receptive endings which clasp muscular fibres, the active contraction of the muscle might be expected to evoke reflex reactions, and to furnish a " contraction " datum for perception of active postures and movements.

IX

ON THE MOTOR AREA OF THE CEREBRAL CORTEX

[*Observations relating to point-to-point localisation within the motor area of the anthropoid cerebral cortex, its instability, the special features relating to the movements of the eyes, face, and tongue, and representation within the central fissure. Experiments concerned with the manner of restoration of spontaneous movements after cortical ablations were made. Only a few of the many original observations incidental to these experiments are reprinted here.*—ED.]

INTRODUCTION[1]

THE investigation the results of which are here recorded arose from an observation, which chance opportunity afforded us, of examining by stimulation the cerebral cortex of a chimpanzee. That anthropoid species had not at that time come under experimental examination. On faradising the cortex we found, contrary to our expectation, that, although the gyrus centralis anterior yielded motor responses readily, we obtained none such from gyrus centralis posterior. A second similar opportunity arising, we repeated our experimental tests, and the results confirmed our former ones. Obtaining then a specimen of gorilla, an anthropoid also not previously experimented on, results were again met confirmatory of our first. It was therefore decided to carry out an inquiry into the motor cortex of the anthropoid apes, more especially from the "localisation" aspect. The following paper is based on the experimental examination of twenty-two chimpanzees, three gorillas, and three orang-utan. The methods[2] employed have included both stimulation and ablation, but chiefly the former.

At the time our observations were begun the only recorded experiment on the cerebral cortex of the anthropoid ape was one of stimulation of the cortex of an orang by Beevor and Horsley (1890).[3] The results they arrived at will be referred to later in the present paper; an excellent diagram summarising them is given by Schäfer in his *Textbook of Physiology* (1900).[4] More recently, observations on localisation in the anthropoid have been (taking them in their successive order of date of publication) two preliminary notes by ourselves;[5] observations on the orang by Roaf and Sherrington[6]

---

[1] This and subsequent extracts in this chapter are from "Observations on the Excitable Cortex of the Chimpanzee, Orang-utan, and Gorilla," published with A. S. F. Leyton (formerly Grünbaum), *Quart. J. exp. Physiol.*, 1917, **11**, 135-222.

[2] Details of methods are given in the original paper.—ED.   [3] *Philos. Trans.*, 1891, **181B**, 129.

[4] Schäfer, E. A., *Textbook of Physiology*, Edinburgh, 1900, **2**, p. 747.

[5] Grünbaum and Sherrington, *Proc. roy. Soc.*, 1901, **69**, 206, and 1903, **72**, 152.

[6] *J. Physiol.*, 1906, **34**, 315.

and by the Vogts;[1] on the gibbon by Mott, Schuster, and Sherrington;[2] on the chimpanzee by T. Graham Brown and Sherrington;[3] and on the chimpanzee by T. Graham Brown.[4]

The main object in view being to "localise" the motor function of each cortical point yielding motor responses, the stimuli applied were systematically kept of weak strength and not far above threshold value, and each stimulus was applied usually quite briefly—e.g., one to two seconds or little more. The sequences of movement are therefore short, our intention being to determine chiefly the primary movement yielded by the cortical point.

We had supposed at commencement of our experiments that the identification of exactly corresponding points in the two hemispheres of an individual and in the hemispheres of different individuals could be much more nearly possible than our experience has left us with the impression that in fact it is. The dissimilarity of the convolutional pattern of the hemispheres even in individuals of the same species (*Troglodytes niger*), and the seemingly variable relation of analogous functional points to sulci of corresponding name, makes it practically impossible to decide with sufficient exactitude what point on the hemisphere of one individual is identical with a given point upon another hemisphere. But in spite of this inability to determine what point on one hemisphere is anatomically identical with some particular point on another hemisphere, our series of experiments as they proceeded, each resulting in a detailed localisation map, showed us clearly that in very many cases, probably in most, the corresponding anatomical points in different individual hemispheres did not, as examined by faradisation in the course of experiment, yield motor responses so nearly similar as to be noted as the same movement in our movement list. Of this many illustrations can be found if the maps with number references furnished in this paper are turned to. The movements so obtained were related movements, often or indeed usually closely related movements, but not identical, not rarely movements of opposite sense, although of the same part. And many instances may be found in the maps where one and the same movement, as noted by the observer, was obtained in one hemisphere from some point which was clearly not that at which it was obtained in another hemisphere, either the opposite hemisphere of the same individual or the hemisphere of the corresponding side in another individual. Our experience is thus clearly in harmony with that of Shepherd I. Franz[5] on the Macaque. Summarising the observations described in Section II of his paper, he writes: "The data show in different animals"—i.e., different individuals of the same species, *Macacus rhesus*—" and in different hemispheres a variety of distribution of the areas concerned with the movements of the individual segments of the leg and arm."

[1] *J. Psychol. Neurol. Lpz.*, 1906-7, **8**, 277.   [2] *Proc. roy. Soc.*, 1911, **84B**, 67.
[3] *Proc. roy. Soc.*, 1912, **85B**, 250, and *Proc. Physiol. Soc.*, *J. Physiol.*, 1913, **44**, xxii.; *Brit. Med. J.*, 1913, **2**, 751.
[4] *Quart. J. exp. Physiol.*, 1915, **9**, 81, 101, 117, and 131; *Proc. Physiol. Soc.*, *J. Physiol.*, 1914, **48**, xxix., xxx., xxxiii.   [5] *Psychological Monographs*, 1915, **19**, No. 1, p. 80.

And it was clear, in our experience, that the motor cortex of an individual hemisphere and of both hemispheres in one individual does not, as its surface is gone over point for point in a systematic localisation experiment, yield the whole series of movements that can be yielded by similar examination of a series, even a small series, of hemispheres. Movements will appear in one hemisphere which do not appear in another, or, putting it in another way, will appear in one experiment which do not appear in another experiment. We think that this is probably largely owing to " facilitation." When the motor cortex in any individual hemisphere is systematically explored point to point by the electrode, particular motor responses when once evolved tend to reappear from adjacent cortical points. These cortical points form groups, each group occupying a small cortical area whence the same motor response is elicited. Such an area is probably partly the result of the facilitation exercised in regard to the response characteristic of it by the influence of one point upon another in it. This facilitation of one response would act in the direction of restricting the appearance of other responses which nevertheless might be latent in the cortex: it would tend to deviate the response (*v. infra*).

FUNCTIONAL INSTABILITY OF CORTICAL MOTOR POINTS

This raises the question of the functional instability of a motor cortical point.[1] In addition to the influence of depth of narcosis, freedom of blood supply, local temperature, and such effects of experimental exposure of the cortex as " drying " or inspissation of applied Locke's solution, the motor responses of a cortical point may be easily and greatly modified by precurrent, especially closely precurrent, stimulation either of itself or of neighbouring, especially closely adjacent, cortical points. The motor response from a given point, though it may, as the maps of cortical localisation usually depict, remain approximately the same throughout a lengthy experiment, even from hour to hour, when similar stimuli are repeated at intervals not too brief, may yet vary considerably in result of precurrent stimulations not too distant in time and place. Experiments in which a large field of cortex is examined systematically point for point by electrical stimulation to determine the functional localisation are likely to display the influence of previous stimulation of one point upon another.

Three phenomena of this kind, presumably all closely akin, make themselves evident in an examination of the motor cortex—namely, *facilitation of response, reversal of response, and deviation of response.* Of these the first, noted by various observers,[2] and particularly fully studied recently by T. Graham Brown[3] in the chimpanzee as well as in Macacus and other monkeys, is characterised by a change of the cortical point's response in the direction

[1] See Graham Brown, T., and Sherrington, C. S., *Proc. roy. Soc.*, 1912, **85B**, 250.
[2] Franck, F., *Fonctions motrices du cerveau*, Paris, 1887, p. 380; also Carville et Duret, *Arch. de Physiol.*, Paris, 1875, p. 437. [3] *Loc. cit., supra*, p. 398.

of increase, with or without other modification. It may be induced by stimulation of the point itself or by stimulation of other points. Reversal of response[1] is a change supervening which may culminate in complete reversal of the sense of the movement of the response—*e.g.*, extension of a joint may become flexion of that joint. Deviation of response is a change which alters the character of the response, so that instead of the original movement appearing, some other movement—*e.g.*, of another joint or part—appears in place of the original. All these changes are temporary. They may be taken as expressions of what has been termed the functional instability of a cortical motor point.

1. *Facilitation of Response.*—Facilitation of response has been a usual accompaniment of our observations on the anthropoid motor cortex. Comparing our experience of it there with our experience of it in Macaque and Calothrix, facilitation seems to be somewhat more extensive in the anthropoid than in the lower forms of monkey. Thus, as was remarked in our preliminary communication, it affects the delimitation of the whole of the anterior border of the motor field. That border is not of sharp and abrupt edge, but seems to fade off forward rather gradually. Facilitation makes it extend farther forward than it does without facilitation. Thus if the anterior border is delimited by stimulating series of cortical points in succession from behind forward, the anterior limit of the field is found to lie farther anterior than if determined by stimulating a series of points starting well in front of the limit and followed from before backward. In a similar way the boundary of the area for any particular movement may by facilitation be extended beyond its average limit; in this latter case, deviation of response comes in as well.

2. *Reversal of Response.*—The mutual influence exerted by points moving the same joint but in opposite directions was dealt with in the paper by T. Graham Brown and one of us.

3. *Deviation of Response.*—A cortical point can also influence the motor response of another whose response is neither diametrically opposed to nor identical with or very closely similar to its own. Thus, chimpanzee, left hemisphere (Fig. 64), leg area. Point 319 gave regularly as response plantar flexion of ankle, followed by flexion of all toes except hallux, followed further by adduction of hallux. That was its response when first stimulated in the experiment. It was the fifth point stimulated in the experiment, and was then stimulated next after a point 41 in face area, which yielded movement 41 (see list on p. 404); and point 41 had been stimulated next after one in arm area, which yielded movement 232. From time to time in the course of the experiment point 319 was returned to from distant points, and gave as response regularly movement 319 and no other.

Point 342, similarly stimulated, was giving with like regularity movement 342, flexion of hip followed by adduction of hip. When point 319 was stimulated immediately after point 342 had been stimulated, time being

---

[1] Graham Brown, T., and Sherrington, C. S., *Proc. roy. Soc.*, 1912, **85B**, 250.

allowed, however, for the movement evoked from 342 to subside completely, the movement given by 319 was no longer movement 319. It then gave instead flexion of hip followed by dorsal flexion of ankle and flexion of knee, followed further by flexion of all toes except hallux, movement 363.

Again, in the same animal and same hemisphere, point 306 gave regularly, when stimulated after points relatively indifferent to it, the response: flexion of little and fourth toes rapidly followed by flexion of third and second, and then followed by plantar flexion of angle, and later adduction of hallux. When stimulated next and quickly after point 306, but with allowance of time for the movement from 306 to subside completely, point 319 evoked no longer movement 319, but the following: flexion of toes without hallux, followed by plantar flexion of ankle, followed by adduction of hallux, movement 298.

Again, point 268 gave as its regular response flexion of hallux, followed by flexion of toes, followed by plantar flexion of ankle. Point 319, when stimulated next and soon after 268, evoked as response simultaneous flexion of toes and hallux, followed by plantar flexion of ankle.

Again, point 331, which evoked flexion of knee when stimulated in quick succession to point 342, evoked when stimulated in quick succession to point 263 extension of hallux, the regular response from point 263 itself being extension of hallux, followed by extension of the remaining toes, followed further by dorsal flexion of ankle, and finally by flexion of hip.

Again, point 232 in the same experiment, in arm area, yielding ordinarily flexion of elbow, yielded when stimulated quickly next after point 127, which was yielding flexion of thumb, flexion of thumb followed by flexion of elbow, 140.

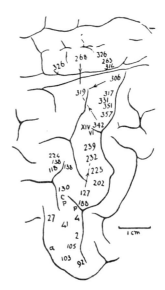

FIG. 64.—EXAMPLES OF "DEVIATION OF RESPONSE" FROM A CHIMPANZEE HEMISPHERE, CHIMPANZEE 19

Some only of the responses obtained are mapped. Left hemisphere. Mesial surface shown above. List of responses on p. 404

Again, in another animal, the following " deviation " occurred. The examination of the motor area had in this experiment been begun at the top limit of the arm area in shoulder region, and proceeded systematically from point to point in the downward direction. Followed in this manner, elbow flexion soon became the leading (primary) movement, and continued so very nearly or even quite down to the inferior genu of sulc. centralis. Beyond a certain point, which was minutely and precisely marked on the map made, elbow flexion disappeared abruptly, and facial movements appeared in the form of closure of opposite eyelids. The lower margin of arm area having thus evidently been reached, we turned to the delimitation of the face area. The examination of this area we started at the lower (Sylvian) end of sulc. centralis, and thence proceeded point by point upward along the precentral gyrus not far in front of sulc. centralis. In due course the point yielding closure of opposite eye was again reached, and it was found that then on proceeding farther upward to the point that had previously yielded elbow flexion as its primary movement, that point now yielded adduction of thumb as its primary movement, and a little farther upward movement of index, chiefly extension, was added to that of thumb; and movements of thumb and index continued to be the primary movements right up through the region which previously had given elbow flexion as primary response, and thumb and index movements as primary responses trespassed actually into the area that had previously yielded shoulder movements as the primary response. Here the "deviation of response" was seen to affect a whole series of points, influencing in its special direction a not inconsiderable fraction of the whole arm area.

Again, in an experiment on a gorilla, a point 172 which had been yielding regularly flexion of all fingers without thumb, on being stimulated next after a point 142, which yielded extension of index finger alone, yielded extension of index alone without movement of the other fingers (Fig. 71, A, p. 432). Later, when stimulated after an interval of some two minutes, it yielded flexion of fingers as at first.

Again, in the same experiment, a point 176, which yielded regularly extension of fingers without thumb, on being stimulated in next succession to point 172, yielded flexion of fingers instead of extension of them. It was, however, not found possible by stimulating point 172 in next succession to point 176 to obtain movement 176 from point 172. Further, on stimulating the two points by separate electrodes concurrently it was found that a stimulation of 172, weak as judged by the induction scale and also by its nearness to threshold value of excitation, caused flexion of fingers in spite of concurrent stronger stimulation of 176. Also an extension of the fingers already brought about by stimulating 176 alone was broken down and converted into flexion by weak stimulation then applied to 172, although the stimulation of 176 was continued unremitted. Indeed, the extension of fingers produced by stimulation of 176 seemed more readily broken down and changed to flexion by stimulation of 172 when the stimulation of 176 had been in progress for some little time than when stimulation of 172 was introduced earlier. When, conversely, flexion of fingers was in progress under stimulation of 172, the application of strongish stimulation to 176 broke down the flexion and changed it to extension; but for this the stimulation of 176 had to be strongish. Also when the stimulation of 172 and 176 was commenced concurrently, but the stimulation of 176 was strong and that of 172 very weak, the result obtained was extension, not flexion— that is, 176 overpowered 172.

Again, we have in several hemispheres observed that a cortical point which ordinarily evoked as its primary response flexion of the elbow would evoke, when stimulated next and soon after a distant point giving adduction of thumb, flexion of elbow and adduction of thumb.

Again, on the opposite hemisphere of the same gorilla referred to above a point 218, which yielded regularly flexion of wrist followed by flexion of elbow, yielded on being stimulated after stimulation of a point 251 yielding rotation of shoulder, rotation of shoulder and not flexion of wrist or elbow. It yielded these latter, however, as secondary movements if the stimulation were prolonged, and it yielded them again as its primary response after a time interval had been allowed (Fig. 71, B, p. 432).

The distances across which " deviation of response " may be exerted by one point on another vary. Though usually the space intervening between the points is short—e.g., less than 5 mm.—it is sometimes double or treble that. It is not equally developed in all directions; thus it tends to occur more readily between two points situate in one and the same functional area—e.g., leg area—than between two points situate in different functional area—e.g., one in leg area and one in arm area. It seems to occur more readily between points which under stimulation give rise, in the " march " (Hughlings Jackson) elicitable from them, to similar motor responses. Thus in the march elicitable from " abdominal wall " points movement of anus is prone to occur, and, vice versa, in the march elicitable from " anus " points there is a proneness for abdominal wall response to appear; and similarly between anus points and abdominal wall points, though their foci are situate quite far one from the other, we have seen deviation of response exerted.

Again, in an experiment a portion of the leg area was ablated, leaving below the ablated portion a small transverse slip of cortex which the faradic stimulations prior to the ablation allocated to hip area, but abutting upon the abdominal wall area. The whole of this strip on being faradised twenty minutes after completion of the ablation yielded no trace of limb movement, but evoked instead vigorous contraction of the abdominal wall. Prior to the ablation it had yielded as movement chiefly flexion of hip; after the ablation it yielded contractions of the contralateral abdominal wall without any movement of hip.

Again, in a chimpanzee, at the region of the gyr. cent. anterior, opposite the brachio-facial genu of sulc. centralis, the following was noted: The lower limit of hand area was determined, care being taken to avoid as far as possible deviation of response by near precurrent stimulation of adjacent points. Similarly the upper limit of angle of mouth area was delimited. Then the lower limit of hand area was obtained by stimulation in serial succession of a number of points descending in order from upper part of arm area downward. The lower border of hand area as thus examined trespassed into face area according to the upward limit of the latter as demarcated previously. The responses of hand given by the hand area points thus trespassing were always similar to the last hand responses obtained from the portion of the hand area above them; and they were accompanied by " angle of mouth " movement, either simultaneous with them or almost so. Conversely, on determining the upper limit of angle of mouth area by following that area upward along a series of points stimulated in it in turn, the upper limit trespassed over into hand area. The responses of mouth movement from these trespassing points always resembled the mouth responses last obtained from points lower down in mouth area, and were accompanied by movements of hand. Similarly, at lower edge of closure of eyelids area that area could by serial stimulation of it be made to encroach on " angle of mouth " area, which lay lower down and rather posterior to it; and the upper and posterior edge of closure of eyelids area could be made to encroach over into hand area, which lay above and rather behind it.

List of Motor Points Shown in Figures 64-71

Numeral or Letter indicating Response.	1st Movement.	2nd Movement.	3rd Movement.
1	Contralateral angle of mouth retracted		
2	,, ,, ,, ,,	Contralateral nostril wrinkled	
4	,, ,, ,, ,,	,, pinna retracted	
21	Upper lip lifted and its edge inverted		
27	Both lips retracted but the lower much the more		
37	Lower lip pouted, more on contra-lateral side	Twisting of contralateral nostril	
41	Upper lip protruded with slight protrusion of lower		
47	Upper lip retracted to contralateral side	Jaw opened	
54	Contralateral angle of mouth retracted	Contralateral eye closed	Contralat. pinna retracted and raised
56	,, ,, ,, ,,	,, ,, ,,	Neck turned away
65	Tongue heaped up and twisted, bringing dorsum to contralateral cheek		
79	Tongue tip turned to contralateral side		
92	Hollowing of tongue tip		
96	Tongue tip protruded with narrowing of tongue		
103	Lower jaw depressed without lateral deviation	Tongue tip turned to ipsilateral side	
105	,, ,, ,, ,,	Tongue protruded straight	Tongue retracted to contralat. side
110	Sucking action of the cheeks		
114	Chewing movement		

List of Motor Points Shown in Figures 64-71 (continued)

Numeral or Letter indicating Response.	1st Movement.	2nd Movement.	3rd Movement.
118	Thumb extended		
120	,, adducted		
122	,, extended	Index extended	Other fingers extended
125	,, adducted	Fingers and wrist moved together	
127	,, flexed		
128	,, ,,	Fingers flexed	
130	,, ,, and adducted		
134	,, extended	Fingers extended	Wrist extended
138	,, ,,	Wrist flexed	
142	Index extended		
144	,, ,,	Wrist extended	
147	,, ,,	,, supinated	
148	,, ,,	Middle finger extended	
150	,, flexed		
152	,, ,,	Wrist flexed	
169	Little finger and ring-finger flexed		
172	All fingers flexed without thumb		
176	,, extended without thumb		
186	,, flexed without thumb	Wrist extended	
187	,, ,, ,, ,,	,, flexed	Wrist supinated
202	Closing of whole hand	,, ,,	
205	,, ,, ,,		
215	Wrist extended	Fingers flexed	
216	,, ,,	,, extended	Thumb adducted
218	,, flexed	Elbow flexed	
223	,, ,,		
224	,, supinated		
225	,, ,,	Elbow flexed	Shoulder raised
229	,, ,,	Thumb flexed	
232	Elbow flexed		
234	,, ,,	Wrist flexed	
238	Shoulder raised		
239	,, retracted		
240	,, ,,	Elbow flexed	
241	,, ,,	,, ,,	Wrist flexed
248	,, raised and protracted		
251	,, rotated outward		
253	,, and muscles of front of chest moved (contralateral)		
256	,, and elbow flexed simultaneously		
263	Hallux extended		
268	,, flexed	Other toes flexed	Ankle flexed
306	Two outermost toes flexed	3rd and 2nd toes flexed	,, plantar-flexed

LIST OF MOTOR POINTS SHOWN IN FIGURES 64-71 *(continued)*

Numeral or letter indicating Response.	1st Movement.	2nd Movement.	3rd Movement.
314	Ankle flexed dorsally	Toes extended	
317	,, ,, ,,	Ankle rotated outward	
319	,, plantar-flexed	Toes flexed except hallux	Hallux adducted
326	,, ,, ,,	,, flexed	Knee flexed
331	Knee flexed		
342	Hip flexed	Hip rotated inward and adducted	
350	,, rotated inward	Contralateral wall of abdomen	
351	,, extended		
359	,, adducted	Contralateral wall of abdomen contracted	
370	Conjugate deviation of eyes toward contralateral side		
372	,, ,, ,, ,,	Both eyes opened	Neck turned to contral. side
373	,, ,, ,, ,,	,, ,, ,,	
379	Ipsilateral eye turned toward contralateral side		
380	Upper eyelids of both eyes raised		
382	Opening of both eyes	Conjugate deviation of eyes to opposite side	Face turned to opposite side
383	,, ,, ,,	Face turned to contralateral side	
385	,, ,, ,,		
386	,, ,, ,, and converging of eyeballs		
a	Contralateral eye closed		
c	Closing of both eyes, contralateral the more		
f	,, ,, ,, ,,	Retraction of contralateral nostril	Retraction contralat. angle of mouth
g	,, ,, ,, ,,	Fingers flexed	
m	,, ,, ,, ,,	Face turned to opposite side	
p	,, ,, ,, ,,	Elevation of contralateral pinna	
P	Contralateral pinna retracted		
VI.	Chest muscles of contralateral side contracted		
XII.	Muscles of contralateral side of abdominal wall, and contralateral loin and anus		
XIV.	Muscles of contralateral side of lower abdominal wall	Anus protruded	

The above instances are cited as typical and somewhat outstanding examples of what in a similar and less pronounced manner was frequently met by us. As to how far such deviations, as also the reversals and facilitations, are traceable to shuntings of route in the cortical structure itself, or how far they are referable to shuntings in subcortical paths and centres, that is a question towards whose solution our observations contribute little or nothing. The diagram furnished by Franz[1] (Fig. 16, p. 148 in his paper) indicates the manifold possibilities in that respect, and Graham Brown[2] has published direct observations in regard to " facilitation " which throw light on the problem as concerns that phenomenon. The main point that we wish here to emphasise in preface to the subjoined list of motor responses and maps of cortical points belonging to them as observed in our experiments is that in looking through such data we would wish the reader to bear in mind that the fixity of such localisations is as regards minutiæ to some extent probably a temporary one—*i.e.*, obtained at the time of observation—but in our opinion might not be precisely the same were examination possible at a number of different times and in a number of different experiments. As regards minutiæ of localisation in the motor cortex, our experience agrees with that of those[3] who find, as Shepherd Franz expresses it, that the motor cortex is a labile organ.[4]

ON THE PORTION OF THE MOTOR CORTEX BURIED IN THE FISSURE OF ROLANDO[5]

A good deal of the excitable motor cortex lies tucked away from the free surface of the hemisphere, buried in the fissures adjoining gyrus centralis anterior. The results of our various experiments[6] on this taken altogether revealed no movement from the buried motor cortex which was not elicitable

[1] *Psychological Monographs*, 1915, **19**, No. 1, p. 80.

[2] *Quart. J. exp. Physiol.*, 1915, **9**, 81, 101, 117, and 131; *Proc. Physiol. Soc., J. Physiol.*, 1914, **48**, xxix., xxx., xxxiii.

[3] Roaf and Sherrington, *J. Physiol.*, 1906, **34**, 315; Graham Brown and Sherrington, *Proc. roy. Soc.*, 1912, **85B**, 250; Graham Brown, *loc. cit.*; Franz, *loc. cit.*

[4] The intimate commingling and overlapping of the cortical areas for different movements is well illustrated in a study of the motor cortex of the baboon (T. Graham Brown and C. S. Sherrington, *J. Physiol.*, 1911, **43**, 209). The reversal of the representation of movement by the action of tetanus toxin was studied in detail with H. E. Roaf (*J. Physiol.*, 1906, **34**, 315). A further discussion of the instability of the reaction of a cortical point to repeated stimulation at short intervals will be found in Graham Brown and Sherrington, *Proc. roy. Soc.*, 1912, **85B**, 250-77. Records of the contraction of an antagonistic muscular pair, supinator longus and triceps in the monkey, showed inhibitory and excitatory effects often independently exhibited. The outcome showed effects suggesting both single and double reciprocal innervation. Lasting effects from the immediately preceding response, both in the cortex and from afferent sources in the limb, were thought to result in the instability of reaction.—ED.

[5] From " Observations on the Excitable Cortex of the Chimpanzee, Orang-utan, and Gorilla," with A. S. F. Leyton, *Quart. J. exp. Physiol.*, 1917, **11**, 155 *et seq.* The wealth of detail as to localisation in the motor area of the higher apes given in this paper is its most important feature. Limitation of space unfortunately forbids republication of all the maps and tables here, and only the following extracts of some of its less well-known chapters are reprinted.—ED.

[6] Some are reported in Grünbaum and Sherrington, *Proc. rov. Soc.*, 1901, **59**, 206.

at one time or another in one specimen or another from the free surface of centralis anterior itself. The buried portion in sulcus centralis extended along the whole length of the anterior wall of that fissure except for its extreme upper tip, where motor cortex leaves the fissure and lies a little forward to it. In some places the motor cortex seems to pass down the whole depth of the anterior wall of the fissure, and not far below the inferior genu it seems in some individuals to occupy the deeper portion of the fissure's posterior wall also. It seems to extend less deeply than elsewhere into the fissure at two places, one of these being the lower part of genu inferius, the other lower part of genu superius, the shallowing being more marked and sharper at the former. The former of the two corresponds approximately with the region for neck lying between arm area above and face area below. The latter corresponds with the region for abdominal wall and chest wall lying between arm area below and leg area above. And we have obtained movements of neck and trunk respectively by actual faradisation of the anterior wall of the fissure at those two places.

The fissure being of considerable depth, exceeding 12 mm. in several places both in the chimpanzee and orang (we have not explored it in the gorilla), the amount of excitable area contributed by it to the motor field of the cortex in the anthropoid is quite large. Fig. 65 illustrates this. It is schematic, but not wholly so; it was prepared from a chimpanzee hemisphere, in which a number of points of the buried motor cortex were actually determined by faradisation, and the depth to which the fissure was excitable was tested at a series of places. With these as a basis, the rest of the deep contour is given by interpolating determinations obtained in other chimpanzee hemispheres. In our observations the posterior boundary of the motor cortex lying hidden in sulcus centralis seems to be more abruptly and sharply delimited than is the anterior margin of it, lying largely on the free surface of the hemisphere.

The motor responses yielded from points buried in sulcus centralis corresponded for the most part rather closely with the motor responses yielded by the free surface of centralis anterior of about the same horizontal level. A good deal of the local area for pinna seems to lie buried in the sulcus close below inferior genu, and we have obtained pinna movements from the anterior wall of the sulcus at that place in specimens where we could not elicit them from the free surface of the gyrus. The precentral sulci, superior and inferior, also contain portions of the motor cortex. These sulci are far more variable in their extent and position in the anthropoid than is sulcus centralis, so that it is not easy to make a general statement as to the amount of motor cortex they contain that can apply strictly to all cases. In Fig. 65, from a chimpanzee, is represented the amount buried in them in that specimen as experimentally determined. Moreover, the determination of the exact position of the anterior limit of the motor cortex is even on the free surface a matter of some artificiality, because in the anterior direction the motor field as examined by faradisation seems to fade off graduatim, so that a prolonged series of stimulations in that neighbourhood produces, by inducing "facilitation," a limit set farther forward than under a brief decisive examination by faradisation at a restricted number of selected points.

In his *Localisation of Cerebral Function* Campbell[1] has furnished an admirable and full account of the structural types of cerebral cortex and their topographical distribution not only in man, but in the chimpanzee and orang. It is instructive, therefore, to compare the limits of the motor

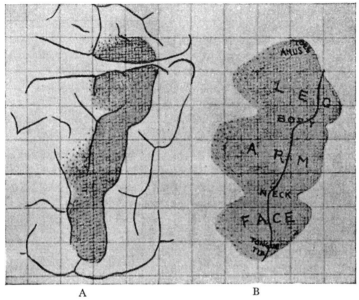

A   B

FIG. 65.—DIAGRAMS TO ILLUSTRATE THE SIZE AND SHAPE OF THE " MOTOR " CORTEX
OF THE CHIMPANZEE AS DETERMINED BY FARADIC STIMULATION

A shows the extent as observed on the free surface; B shows the extent and shape as observed when the portions buried in the sulci are added to that on free surface. The line running through B marks the position of the sulcus centralis; all the shaded area behind that line represents the part of the " motor " surface buried in that fissure. The stippling to left of the shaded area in each diagram indicates the gradual fading off of excitable area in the anterior direction, making the actual demarcation of the motor field in that direction a somewhat arbitrary one. The smallest squares on the map represent sq. mm. of actual cortex surface in the specimen mapped

field as determined by faradisation in those anthropoids with his " precentral " area determined by cell and fibre lamination. The posterior borders of the two as delimited by these two different methods seem to agree so closely that there can be little doubt that as regards that limit the two fields or areas are the same. In regard to the anterior border, the motor field's boundary seems to lie, especially in its lower two-thirds, farther forward than does that of Campbell's precentral area. The anterior boundary, as determined by faradisation, is, however, not a sharp one, and

[1] *Histological Studies in the Localisation of Cerebral Function*, London, 1905.

its situation seems to vary somewhat from specimen to specimen. As placed by us, it certainly appears to lie for the most part in the intermediate precentral area of Campbell. Opposite the " arm area " it lies not far behind the anterior boundary of the " intermediate precentral area," but opposite the " leg area " more considerably so. Opposite the " face area " it lies very much farther behind the anterior limit of " intermediate precentral area," although in front of anterior limit of the pure " precentral area " of Campbell. Campbell in his original description furnishes a number of arguments in favour of his " intermediate precentral type " of cortex possessing motorial functions, though differing from the precentral type or motor cortex pure. The gradual shading off of the pure motor field in the anterior direction, as experienced in our observations, and the variability of its anterior edge, as mentioned above when faradised under different experimental conditions, seem to us to lend support to his contention, although the latter is put forward on other evidence.

On the whole, we should estimate that in the anthropoid brain the portion of the motor region which lies buried in the sulcus centralis and other fissures amounts to not less than about 35 per cent. of the whole motor region.

REMARKS ON THE GROUPING OF THE RESPONSES OF THE MOTOR CORTEX

An occurrence met in some of our experiments was that in the course of examination of gyrus centralis anterior some small area of its surface might exist whence the faradisation failed to evoke responses. An instance is figured close to the genu inferius of sulcus centralis. The appearance of the cortex at such a place would reveal to inspection no obvious circulatory disturbance; nor so far as we were aware had any damage been inflicted there. But in many experiments systematic exploration of the whole motor field revealed no obvious gap in it. Beevor and Horsley in the brain of the orang they stimulated met with relatively large and numerous gaps of this kind, and supposed them characteristic of the motor area of the anthropoid brain. Franz records meeting with small areas not yielding responses in the motor field of the Macaque monkey. In our experience, a return later in the experiment to the small area which had not yielded responses found it still unyielding of response. Such an area was on several occasions ascertained to have no counterpart that we detected in the hemisphere of the opposite side. Nor were the places of occurrence of such seemingly non-stimulable gaps the same in hemispheres of different individuals, a finding in conformity with that of Franz in Macacus. In our experience, such a gap was perhaps more frequent than elsewhere about the region where face area meets arm area.

It may be noted that among the chimpanzees we examined were two very young ones, the younger of them, though in good nutritive condition, weighing only 2·240 kilograms. In one of these we found a cortical differentiation of the finger movements at least as great as in any other of the anthropoid brains we explored. In this animal we obtained from appropriate points in the cortex isolated movements of the little finger, both isolated flexion and isolated extension; also isolated movement of the second toe, both of flexion and of extension; also movement of the second and third toes without movement of the other toes. The animal was so young as to be infantile; it was fed from a sucking-bottle, and had the petulance and habits and cries of a very young animal.

Epilepsy.—Prolonging the faradisation, especially strong faradisation, of a spot in the motor surface usually induces not only a considerable " march " or sequence of responsive movement, but also, as is well known, an epileptiform convulsion. Our experiments were not directed toward observation of these, but we induced such effects from time to time. We found them easily provoked in the anthropoid, but not obviously more readily than in small monkeys such as Macacus and Calothrix. A difference in the two cases seemed the greater relative ease with which in the anthropoid an epileptiform convulsion could be evoked in this or that small region of musculature without the convulsion spreading beyond that part. Thus it could be evoked in the index finger, in the angle of the mouth, or in the toes, and remain confined to the field in which it started; such restriction is, in our experience, quite uncommon in Macacus or Calothrix.

" Epilepsy " was evoked readily in the " baby " chimpanzees coming under observation; it seemed neither more nor less readily obtained in them than in the grown specimens. On the other hand, the ease with which it was evoked, and the tendency for it to occur in the course of an experiment, appeared to us to vary distinctly in different individuals; in some individuals stimulation of duration and intensity too small to evoke it usually tended to evoke it from the very beginning of the experiment, and that tendency continued throughout the experiment.

It may be of interest to remark that in ablation experiments with small monkeys we have sometimes found a collodion dressing applied to the scalp over the area of removal of bone produce severe epileptiform convulsions, which ceased at once on removal of the dressing. The shrinkage of the collodion in such cases caused the dressing to press upon the scalp and underlying brain, the surface of the dressing over the region of the opening becoming flat or slightly concave outward.

A few general remarks may be offered in regard to certain of the movements evoked and the representation of separate motile parts in the cortex. We follow for convenience the order taken in the foregoing index to the motor responses listed.

1. *Face Area*   (See Figs. 67 and 68)

Face area so called might be better termed head area, since it includes not only the face, but tongue, palate and fauces, and larynx. Its upper boundary is usually with close accuracy marked by the level of the genu inferius of sulcus centralis. In some chimpanzees and gorillas, and especially, in our experience, in the orang, there is a tendency to the appearance of a third genu of the fissure below the ordinary genu inferius. And this third genu indicates approximately the level of subdivision of the so-called face area into an upper part in which movements of face proper predominate, and a lower part in which are represented tongue movements and movements of fauces, vocal cords, and palate. This third genu might be called a labio-lingual genu, because at it the area where lip movements predominate as primary responses meets the area where tongue movements as primary predominate. In the upper part of the face area the movements elicited can bear for the most part an interpretation as being partial movements in mimetic acts. In the lower part of the face area the movements suggest for the most part their being parts of acts subserving feeding —e.g., chewing, mastication, deglutition, etc.

Lips.—The upper lip movements are rather closely associated with movements of the nose, but the lip has a much wider focal field than has the nose. The lips are represented largely together, but independent movements of both upper and lower lips were seen. The field of representation of the lower lip seems somewhat larger than that of the upper. The areas for the lips are much commingled, but the representation of the lower lip seems to extend or to have its chief seat rather lower down the centralis anterior than does the upper. Pouting of the lips was distinct and not uncommon. Retraction of contralateral angle of the mouth, either primary or secondary, seemed the most common of all the lip movements.

Nose.—Movements of the nose seemed better developed, and to have a wider cortical representation in the orang than in chimpanzee or gorilla. They were not so marked in the orang, however, as they were found to be in the baboon.[1]

Pinna of Ear.—Movements rarely alone, almost always associated with other movements of the face; focal area lies partly buried in sulcus postcentralis. The area seems larger in the chimpanzee than in the orang.

Cheek and Chin.—Movements were elicitable, but not common.

Eyebrow and Frontalis.—Movement always contralateral; field in upper part of facial area.

Tongue.—Movements of tongue were obtainable from a very large area, in which they were usually the predominant primary movements. They were extremely varied in their form and sequence, almost baffling verbal description. For the most part they could be grouped under the headings retraction, protrusion, rolling on long axis, upcurving of base or tip, and hollowing of upper surface from side to side.

Protrusion very rarely carried the tongue tip beyond the lips. The appearance of the movements frequently suggested that they were part actions in mastication, licking, lapping, and swallowing. Thus one not infrequent was a thrusting of the tongue against the inside of the cheek-

[1] *J. Physiol.*, 1906, **34**, 315; *ibid.*, 1911, **43**, 209.

pouch as though to remove food thence; again, a rhythmic movement of licking or lapping; again, a heaping of the back of the dorsum against the back of the palate, followed by contraction of the faucial opening as though in swallowing. Occasionally the tongue was drawn back or thrust forward straight; much more commonly the retraction or protrusion was deviated, the deviation being sometimes to the ipsilateral, sometimes to the contralateral side. Retraction and protrusion were evidently much commingled

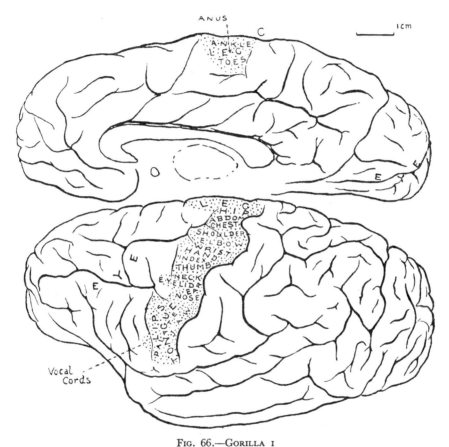

FIG. 66.—GORILLA I

Perspective view traced from a photograph; responses grouped diagrammatically. C, opposite the end of the sulcus centralis

in their representation in the cortex, but on the whole protrusion seemed situated lower down the convolution than was retraction. Sometimes the protrusion of tongue was accompanied by closing of jaw, and then occasionally the tongue was nipped by the teeth, recalling the biting of the tongue in epilepsy. On many occasions the points of excitable cortex farthest down of all in the convolution evoked movement confined to the tongue tip.

Jaw.—Opening and closing were both elicitable, but the former has a considerably larger field of points than has the latter; the latter's field seems to lie the farther forward and not to extend nearly so far down, at least as a primary movement, although in sequence to opening it extends far downwards. Rhythmic chewing, a movement observed by Ferrier as readily elicitable from the cortex of the cat, dog, and monkey, was observable in the anthropoids, and was got from points low down and far forward at the foot of the convolution. The jaw was not infrequently deviated towards the contralateral side as well as opened or closed. By dividing the symphysis it was found that the cortical representation is mainly unilateral, although when the two lateral halves are normally conjoined by the symphysis the unilateral representation in the hemisphere is mechanically obscured.

Hyoid.—Lifting of hyoid from a restricted part of lingual area.

Fauces.—Movement usually bilaterally symmetrical in appearance; generally from posterior part of lingual region about half-way down and from a quite restricted region often in association with heaping up of tongue at the back of the mouth.

Vocal Cords.—Movement almost always adduction, bilateral, but sometimes clearly more marked on contralateral side. Focal field small in the anterior and lower part of the face area—*i.e.*, adjunct to the lingual field.

Movements of the Eyelids and Eyeballs.—Cortical stimulation draws a sharp distinction between eyelid movements of closure and of opening respectively. This is the more striking because movements of opposite sense implicating one and the same part—*e.g.*, thumb, index, ankle, wrist, tongue, lips, even elbow and jaw—are not easily or even commonly separable in the cortex by reason of their foci of representation lying considerably remote one from the other. But the fields for eye-opening and eye-closure respectively do lie considerably separated apart (see Fig. 71, p. 432).

The great field of excitable cortex which lies open to examination in the free surface of gyrus precentralis may be termed the precentralis motor field; and we may include under that term the whole of the seemingly continuous field of motor points which occupies as well as the free face of gyrus precentralis the adjoining portions of sulcus centralis and of sulci precentrales and parts of the free faces of the gyri annectantes connecting gyrus precentralis with the frontal convolutions. Among all the numerous and varied movements which faradic stimulation applied at the appropriate points evokes from this great field, opening of the eye does not appear to be included, neither do movements of the eyeball. But closure of the eye is well and definitely included among the movements elicitable from precentralis field.

Closure of Eye.—The place in that field which yields eye-closure lies at the level of, and extends a little above, and to a wider extent below, *genu inferius* of *sulc. centralis*. It meets, as examined by the electrode, the lowest points of hand area (thumb) above; it is intimately adjunct to areas for ear, nostril, neck, and lip, occupying part of the upper portion of face area, and is traceable with the electrode into tongue area. The eye-closure is obtainable with faradic stimuli of the same strength as suffice for other motor responses from precentralis and with the same readiness. The movement may be (e.g., with weak stimuli) restricted to closure of opposite eye only, or even to isolated movement of the upper or lower lid only of that eye. With moderate stimuli the closure is of both eyes, but practically always is more vigorous in the opposite eye. The closure sometimes has the appearance, when the animal is not too deeply narcotised, of being executed against the animal's will, for it occurs while the other eye remains almost open, and on withdrawal of the cortical faradisation the contralateral eye, as also the less closed ipsilateral, re-opens again immediately and quickly.

Opening of the Eye.—This movement is observable under stimulation of the cortex in various widely separated regions. It may occur, so to say, in a desultory manner, and, in our experience, is prone to crop up unexpectedly. But in two regions it occurs fairly regularly; these regions are a frontal area anterior to the lower half of precentralis gyrus, and an occipital region including the calcarine area and the occipital pole.

Taking the second region first, the opening of eyes elicitable thence is clearly associated with a turning movement of the eyeballs toward the opposite side. The eye-opening, like the eye-turning which it accompanies,[1] is elicitable from this region much less easily and regularly than are the ordinary motor responses evocable from the precentralis motor field. Moreover, the points which here yield it seem, as tested by the electrode, to lie in a scattered manner, not constituting a continuous field of excitable points. Examination of the region shows that reacting points are most numerous along the area bordering the posterior part of calcarine fissure, and therefore on the mesial face of the hemisphere, but both in chimpanzee and gorilla the response was obtained also from a few points of the lateral face of the hemisphere at its occipital pole; the experiments giving this were on quite young animals, except in the case of one adolescent chimpanzee.

The other region whence eye-opening is elicitable, the frontal, is a large one. It embraces a considerable part of the 2nd and 3rd frontal convolutions, and seems separated from the " precentralis motor region " by an intervening strip of " silent " cortex, although this strip is sometimes encroached on almost to extinction. Elicitation of eye-opening from this region, like its elicitation from the occipital field, though apparently in a less degree, is irregular, and requires stronger faradic currents than are required for exciting motor responses from precentralis region. The movement when evoked has commonly a more deliberate execution, and the points which yield it are in any one experiment scattered in discrete fashion, instead of forming a seemingly continuous excitable field—as obtains, for instance, with the points yielding eye-closure in precentralis. The move-

[1] *J. Physiol.*, 1906, **34**, 315.

ment is practically always bilateral, often without obvious trace of pre-ponderance of vigour for the contralateral eye. With it is associated turning of the eyeballs—almost always conjugately away from the side stimulated, occasionally, however, convergently, and then sometimes toward a plane continuous with sagittal plane of head. Sometimes the eye-opening precedes the turning of the eyes, sometimes it follows it. In our experience the former is more frequently the case with the lower part—*e.g.*, 3rd frontal gyrus—of the frontal region, the latter with the upper part of the region. The opening of eyes tends to be followed, especially after reiterated stimu-lation, not only by eyeball-turning, but by turning of the neck and head in addition. This secondary and tertiary movement is always directed so as to turn the face away from the side stimulated.

In some experiments—*e.g.*, young gorilla (Fig. 71, p. 432)—the frontal area yielding eye-opening seemed to be subdivided into two by an in-excitable strip running horizontally across it. But considering the scattered distribution of the points in this field, this subdivision may be one that more extensive experimentation would break down, and certainly in some specimens it did not seem confirmed. Where it occurred the lower of the two sub-fields usually yielded eye-opening precedent to eye-turning, and the upper sub-field eye-turning precedent to eye-opening, and not rarely altogether without the latter.

It was said above that the movement of eye-opening seems absent from the long list of motor items assembled in the large precentralis motor field. Although that, as a broad statement, is true, it requires some modification, inasmuch as occasionally, and, in our experience, very rarely with weak and moderate stimuli, eye-opening is evoked from precentralis. It is not then a primary movement, in our experience, but is secondary to, or developed from, the turning of neck and head elicitable from a restricted area between hand and face regions; and with it sometimes occurs move-ment of eyeballs to opposite side, also not a primary movement from pre-centralis. More usually this neck movement, which is a movement carrying the face away from the side stimulated, is associated with movement of eye-closure, as mentioned above. From the evidence of our experiments in anthropoids, we infer that the eye-opening sometimes elicited from this part of precentralis region is not to be taken as evidence of the existence in precentralis of motor foci there situate and directly executive of eye-opening, but rather of secondary connections of the precentralis neck focus with foci for eye-opening situate extrinsic to precentralis motor region proper.

In addition to the instances of eye-opening coming under one or other of the three groups in the above category, there are instances of its occur-rence under faradic stimulation of still other regions of cortex. Such instances as these latter are those we had especially in mind in the opening paragraph as desultory, unexpected, and unreliable of repetition even at one and the same period of an experiment. When they have occurred they

GROUPING OF RESPONSES 417

have been noted by us, and the places of their occurrence have variously included points in the first temporalis, calloso-marginalis, and post-centralis, as well as various parts of precentralis. In regard to the whole of this group of " desultory " eye-opening responses, it is to be borne in mind that the movement of eye-opening is one commonly accompanying an awakening from sleep, and that the grade of narcosis under which the faradic examination of the cortex has to be carried out is one which in its depth somewhat resembles natural sleep. Any stimulus which arouses the animal is likely to evoke an opening of the eyes. For instance, the application of the faradic stimulus to the dura mater instead of to the cortex commonly does so. The eye-opening has therefore to be accepted with much caution as evidence that the stimulus which evokes it is one really playing in a direct manner upon a " motor " eye-opening centre of the cortex.

Movement of Eyeballs.—This, as obtained from cortex cerebri in the anthropoids, is, as in the small monkeys, almost always lateral conjugate deviation to the side away from the stimulus. It is obtainable from (1) the calcarine region and occipital pole in the same area as that already mentioned under eye-opening; (2) a frontal area embracing a considerable part of the surface of the 2nd and 3rd frontal gyri, corresponding fairly well with the frontal area above mentioned under eye-opening. The conjugate deviation of the eyeballs to the opposite side seems usually purely lateral, but sometimes the deviation is partly downward or partly upward as well as lateral; a partly downward deviation has, in our experience, been more common than a partly upward one. To evoke these eyeball movements, whether purely lateral or not, requires, in our experience, stronger stimuli than are required for motor responses from precentralis motor area, and the responses even under these stronger stimuli are not so regularly obtainable as are the responses from precentralis area.[1] Nor do the points yielding them form, in our experience, a seemingly continuous field of excitable surface either in the occipital or in the frontal regions. The movements when obtained have further a slow deliberate development[2] usually, distinguishing them somewhat from the limb, face, and eyelid-closure movements evocable from precentralis region. The movement is usually bilaterally symmetrical, but not rarely the ipsilateral eyeball lags somewhat behind the contralateral. Very occasionally we have seen convergence of the eyeballs occur, sometimes very markedly, and as though to fixate a point approximately in a plane continuous with the sagittal plane of the head. After the lateral conjugate deviation has been obtained it has been usual for the eyes to remain for some time in the posture thus assumed, and to return very slowly toward the primary straightforward posture after the stimulus has been withdrawn.

Quite exceptionally we have seen movement of the eyeballs produced by stimulation of the precentralis motor field. The movement has not

[1] Mott and Schäfer, *Brain*, 1890, **13**, 164.
[2] Schäfer, *Internat. Monthly Journ. Anat. and Physiol.*, 1888, **5**, 149.

been primary; it has accompanied turning of the neck, carrying the face to the opposite side, and the region which has yielded it has been that of genu inferius, which contains representation of the neck. The eyeball movement has always been conjugate deviation of both eyes to the opposite side. It has, in our experience, almost always been accompanied by eye-opening. Our inference from our experience of it is that in the anthropoid cortex there is no focus in the precentralis motor field which represents eyeball movements in the same relatively direct way as do foci therein represent movements such as those of hand, face, neck, etc., regularly elicitable from the precentralia. We regard the eyeball-turning movement occasionally elicitable from the inferior genual portion of precentralis as secondary to the neck-turning foci, in the same way as we regard the eye-opening elicitable from the same portion as secondarily associated with the neck-turning foci.

As regards the eyeball-turning movement obtainable from the frontal region, this may be unaccompanied by eye-opening, especially so in the upper part of the region, in our experience. The eyeball-turning is easily detectable, although the lids remain closed, the movement of the balls being obvious under the shut lids.

We are disposed to regard the neck-turning elicitable from precentralis motor region as a protective movement mainly associated with closure of the eyes. The neck-turning movement elicitable from frontal region and from occipital region seems connected with the management of the direction of the gaze.

2. *Neck Area*

The area in which neck movements as primary or isolated responses are elicitable is, in our experience, small. The movements are closely associated with that of closure of opposite eye, and the movement is almost invariably one which turns the face away from the side to which the stimulated hemisphere belongs. We have not met with indubitable " retraction " of the neck, although in an orang in which tetanus had been induced by inoculation with tetanus toxin, H. E. Roaf[1] and one of us observed " retraction," which suggests that the observed retraction in that case was a deviated response due to the disease, and probably symptomatic of tetanus. To the small neck field lying on the free surface of the centralis anterior, our observations show that, at least in some specimens, a part of the cortex buried in sulcus post-centralis has to be added. Neck field lies between arm area and face area, and seems to mingle more with the latter than with the former. Occasionally the turning of neck is towards the ipsilateral side.

3. *Arm Area*

Thumb.—Movements of thumb are among the movements obtained from the lowest part of arm area, and usually the predominant ones there. Their field abuts on, but mingles relatively little with, eyelids, neck, and " pinna of ear " fields.

[1] *J. Physiol.*, 1906, **34**, 315.

Index Finger.—The field for primary movements of this digit appeared in some of our specimens to be larger even than that for thumb. Extension was a much more common movement than flexion, but isolated flexion was sometimes evoked. Extension of index as an isolated movement without any motion in thumb or other fingers was on very many occasions readily obtained. A not infrequent response from cortex when the resting posture happened to be one with adducted thumb and semi-flexed index was simultaneous abduction of thumb and straightening of index as if to let go an object that had been picked up. Occasionally isolated extension of the terminal and second phalanx only of index was evoked. In some chimpanzees we noted the using the singly extended index finger for various purposes to be habitual; thus, for picking the teeth after eating, for getting up a rice or maize grain between boards of the cage floor. The marked individuality of this finger's representation in cortex stands in harmony with such habituation. As an occasional response from cortex we saw extension of index finger accompanied by flexion of the three other fingers, no movement at all occurring in thumb.

Other Fingers.—Isolated movements of other individual fingers were, as might be expected, much less elicitable. Isolated flexion of middle finger alone was, however, obtainable occasionally, and notably in two very young chimpanzees. Isolated movement of annulus was never obtained. Closure of the whole hand was usually easily obtained, but the degree of separateness of the representation of the fingers as a group from that of thumb was marked. Over and over again all the fingers were extended or flexed without accompanying movement of thumb.

Wrist.—The motor field for wrist is extensive, and both flexion and extension are readily elicitable, the foci for the two lying not together, although near one another. The responses of wrist are closely bound up with those of fingers, but the former's focal field lies higher up the convolution. Wrist responses sometimes were obtainable from points very far forward, in front of precentral sulci, and then commonly in association with index and thumb; but there also the wrist tended to have its representation higher upon the face of the hemisphere than either thumb or index. There appears no great predominance in representation of flexion over extension or extension over flexion in regard to wrist when observations made in a number of hemispheres are taken together, although in a single experiment on a single hemisphere one or the other may appear to predominate.

Elbow.—Elbow has a large focal field, situate higher up centralis anterior than is wrist's, and below the shoulder's. Flexion of elbow predominates over extension in its representation. The two focal fields are commingled, but the smaller extension focus, in our experience, lies posterior to that for flexion; some of it lies buried in sulcus centralis.

Shoulder.—These movements are, as was to be expected, represented in a wide focal area, occupying their well-known position at the top of arm area. Their area extends into both central and precentral sulci. Genu superius varies much in prominence, and not rarely a small spur fissure, generally cutting into centralis anterior from behind, but sometimes from in front, lies partly, or rarely wholly, across the convolution at level of the

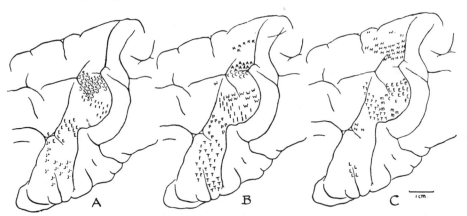

FIG. 67.—DIAGRAMS OF THE FOCAL REPRESENTATION OF SOME OF THE MOTOR RESPONSES IN THE CORTEX OF THE CHIMPANZEE

Illustrated on gyrus centralis anterior of one specimen, chimpanzee 6, but deduced from four specimens of fairly similar convolutional pattern

A.—S, primary movements of shoulder; F, primary movements of flexion of all fingers; L, primary movement of little finger alone; E, primary movement of closure of opposite eye; J+, primary movement of closure of jaw; J−, primary movement of opening of jaw

B.—K, primary movements of knee; A, primary movement of contralateral side of abdominal wall; C, primary movement of contralateral side of chest; W, primary movement of wrist; I, primary movement of index-finger by itself; P, movement of pinna of ear primary but usually concurrent with movement of other parts, generally facial; T, primary movement protrusion of tongue; t, primary movement retraction of tongue

C.—H, primary movements of hip, not always alone; E, primary movement flexion of elbow; e, primary movement extension of elbow; M, primary movement of middle finger alone; T, primary movement of thumb; N, primary movement of nose; L, movement of lapping (or licking) with the tongue

genu. Into the lower wall of this spur fissure shoulder area sometimes dips. Shoulder area merges somewhat gradually into elbow area below and into a chest-wall area above.

4. Trunk Area

Chest Wall.—There is a small area focal for movements of the contralateral chest wall. This lies opposite or close below genu superius of sulcus centralis. It lies partly buried in anterior wall of that sulcus, and in the spur fissure usually when that is present. It merges upward quickly into an area focal for movements of the abdominal wall.

Abdominal Wall.—Movements of the contralateral abdominal wall are very regularly elicitable from a small area situate at the genu superius level. The area merges in chest-wall area below and hip area above. The movements are, in our experience, always unilateral and contralateral. Some of the area commonly lies buried in sulcus centralis, and in the spur fissure when that is present. Over the area one or more large veins commonly traverse the face of the convolution, rendering the experimental examina-

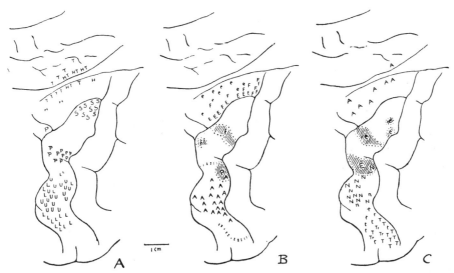

FIG. 68.—DIAGRAMS OF FOCAL REPRESENTATION OF SOME OF THE MOTOR RESPONSES IN THE CORTEX OF THE ORANG, FIGURED ON THE GYRUS CENTRALIS ANTERIOR OF ONE SPECIMEN (ORANG 3), BUT DEDUCED FROM OBSERVATIONS ON THREE ORANG HEMISPHERES OF FAIRLY SIMILAR CONVOLUTIONAL PATTERN

A.—T, primary movement of toes without hallux; H, primary movements of hallux alone; HT, primary movements of toes and hallux together; S, primary movements of shoulder; P, primary movements of thumb alone; *p*, primary movements of thumb along with other digit or digits; L, movements of lower lip without upper; U, movements of upper lip without lower

B.—F, primary movement flexion of hip; E, primary movement extension of hip; *e*, primary movement extension of hip concurrently with some other movement in leg; *f*, primary movement flexion of all fingers; P marks a point whence was sometimes obtained primary isolated movement of contralateral pinna; the shaded area surrounding it shows a field in which pinna movement was often primary; A, movement of angle of mouth (contralateral), almost always retraction and primary. The double-dotted lines above and below the group of A's indicate the upward and downward limits of the area whence angle of mouth movement was obtained secondarily or concurrently with other movements of face or tongue. One of the A's lies in the area focal for pinna movements

C.—A, primary movements; *e*, areas where the primary movement was flexion of wrist and extension of fingers; E, primary movement closure of opposite eye; N, movement of contralateral nostril alone; N (this is distinguished on map by being a smaller capital N), primary movement of nose, but concurrent with movements of other parts; *n*, movement of nostril closely secondary to other movements; *t*, retraction of tongue as primary movement; T, protrusion of tongue primary movement; Tr, twisting of tongue round its long axis as primary movement

tion of the area somewhat difficult. From the abdominal wall area anal movement is sometimes elicitable secondary to movements of the abdominal wall.

5. *Leg Area*

Leg Area.—The movements of the several parts of the limb seem more commingled in this area than are those of the separate limb parts in the arm area. Nevertheless, a general sequence of foci of main representation is recognisable; as the area is examined from below upwards this sequence runs hip, knee, ankle, and digits. The leg area extends over the mesial border of the hemisphere, and dips into the mesial surface for about one-third of the depth toward corpus callosum (Figs. 64, 66, 68). The area does not usually follow sulcus centralis to the extreme end of the sulcus, but leaves it a few millimetres below that, and slants obliquely forward over the mesial edge of the hemisphere.

Hip.—The movements have a wide focal field; in our experience, the lowest situate of the movements is flexion. On the whole, extension of hip lies farther anterior than does flexion. In some specimens, notably in one orang, extension of hip was represented as a primary movement over a much wider field than was flexion, but the reverse is more usual.

Knee.—Extension of knee as the sole movement of a response is rare, much more so than is flexion.

Ankle.—Movement of ankle occurs often as a leading movement, but tends to be rapidly followed by movement of some other part of the limb.

Digits.—Isolated movement of individual digits is not uncommon, as the " list of movements " shows. Some of the movements obtained from cortical stimulation of the anthropoid are such as we find difficult of execution ourselves. This was notably so with the foot area. Flexion of digits along with dorsal flexion of ankle we observed under cortical stimulation both in chimpanzee and orang. Extension of the second toe isolatedly from the other toes was also seen.

6. *Perineum Area*

Anal movement, usually protrusion, was elicitable fairly regularly and readily from a small area near the mesial border of the hemisphere in the anterior part of leg area, and apparently surrounded by this latter. The movement often seemed bilaterally symmetrical, but with weak stimuli was usually quite clearly unilateral and contralateral. Associated with it secondarily was movement of abdominal wall, as has been noted in the smaller monkeys by Schäfer[1] and by Jolly and Simpson.[2]

INFERENCES REGARDING FUNCTIONS OF THE MOTOR CORTEX

Franz[3] has recently obtained experimental evidence indicating that the functional topography of the motor cortex exhibits in *Macacus rhesus* demonstrable variation from individual to individual. The larger scale on which the motor cortex presents itself in the anthropoid, and the greater degree to which isolated movements of separate motor parts are elicitable from it, favours examination of the question, although our observations were not specially directed toward it when they were made. Compared one with another, the charts obtained from our anthropoid specimens of the

[1] *Textbook of Physiology*, Edinburgh, 1900, **2**, p. 747.
[2] *Proc. roy. Soc. Edinb.*, 1907, **27**, 63.
[3] *Psychological Monographs*, 1915, **19**, p. 80.

same species exhibit, as said above, differences in detail; the amount of difference varies very greatly, as reference to those of the charts reproduced will show. The differences are present even in those brains in which the convolutional pattern is less dissimilar than usual, and are then for that reason better recognisable. One difficulty for such comparisons is the fluctuating character of the sulci as landmarks for evaluating the topography. Since we must suppose that the sulci have some functional significance, this fluctuation may itself be taken as an indication of individual variation of function. And certainly variation of convolutional pattern from individual to individual is, in our experience, one of the most salient structural features of the anthropoid cerebrum. Another difficulty in making the comparison from individual to individual is the fact, illustrated above, that the cortical motor points, or many of them, are within limits functionally unstable. The chart obtained from a motor region examined at one time and by one series of stimulations may not agree in detail with that obtained from the same motor region at another time and under another series of stimulations. But the differences between the charts from different individuals in our experiments seem too wide in most instances to be accounted for by merely temporal fluctuations of response, such as localisation experiments somewhat differently conducted might evoke from one and the same hemisphere. Inspection of the charts reproduced exhibits the scale of difference observed better than can verbal description. We regard them as indicating that individual variation of the functional topography of the motor cortex, as found by Franz[1] in *Macacus rhesus*, is demonstrable in the anthropoid species examined by us, and in at least as liberal measure.

The list of motor responses taken as a whole shows that a very considerable number of different movements are obtainable from the motor cortex of the anthropoid, far more than can be obtained from the dog or Macaque. Although of these a very large proportion may crop up in any single systematically conducted point-to-point examination of a single hemisphere, many of them do not. From our experience we imagine that had our experiments extended to a larger number of hemispheres, the list, which continually slowly grew in length as our experiments proceeded, might have grown a great deal farther. Another point obvious from the bare memoranda in the list, but still more obvious to inspection of the movements as they occurred at the time, is that the individual movements, elicited by somewhat minutely localised stimulations, are, broadly speaking, fractional, in the sense that each, though co-ordinately executed, forms, so to say, but a unitary part of some more complex act, that would, to attain its purpose, involve combination of that unitary movement with others to make up a useful whole. In evidence of this " fractional " character it is only necessary to note the predominantly unilateral character, as elicited from the cortex, of movements that under natural circumstances are

---

[1] *Loc. cit.*

symmetrically bilateral. Thus under cortical stimulation even such movements as contraction of the fauces, adduction of the vocal cords, closing and opening of the jaws, protrusion of anus, were often, indeed usually, detectably asymmetrical, the execution being chiefly or wholly in some cases by the muscles of the contralateral side. A further point evident from the list is the considerable variety of combination into which these fractional movements were welded in the movement sequences noted. Our main purpose being " localisation " of the primary movement, we did not usually, by pressing and prolonging any single stimulation, develop these sequences in our observations. Had that been done, the listed variety of them would doubtless have been greatly increased. Their variety, however, even in the list obtained, indicates that a property possessed by the cortex is the combining of a large, though exhaustible, number of movements, belonging to this and that restricted portion of limb, face, or other motile part, into sequences of very great variety, sequences in which members of the same group of elementary movements follow now in one order, now in another, according as the point of cortex stimulated is chosen now at one place or now at another not too far apart, and influenced also by the stimulations that have been more immediately precurrent. It is the isolated and restricted character of the primary movements elicited by punctate stimulation of the cortex, or, to repeat the term introduced above, their fractional character, which makes so equivocal any purpose that an observer, who would interpret their purpose, can assign to them. Such a movement as the extension of the index finger can serve many purposes, so, again, a closure of the lips, or a retraction of the tongue, or flexion of the ankle. Some of the facial movements observed suggest mimetic acts, some the acts concerned with feeding; some, such as the narrowing of the glottis, might be mimetic on one occasion, deglutitional on another. But the combinational sequences are, so to say, eloquent of purpose in most instances. The large variety of partial, though discrete and in themselves perfect, movements of separate portions of the bodily framework, evocable by localised point-to-point stimulation of the motor cortex, and the multiform combinations which these assume under cortical reaction and the rich mutual associations of the cortical motor points which the physiological phenomena of " facilitation " and " deviation of response " reveal, are suggestive. They lead to the supposition that from movements of locally restricted parts—e.g., movements of a finger or of a limb-joint (movements themselves discrete and individually separable in the motor cortex)—the upbuilding of larger combinations varied in character and serviceable for purposes of different and varied kind, prehensile, defensive, locomotor, mimetic, masticatory, deglutitional, orientational (in von Monakow's sense[1]), etc., is one of the main offices performed by the motor cortex. The functional properties of this cortex seem specialised for that end. It appears at first sight surprising that a motor nervous organ relatively so

[1] *Die Localisation im Grosshirn*, 1914.

high as is the cerebral cortex in the nervous hierarchy, where the power to deal with large integrated complexes of the motor machinery might be expected, exhibits on actual examination a representation, still more or less discrete, of relatively small and " partial " movements. And in the motor cortex this discrete " representation " of small local items of movement, each highly co-ordinated with others yet separably elicitable, instead of becoming less evident with ascent to the higher types of hemisphere, becomes more so. Thus, it is more evident in cat and dog than in rabbit, more evident in the Macaque than in cat or dog, in baboon than in Macaque, in gibbon than in baboon, and in the chimpanzee, orang, and gorilla than in gibbon. It would seem that in order to preserve the possibility of being interchangeably compounded in a variety of ways, successive or simultaneous, these movements must lie, as more or less discrete and separable elements, within the grasp of the organ which has the varied compounding of them. To draw an analogy merely illustrative, the synthesis of the proteins of the body requires that certain metabolic organs must have, lying at their hand, the numerous amino-acid constituents of proteins; for that purpose the food proteins, split up into constituent chemical sub-groups, more or less freed one from another, are presented to the synthetic organs for varied re-grouping in the re-synthesis which follows. The motor cortex appears to be *par excellence* a synthetic organ for motor acts. How does the motor cortex obtain these fractional and partial movements on which work its powers of varied synthesis ? Simpler co-ordinated elements, such as flexion of a single joint—*e.g.*, knee or elbow—can be safely assumed to lie ready to its hand in the bulbo-spinal mechanisms. But the higher of the compounded movements which those mechanisms give tend, if judged from the spinal and decerebrate dog and cat, to be compounds exhibiting total flexion or total extension of a whole limb. In the limb movements evoked from the anthropoid motor cortex, flexion of one joint may go either with flexion or with extension of another. The motor cortex may therefore obtain the partial and fractional movements it so variously weaves together by, to a certain extent, breaking up compounds already constructed by lower centres. Such analytic power may be a property of its own, or of some other, perhaps subcortical, organ with which it keeps close touch. Such synthesis involves time adjustments as well as spatial adjustments. The bulbo-spinal axis also, of course, synthesises motor acts. But the difference between the constructive planes of the two is considerable. Bulbo-spinal synthesis constructs in the main those locally restricted but co-ordinate movements which the cortical synthesis finds ready to hand as elements for it to work with. The bulbo-spinal organ taken as a whole does, even in types so high as dog and cat, synthesise in addition to the local elementary movements a not inconsiderable number of more complex ones, such as respiratory, defensive, and even locomotory. But comparison of the synthetic capacity of the bulbo-spinal organ with that of the motor cortex reveals a great excess of synthetic capacity in the latter, as evidenced by the variety and multiform scope of the motor acts and sequences it builds up. Especially is this so when it is borne in mind that many acts which, when naturally performed, are bilateral, are, when excited by stimulation of one motor cortex, essentially unilateral, indicating that the two motor cortices have to be regarded as in many respects a single organ when in natural operation. Together they form, in such an animal type as the anthropoid ape, an organ for synthesis of movements—and of postures— on a vast scale. Phenomena, such as " reversal of response," " facilitation," and " deviation of response," prominent in cortical responses, and accounting for the functional instability of cortical motor points, are indicative of the enormous wealth of mutual associations existing between the separable motor cortical points, and those associations must be a characteristic part of the machinery by which the synthetic powers of that cortex are made possible. The motor cortex seems to possess, or to be in touch with, the small localised movements as separable units, and to supply great numbers of connecting processes between these, so as to associate them together in extremely varied combinations. The acquirement of skilled movements, though certainly a process involving far wider areas (cf. v. Monakow) of the cortex than the excitable zone itself, may be presumed to find in the motor cortex an organ whose synthetic properties are part of the physiological basis which renders that acquirement possible. What has been termed above the " functional instability " of cortical motor points seems but one aspect, revealed to experiment, of the many-sided motor synthesising which this cortex can effect. Such " instability " may be a means used in those cortical readjustments which the experiments of Osborne and Kilvington[1] and of Robert Kennedy[2] prove to take place where, after the experimental crossing of nerve-trunks, willed movements of normal effect are practically restored. As Franz and Bayliss[3] point out, the " instability " may serve as part of the basis on which is founded the educability of the cortex.

EXPERIMENTS BY ABLATION

Experimental Ablation of Arm Area of Left Hemisphere, Chimpanzee[4]

Troglodytes niger, ♂, strong, adult; tame. Not infrequently walks erect. Accepts fruit, etc., with either hand; no apparent preference of right. After food picks teeth with extended index of either hand. Generally walks quadrupedally; a common posture is the semi-erect, the support from front-limbs being given by knuckles touching floor. Shakes hands with either hand, and occasionally the grip of the hand is then felt to be very powerful. Picks up nuts with deftness, but the thumb is less used in such movement than might be expected; it seems too short to help the fingers

---

[1] *Brain*, 1910, **33**, 261.   [2] *Philos. Trans.*, 1914, **205B**, 27.
[3] *Principles of General Physiology*, London, 1915, p. 480.
[4] From same paper, p. 180. This is the first of seven ablation experiments reported in detail in the original.

for things requiring the finger tips. Sleeps with arm under head for pillow, generally with body not on side, but fully supine. When wanting to attract notice it has a habit of stamping one foot or both feet on the floor.

March 26, Forenoon.—Under deep chloroform anæsthesia the left hemisphere exposed through enlarged trephine hole over lower part of centralis region. The lower part of arm area of cortex and the upper part of face area explored by unipolar faradisation. The stimulation results mapped (Fig. 69) and recorded. Then the whole of the area yielding primary movements of thumb, index fingers, wrist, and elbow excised to a depth of about 7 mm. The excised field included the anterior wall of centralis fissure, but not the posterior wall, because no motor responses were elicited from it or from the free face of post-centralis gyrus. Wound closed aseptically.

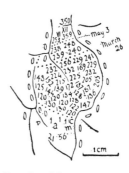

Afternoon.—The animal since recovering from the operative narcosis has eaten two bananas, and is lively. The right arm, which it seems surprised to find disability in using, shows marked wrist-drop. It moves right elbow and shoulder imperfectly, but with less imperfection at shoulder than at elbow. It moves right fingers little, and thumb and index hardly at all. There is a frequent twitching adduction of right thumb. Animal seems unable to grasp with right hand; the right hand slips on the vertical bars of the cage when animal tries to hold them by it.

FIG. 69.—MAP SHOWING THE CORTEX AREA ABLATED IN ABLATION EXPERIMENT I

The numerals indicate the responses obtained from it and its neighbourhood. Dotted lines indicate the edges of the ablation, the top one that of May 3, the others those of March 26. The numerals refer to the " list of motor responses," p. 404. o denotes that at no time did stimulation of the point so marked evoke any response

March 27.—The movement of right shoulder is obviously defective. The condition of right hand and elbow is the same as yesterday; but the animal rarely now attempts to use the hand for grasping, etc.; it seems to have learnt its disability in regard to that hand, and to do without it. Animal seems very well otherwise, and is active. Wound looks well.

March 30.—The movement of right shoulder has improved, but otherwise the condition of right arm remains apparently the same as on the day after operation. The animal was seen sleeping with its head pillowed on right arm, as was not unusual with it before the operation.

April 26.—Right shoulder seems perfect in all movements, so also elbow. Animal often supports itself in the quadrupedal posture by one fore-limb, while the other is used for feeding, etc.; for such support the right arm is employed seemingly as often as the left, the hand resting on the knuckles, and the support involving fixation of elbow in extension and of somewhat protracted shoulder. Wrist is moved well, and if any wrist-drop is present it is slight, although that wrist is often postured in a somewhat drooping pose, but questionably more so than usual. The three ulnar fingers seem perfectly strong and good in all actions. Index is imperfectly moved; it is generally flexed along with flexion of the ulnar three fingers, but without much strength. Nor does it follow the flexion of the ulnar three digits perfectly, for occasionally when the vertical bars of the cage are grasped by this hand the ulnar three fingers clasp the bar, but the index, although incurved, is curved not round the bar, but between the bar and the palm. This does not happen with the sound left hand. Neither is index of right hand ever seen to be moved independently of the other digits, although that is frequently the case in the left hand. In the left hand index is often both extended and flexed independently of the other fingers, but never in right. Thumb: this digit in the normal (left) hand is used less than might have been supposed; as mentioned above, the thumb seems too short to be very competent for opposition to the other digits, at least for many purposes. In the paretic right hand the thumb slightly but indubitably combines with the other digits in a general grasp with the hand, but this grasp movement is in reality less abnormal to inspection than it proves to be when the grasp is felt. The animal had been taught to shake hands, and with either hand. When one shakes hands with its right hand, one feels that it exerts very little compression or force with thumb of that hand; whereas, when one shakes hands with its left hand, the compressive force of the left thumb is felt to be good and considerable. Yet the right thumb is employed by it to a far from negligible degree. Thus it frequently employs the thumb of right hand in holding a banana, an apple, etc., with that hand; also in peeling a banana, the fruit itself being held in the left hand. Occasionally when eating fruit it holds the fruit with both hands, the right contributing seemingly an equal share of manipulation with the left. Thus, on one occasion, the right thumb was clearly seen to be employed with successful force to break a banana open, the ends of the fruit being held each with one hand, the thumb of each hand pressing down on the convexity of the banana from above, and so breaking the fruit. Sometimes the animal feeds from fruit held to the mouth by right hand alone. The ulnar three fingers of right hand are well used, not only for grasping, but apparently for all their full variety of movements.

May 3.—Condition of right arm appears the same as when last note was written. Animal lively and well. The scalp wound has been completely healed for more than a fortnight.

Animal anæsthetised, and the left hemisphere re-exposed in the same situation as before. Faradisation of the old lesion yields nothing. Stimulation of cortex adjoining it in front and behind yields nothing. Faradisation of post-centralis for the whole exposed extent of it yields nothing. Faradisation of precentralis adjoining the lesion above evokes brisk and strong retraction of shoulder, but no movement of wrist or hand, and questionably any of elbow. Faradisation of precentralis adjoining lesion below evokes retraction of opposite angle of mouth, especially of upper lip.

The old lesion was re-excised and slightly extended in depth, and the cortex adjoining its upper edge was excised for a 3-mm. strip. The wound was then closed aseptically.

May 4.—Animal very well and active; feeds eagerly, dances about and stamps on floor to attract notice; climbs about, coos, and calls, etc. Face perfectly normal. Right arm, including hand, is used as freely and well as before the last operation, but there seems somewhat less free use of the shoulder. The limb is, however, used for climbing, swinging, holding food, etc., apparently just as before.

May 5.—Same condition.

May 10.—Right shoulder seems to be fully used now; the second operation had seemed to impair its movement to some extent. Hand, etc., used freely, and seem to have been in nowise impaired by second operation: they seem in the same condition as recorded in the note written on April 26, certainly no worse.

May 14.—Animal well. Wound is practically healed. Animal deeply narcotised with chloroform; whole centralis region of left hemisphere exposed, faradised point for point, mapped, and results recorded. Results of stimulating cortex adjoining borders of lesion same as before. Lesion measured 10 mm. along lower horizontal border, 13 mm. along upper horizontal border, and has a vertical length of 14 mm. While the animal was being put under the anæsthetic it was noticed that it clenched its right hand vigorously on several occasions, exerting considerable force with fingers and thumb.

Left hemisphere's centralis region then exposed and explored. Animal then killed with chloroform.

Bulb and cord examined by Marchi method revealed a heavy degeneration in the left pyramidal tract (Fig. 70). In the pyramids the degeneration was entirely confined to the left pyramid. At the region of the most anterior part of the pyramidal decussation some of the degenerated fibres are seen to be among the very first to decussate. In the left pyramid the degenerated fibres, although scattered over the whole cross area of the pyramid, were somewhat less numerous, in comparison with normal fibres, at the ventral lateral angle than elsewhere. In regions of the decussation, where the decussation is in full progress and the degenerating fibres are undergoing that rearrangement in large bulk, it can be clearly seen that a certain few of them pass slanting dorsally and toward the left into the dorsal part of the lateral column of the ipsilateral side,[1] although the vast majority cross to the lateral column of contralateral side. In the upper cervical region (Fig. 70) the degeneration consists of a heavy crossed pyramid field, occupying most of the contralateral lateral column except for a well-marked border zone and for a ventral area. In the 2nd and 3rd cervical levels a few degenerated fibres lie at the extreme edge of lateral column for a short

[1] W. Muratoff, *Arch. Physiol.*, 1893; C. S. Sherrington, *Lancet*, February 3, 1894, **1**, 265; and E. L. Mellus, *Proc. roy. Soc.*, 1894, **55**, 208.

strip about midway between the dorsal and ventral roots.   Many degenerated fibres lie in the reticular formation at the base of the dorsal grey horn.   In the ipsilateral half of the cord there exists a slight and scattered degeneration in lateral column, occupying about the same area as that of the crossed pyramidal of the contralateral side[1] [2].   In the ipsilateral ventral column there is a well-marked ventral pyramidal tract[3] degeneration bordering the whole length of the cross-section of the lip of the ventral fissure.[4]

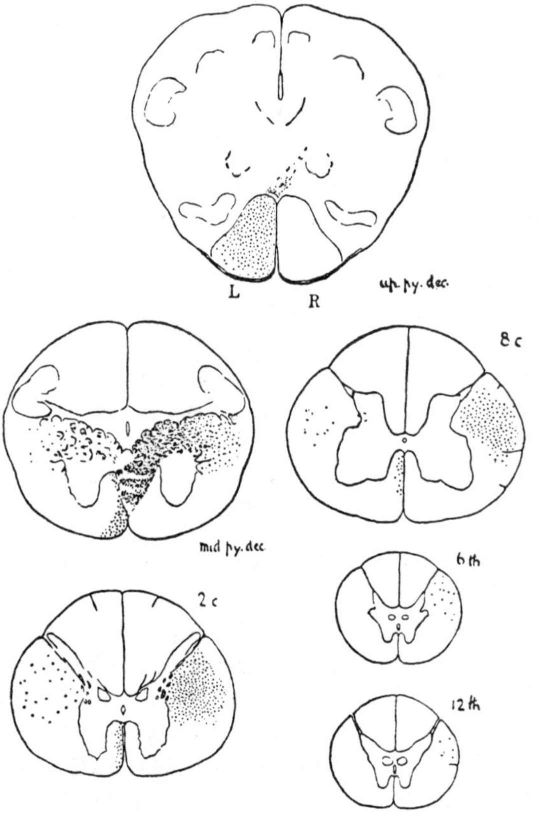

In lower cervical region the crossed and uncrossed lateral column degenerations have become very distinctly less heavy, although their areas relatively to that of the lateral column remain about the same as higher up. They also retain about the same proportions relatively each to the other. In the ipsilateral ventral column a " direct pyramidal tract " degeneration is still marked, but its area is smaller, and is confined to the deeper part of the side of the ventral fissure. Below the brachial enlargement the degenerations are seen to have become much smaller. In the mid-thoracic region no degeneration is detectable in the ipsilateral lateral column, but in ipsilateral ventral column a few degenerated fibres are still

FIG. 70 —OUTLINES (× 3 nat. size) OF CROSS-SECTION OF THE BULB AND SPINAL CORD OF CHIMPANZEE, SHOWING THE PYRAMIDAL-TRACT DEGENERATIONS AFTER LESION IN THE ARM AREA OF THE LEFT HEMISPHERE, IN ABLATION EXPERIMENT I

obvious near the ventral lip of the fissure.   In the contralateral side a faint scattered degeneration is still obvious occupying the usual pyra-

---

[1] W. Muratoff, *Arch. Physiol.*, 1893; C. S. Sherrington, *Lancet*, February 3, 1894, **1**, 265; and E. L. Mellus, *Proc. roy. Soc.*, 1894, **55**, 208.

[2] F. Franck and Pitres, *Gaz. méd.*, Paris, Mars, 1880, and Sherrington, *J. Physiol.*, 1889, **10**, 429.

[3] Grünbaum and Sherrington, *Proc. roy. Soc.*, 1901, **69**, 206, and 1903, **72**, 152, and Sherrington, *Integrative Action*, 1906.

[4] In the original paper this is illustrated by a photomicrogram showing the Marchi degeneration, the first demonstration of this tract in the anthropoid.—ED.

midal tract area. This latter degeneration is still detectable, although much less, at the 13th thoracic level, but lower than that is not recognisable with certainty. In the lumbar enlargement no degeneration can be detected.

The ventral horn of grey matter in the lower part of the brachial enlargement shows, especially in 7th and 8th cervical segments, a marked difference between the right and left sides. On the right side, the whole of the cross-area of ventral horn has scattered through it many degenerating fibres of very minute size; they give a " peppered " appearance to the grey matter there, in contrast to the ordinary clean appearance of the corresponding grey matter of the left half of the cord. The peppering is perhaps most marked in the dorsolateral and ventrolateral cell-group regions. It is certainly least in the medio-ventral cell-group. Sections stained with Marchi show these degenerated fibres in the grey matter but slightly, although, when aware of them, one can detect the presence of a number of them by that method. The degeneration in the ventral horn is, however, much better revealed by the Schäfer[1] combination of the Marchi and Kulschitzky methods; the minute blue-black ring surrounding the pale axis cylinder, which many of the very small fibres in the grey matter give by that method, when seen in cross-section, is altered to a minute blob containing no axis cylinder. In other words, the fine collaterals are degenerated, and their sheaths, with that element of it which the hæmatoxylin stain after the mordant tinges deeply, is broken up, and the axis cylinder also; and this kind of minute degeneration is scattered widely and liberally through the ventral horn. Our sections have not detected changes in the perikarya of the motoneurones, even where the minute nerve-fibre degeneration is most heavy.[2]

Experimental Ablation of Area yielding Closure of Eyelids from both Hemispheres[3]

December 2.—Gorilla savagei, young, ♂. Under deep chloroform narcosis trephined over the left hemisphere, lower centralis region. With strict aseptic precautions the centralis from superior genu downward and the frontal region anterior to it exposed and explored. Closure of eyelids extremely readily and regularly elicited as a primary movement from a small area which was made up of a seemingly continuous field of points, each of which evoked closure of eyelids, especially of contralateral eye, usually accompanied or followed immediately by some other secondary movement. In this area, on some occasions, from a small part of it the eyelids-closure was not primary, but followed upon a briefly precedent

[1] *Essentials of Histology*, London, 1901.
[2] For further observations on the degeneration of the pyramidal tract the reader is referred to the other ablation experiments reported in the same paper (*Quart. J. exp. Physiol.*, 1917, **11**, 135). See also Schäfer's *Textbook of Physiology*, 1900, **2**, pp. 808-9; *J. Physiol.*, 1893, **14**, 264, 281, 282; *ibid.*, 1890, **11**, 121 and 390; *ibid.*, 1889, **10**, 429. The bifurcation of fibres in the pyramidal and other tracts in their passage along the cord (" geminal fibres ") was described in *J. Physiol.*, 1892, **13**, *Proc. Physiol. Soc.*, xxi., and 1893, **14**, 295.—ED.
[3] Ablation experiment 5 of original series, from same paper, p. 200.

movement of mouth (retraction of angle of mouth contralateral to stimulus). The map (Fig. 71, A) illustrates with simplification of details the condition and area found.   The area's general position in the functional topography of centralis anterior was determined carefully by test stimulations of points above and below it.   The centralis anterior was found to yield a seemingly continuous field of motor points from genu superius above to the very tip of the centralis fissure below.   Characteristic localising points, as found in it, are entered on the map (Fig. 71, A).   Centralis posterior was nowhere found excitable.

Forward of the centralis anterior, in the region exposed, two fields were found, giving eyelid movements, in addition to the area yielding closure of lids in the precentral gyrus itself.   Both these frontal fields yielded open-

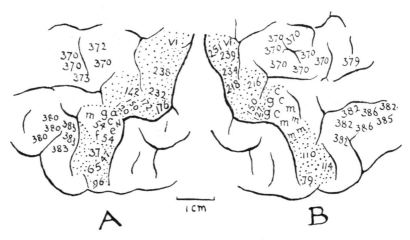

FIG. 71.—GORILLA 2, VERY YOUNG

A, left hemisphere; B, right hemisphere. The extent of the excitable area indicated by stippling, and its gradual merging forward into excitable indicated by decrease in density of stippling. Only some of the responses are mapped.   The areas enclosed in the heavier dotted lines indicate the portions ablated. See list on p. 404 for responses corresponding to numbers and letters

ing of eyes, and were functionally characterised by other distinctions, also from the eyelid region in precentralis.   These distinctions were that (1) the responsive movement could be evoked only by stronger faradisation than that sufficing to evoke motor response, including eyelid-closure response from precentralis—e.g., precentralis, eye-closure at 12·5 cm. of second coil; eye-opening from frontal regions at 10·5 cm. of second coil; (2) neither of the frontal fields yielding eye-opening offered a seemingly continuous field of excitable points, but consisted of scattered points which were excitable, yet even these were not excitable so regularly as were the eye-closure points in the precentralis; (3) the eye-opening movement was usually to all appearance fully symmetrically bilateral, sometimes it seemed slightly quicker or stronger contralateral to stimulation, but on the whole its bilateral equality was in marked contrast to the decided asymmetry of the eyelid-closure movement evoked for precentralis; this latter was never observed to be fully equal in both eyes, there being always a detectable preponderance of the movement on the contralateral side. Not rarely the eyelid-closure from precentralis was confined to the contralateral eye, and, when weak, was observed on one occasion to be confined to the contralateral eye's lower lid only, and on more than one occasion seemed to be confined to the upper lid of crossed eye only.

The movement of opening of eye responsive to faradisation of frontal cortex anterior to precentralis occurred, as mentioned above, in relation to two seemingly separable fields. Of these the lower one (Fig. 71, A) lay with sulcus precentralis inferior not far behind it. From this region the scattered points evoked eye-opening, often quickly followed by lateral deviation of the pupils towards the contralateral side. The other and higher field lay with the superior spur of sulcus precentralis medius behind it, and the inferior spur of sulcus precentralis superior farther behind it still. In this upper field the scattered points yielded eye-opening seemingly secondarily to turning of the eyeballs to contralateral side.

After the exposed region of cortex had been carefully explored and these results noted and mapped, the whole of the small field yielding eye-closure was carefully excised, the limits of the excision being shown in the map (Fig. 71, A) by a dotted line.

The dura was then replaced, stitched, and the whole wound closed. On recovering from the operative narcosis the animal revealed no indication whatever, so far as could be detected, of this lesion in regard to the eyes or eyelids. There was, however, distinct, though slight, drawing of the mouth toward the left side, and a slight flattening of the nasal fold on the right side—i.e., some slight paresis of lower part of face on right side. These symptoms were obvious the same evening and the next morning, and no others were observable. Two days later the slight facial paresis was no longer observable, and no abnormality of eyelids had been noted at any time.

December 6.—Under deep chloroform narcosis trephined over the lower centralis region of right hemisphere. Centralis fissure exposed from genu superius downward, also the frontal region anterior to it for some distance. Precentralis carefully explored with unipolar faradisation, with especial reference to eyelid-closure area. A small continuous field of excitable points giving this movement as its primary response was made out, as indicated on map (Fig. 71, B). Precentralis above and below also offered a seemingly continuous field of motor points; characteristic landmark points in the field as noted among others at the time are inserted in the map. It was noted that the eye-closure obtained from precentralis seemed rather more markedly contralateral than usual—i.e., that the associated closure of right eye accompanying closure of left seemed rather weaker than usual. As with the left hemisphere explored five days previously, so here with the right, a wide field yielding eye-opening was met with, and this field seemed separable into a lower and an upper, as in the left hemisphere, and the characters of its reaction resembled those already mentioned for the corresponding area of left hemisphere. It was noted, however, that from two points in the lower field the movement of eye-opening was followed by distinct convergence of the eyeballs, the convergence being directed toward a point not far aside from a plane continuous with mid-sagittal plane of head.

The eyelid-closure area was then carefully ablated within the delimitations marked in the map (Fig. 71, B). The dura was replaced, stitched, and the whole wound closed with aseptic precautions. On recovering from the operative narcosis the animal was noticed not to close the eyelids fully when blinking. Blinking was as frequent apparently as usual, and could be elicited by suddenly approaching the hand to the animal's face. Stronger eyelid-closure was elicited by touching the eyelids or conjunctiva, but even then the eye-closure was not tight, and seemed distinctly less vigorous than normal. The eyelid-closures which the animal now showed were clearly much less tight and vigorous than had been the closures evoked by many of the stimulations applied to the cortex. In these latter the skin of the eyelids themselves often was actually wrinkled by the closure, but this was never the case now with the closures produced by the animal itself, even in response to touching the conjunctiva.

The next day the condition remained the same as regards eyes. Some paresis of the lips was obvious.

December 8.—" The closing of the eyes seems now better; paresis in face quite as marked as yesterday; wound puffy."

It was then determined to open up the cortex; this was done under deep anæsthesia. The whole of the central region of both hemispheres was then systematically examined by unipolar faradisation. Nowhere in either precentralis were any further points found yielding eye-closure. The eye-closure area of both sides appeared to have been completely extirpated. The " motor " area otherwise gave under the analysis results' in harmony with the results obtained on the two previous gorillas. The results were mapped and recorded, but as the observations on the other two animals have been given in some detail, and these on this animal presented no obvious departure from those, the details are not reproduced, although incorporated in the general list of movements recorded in the anthropoids examined by us.

Remarks on Ablation Experiments : Recovery of Function after Ablation of the Cortex[1]

Owing to their lesser remoteness from human type it seems more possible, in regard to the anthropoid than to monkeys such as Macacus, to infer the animal's mental attitude at various times. A point which impressed

[1] From same paper, p. 206.

us repeatedly was the seeming entire ignorance on the part of the animal, on its awakening from an ablation experiment, of any disability precluding its performance of its willed acts as usual. Surprise at the failure of the limb to execute what it intended seemed the animal's mental attitude, and not merely for the first few minutes, but for many hours. It was often many hours before repeated and various failures to execute ordinary acts contributory to climbing, feeding, etc., seemed to impress gradually upon the animal that the limb was no longer to be relied upon for its usual services. The impression given us was that the fore-running idea of the action intended was present and as definitely and promptly developed as usual. All the other parts of the motor behaviour in the trains of action coming under observation seemed accurate and unimpeded except for the rôle, as executant, of the particular limb whose motor cortex was injured. And there seemed to be, and to persist for some time, a mental attitude of surprise at the want of fulfilment of that part of an act which had been expected to occur as usual. The surprise seemed to argue unfulfilled expectation, and defect in the motor execution rather than in the mental execution of the act, raising the question whether the function of part of the cortex ablated in such cases be not indeed infra-mental.

We would not by this suggest that the part of the cortex in which the motor zone is situate may not be involved in processes of synthesis of sensation as well as in that of motor and postural action. The recent experiments by Dusser de Barenne,[1] by minutely localised application of strychnine to the cortex of the " motor " zone, as well as to other adjoining parts of the cortex, clearly give grounds in support of the view that the cortex of the motor zone influences sensation.

The paresis of the limb whose corresponding motor cortex area had been heavily damaged by ablation was severe, as evidenced by imperfection of willed movements attempted to be executed by it in the early days following upon the inflicting of the lesion. But this paresis was largely temporary. Improvement in the willed actions of the limb set in very early, and progressed until the limb was finally used with much success for many purposes even of the finer kind. Thus after destruction of the greater part of the arm areas of both hemispheres the two hands were freely and successfully used for breaking open a banana and bringing the exposed pulp of the fruit to the mouth. And again, after considerable destruction of one leg area the foot was successfully used for holding on the bars when climbing about the cage. As we said in our preliminary communication, the absence of recrudescence of the hand paresis on ablating the remaining intact part of the arm area showed that that latter part of the cortex had not taken over the functions, at least not to any marked extent, of the ablated portion. " In accord with the absence of recrudescence of the hand paresis on ablating the remaining intact part of arm area was the finding that faradisation of that part (elbow and shoulder)

[1] *Quart. J. exp. Physiol.*, 1916, **9**, 355.

provoked as usual movements of elbow and shoulder, but not of hand itself, or only of hand late in a general arm movement, and that very rarely. In short, neither the ablation nor excitation methods gave any evidence that the remaining part of the arm area had taken on the functions of the ablated hand area.   Neither was the gyrus centralis posterior appreciably altered under exploration, and had not become a stimulable area for arm, hand, or other movements." And recently it has been found by T. Graham Brown and one of us, and by the former in independent observations, that subsequent ablation of the adjoining centralis posterior does not cause recrudescence of the arm paresis.   Further, as pointed out in our preliminary communication, the double arm area lesion showed clearly that the regaining of ability to use the limb could not be attributed to the arm area of one hemisphere taking over the functional powers of the arm area of the other hemisphere after the latter's ablation.   This confirms for the anthropoid the result obtained in the dog by François Franck,[1] and is itself confirmed by an experiment on the chimpanzee published by T. Graham Brown and one of us[2] much more recently.   On the other hand, that in the movements of some parts the motor cortex of one hemisphere is supported in its function by the corresponding part of the motor cortex of the other hemisphere is indicated by our ablation experiment on the eye-closure area.   In it the ablation of the area from one hemisphere produced very little paresis of the movement, but a rapidly successive ablation of the corresponding area from the other hemisphere brought about distinct paresis.   In this instance the movement impaired tends usually to be a bilateral one, and that seems the main factor accounting for the different result.

The absence of obvious symptoms resulting from destruction of a large part of the left inferior frontal gyrus in a very vociferous chimpanzee has probably not much weight in regard to the possible functions of that convolution in man.   The experiment and its negative result were mentioned in our preliminary communication, at a date prior to the interesting and important controversy as to the functions of that gyrus which has led to so much recent inquiry in regard to human material.

As regards the secondary degeneration in bulb and cord, they show that the pyramidal tract in the anthropoid (chimpanzee) more closely resembles the human than does that of any other animal so far examined.   In the chimpanzee, as in man, there is a well-marked uncrossed ventral column bundle belonging to the tract, and as in man, so in the chimpanzee, to judge from our experiments, though they are few, much individual variety exists in the relative size of that bundle to the rest of the tract.   The uncrossed ventral column bundle shows degeneration after arm area lesions as well as after leg area lesions, but in the latter case its degeneration is traceable into the lumbar region, whereas in the former it ceases much higher up the cord, although there it may be large.   The degeneration at the region of the pyramidal decussation shows, in addition to the main mass of fibres

---

[1] *Fonctions motrices du cerveau*, Paris, 1887.   [2] *J. Physiol.*, 1911, **43,** 209.

crossing to the contralateral lateral column, a small number of fibres sloping backward towards the ipsilateral column, as has been shown for the smaller monkeys, and presumably holds also for man. It is this uncrossed pyramidal tract slip entering ipsilateral lateral column which probably accounts for the scattered slight degeneration in the pyramidal tract area of the lateral column of the cord ipsilateral with the cortical lesion, an ipsilateral degeneration observed in all of our experiments. The pyramidal-tract degeneration after the arm area lesions was traceable to much below the brachial enlargement (cf. Sutherland Simpson and W. A. Jolly), but did not reach the lumbo-sacral. In the grey matter of the ventral grey horn of the side contralateral to the cortical lesion a heavy degeneration in the minute fibres was evident, in the brachial segments after arm area lesion, in the lumbo-sacral enlargement after leg area lesion.

FUNCTIONAL GROUPING OF PYRAMIDAL-TRACT FIBRES IN CRURA AND PONS[1]

The size of the pyramidal tract in the anthropoids is large enough to offer a better chance than in animals which are smaller or in which it is less developed for testing by faradisation the degree to which the various fibre groups from the various fields of the motor cortex lie separate or commingled in the tract at various levels. In the largest of our orangs we removed the whole brain in front of a transection through the posterior part of the anterior colliculi, and examined by faradisation the cross-section of the crusta. As so exposed, the pyramidal-tract fibre bundles run, of course, perpendicular to the plane of the transection. With fibres thus exposed the unipolar method of faradisation gives better opportunity than does the bipolar for minutely localised stimulation. With the former method the current lines converge in a direction more nearly parallel with the lengthwise direction of the fibres it is devised to excite. Examined by unipolar faradisation, the results obtained from the orang's crusta were as follows: The most lateral third of the cross-section gave no detected responses at all, neither did the most mesial fourth. The intermediate portion gave responses which, taken in sequence from its lateral edge to its mesial, were in the following order: toes, ankle and knee, hip, trunk, arm, face, and tongue (Fig. 72, A). There was very great overlapping of the areas yielding these results; thus it was easy to obtain from some points concurrent movement in leg, trunk and arm, or again of arm, face, and tongue.

The severity of the operation necessary for exposing such a cross-section did not allow a repetition of the observations at a lower level in the same

[1] From same paper, p. 216. Chapters on the effect of stimulating the insula, the effect of heat and cold applied to the scalp in changing the temperature of the cortex, the relative excitabilities of the cortex of cat, monkey, and chimpanzee, and the effect of carotid ligature are omitted here. See also note on arterial supply to the brain in apes, *Brain*, 1902, **25**, 270.—ED.

animal. But in the largest of our gorillas we removed the whole brain in front of a transection through the highest part of the pons, and examined by faradisation with the unipolar electrode the cross-section of the pyramidal tract at that level. The results obtained in both right and left pyramidal tracts were similar, confirming each other. They were that, although facial, lingual, brachial, and hind-limb movements of the contralateral side were evoked together by stimulation anywhere in the cross-section of the tract at that level, the movements in face and tongue predominated greatly when the electrode was applied to the mesial portion of the cut face of the tract, and movements of toes when the application was to the outer lateral portion of the tract, while, when the electrode lay about midway between the mesial and lateral borders of the tract, there was marked predominance of the finger movements (Fig. 72, B). The inference is therefore that

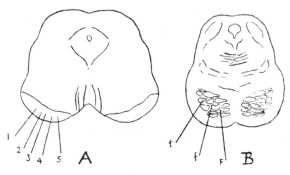

FIG. 72

A, outline of cross-section of the crura cerebri in a large orang, to show the position of the spots in the crusta whence unipolar faradisation elicited separable movements of opposite side

1, movement of toes and ankle; 2, hip and knee; 3, abdominal wall and chest wall; 4, fingers, thumb and wrist; 5, face and tongue; between 3 and 4, movements of elbow, wrist, and shoulder

B, outline of cross-section of anterior part of pons of gorilla, to show points whence movements predominating in toes (t), in fingers and thumb (f), and in face (F) respectively were elicitable by unipolar faradisation

although by that level the pyramidal-tract fibres from face, arm, and leg areas have become a good deal commingled, those for face predominate toward the mesial side of the tract, those for leg towards the lateral, and those for arm in the middle part of the tract's cross-area.

Along with these observations may be mentioned a feature observed in the pyramidal-tract degeneration following on destruction of the arm area in the chimpanzee (v. supra, Fig. 70). In the cross-section of the degenerated pyramid the degenerated fibres are somewhat less numerous in the ventro-lateral part than elsewhere.

And the same case showed that some of the fibres from arm area are among the highest of the fibres which decussate to the contralateral side in the pyramidal decussation.

In another of the orangs we made the following observations: After the hemispheres had been systematically explored with the electrode, and were still responding well, the spinal cord was exposed at the 4th thoracic segment, and the right lateral half carefully severed. Subsequent microscopic examination of the semi-section proved it to have been an accurate one, the whole right half being severed, with a slight trespass only into the left side on the dorsal column. Stimulation of the left cortex evoked after this lesion unaltered responses from face and arm area, but no response at all from trunk area or leg area. Responses from right cortex as before the semi-section. A second right side semi-section of the cord midway between 3rd and 4th cervical roots was then made. Microscopic examination subsequently showed that in this semi-section the mesial part of right ventral white column escaped severance. Stimulation of the left hemisphere's face area after this second semi-section evoked facial movements as before, but stimulation of the arm area evoked no intrinsic arm movements, although responses in trapezius and rhomboids were obtained from it. Responses from right hemisphere remained unaltered.

X

ON THE NATURE OF EXCITATION AND INHIBITION

[*The observations of Cajal had, by 1889, dealt a severe blow to the then prevalent hypothesis that the propagation of nervous impulses from cell to cell in the central nervous system took place through a continuous network of anastomosed dendritic branchings. With the appearance of the " neurone theory " the irreversible conduction of the reflex nervous mechanism, already stressed by James (1880), was first thought to indicate some " dynamic polarisation " of the whole nerve-cell. Sherrington (1897) preferred to regard the transmission by nerve-fibres within the central nervous system as being of the same nature as that in peripheral nerve, and to relate phenomena of selective transmission along this or that channel to properties of the place of contact between neurone and neurone, which he named the " synapse."*[1]

The principle of the " final common path " (1904) was introduced to account for the mode of interaction of different reflexes, and cleared the ground for a new conception of the interaction of inhibition and excitation. The manner in which one process neutralises the other, and the particular qualities of summation, after-discharge, and successive induction shared by all kinds of reflex activity were shown in a series of studies, particularly of the scratch-reflex and flexion-reflex, summarised in the Integrative Action of the Nervous System (1906).

In 1925 the hypothesis of nervous states existing at the synapse, " E " and " I," themselves mediators of the conditions excitation and inhibition of the neurone, was put forward to stress the occurrence of reflex effects which fell short of actual discharge of the motoneurone, and yet when intense could persist and cause discharge or inhibition for a period of many seconds. The hypothesis drew sharp distinction between " E " and " I," two processes of like physical behaviour but of opposite effect on the neurone. It was in direct conflict with that view by which others had supposed inhibition to occur as a result of a physical interference-effect between two trains of excitatory impulses.

The introduction of more accurate recording methods allowed the convergence of allied reflexes to be studied quantitatively. The result of interaction of two allied reflexes converging on the same final common path was found to be not inhibition as some had postulated, but " occlusion " (1927), the full saturation of the effector mechanism concerned. This had been predicted by the " E " and " I " hypothesis. Further work revealed the wide extent of reflex effects which influenced the state of neurones without actively provoking discharge (" subliminal effects "). Renewed study of the convergence of two single-volley flexion-reflexes with improved technique now enabled the relative intensity and duration of the two processes " E " and " I "

[1] Foster's *Textbook of Physiology*, London, seventh edition, 1897, **3,** 929.

440

(*now renamed " central excitatory state " and " central inhibitory state ") to be charted with exactitude.   The nature of these states is thought to be a physico-chemical change.—*Ed.]

1. The Final Common Path

If[1] we regard the nervous system of any higher organism from the broad point of view, a salient feature in its architecture is the following : At the commencement of every reflex arc is a receptive neurone, extending from the receptive surface to the central nervous organ.   That neurone forms the sole avenue which impulses generated at its receptive point can use whithersoever may be their distant destination.   That neurone is therefore a path exclusive to the impulses generated at its own receptive points, and other receptive points than its own cannot employ it.

But at the termination of every reflex arc we find a final neurone, the ultimate conductive link to an effector organ, gland, or muscle.   This last link in the chain—*e.g.*, the motoneurone—differs obviously in one important respect from the first link in the chain.   It does not subserve exclusively impulses generated at one single receptive source alone, but receives impulses from many receptive sources situate in many and various regions of the body. It is the sole path which all impulses, no matter whence they come, must travel if they would reach the muscle-fibres which it joins.   Therefore, while the receptive neurone forms a private path exclusive for impulses from one source only, the final or efferent is, so to say, a public path, *common* to impulses arising at any of many sources in a variety of receptive regions of the body.   The same effector organ stands in reflex connection not only with many individual receptive points, but even with many various receptive fields.   Reflex arcs arising in manifold sense-organs can pour their influence into one and the same muscle.   A limb-muscle is the *terminus ad quem* of nervous arcs arising not only in the right eye but in the left, not only in the eyes but in the organs of smell and hearing ; not only in these but in the geotropic labryinth, in the skin, and in the muscles and joints of the limb itself and of the other limbs as well.   Its motor nerve is a path common to all these.

Reflex arcs show, therefore, the general feature that the initial neurone is a private path exclusive for a single receptive point; and that finally the arcs embouch into a path leading to an effector organ, and that this final path is common to all receptive points wheresoever they may lie in the body, so long as they have any connection at all with the effector organ in question. Before finally converging upon the motoneurone arcs usually converge to some degree by their private paths embouching upon internuncial paths common in various degree to groups of private paths.   The terminal path may, to distinguish it from internuncial common paths, be called *the final*

[1] From " Correlation of Reflexes and the Principle of the Common Path," *Brit. Ass. Rep.*, 1904, p. 730.

common path. The motor nerve to a muscle is a collection of such final common paths.

Certain results flow from this arrangement. One seems the preclusion of qualitative differences between nerve impulses arising in different afferent nerves. If two conductors have a tract in common, there can hardly be qualitative difference between their modes of conduction.

A second result is that each receptor being dependent for communication with its effector organ upon a path not exclusively its own but common to it with certain other receptors, that nexus necessitates successive and not simultaneous use of the common path by various receptors using it to different effect. [1]Were there to occur at the final common path summation of the impulses received from two unlike receptors there would result in the effector organ an action useless for the purposes of either. When two stimuli are applied simultaneously which would evoke reflex actions that employ the same final common path in different ways, in my experience one reflex appears without the other. The result is this reflex or that reflex, but not the two together.

Suppose stimulation at the left shoulder evoking the scratching movement of the left leg, and the right shoulder then appropriately and strongly stimulated. This latter stimulus often inhibits the scratching movement in the opposite leg and starts it in its own. In other words, the stimulus at the right shoulder not only sets the flexor muscles of the leg of its own side into scratching action, but it inhibits the flexor muscles of the opposite leg. It throws into contraction the extensor muscles of that leg. In the previous example there was a similar co-ordination. The motor nerve to the flexor muscle is therefore under the control not only of the arcs of the scratch-reflex from the homonymous shoulder, but of those from the crossed shoulder as well. But in regard to their influence upon this final common path the arcs from the homonymous shoulder and the opposite shoulder are opposed. The influence of the latter depresses or suppresses activity in the common path.

Experiments by Verworn disallow any view that this kind of depression has its field in the motor nerve itself. Many circumstances connect it with the place where the converging neurones come together in the grey matter at commencement of the common path. The field of competition between the rival arcs seems to lie in the grey matter, where they impinge together upon the final or motoneurone. That is equivalent to saying that the esssential seat of the phenomenon is the synapse between the motoneurone and the axone-terminals of the penultimate neurones that converge upon it. There some of these arcs drive the final path into one kind of action, others drive it into a different kind of action, and others again preclude it from being activated by the rest.

My diagram treats the final common path as if it consisted of a single individual neurone. It is, of course, not so. The single neurone of the diagram stands for several thousands. It may be objected that in the

[1] *Ibid.,* p. 731.

various given actions these motoneurones are implicated in particular sets—one set in one action, one set in another. That view seems unlikely. In the scratch reflex, I think we can exclude it.[1]

2. On the Nature of Reflex Excitation and Inhibition of the Motoneurone, with Particular Reference to Variations in Quantity and Duration of Effect in Different Motoneurones from one and the same Stimulus[2]

[A reflex movement is the result of nervous discharge from motoneurones. There are grades of reflex effect in which the neurone is excited to a degree short of provoking actual discharge—sub-threshold (subliminal) effects. On the other hand discharge is often very prolonged after stimulation. In any diagrammatic, theoretical consideration of the central nervous process it is necessary to account, not only for variations in quantity and duration of the excitatory effect on the motoneurone, but also that the same afferent stimulus has different potency in its effect in different neurones in the same motor centre.

Similarly, consideration of the process of inhibition must take account of different quantities of inhibitory effects in different motoneurones from the same stimulus, and the capacity of the effect to persist a measurable time. The inhibitory effect " I " requires to be pictured as separate from that of excitation " E." It is a negation actively and extremely rapidly performed, and requires a positive mechanism.—Ed.]

If the following remarks venture to devise for reflex inhibition yet another schema additional to the several existent, they do so with full recognition of the value and service of schemes already ([3, 4, 5, 6, 7, 8]) in the field. A complex problem, however, may be helped by offer of alternative suggestions.

Dealing with the well-known schema originating from Keith Lucas,[3] and developed with such notable advantage to the subject by Adrian and Forbes, Adrian himself has very recently[6] summarised the present position of the problem and main views obtaining on it. Here, therefore, it may be permitted to proceed without further preface to the scheme which it is sought to offer for consideration.

The statement of the schema involves some preliminary account of the view which it implies of an excitatory reflex, since against that latter the reflex inhibition operates.

I. Excitatory Reflex

The scheme representing this can be given most concisely by describing the diagram (Fig. 73, p. 449) and stating the meaning attached to its features.

---

[1] In the original paper there follows an argument based on the results of conflict of the rhythm of two opposed scratch-reflexes, p. 734. Also discussed in *Integrative Action*, 1906, pp. 55-60 and Fig. 13.—Ed.

[2] From " Remarks on Some Aspects of Reflex Inhibition," *Proc. roy. Soc.*, 1925, **97B**, 519-45.

[3] Lucas, K., *The Conduction of the Nervous Impulse*, London, 1917.

[4] Forbes, A., *Physiol. Rev.*, 1922, **2**, 361.   [5] Brucke, E. T., *Z. Biol.*, 1922, **77**, 29.

[6] Adrian, E. D., *Brain*, 1924, **47**, 399.   [7] Brown, T. Graham, *Quart. J. exp. Physiol.*, 1924, **14**, 18.

[8] Cooper, S., and Adrian, E. D., *J. Physiol.*, 1924, **59**, 78.

A, A', A" represent the collection of the fibres of a purely excitatory afferent nerve, stimulation of which evokes contraction of the muscle M, M', M", through the central organ of C, C', C". A represents the afferent fibres of lower threshold than those represented by A', and A" the afferent fibres of higher threshold than A'. The fibre A acts on a unit C of the central organ by a main terminal, and has also a subsidiary terminal on a unit C' of that organ. Fibre A' acts by its main terminals on C' and C, and has also a subsidiary terminal on C". Fibre A" acts on C", C' and C. M, M' and M" represent the collection of the " motor-units " engageable by the reflex in regard to a muscle (or muscular group) excited by the reflex. The term " motor-unit " includes, together with the muscle-fibres innervated by the unit, the whole axon of the motoneurone from its hillock in the perikaryon down to its terminals in the muscle.[1] For the motor-unit the " all-or-none " principle of reaction is accepted, in accordance with the views established by Adrian, Lucas, Forbes, etc. That the unit contains further an " all-or-none " effector in the muscle-fibre itself (Lucas, Adrian, Pratt, etc.) is, for avoidance of complication, not indicated in the diagram. A more important omission is that although the thresholds of motor-units M, M', M" cannot, as is known from experiment, be equal, the diagram, again for simplicity, neglects that complication. To include it would give greater pliability to the diagram, but at impairment of facility for the textual description which follows. The " all-or-none " principle of reaction is also, in accordance with Forbes and Adrian,[2] accepted for the fibres of the afferent nerve, A, A', A". The excitation which stimulation of these fibres sets up in the central organ at C, C' and C" will be referred to in the textual description as E. Certain features are implied for it which, though not absolutely essential to the scheme, require mention as of importance for it.

[1] The use of an isometric myograph of the Blix pattern, with optical recording of the movement and consequent reduction of shortening of the muscle during contraction (*Proc. roy. Soc.*, 1921, **92B**, 245, and *ibid.*, 1926, **100B**, 266), allowed the assumption that at comparable rates of neurone discharge a rise or fall in the contraction-tension meant a corresponding quantitative rise or fall in the number of muscle-fibres in action. From the all-or-none law, it followed that this was directly translated into the proportionate number of motor nerve-fibres, and so motoneurones, which had entered or ceased discharge. As it was not at first known how rapidly the motoneurones discharged in reflexes, quantitative deductions were made only with maximal reflexes or break shock discharges (*Proc. roy. Soc.*, 1921, **92B**, 245; *ibid.*, 1923, **94B**, 142, 299, and 407; *ibid.*, 1925, **97B**, 488; *ibid.*, 1926, **100B**, 448). The isometric myograph thus improved and introduced into reflex analysis by Sherrington proved an extremely accurate instrument, and he later perfected (*J. Physiol.*, 1930, **69**, i, and *ibid.*, 1930, **70**, 101) a frictionless bearing to allow motor twitch curves to be recorded faithfully.

For this type of analysis of reflexes the term " *motor unit* " was coined, to represent the neurone in terms of muscular contraction (Liddell and Sherrington, *Proc. roy. Soc.*, 1925, **97B**, 488, Sherrington; *ibid.*, 1929, **105B**, 332). Later the numbers of motor units represented by many sample muscles, and the amount of contraction performed by one motor unit, were worked out (Eccles and Sherrington, *Proc. roy. Soc.*, 1930, **106B**, 326), and single motor units in reflex activity were recorded myographically. The latter paper also contains much information relating to the sizes and branching of motor nerve-fibres.—ED.

[2] Forbes, A., and Adrian, E. D., *J. Physiol.*, 1922, **56**, 315.

Following the view that with the nervous impulse a short-lived local change in the lateral membrane limiting ions in the axis-cylinder is propagated along the course of the nerve-fibre, it may be supposed that the arrival of that change at the central terminals of the afferent fibre is an essential element in the central excitation process. Along the course of the fibre the membrane separates nervous conducting substance from material which, in so far as it is not in that sense conducting, may be thought of as indifferent. But at the end of the terminal the intervention of the membrane is between a conducting substance and a conducting substance, namely, of one neurone and the next. There the membrane-change and the local ion-concentration it affects become significant for excitation of a trans-membrane conductor. There the nervous impulse resulting directly from the external stimulus may be regarded as ending, for there through an intermediary process and mechanism it generates, not inevitably though commonly, a new impulse located in, and conditioned by, the state and circumstances for the time being of the next down-stream neurone, a self-centred entity in many ways independent. Here, with other changes, may rise change in impulse-frequency, though that be still related to the centripetal. Lugaro[1] has proposed restricting the term " conduction " to intracellular propagation of the excited state, and employment of the term " transmission " for intercellular transference of the excited state.

In the Nernst theory developed by Lapicque,[2] Hill,[3] and others the rise in concentration for effective excitation must be in amount and rate above a certain critical value. And the theory takes account of a process, inherent in the conditions attending the establishment of the local ion-concentration, which tends to take those ions out of the sphere of action, a process for which diffusion and adsorption have been assigned as probable causes. This process, when the production of further excitation-ions ceases, removes the local concentration, the excitation ceasing. Suppose that, in result of an impulse transmitted up A, a change with these features at C form an exciting agent for the down-stream neurone leading to motor-unit M. The exciting-agent produced by the single impulse up A, after a short period of e.g. supraliminal intensity, will by deconcentration fall below threshold value and cease to be effective excitation.

But in any scheme of reflex action account has to be taken of the circumstance that mere prolongation—e.g., by repetition—of a brief external stimulus of the afferent nerve has usually the effect that a stimulus, which when brief is subliminal, becomes by prolongation—e.g., repetition— liminal or supraliminal. " Mere duration of the stimulus comes to be equivalent therefore to intensity."[4] And this result is intra-central. This result is explicable if at some central situation there be a structure which is something other than a nerve-fibre, and has, unlike nerve-fibre, no abso-

---

[1] Lugaro, E., *Revista d. Patologia Nerv. e Ment.*, 1917, **22**, fasc. 3.
[2] Lapicque, L., *J. de Physiol. et Path. gén.*, 1909, **11**, 1009 and 1035.
[3] Hill, A. V., *J. Physiol.*, 1910, **40**, 190.   [4] Sherrington, *Quart. J. exp. Physiol.*, 1908, **1**, 67.

lute refractory phase, and has, as have many other cell-structures including skeletal muscle-fibre itself, a property of summating its successive reactions when these are not too far apart in time.   In such a structure the production of an exciting agent, in response to a previous stimulus, would on receipt of a second stimulus before subsidence of it be augmented by further production, so that its amount would be increased.   In this way the central exciting state might by repetition of successive stimuli to the afferent nerve-fibre arise from below liminal amount or concentration to above liminal value.   The exciting state or agent, denoted E, is in the working of the diagram taken to be multiplied twofold by temporal summation.   Further, at such a structure the greater the amount of concentration of the exciting state or agent beyond the threshold value rendering it effective for excitation, the longer, other conditions equal, the time required for it to fall, by diffusion or adsorption, to below threshold value again; therefore persistence of the central excitation, after withdrawal of the stimulation of the afferent nerve, would occur, and the duration of that persistence would be, in so far, a measure of the degree of amount or concentration reached at the central unit by the exciting state or agent.

Further, account has to be taken of the experimental datum that with a single brief stimulus—e.g., a single-shock stimulus exciting fibres of the afferent nerve—increase of the strength of that stimulus so as to excite more fibres of that nerve, increases the after-discharge, not only as to number of motor-units evidencing it, but also as to the duration of the after-discharge in individual units.   From the principle of " convergence "[1]— shown as a histological feature of the central organ—it is a near inference that with the stronger stimulus of the afferent nerve, exciting more fibres in it than does the weaker, not only is the number of downstream neurones affected increased, but also that, even when the centripetal impulses from the afferent nerve consist of one single volley only, some of those neurones receive per individual affluent impulses by way of more terminals than they do under the weaker excitation of the afferent nerve.   It has been pointed out by Forbes[2] that, since the distance of travel of the centripetal impulses in reaching different terminals cannot be equal for them all, the receipt by one and the same downstream neurone of impulses *via* different terminals will involve asynchronism of that receipt, and some time-succession of arrival of the impulses at the neurone.   In this way, as Forbes points out, the excitation at the neurone will tend to last somewhat longer than when only one or fewer terminals act on it.   But the duration of after-discharge is commonly too prolonged to be, in my judgment,[3] explicable adequately by this datum only.

The increased duration of after-discharge produced by increase of strength of the single-shock stimulus of the afferent nerve would be explicable, however, if the several afferent terminals convergent upon the same

[1] *Brit. Ass. Rep.*, 1904 (p. 441 above).   [2] Forbes, *Physiol. Rev.*, 1922, **2**, 361.
[3] Sherrington, *Arch. int. Physiol.*, 1921, **18**, 620.

downstream neurone summate their several individual productions of the exciting state or agent in some central structure where their effects are confluent. If they there obtain a combined quantitative result in the amount or concentration of the exciting state they produce, then the argument above used holds here too—namely, that the local exciting state will, in proportion as it has risen above threshold value, take more time before it declines to below threshold value once more. In this way the prolongation of after-discharge would not be confined to the brief period measured by difference of distance of travel of centripetal impulses ere arrival at the central neurone; it becomes extended by the greater period involved in subsidence of the exciting state from supraliminal to liminal value, and that extension of period is greater for a greater supraliminal amount or concentration than for a smaller.

The after-discharge contraction is therefore in the working of the diagram regarded as the response of an all-or-none motor-unit during the period in which a centrally seated supramaximal stimulus exciting it is waning from supramaximal to threshold value, and so similarly the after-discharge efflux of impulses in the motoneurone axon supporting that contraction. The notion meant to be conveyed is not that of a continuous level of intensity of E, persisting—e.g., at C—after a single-shock stimulus or during a tetanic one. It is that in response to a single centripetal impulse there results, to use a term already suggested,[1] a " charge " of E, which shoots up to a certain amount (intensity) and then, less rapidly, declines. How brief may be the period during which the single charge remains supraliminal is seen from the observations of Forbes and Gregg,[2] and of Forbes and Adrian,[3] which show that a single charge may give one single impulse volley in the motor-units. Similarly the knee-jerk contraction is often equivalent only to a twitch contraction. Not uncommonly, however, the action of a single-shock " charge," as evidenced by the motor-units, lasts longer than in the cases mentioned above, and occasions in some of the motor-units a short tetanic response,[4, 5], owing to after-discharge appending itself to the initial effluent volley.

With a tetanic stimulus a succeeding individual stimulus arriving before a previous charge has fully subsided causes a second charge, which shoots up from the level of the residuum of the previous charge and again subsides, and so forth. Thus, with a tetanic stimulus at 30 per second the valleys, so to call them, between the successive rises of charge will be deeper than with a tetanic stimulus of equal strength, as regards its individual stimuli, but of 90 per second frequence. The fluctuating intensity of E may drop to below threshold value for M″ (through C″), or for M′ (through C′), while not for M (through C), between the successive stimuli, though above

[1] *Idem, Proc. roy. Soc.*, 1921, **92B,** 245.

[2] Forbes, A., and Gregg, A., *Amer. J. Physiol.*, 1915, **37,** 118, and **39,** 172.

[3] Forbes, A., and Adrian, E. D., *J. Physiol.*, 1922, **56,** 315.

[4] Sherrington, *Proc. roy. Soc.*, 1921, **92B,** 245.   [5] *Idem, Arch. int. Physiol.*, 1921, **18,** 620.

threshold immediately after each centripetal impulse (Fig. 73). The production of E, though a discontinuous process, can by repetition, especially of frequent and of strong centripetal impulses, lead to a continuous supra-liminal residuum of E, above which runs a fluctuating intensity with fluctuations corresponding in rate of frequence with the frequence of the external stimulus. The individual fluctuations will be smaller, and the mean intensity higher, in proportion, other conditions equal, as the frequence of the stimulus is rapid. Placed upstream from the motor-unit itself, the kind of temporal summation in view would, though in a different, so to say less sluggish, material, have likeness to that exhibited by the muscle-fibre lower down the arc.

On this view the central fluctuations in amount (intensity) of E corresponding with delivery of the external stimuli cease on withdrawal of that stimulus, and E's residuum which, after that withdrawal still causes, if above threshold value, after-discharge, dwindles steadily and is unsubjected to fluctuations such as the external stimulus produced. Hence, " after-discharge " contraction will exhibit no rhythm corresponding, as does that of the stimulation contraction-period, with that of the external stimulus. In this the scheme conforms with the experimental data.[1] Also with the fact that after-discharge contraction irregularities are, with a good myograph, all of them descents not ascents.

Looked at in the above way the phenomena of after-discharge, thus indicating that the quantities of exciting state or agent due to the individual afferent terminals convergent upon one and the same central unit C there reinforce one another, have a bearing upon the location of that central unit. Of the terminals themselves histological evidence (Cajal[2] and others) shows them as severally discrete.[3] But those convergent upon the same perikaryon and dendrites, although themselves discrete, reach a surface or synaptic membrane which, since it is that of one and the same cell, is in so far a single entity and is at the same time an arrival place common to the several terminals. And the same applies to perikaryon-dendrite substance proper as well as to their membrane. The locus of the mutual reinforcement of action of the terminals would therefore be assignable, not to the actual terminals themselves, but to the structure upon which they impinge in common. In the diagram, C, C', and C" represent loci of those common impingements, which must of course lie downstream from the afferent terminals themselves. Of the motoneurone itself those portions upstream from its axon presumably constitute one or more loci of this kind. But in the central field, extending between the terminals of the fibres of the afferent nerve and the emergent motor axon toward which they conduct, there are probably various other such loci, some at successive

[1] Liddell, and Sherrington, *Proc. roy. Soc.*, 1923, **95B**, 299.
[2] Cajal, Ramon y, *Histologia Normal*, Madrid, 1914, p. 612.
[3] In Cajal's figures two " boutons terminaux " are given occasionally to the same perikaryon by one and the same terminal fibre.

levels. The diagram does not attempt to enter upon representation of these. Each C stands, however, for a number of such convergence loci in the central organs, and some of them set " in parallel," but also some of them set " in series."

It is with these implications that E is used as a symbol for the central exciting state or agent, and numerals are attached to E for rough quantitative expression of its amount or concentration. C, C′, and C″ in the diagram indicate places at which the amounts or concentrations of E occur. When E at C in what follows has a quantity 1, its quantity is supposed to be of threshold value for the motor-unit M to which C leads. And similarly for E at C′ and C″. Stimuli delivered to the excitatory afferent are denoted by S when above threshold for A, but below for A′ and A″, by S′ when above for A and A′, but below for A″, by S″ when above threshold for A, A′, and A″. A, A′, and A‴'s main terminals provoke individually E of value 1; their subsidiary terminals (broken lines, Fig. 73) provoke individually E of value 0·5.

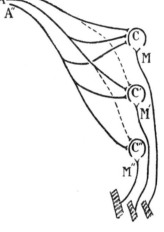

Fig. 73.

The diagram attempts to satisfy certain experimental facts:

1. With increase, within limits, of strength of a single-shock stimulus applied to the afferent nerve there occurs increase of the muscular response.[1]

[a] Stim. S, above threshold for A but below for A′ and A″, produces at C an E of value 1, at C′ by A's subterminal an E value 0·5. M's muscle-fibres contract, but M′'s do not, nor M″'s.

Stim. S′, above threshold for A and A′ but below for A″, evokes at C an E of value 2, at C′ an E of value 1·5, at C″ an E value 0·5. M's and M′'s muscle-fibres contract therefore; M″'s fibres do not respond.

Stim. S″ above threshold for A, A′, and A″ evokes at C an E value 3, at C′ an E value 2·5, at C″ an E value 1·5. M's and M′'s and M″'s muscle-fibres contract. Hence there is grading of the motor-responses in accordance with grading of the single-shock stimulus of the afferent nerve.

2. The single-shock reflex exhibits after-discharge.[2] With increase, within limits, of the strength of a single-shock stimulus of the afferent nerve, the reflex after-discharge is increased and prolonged.

[β] Stim. S (v.s.) evokes E of value 1 at C; stim. S′ (v.s.) evokes E of value 2 at C; stim. S″ (v.s.) E value 3 at C. E value 1 was taken (v.s.)

[1] Cf., for example, *Quart. J. exp. Physiol.*, 1908, **1**, 67, Figs. 1, 2, 3; *Proc. roy. Soc.*, 1921, **92B**, 245, Figs. 1, 2, 3.
[2] *Proc. roy. Soc.*, 1921, **92B**, 245; *Arch. int. Physiol.*, 1921, **18**, 620; *Proc. roy. Soc.*, 1923, **95B**, 299.

as liminal for obtaining response of M; therefore, after S″ E's value will take longer in subsiding to liminal than it takes after S′, and after S′ longer than after S.

Stim. S evokes E of value 0·5 at C′; S′ evokes there E 1·5; S″ evokes there E value 2·5; therefore the after-action at C′ effective for after-discharge in M′ is likewise longer after S″ than after S′, and after S′ than after S, which provokes none. At C″ similarly the after-discharge is longer after S″ than after S′, which provokes none.

Further, the diagram satisfies the requirement that the after-discharge is greater—i.e., effective on more motor-units after the stronger stimulus S″ than after the weaker stim. S′, and still more so than after the still weaker S.

The diagram, which is based chiefly on the crossed reflex of the knee-extensor, also indicates further that, other conditions equal, those motor-units which, as regards stimulation of the afferent nerve, offer a higher threshold are those in which after cessation of stimulation of that nerve the after-discharge will cease the earlier; and this is in conformity with the experimental data.[1]

3. In many excitatory reflexes mere prolongation of the otherwise unaltered stimulation of the afferent nerve increases the reflex contraction.[2] The process underlying this has been termed[3] " recruitment," meaning by that the activation of additional motor-units, within limits, under simple prolongation of the stimulus.

[γ] The diagram deals with this. By temporal summation (v.s.) suppose that the value of E can be increased twofold from that which it has without temporal summation. Then: under stim. S if tetanic in form value of E by temporal summation becomes 2 at C, at C′ becomes 1; therefore S which, when a single-shock stimulus, excites M but not M′, when repeated—e.g., as a tetanic series—excites M′ as well as M. Again, when tetanic, S′ gives, at C, E 4; at C′, E 3, and at C″, E 3—i.e., in virtue of prolongation S′ activates all the motor-units, whereas as a single-shock stimulus it activated (v.s.) M and M′ only; and this result complies also with the requirement that motor-unit M shall show after-discharge longer than the others.

The recruitment obtainable by prolonging a given stimulus of the afferent nerve does not, if that stimulus be below a certain intensity, proceed so far as to enlist all the motor-units of the whole motor-unit aggregate, however long the duration may be extended.[4] Conformably with this requirement, S, by prolongation in time, succeeds in exciting M′ in addition to M, which latter it can, without recruiting, excite. But by no prolongation can it extend its recruitment to C″ and so through it excite M″. The experimental fact would thus be taken to mean that the afferent fibres do not each one of them supply terminals to the central mechanisms corre-

[1] *Proc. roy. Soc.*, 1925, **97B**, 488.

[2] *Cf.*, for example, *Integrative Action*, 1906, Fig. 12; *J. Physiol.*, 1915, **49**, 346, Fig. 6; *Proc. roy. Soc.*, 1923, **95B**, 299, Figs. 12, 13.

[3] Liddell and Sherrington, *Proc. roy. Soc.*, 1924, **96B**, 212.   [4] *Ibid.*, 1923, **95B**, 299.

sponding with each one of all the individual motor-units. Conformably with this, strychnine, although favouring recruitment, does not increase it indefinitely—*i.e.*, convert every "partial" excitation of the whole moto-neurone aggregate into a "total" one, in the sense of enabling every effective afferent nerve stimulus to activate the whole aggregate of the motor-units.

4. Increase of strength (within limits) of the stimulus applied to the afferent nerve shortens the initial latent interval of the reflex.[1]

[δ] With stimulus S, in single-shock form, the value 1 is reached by E at C, exciting M. With stimulus S', in similar form, the value 2 is developed by E at C; presumably, therefore, E reaches its threshold value for C—namely, 1—earlier under stimulus S' than under stimulus S—*i.e.*, the latency of the response of M is shorter for stimulus S' than for stimulus S. In the same way, with stimulus S" as a single shock, the value developed by E at C is 3; and E will reach threshold value for C more quickly still. The reduction of initial latency under increase of strength of stimulus is found, experimentally, by recruitment, for the motor-units which in regard to stimulation of the afferent nerve have higher thresholds to be relatively greater than for those which have lower. Conformably with this requirement, under recruitment, S in its tetanic form gives E of value 1 at C', but S' gives E 3 at C'—*i.e.*, a value sixfold that of S at C' without recruitment—whereas at C it gives E 4—*i.e.*, only a fourfold increase of that which S without recruitment has at C. Therefore, the shortening of the latent period of response will be relatively greater at C' than at C.

5. Increase, within limits, of strength of stimulation of the afferent nerve increases the muscular response, not only when the stimulus is a single shock, but also when it is tetanic.[2]

[ε] The diagram evidently meets this. It satisfies also the further requirement, already shown for [β] the single-shock stimulus, that after cessation of the stronger stimulus, other conditions equal, more after-discharge will ensue than after cessation of the weaker.[3] Even with a reflex which does not "recruit," temporal summation will yet, under prolongation, within limits, of the otherwise unaltered external stimulus, increase the duration of the after-discharge.[4] And in no case will the "after-discharge" contraction exhibit the stimulus rhythm.[5] The diagram further meets the requirement that, *e.g.*, in the crossed reflex of the knee-extensor the after-discharge will be of longer duration in these motoneurones which, as regards the stimulation of the afferent nerve, are of lower threshold than in those which are of higher threshold.[6]

6. Persistence of after-discharge, both under single-shock[7] and tetanic stimuli, attaches in one and the same reflex-sample very unequally to

---

[1] *Cf.*, for example, *Ibid.*, 1905, **76B**, 269, Figs. 1, 2; *Integrative Action*, 1906, Figs. 2, 9, 16, 30, 31.
[2] *Cf.*, for example, *Integrative Action*, 1906, Fig. 5; *Proc. roy. Soc.*, 1910, **83B**, 456, Fig. 6.
[3] *Cf.*, for example, *Proc. roy. Soc.*, 1905, **76B**, 269, Fig. 8; *Integrative Action*, 1906, Figs. 5, 6, 7, 9.
[4] *Cf.*, for example, *ibid.*, Fig. 8.   [5] *Proc. roy. Soc.*, 1923, **95B**, 299.
[6] *Ibid.*, 1925, **97B**, 488.   [7] *Quart. J. exp. Physiol.*, 1913, **6**, 251.

different individuals of the " motor-unit " group engaged. This is so both with the flexion and the extensor reflex-types; in the former as a spinal reflex the after-discharge is rarely " total,"[1] even with strong external stimuli—*i.e.*, in some of the motor-units there is virtually no after-discharge, while in others there is lengthy after-discharge.

The scheme and diagram are obviously in conformity with this requirement of inequality in after-discharge, and various examples have been given above.

II. *Inhibitory Reflex*

Proceeding to the inhibitory reflex, the scheme offered is on lines similar to those suggested for the excitatory, but with replacement of E (v.s.) by I, this latter standing for a state or agent which produces lessening or

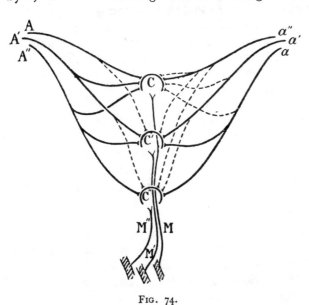

total disappearance of E. It will be noticed that in the diagram (Fig. 74) the terminals of a, a', a'', which stand for collections of fibres representing different threshold grades of a purely inhibitory afferent, are not in regard to the central mechanism, C, C', C'' disposed fully symmetrically with those of the excitatory afferent A, A', A''. It seems significant that if symmetrically disposed the diagram, though less clumsy of appearance, fails to comply as competently with the experimental data by which it is tested. If still less symmetrically disposed than as offered, the diagram would in some respects comply with the facts more fully, but becomes less simple for textual description.

Fig. 74.

Regarding the presumed state or agent I the following considerations are taken into account:

(1) The Nernst theory of excitation, and the development of it by Lapicque, Hill,[2] and others, recognise the existence of a process counter to the local accumulating of excitatory ion-concentration, a process which after cessation of the external stimulus—*i.e.*, in excitatory reflexes the stimulus applied to the excitatory afferent nerve-effects the disappearance

---

[1] *Proc. roy. Soc.*, 1923, **95B**, 299.   [2] *Loc. cit.*, p. 445.

of the local concentration. Suggestions offered as to the nature of this counter process responsible for the deconcentration have been that it consists in diffusion or absorption, or both, of excitation-ions. It might likewise conceivably be of the nature of a neutralisation of them, chemical or electrical.

(2) Inhibition in many respects resembles the subsidence and disappearance of excitation such as ensues on cessation of an excitatory stimulus; a difference is, however, the speed, often the much greater speed, of inhibition than of automatic post-excitatory subsidence. Hence arises an inference that inhibition may be essentially an active acceleration of the spontaneous dissipation of an exciting agent or state—e.g., an acceleration and augmentation of that deconcentration process already taken account of in the Nernst theory of excitation. Such acceleration might occur conceivably in several ways—e.g., by dilution of the medium, or by raising the local temperature, or by secretion of a catalyst, or by increasing the local conditions for chemical or electrical neutralisation of the excitation-ions, or by change in the membrane confining the concentration. Of these the two last mentioned seem to have the greater probabilities. Neutralisation is easier quantitatively pictured than is membrane change, and seems preferable further for a reason more conveniently stated later. The assumption followed, therefore, is that the impulses from the inhibitory afferent mediately or immediately evoke at C the production of an agent I which neutralises less or more of the exciting agent E and so lessens the amount or concentration of it. An analogy which rises to mind is the neutralisation of acid by alkali or of kations by anions.

(3) The inhibitory process not only accelerates the disappearance of a state of excitation, it also carries the condition of the excitable structure to a state farther removed from excitation than is its normal resting one. It resembles in so far the anodal effect of a galvanic current upon nerve; or, turning to another analogy, if we picture the excited state as one of acidity contrasted with a normal resting one of neutrality or faint alkalinity, then by inhibition a state can be arrived at which would be pictured by alkalinity of higher grade than the normal resting one. And observations by Adrian[1] illustrate the influence of pH on the nerve-impulse reaction itself.

(4) The procedure usually followed for observation of reflex inhibition is elicitation of its effect against an excitation already evoked and in operation. Stimulation of the inhibitory afferent when the excitatory reflex is not in operation may often seem to produce no central effect. That this absence of central effect is, however, only semblance can be shown in several ways. Thus precurrent brief stimulation of the inhibitory afferent will lengthen the latency and diminish the result of a closely following stimulus of the excitatory afferent. Again, stimulation of the inhibitory afferent begun precurrently and continued concurrently with a stimulation of the

[1] Adrian, E. D., *J. Physiol.*, 1921, **55**, 214.

excitatory afferent can prevent altogether or diminish the reflex result of the latter. The latter's effect will then not occur, or will not do so until the inhibitory nerve's stimulus has been withdrawn, or will before and for a brief period after that withdrawal do so only in diminished measure. Again, although no excitatory stimulus be present, stimulation of the inhibitory afferent. while producing no relaxation of the resting muscle may yet be followed, at some interval after cessation of the inhibitory stimulus, by " rebound "[1, 2] contraction of the muscle. This rebound contraction, of central origin as it is,[3] is post-inhibitory, and its occurrence documents a precurrent inhibition-state in the centre. It thus shows that the stimulation of the inhibitory afferent produced an inhibitory state even in absence of an excitatory state.

Therefore the state or agent immediately responsible for the central inhibition does not draw its source directly from a co-existent state of excitation. It does not arise from something furnished by the state of excitation or by the exciting agent. To establish it the co-existence of excitation or of the excitatory agent is not necessary. An analogy which rises to mind is the buffering of a medium against addition of acid. And just as a degree of central inhibition can be established which can preclude and prevent a certain strength of excitatory stimulus from provoking any muscular response at all, so conversely a degree of central excitation can be provoked which will prevent a given inhibitory-afferent stimulus from evoking in the reflex contraction any relaxation at all.

That I substance can arise and exist apart from co-existent E is yet compatible with the well-established fact that post-inhibitory " successive induction "[1] and " subsequent augmentation " (Forbes[4]) of excitatory discharge commonly occur, especially after strong inhibitory stimuli. These seem comparable with the phase of super-excitability ensuent in nerve after the anelectrotonus obtained in the anodal region of a galvanic current. Post-inhibitory rebound contraction is a common sequel to strong inhibition, and can be viewed as essentially analogous, although in terms of reflex action, to the " break-contraction " arising in nerve at the seat of the anode on cessation of a strong galvanic current. And post-inhibitory " successive induction " and " augmentation " have their counterpart in the favouring[5, 6] of inhibition by the so-called " fatigue " consequent on strong excitation. Though, therefore, it is assumed that the I state or agent can be produced independently of E, just as it is universally accepted that excitation can arise and exist independently of I, that assumption regarding I does not indicate that excitation has no relation to or consequences for the production of I, and *vice versa*.

(5) The phenomena of reflex action show central inhibitory after-action

[1] Sherrington, *Proc. roy. Soc.*, 1905, **76B,** 160.   [2] *Idem, ibid.,* 1907, **80B,** 53.
[3] *Idem, Quart. J. exp. Physiol.,* 1909, **2,** 109.   [4] Forbes, A., *ibid.,* 1913, **5,** 149.
[5] Sowton and Sherrington, *Proc. roy. Soc.,* 1911, **84B,** 212.
[6] Brown, T. Graham, *Quart. J. exp. Physiol.,* 1914, **7,** 210.

just as they show central excitatory after-action. The former evidences itself by, for instance, suppression of after-discharge, by retardation of return of contraction, by the long latency of rebound contraction, and so forth. There is therefore implied here in regard to I, the inhibitory state or agent, that like E its quantity or concentration after cessation of the stimulus of the inhibitory afferent, automatically subsides or deconcentrates, and that its amount or concentration and its persistence exhibit various degrees, one factor in them being production or presence of E, which tends to neutralise it. Thus, there may be present at a central locus, such as C (or C′, or C″), more of I than is sufficient to neutralise there the amount or concentration of E or enough just to do so, or only to do so partially. Where a numeral is attached to I in what follows, that indicates an amount or concentration of I just sufficient to neutralise E of quantity or concentration expressed (v.s.) by the same numeral. Since reflex inhibition in tetanic form is resoluble into successive brief units of inhibition,[1, 2, 3] just as reflex excitation in its tetanic form is resoluble into successive brief units of excitation, what was said previously (p. 447) as to the time-relations of the production and disappearance of E under single and tetanic forms of external stimulus is meant *mutatis mutandis* to hold for I. Reflex inhibition having its source in nervous impulses which themselves are individually short-lived events separated by intervals of refractory phase, the primary source of the inhibitory state is in so far a discontinuous process.

(6) As to time-relations of a single temporal inhibition-unit, they seem, as the view taken here would expect, closely like those of the excitation-unit. Thus, thanks to the work of Beritoff,[4] and of Adrian,[5] we know that the period for which a single inhibition-unit may make co-existent " excitation "—*i.e.*, E—subliminal may be as brief as to precede one single volley only of the centrifugal discharge. Beritoff, observing muscle action-currents, finds inhibitory pauses as short as 0·004 second; and with the myograph an inhibitory " relaxing " of the muscle from a single-shock stimulus of the inhibitory afferent can be as brief as 0·01 second,[6] and the entire inhibitory influence be finished and recovered from in 0·04 second. With stronger single stimuli, however, the central inhibition-state, like the central excitatory, lasts longer, its persistence being evidenced by after-action analogous with the " after-discharge " from persistence of E.[7]

When the repetitions of the centripetal impulses provoking the inhibition lie spaced too far apart in time for coalescence of the successive inhibitional units, the inhibition is discontinuous. And with weak, not too rapid, tetanic stimuli of this inhibitory afferent discontinuous—*i.e.*, tremulous—inhibitions are very usual.[8, 9] By completer fusion of the successive inhi-

[1] Sherrington, *Proc. roy. Soc.*, 1905, **76B**, 269.   [2] *Idem, ibid.*, 1908, **80**, 552.
[3] *Idem, Quart. J. exp. Physiol.*, 1908, **1**, 67.   [4] Beritoff, *Z. Biol.*, 1924, **80**, 173.
[5] Adrian, *Brain*, 1924, **47**, 399.   [6] Liddell and Sherrington, *Proc. roy. Soc.*, 1925, **97B**, 488.
[7] Sherrington, *Proc. roy. Soc.*, 1921, **92B**, 245.
[8] *Idem, Quart. J. exp. Physiol.*, 1908, **1**, 67, Fig. 6.
[9] *Idem, Proc. roy. Soc.*, 1909, **81B**, 256, Figs. 1, 9, 10.

bition-units—*e.g.*, under more frequent repetition—the inhibitory state becomes more fully continuous, and the effect consequent in the motor-unit can be a perfectly continuous one, since in the nerve-fibre and muscle-fibre the state of rest, unlike the nerve-fibre's activity, can be uninterruptedly continuous. That reflex tetanic inhibition commonly arrives at this continuity of expression is evidenced in the muscle (1) mechanically by perfectly continuous relaxed state,[1] and (2) electrically by unbroken absence of action-currents.[2]

A given single-shock stimulus of the inhibitory afferent will therefore be more effective in result on M (or M', or M") when it falls later after a single-shock E stimulus than when it falls earlier; and a stimulus of the excitatory afferent will be more effective in result upon M (or M', or M") when it falls later after an I stimulus than when it falls earlier. Hence, with tetanic stimuli the I will notch the reflex contraction more deeply when the individual I stimuli fall late in the intervals between the stimuli of the excitatory afferent, and conversely the stimuli of the excitatory afferent will better break through the effect of the inhibitory tetanic stimulus when they fall late in the I intervals. Also a rapid weak tetanic stimulation of the inhibitory afferent will leave contraction " teeth,"[3] or accentuate the contraction teeth, of a tetanic contraction caused by a tetanic stimulation of relatively low frequency applied to the excitatory afferent. The results of the " beat " experiments of Brucke[4] seem explicable in this way. The tremulous inhibitions[5] commonly met where two ordinary spring-hammer inductoria are used for tetanising the excitatory and inhibitory afferents concurrently, seem due to a like cause, mutual effect fluctuating according as the mutual incidence of the individual stimuli shifts. Such discontinuous inhibition changes to a fully continuous on strengthening the inhibitory stimulus.

In the diagram the several effects of the separate inhibitory terminals at C (or C', or C") upon which they are convergent are regarded as being confluent and mutually reinforcing, just as were those of the excitatory terminals; and also of being confluent there with those of the excitatory terminals, so that there results an algebraic summation of E and I. " The condition of the material of the common locus seems altered in two diametrically opposite ways by the two antagonistic arcs."[6]

The central seat of the reflex inhibition cannot lie farther up-stream than the intra-central seat of the excitatory after-discharge.[7] In the perikaryon (or dendrite) which the convergent though discrete terminals reach,

[1] *Idem, Trans. Med.-Chir. Soc.*, London, 1899, **82.**
[2] Dusser de Barenne, J. G., *Zbl. Physiol.*, 1911, **25**, 334; Einthoven, W., *Arch. néer. Physiol.*, 1918, **2**, 489; Beritoff, *loc. cit.*; Adrian, E. D., *Brain*, 1924, **47**, 399.
[3] Liddell and Sherrington, *Proc. roy. Soc.*, 1923, **95B**, 142.
[4] Brucke, E. T., *Z. Biol.*, 1922, **77**, 29.
[5] Sherrington, *Proc. roy. Soc.*, 1909, **81**, 256, Fig. 1.
[6] Sherrington, *Proc. roy. Soc.*, 1908, **80B**, 552; p. 269 this volume.
[7] Sherrington, *ibid.*, 1905, **76B**, 269; *Integrative Action*, 1906; *Quart. J. exp. Physiol.*, 1913, **6**, 251 (here p. 269); Liddell and Sherrington, *Proc. roy. Soc.*, 1923, **95B**, 142.

not only is its surface a structure common to those terminals in the sense that though they each reach a separate point of it, it yet is one surface underlying them in common; but so likewise is the subsurface. Cytological evidence as well as physiological consideration teaches that the perikaryon substance presents differences (of staining, etc.), from point to point. For the terminal " boutons " themselves evidence of such differentiation one from another is strikingly lacking. These data suggest that two terminals, though themselves essentially similar, may yet act in the perikaryon on subsurface material of different kind, so that one may cause there an excitatory, the other an inhibitory response. Separate intra-central terminals of one and the same (e.g., afferent) nerve-fibre may thus produce some of them excitational response in perikarya they reach, while others in other perikarya produce inhibitional response. J. N. Langley's[1] results demonstrating exchange of function in regenerated nerve-fibres in peripheral ganglia and other effector structures can be adduced in support of such a view, for in this case, as in those, the terminal effect is determined not by the afferent fibre and process, but by the seat and nature of the material receptive of them.

In diagram 2 main terminals of a, a', and a'' provoke individually I of value 1, the subsidiary terminals (dotted lines) provoke individually I of value 0·5. Stimuli delivered to the pure inhibitory afferent are denoted by s, s', and s'', s meaning a stimulus supraliminal for a but subliminal for a' and a'', s' a stimulus supraliminal for a and a' but subliminal for a'', s'' a stimulus supraliminal for a, a', and a''.

The diagram, as said above, envisages chiefly the kind of effects given at the knee-extensor under opposed play of its excitatory and inhibitory afferents. The power of the inhibitory afferent in respect of a given functional group of motor-units as contrasted with that of the excitatory afferents on that group is, as is well known, less in some instances than in others; and conversely. Thus, with the hind-limb, the inhibitory power of the ipsilateral afferents over knee-extensor's motor-units is as compared with the excitatory power of the contralateral afferents strong, while with knee-flexor[2] the inhibitory power of the contralateral afferents is weak as compared with the excitatory power of their opponents. An afferent, adequately and purely representing a natural receptive function,[3] will, if it in one " half-centre," to use Graham Brown's[4] useful term, have inhibitional upper hand, in the fellow half-centre have excitational upper hand. This seems clear from the case where two symmetrical stimuli, one right, one left, each evoking inhibition and excitation respectively in its two pairs of half-centres, but as regards its fellow stimulus antagonistic in effect on those half-centres, yet evoke, when concurrent, symmetrical muscular

[1] Langley, J. N., *J. Physiol.*, 1897, **22**, 215, and 1898, **23**, 240.
[2] Sherrington, *Proc. roy. Soc.*, 1909, **81B**, 256.
[3] Liddell and Sherrington, *Proc. roy. Soc.*, 1925, **97B**, 268.
[4] *Quart. J. exp. Physiol.*, 1911, **4**, 350.

effect—*e.g.*, flexion—of the limb-pair.[1] To deal with such differences between type-reflexes the diagram, without change in qualitative principle, would require quantitative adjustment—*e.g.*, in number of afferent terminals represented and in values of E and I attaching to them. A striking illustration of the complex and independent distribution of such terminals is the experimental datum[2] that the ipsilateral and popliteal nerves each cause commonly some contraction of knee-extensor which their greatly preponderant inhibitory effect on that muscle is unable to quell and seemingly leaves untouched. The searching quantitative analysis recently given by Graham Brown[3] of the interplay between inhibition and excitation at the ankle-antagonists under rapid tetanic stimuli, explaining the various results of concurrent summation there, brings out, among other things, the weight and upshot of non-coterminous distribution of the points of action, at each " half-centre," of inhibitory afferent with excitatory afferent. For adequate expression of this the above diagram, limited for simplicity to three central units only, is at disadvantage. The meagre extent to which it does so is, however, eked out further by allowing half-power only to " subsidiary " afferent terminals. Were the conditions taken as basis of the diagram those of the knee-flexor rather than the knee-extensor, there would have been better opportunity for expressing it. With the relations and proportioning between two half-centres of an antagonistic pair the diagram does not deal; it supposes, using Graham Brown's term, a half-centre only.[4]

III. *Concluding Remarks*[5]

The schema illustrates reflex " inertia " and " momentum," the former as due to temporal summation, the latter as the expression of after-discharge and its converse inhibitory after-action. " Conduction along reflex arcs presents in contrast to that along nerve-trunks characters that may be figuratively described as indicating inertia and momentum."[6] The simple analogy cannot be taken closely, because " reflex inertia " may be practically absent in cases where considerable " reflex momentum " is present, and *vice versa*. In the crossed extensor reflex with the knee-extensor de-afferented by appropriate root-severance, recruitment is markedly present and even exaggerated, while after-discharge is usually greatly reduced.[7, 8] And again, in the ipsilateral flexion reflex recruitment is practically absent, though there may be considerable after-discharge. *A priori* it seems somewhat surprising that a process such as temporal summation should exist

---

[1] Sherrington, Schäfer's *Textbook of Physiol.*, 1900, **2**, p. 840, Fig. 358.
[2] Liddell and Sherrington, *Proc. roy. Soc.*, 1923, **95B**, 407.
[3] *Quart. J. exp. Physiol.*, 1924, **14**, 18.
[4] In the original text the above hypothesis is tested against a series of experimental data, for which it appears to give adequate explanation. The reader is referred to the original if he wishes to pursue this exercise in detail.—Ed.
[5] Extract from the same paper, p. 522.   [6] *Integrative Action*, 1906.
[7] *Proc. roy. Soc.*, 1908, **80B**, 552.   [8] *Quart. J. exp. Physiol.*, 1909, **2**, 109.

as a necessity, dominating reflex action to the extent it does. It is true that it attaches much less to some reflexes than to others. Doubtless it confers advantages for function, but its disadvantages for speed of function might appear to outweigh other advantages. On the other hand, " after-discharge " and inhibitory after-action underlying " momentum " seem inherent to the central nervous system's use of surcharges of stimulus for the working of " all-or-none " mechanisms. Or, conversely put, the instruments of expression of the nervous system being " all-or-none " mechanisms, the nervous system, taking advantage of that safeguard, employs supramaximal stimuli in driving and arresting them, and so gains simplification for the problem of grading its resultant outcome by placing this latter upon the single basis of additive quantity of units engaged. The disadvantages attaching to the supramaximal stimuli as producing after-discharge and inhibitory after-action are, where these are not wanted, cured by counteruse of the two antagonistic processes of inhibition and excitation.[1] And, it may be remembered, in some cases—e.g., in visual phenomena—as long since pointed out by E. Hering, " positive " after-action possesses evident utility; so also in muscular acts it contributes toward smoothness and steadiness of the nerve-discharge underlying them.

From the standpoint which the diagram illustrates, reflex actions offer two discriminable attributes, quantity and intensity, quantity being expressed as the number of neurones engaged—i.e., the number activated in excitatory reflexes, and the number inhibited in inhibitory reflexes; intensity, on the other hand, being the excess of supraliminal state or the " surcharge " exerted from up-stream on the individual down-stream neurones and " all-or-none " mechanisms, whether that " surcharge " be excitatory, or inhibitional, or, as usually, some algebraical resultant of the two together.

Reverting to the schema above proposed, one weakness lies admittedly in its assumption of the existence of an agent simply as inferred from reactions of which that agent could be the cause; and that agent, moreover, one whose existence lies outside the intrinsic properties of pure nerve-fibre and with a, so to say, more chemical mode of origin and function than the nerve impulse *per se*. Nevertheless, reflex arcs always contain and reflex actions always involve, in addition to pure nerve-fibres, other nervous elements—e.g., synapses and perikarya—and these latter lie always in the grey matter; and the contrast between grey matter's wealth of blood-supply and white matter's poverty in that respect allows the inference that a chemical activity of nervous function exists in the former which is lacking to the latter, dealing as this latter does virtually with nerve-fibre reactions alone. Further, despite the low temperature-coefficient of nerve-fibre conduction (Lucas), the frequence-limit of impulse-transmission through spinal grey matter is halved by fall of 10° C. (Cooper and Adrian).[2] Moreover, in the grey matter appear functional features which nerve-fibres of themselves seemingly fail to give, features characteristic of reflex actions,

[1] *Quart. J. exp. Physiol.*, 1909, **2**, 109.   [2] *J. Physiol.*, 1924, **59**, 78.

such as long latency, preclusion of antidrome transmission, temporal summation, lengthy after-action, fatigue.

It may further be objected to the scheme that it reduces the afferent neurone-fibre, and the axons of the down-stream neurones on which that acts, to somewhat the character of secretory nerves. This, however, would be but in accord with recent evidence in favour of a so-called humoral view[1] of the nervous production of peripheral excitation and inhibition. "It appears unlikely that in their essential nature all forms of inhibition can be anything but one and the same process."[2] Thus, to go no farther than the "spontaneous" play of alternating phases of activity of the respiratory "centre"-group with their sensitivity to blood reaction (Haldane, Priestley, Douglas, Barcroft[3] and others), these suggest and seem significant of mutual quantitative "neutralisation" in interplay of opposed agents as argued in the scheme offered above. But the aim of such a provisional scheme can be but "*pour préciser les idées*," so the further and the better to test them against fact.

3. ANALYSIS OF REFLEX EFFECTS IN TERMS OF LARGER NUMBERS OF MOTO-NEURONES. CONVERGENCE OF AFFERENTS ON THE FINAL COMMON PATH, AND THE MANNER IN WHICH AFFERENTS OF SIMILAR REFLEX EFFECT HAVE REPRESENTATION AT THE MOTONEURONES WHICH THEY SHARE

[*The motoneurones which form the final common path of a reflex are numerous, and represented in a number of muscles, where each neurone controls the activity of certain muscle fibres. A reflex does not activate all the muscle fibres in (or moto-neurones for) a given muscle. In the flexion reflex the response from stimulation of one afferent nerve resembles that of stimulation of another, for the field from which the reflex can be obtained is large and is supplied by many nerves. When the response in any one flexor muscle is examined it is found that the muscle fibres (and therefore motoneurones) brought into activity are not exactly the same for the two afferents. Some are available to one, some to another, some are shared. If one set is already active at full rate of discharge, additional stimulation of the other afferent then evokes only the additional discharge of the neurones which are not shared. The others, being already in maximal discharge in response to the first afferent, are said to be "occluded."*

Occlusion increases if the reflexes are more intense. If the reflexes are very weak, the effect of one is added to that of another at the motoneurones where their effects overlap. Thus facilitation occurs in weak effects, where occlusion occurs with strong ones. An afferent stimulus of high frequency is "weak" or "strong" in terms of the number of afferent nerve fibres responding to the stimulus. Each afferent fibre

[1] Howell, W. H., and Duke, W. W., *Amer. J. Physiol.*, 1908, **21**, 51; Loewi, O., *Pflüg. Arch. ges. Physiol.*, 1921, **180**, 30 and 201; Brinkman, R., and van Dam, E., *J. Physiol.*, 1923, **57**, 379.

[2] Sherrington, C. S., *Integrative Action*, 1906.

[3] Douglas, C. G., and Haldane, J. S., *J. Physiol.*, 1909, **38**, 420; Haldane, J. S., and Priestley, J. G., *J. Physiol.*, 1905, **32**, 225; Barcroft, J., *J. Physiol., Proc. Physiol. Soc.*, 1919, **53**, xlviii.

must therefore be arranged so as to produce differing quantities of excitatory effect in different synapses, intense at some, slight at others, in a graded series. Of the fraction of the flexor motor neurones affected by a flexion-reflex-producing afferent, there is a set which is excited, but not sufficiently to provoke discharge. This " subliminal fringe " of the fraction must vary in numbers not only owing to facilitation or the reverse by other reflexes, but also according to the general excitability of the motoneurones.—ED.]

The Reflex Fractions of Muscles

The " flexion reflex,"[1] flexing the limb (hind) at hip, knee, and ankle, is elicitable from any one of a number of the various afferent nerves of the limb. It reveals to inspection little difference whichever be the particular afferent nerve stimulated. That the flexion evoked cannot, however, be strictly the same under excitation of the several different nerves has been already shown.[2] To examine further the differences it thus presents as evoked from the several nerves we have taken simultaneous myograms from paired flexor muscles under provocation of the reflex from various different afferent limb-nerves. The muscle pairs selected have been (1) a hip-flexor and a knee-flexor (tensor fasciæ femoris and semitendinosus) together, (2) a hip-flexor and an ankle-flexor (tensor fasciæ femoris and tibialis anticus) together, and (3) a knee-flexor and an ankle-flexor (semitendinosus and tibialis anticus) together.

The relative amount of contraction concurrently excited in pairs of muscles flexing hip, knee, and ankle, under stimulation of this or that different afferent nerve, is examined and shown to be different and more or less characteristic for each several nerve. Each afferent possesses motor-units, which in regard to itself are of practically similar threshold, scattered apart in separate and even widely distant muscles of the limb; and the latency of mechanical response of these is closely similar.

In the performance of a spinal reflex act therefore the executant muscular entity is not this or that individual muscle, but a set of motor-units made up from parts of various muscles. In carrying out this principle the several afferent nerves, although all severally evoking limb-flexion, combine the component part-contractions of the confederate muscles in proportions and degrees which are different and more or less characteristic for each individual afferent. The flexion-reflex is thus not wholly the same when evoked by different afferent nerves, even under comparable strengths of stimulus. The contraction of these or those particular flexor muscles is stressed according as the elicitation of the reflex is by this or that particular afferent nerve.

The term " flexion-reflex," therefore, just as the term " scratch-reflex," denotes, strictly speaking, a *group* of reflexes all more or less alike and all using approximately the same motor apparatus in approximately the same way, yet from one afferent to another differing in detailed distribution of

[1] Extracts from Creed and Sherrington, *Proc. roy. Soc.*, 1926, **100B**, 258, 264, 265.
[2] This volume, p. 168, and *Integrative Action*, 1906.

the motor-units employed, while yet always conforming to the general type " flexion-reflex."

The contraction values[1] of the reflexes yielded severally by individual afferent nerves, maximally stimulated and capable of activating the test-muscle, give in sum a value largely in excess of that of the muscle's maximal contraction. This we find with each of the three test-muscles. The amount of the surplus in the case of two of them may be instanced as follows:

(1) *Tibialis anticus*—maximal motor tetanus; 2,460 gm.

Afferent Nerve.	*Reflex Contraction.*
	Gm.
Dorsal digitals, 4 at 900 gm. each (sampled from one)	3600
External plantar	1240
Internal plantar	1330
Nerve of quadriceps extensor and sartorius	1190
Nerve of sural triceps	300
Hamstring nerve	515
Small sciatic	680
Obturator	565
	9420

(2) *Semitendinosus*—maximum motor tetanus; 3,000 gm.

Afferent Nerve.	*Reflex Contraction.*
	Gm.
A dorsal digital	2400
Another dorsal digital	2550
Another dorsal digital	1240
Obturator superficial	1270
Obturator, deep	630
Internal saphenous	1900
Nerve of sartorius	1500
Nerve of quadriceps extensor	2800
External cutaneous (groin)	830
Small sciatic	1860
Anterior tibial	2900
Popliteal	2650
	22530

Had the series of afferent nerves taken been a more numerous one and made up from individually smaller branch-nerves the surplus arrived at would have been certainly larger still. In neither of the above series was the afferent nerve of the test-muscle itself explicitly included, although that afferent possibly contributed, owing to stimulation by the contraction itself. The above results suffice, however, to show that the total aggregate of motor-units belonging to the test-muscle is represented several times over in the total collection of the limb afferents which can reflexly activate it. If the

[1] Extract from Cooper, Denny-Brown, and Sherrington, *Proc. roy. Soc.*, 1926, **100B**, 459, 460.

values taken above for the reflexes of the individual afferent nerves be replaced by those obtainable under strychnine, their joint excess over the maximal tetanus contraction becomes much greater; in other words, the overlap of the individual convergent afferents upon the units of their field of effect is seen to be potentially even more extensive yet. The values of the reflex contractions obtained severally, by maximal stimuli, from the individual branches derived from an afferent nerve yield a sum which exceeds the value of the contraction evoked, by maximal stimulation, of the whole parent nerve.

The reflex contractions obtained in certain typical flexor muscles of the hind-limb by stimulation of various afferent nerves of that limb within a few hours after spinal transection have been quantitatively examined, and show that under that condition the great majority of the individual nerves even when their stimulation is maximal activate the muscle only partially.

The fractional size of the reflex obtainable from a given afferent nerve shrinks under " spinal shock " and under " decerebrate shock," and, on the other hand, becomes much enlarged under strychnisation even of sub-convulsive degree.

Inferences drawn are that in its reflex use of a muscle the afferent nerve fractionates it, that the fractionation by different afferent nerves is different, and that the fractions of the muscle proper to the various individual afferent nerves overlap each other in the muscle.

Conclusions drawn from Observation of the Interaction of a Pair of Allied Flexion Reflexes acting on the Same Muscle[1]

Examination of the interaction between a pair of allied reflexes in a muscle which they both excite (the pairs of allied reflexes taken being those constituting the ipsilateral flexion-reflex of the spinal hind-limb) finds that the contraction evoked in the muscle by the two afferents acting concurrently is (apart from some limited exceptions[2]) less than the sum of the contractions yielded by them when not concurrent.

If the missing amount of contraction be referred to as " occluded," the occluded contraction is, with any given pair of afferents, relatively as well as absolutely greater when the reflexes are large as when they are small. In some instances the contraction of the smaller of two concurrent reflexes is occluded totally.

Examination of the features of the occlusion allows the inference that at some structure—e.g., motor-unit—of common approach by the convergent allied afferent arcs (a) tetanic activation at sufficient frequence by one of the arcs precludes additional effective activation by the other of them;

[1] Extract from Cooper, Denny-Brown, and Sherrington, *Proc. roy. Soc.*, 1927, **101B,** 299. See also *Reflex Activity of the Spinal Cord*, Oxford, 1932.
[2] The exceptions stated in the original paper were traceable to antagonisms between two afferents in relation to two of the test muscles. The ipsilateral nerves concerned contained elements capable of exciting the reflex of ipsilateral extension.

and that (*b*) activation in process from one arc is unimpaired by concurrent activity of the other arc. That concurrent stimulation of the two afferent arcs evokes a contraction less than the sum of the contractions observed when the afferents react apart would thus be an expression of the overlap of the two arcs upon motor units which are common to both.[1] The amount of deficit of contraction (occlusion) would measure the degree of overlap.

Convergence and Motoneurones[2]

Over and over again in the arrangement of the conducting paths of the nervous system there are places where two or more such paths converge and run to one. There two or more of the convergent paths when active will interact. Notable instances of such convergences occur in the spinal cord. The convergence point itself is, of course, inaccessible to direct experimental observation, situate in the spinal grey matter and at best a microscopic point. But happenings at the convergence-point, and inter-action there, can be gauged by consequences for the path or organ beyond— *i.e.*, down-stream from the place of confluence itself. One set of spinal convergences lies where the several afferent nerves which excite or inhibit a given muscle converge upon the mouth of the motor channel leading to that muscle. The muscle itself can serve as an index of the interaction. The muscle and its nerve may be thought of as an additive assembly of " motor-units," meaning by " motor-unit " an individual motor nerve-fibre together with the bunch of muscle-fibres it activates. Each such " motor unit " has centrally, of course, a nerve-cell, of which a group or " pool " represents the muscle in the spinal cord. The knee-flexor of the cat, *semi-tendinosus*, a useful muscle for reflex experiments, counts about 480 motor-units, with an average contraction tension of some 7·5 grammes per unit, when the unit is fully tetanised under isometric conditions. Gastrocnemius, a larger muscle, presents about 950 motor-units, but in it the average tension value per unit is some four times greater than in semitendinosus. The same contraction-tension value obtains whether the tetanisation is reflex or direct; it increases little with rate when once the tetanus is fairly completely fused. In the flexion-reflex risk of the tetanus being incomplete is easily avoided, because the tetanising frequency employed for the afferent nerve comes right through to the motor-units it activates, indeed some of them tend to discharge faster than the stimulus fires.[3] The tension-height of the isometric tetanus, reflex or direct, thus indicates the number of motor-units active.

[1] The possibility that individual afferent nerve fibres undergo sufficient branching in the peripheral nerves to account for inclusion of branches of the same fibres in two different nerves is discussed in the original paper. The effects here discussed are from nerves from widely different regions in the same limb, where branches of the same afferent fibre are likely to be few.—ED.

[2] This and the following sections constitute the Ferrier Lecture, " Some Functional Problems attaching to Convergence," *Proc. roy. Soc.*, 1929, **105B**, 332. A preliminary eulogy to Ferrier has been omitted, and the illustrations reduced from 25 figures to 11.

[3] Sassa and Sherrington, *Proc. roy. Soc.*, 1921, **92B**, 108; and Sherrington, *ibid.*, 1921, **92B**, 245, *Arch. int. Physiol.*, 1921, **18**, 620.

I.—*Confluence of Excitatory with Excitatory Path*

When the convergence point is tested by exciting concurrently two of the various afferent nerves converging upon it, the motor-units excited in the test-muscle under the concurrent stimulation are, in a large class of cases, found to be fewer than the sum of units activated by the two afferents when acting singly.[1] The conjoint stimulation then shows a contraction-deficit as against the sum of the contraction-responses of the two nerves taken separately.

This defect might be the result of central inhibition such as at some convergence points commonly occurs by reason of certain afferents, while exciting their own motor-units, inhibiting those belonging to a rival. Or the inhibition might be of the Wedenskii interference type, as has at times been argued for confluent paths in the central nervous system, the two convergent trains of excitatory impulses interfering and so weakening and partly invalidating each the other. Experiment proves, however, that in the class of cases before us here the valid explanation is neither of the above. What in fact happens is illustrated by experiments of the following kind, the actual sample here cited being an extreme instance of its kind.

Occlusion of Contraction

The large afferent A (Fig. 75A, *p'*) produces in the test-muscle a tetanic contraction of which the isometric myograph registers the tension value. Another large afferent B (Fig. 75A, *ei'*) is similarly tetanised and its contraction response in the same muscle is similarly registered. The two afferents are then stimulated in overlapping sequence, A leading. B's excitation is found to be unaccompanied then by obvious mechanical result, until A's excitation is brought to an end, when B's mechanical effect at once appears. Before and after the reflex observations the muscle's motor nerve is tetanised maximally and the maximal contraction obtainable is recorded under conditions the same as those employed during the reflex contractions. This comparison shows that the afferent A in the above instance was evoking the same tetanic tension as is given by direct maximal tetanisation of the whole muscle. That same value of tetanic tension was also maintained throughout the concurrent stimulation of A with B. Therefore under the concurrent stimulation none whatever of the motor-units of the muscle could have been in any way inhibited, for every fibre of the entire muscle was in full tetanic contraction and therefore clearly every one of its motor-units was in full activity. Indeed, the smooth unhesitating emergence of B's mechanical response immediately A's stimulus is remitted, as also the steadying supporting effect of B on A's response where (Fig. 75B) A's contraction is unsteady or begins to fail, indicates that B far from inhibiting really supports the muscle's contraction during concurrence

---

[1] Cooper, Denny-Brown, and Sherrington, *Proc. roy. Soc.*, 1927, **101B**, 262.

with A.[1] The two impulse-trains are, so to say, filtering through each other *via* the convergence-point. A factor determining the freedom with which they do so, and, so to say, the fineness of their filtration, is the duration of the refractory phase. Observation has not so far detected a central refractory phase, at least not one longer in duration than that of the motor-unit itself. But the size of the motoneurone and of its axon differs individually, even within the same motoneurone pool, more than has been thought, and with that the time-relations of the whole conducted disturb-

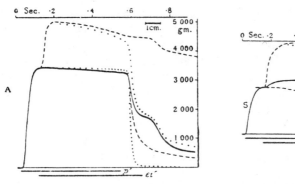
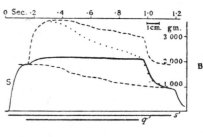

FIG. 75A.—OCCLUSION OF CONTRACTION

Contraction (unbroken line) in response to peroneal stim. (12 cm. coil, 90 per second) during *p'* followed by stim. (12 cm. coil, 80 per second) of both plantar nerves together during *ei'*. Upper broken line shows control reflex of plantars in absence of peroneal; lower broken line shows course of control reflex of peroneal alone. The lower dotted line marks the course of the tetanic contraction from maximal motor nerve stim. (12 cm. coil, 90 per second) during *p'*. The upper dotted line indicates the course of the reflex contraction from *p'+ei'* had their reflexes simply summed. The rhythms of the concurrent stimuli would yield interference beats of 10 a second, but no corresponding waves noticeably break the contraction plateau of the concurrent period, although the occlusion amounts to about 44 per cent. of the resultant contraction. *Semitend.*

FIG. 75B

Contraction S elicited by stim. (13 cm. coil, 95 per second) of int. saphen. n. during *s'*, followed by n. of quad. extensor (13 cm. coil, 88 per second) during *q'*. Upper broken line, control reflex of *q'* alone; lower broken line, control of *s'* alone. Fall after *q'* indicates that during concurrence the motor-units largely changed hands; the concurrent period's plateau shows no undulations at interference rate of the stimuli. *Tens. f. fem.* (Cooper, Denny-Brown, and Sherrington, *Proc. roy. Soc.*, 1927, **101B**, 262)

ance will vary more than was thought from unit to unit. Our immediate concern here is that the convergence-point is letting through a second train of impulses upon muscle-fibres which are already producing under another

[1] The interaction of a large number of flexion reflexes in different muscles and with different afferents was examined (Cooper, Denny-Brown, and Sherrington, *Proc. roy. Soc.*, 1927, **101B**, 262-303). Between some, as might be expected from variation in detail between one flexion reflex and another, there is true inhibition. A large reflex may be prevented or stopped by a small one. On the other hand, it is in the addition of reflexes of like effect that " occlusion " occurs. It is not abolition of one reflex response by another, but previous saturation of part or whole of the reflex effector mechanism by the one, so that the other finds the motoneurones already active. Discharge is not actively prevented, as occurs in inhibition; it is already in progress. It is important to realise that in many kinds of nervous reaction both inhibition and occlusion occur, and are two distinct processes with differing mechanism.—ED.

train their full mechanical tension; and those muscle-fibres can for the time being increase their mechanical tension no farther. Far from being inhibited the central units of the motoneurone pool are more active under the double stimulation than under either stimulus singly.

A functional limit to the mechanical response of the muscle-fibres themselves determines therefore this deficit shown by the conjoint reflex response. A's mechanical response, where it occurs in the same motor-units as does B's, occludes this latter. The central convergence-point is not the seat of the reflex deficit; though the confluence admitted at that point is a condition for the occlusion which results in the muscle and occasions the deficit.

Thus, the occlusion, itself an easily measurable result, serves as measure of the amount of convergence of separate afferents upon the central ends of motor units which they reach in common. Occlusion in short measures the amount of overlap of different afferents upon one and the same motor unit. Examined by occlusion the central overlap of different afferents upon motor units common to them is found to be extremely great, both in kind and degree. On one and the same motor unit there overlap not only skin afferents with skin afferents, but muscle afferents with muscle afferents, and muscle afferents with skin afferents and visceral with both those others, and over and above these the proprioceptives intrinsic to the given test-muscle itself. In the limb no pair of afferent nerves is found which does not when stimulated maximally exhibit overlap between their proper fields of effect in the motoneurone pool of the test-muscle. Examined by occlusion the overlap of the constituent branches of a single large afferent nerve upon its motor-units can be well above tenfold. The picture arrived at by reflex experiment shows a wealth of convergence on a par with that indicated long since by the histological researches of Ramón y Cajal.[1]

Occlusion as Index to Reflex Overlap

Central overlap is measured by deficit due to occlusion. In order to find the extreme limit of the central overlap between a given pair of afferents the stimulation of them has to be " maximal "—i.e., should excite all the afferent nerve-fibres. The central field of excitatory effect will then be at its largest for each of the afferent nerves, and so afford the widest chance of overlap upon the motor-units. The field of excitatory effect of a single maximally excited afferent nerve rarely covers the entire motoneurone pool of a given muscle.[2,3] Practically always the reflex action activates the muscle fractionally; but, other things equal, the fraction is largest when the stimulation of the afferent is maximal.

Is the limit set to this fraction an absolute and structural one? The size of the " maximal " fraction may vary within the course of one and the same experiment. Thus, as spinal shock passes off it becomes larger;

[1] *Trab. Lab. Invest. biol. Univ. Madr.*, 1903, **2**, 129.
[2] Creed and Sherrington, *Proc. roy. Soc.*, 1926, **100B**, 258.
[3] Cooper, Denny-Brown, and Sherrington, *Proc. roy. Soc.*, 1926, **100B**, 448.

an anæsthetic diminishes it before extinguishing it; a subconvulsive dose
of strychnine increases it while still leaving it a fraction—*i.e.*, unable to

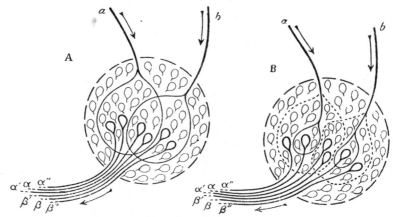

FIG. 76A.—OCCLUSION

Two excitatory afferents, *a* and *b*, with their fields of supraliminal effect in the motoneurone
pool of a muscle. *a* activates by itself 4 units (α′, α, α″ and β′); *b* by itself 4 (β′, β, β″ and α′).
Concurrently they activate not 8 but 6—*i.e.*, give contraction deficit by occlusion of contraction
in α′ and β′

FIG. 76B.—FACILITATION

Weaker stimulation of *a* and *b* restricting their supraliminal fields of effect in the pool as shown
by the continuous-line limit. *a* by itself activates 1 unit; *b* similarly; concurrently they activate
4 units (α′, α, β′ and β) owing to summation of subliminal effect in the overlap of the subliminal
fields outlined by dots. (Subliminal fields of effect are not indicated in diagram A)

cover the pool entirely. The upper limit of the fraction is evidently therefore a functional limit[1]—a functional state sensitive to exaltation and
depression, and within limits capable of rapid fluctuation.

Subliminal Fringe

An experiment which throws some light on this functional limit is the
following.[2] Full tetanic stimulation of the afferent A gives a powerful and
fairly well maintained tetanus in the test-muscle. For another afferent, B,
let the stimulus be a single break shock. This latter evokes a brief twitch-
like reflex contraction. These being the component reflexes they are then
compounded by applying the single shock stimulus to B during the plateau
of A's contraction. B's contraction is in great part occluded by A's, though
a distinct increment is given. But the increment, instead of being as is
B's separate contraction, brief, is after its arrival maintained as long as
A's stimulus continues. The additional motor-units, which B activated,
were, when B's stimulation had ceased, maintained in activity by A. The
motor-units which B brought into activity as an increment must in fact
have belonged also to A, although A did not initially excite them to discharge.
Clearly A possesses in the motoneurone pool, in addition to that fraction

[1] Cooper, Denny-Brown, and Sherrington. *Proc. roy. Soc.*, 1926, **100B**, 448.
[2] Denny-Brown and Sherrington, *J. Physiol.*, 1928, **66**, 175.

which it excites to discharging activity, a further fraction which it excites, though not unaidedly, to actual discharge. In other words, A's field of effect in the motoneurone pool consists of a portion where its excitation is sufficient to cause units to contract and a portion where the excitation though present is of itself insufficient to cause the units to contract. The former portion may be termed the supraliminal field. The latter is the so-called "subliminal fringe." The fractional field of the afferent in the motoneurone pool is therefore not represented in its entirety by those motor units whose muscle-fibres contract. And the experiment shows that the subliminal field coexists with the supraliminal even when the afferent is excited strongly. Therefore, the central overlap of two concurrently excited afferents even under strong stimulation will hardly be measured to the full by occlusion, although occlusion may then be at its fullest.

With weaker stimulation of the afferent nerve—*i.e.*, stimulation which excites a lesser moiety only of its fibres—the reflex contraction of the test muscle is, of course, less—*i.e.*, the central field of supraliminal effect is less extensive. With that restriction goes lessening of the overlap of supraliminal effect between nerves so stimulated and as a consequence a lessening of contraction-deficit arising from occlusion. But as the stimuli to the two afferents

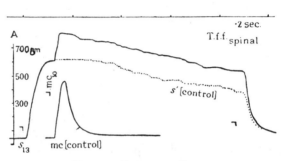

FIG. 77.—SUBLIMINAL FRINGE

Reflex from *s*, int. saph., 13 cm. coreless coil, 2 volts in primary, 50 per second frequency; *s′* (control), without addition of single shock reflex of musculocutaneous at 10 cm. coreless coil. *mc* (control), single shock reflex excited from musculocutaneous alone at 10 cm. coreless coil as control for incremental contraction in the tetanic reflex. (Denny-Brown and Sherrington)

are progressively reduced, the result of their concurrence exhibits further not merely a reduction of the deficit but a replacement of the deficit by a surplus.[1] The contraction value of the conjoint response instead of being less than the sum of the two separate responses is in excess of their sum (Fig. 76).

Summation of Subliminal Excitation

This surplus of response would be accounted for if in the overlap of the fields there were summation of subliminal effect. As to this, there can be no doubt that the fields of subliminal excitation of the two afferents in the motoneurone pool do overlap. Occlusion has proved that their fields of supraliminal effect overlap, and under progressive weakening of the stimulation what has been excited supraliminally becomes in turn excited subliminally. With weaker stimulation of each afferent its central exci-

[1] Cooper, Denny-Brown, and Sherrington, *Proc. roy. Soc.*, 1927, **101B**, 262, and Eccles and Granit, *J. Physiol.*, 1929, **67**, 97.

tatory effect on its individual motoneurones passes through stages of successive decline so that many which had been excited supraliminally become, under the weaker stimuli, excited subliminally (Fig. 76B). Since the supraliminal fields of the two afferents overlapped at least in part, so at least in part must their subliminal fields.

The other factor explaining the " surplus " contraction is that central excitement is a process which can sum on the individual motoneurone. There is specific proof that it does so. That it should do so in its subliminal grades as in these fields of effect, thence termed subliminal, accords with much else known of it. The " surplus " is therefore an outcome of central summation of subliminal excitements; and central summation of subliminal excitements, though most obvious with weak stimuli, must occur under stronger stimuli as well, for under those stronger stimuli subliminal fringe, as shown (*v.s.*), occurs. The subliminal portion of the central field of excitement produced by the afferent nerve in the motoneurone pool can relatively to the supraliminal portion be greater under weaker than under stronger stimulation of the afferent. To stimuli of above threshold value, however, throughout a whole gamut of intensities, the reflex response of the muscle under concurrence of the two afferents A and B is the net result of an AB admixture of " contraction-occlusion " (subtracting) and " central summation " (adding) along with further, ordinarily, some separate individual effect of A and of B acting independently each of the other. The greater amount of occlusion occurring under stronger stimuli will tend to obscure summation-increment in the net result; under weaker stimuli the lesser amount of occlusion will tend in the net result to be minimised further or wholly hidden by summation-increment.

In its application the above carries further. The individual afferent nerve A or B differs from the nerve pair AB only in that it itself is a smaller collection of convergent fibres. The considerations above apply then to it and to any afferent nerve. The reflex action evoked from such a nerve connotes therefore concurrent central excitations of various grade, subliminal and supraliminal, operating upon the various central units of the muscle. These various degrees of excitation of the various simultaneously operated motoneurones are not distinguishably indexed by the corresponding motor-units themselves. These last are activated or non-activated and so draw only the broad distinction between central excitation which is supraliminal and central excitation which is subliminal. But *shades* of grading of subliminal central excitement are not indicated by the motor-unit; to the whole scale of them it, by definition, does not respond. Again, to supraliminal excitement of whatever grade it responds, and, aside from iterative frequency (*v. infra*), with the undifferentiating character of all-or-none response.

Recognition of central excitation existing in subliminal intensity brings with it a question, " of what nature is the threshold stimulus ? " meaning by threshold stimulus the least stimulus which applied to the afferent nerve evokes contraction in the test muscle. On this some light is thrown by observations such as the following:

An afferent nerve is armed with two pairs of stimulating electrodes, one distal and one proximal, about 2 cm. apart. The nerve chosen is without branches for the interval between the electrode pairs, and is one which lends itself to being split into two fairly equal lengthwise subdivisions α and β in the region where the electrodes are applied. The nerve is carefully so split. The threshold value of the single-shock stimulus for reflex action on the test muscle is then determined for the distal electrode pair d, and similarly for the proximal electrode pair p. With a sensitive optical myograph magnifying tendon movement highly—e.g., 900-1,000 times—we can detect contraction due to even a single motor-unit. The observation proceeds by determining the threshold stimulus at d before and then after cutting at mid-distance between d and p one of the lengthwise subdivisions —e.g., α. The section causes the previously threshold strength of stimulus at d to be ineffective. To re-obtain the minimal reflex from d the strength of stimulus applied there has to be notably increased. The threshold strength of stimulus at p has remained unaltered. The rise of threshold at d might mean that the previous low threshold strength of stimulus there had been conditioned by the fibres of lowest threshold in the afferent nerve and that these fibres (or fibre) ran in the subdivision α and not in β of the nerve; when α was severed proximal to d but distal to p the previous threshold strength of stimulus became ineffective at d but persisted unchanged at p. Continuing the experiment by comparing the threshold strength of stimulus obtaining at p before and after cutting sub-division β proximal to p the threshold of stimulus for p rises just as previously it had at d after cutting α. Clearly therefore the above explanation cannot hold. The lowness of the threshold stimulus obtaining for the whole nerve, both at d and at p, must result from summation of the effects of two stimuli each in itself subliminal (as regards reflex effect), the one from the α half the nerve, the other from the β half; and such summation can only be central.

Thus the liminal stimulus consists of two or more subliminal ones (cf. p. 469 above). The central liminal reaction is built from subliminal; and this in one of the most simple of all reflexes, the ipsilateral flexion reflex. An inference hardly avoidable is that even at threshold no reflex is ever effected by a single afferent fibre working alone. It is not surprising then that compounded as it is from individually subliminal reactions, the reflex threshold, as measured by the amount of afferent nerve stimulus corre-sponding with it, is notoriously, and to the experimenter exasperatingly, variable. One clear outcome is that each group, even small, of afferent fibres makes its own degrees of threshold for its motor-units—the threshold being determined by density of afferent terminals on the motoneurone. The motor-units of lowest threshold for one afferent will not be those of lowest threshold for another. Nor need the low threshold motor fibre as tested by electrical stimulation of the motor nerve correspond with the low threshold motor-units under a reflex action.

Time-relations of " Central Excitatory State "

The experimenter can fairly regularly produce a supraliminal reflex effect from two " subliminal " stimuli, employing central summation. Thus a favourable opportunity is given for studying the time-relations of the central excitatory process.   The duration and intensity of the subliminal central effect of a just subliminal afferent nerve stimulus can be tested by noting the effect of a further subliminal stimulus applied at increasing interval to some other afferent nerve which overlaps centrally upon motor-units belonging to the first.   In making the observations care has been taken[1] to simplify as far as possible the reflex circumstances.   An ideal would be complete isolation of the centre from all disturbance and activity except those of the two interacting minimal excitations.   The spinal cord has been cut near above the segmental level of the reflex.   The reacting muscle itself has been de-afferented by severance of the appropriate dorsal spinal roots, and other afferent roots except those containing the fibres of the two selected afferent nerves have also been cut.   The nerves selected have often been the twin pair innervating the twin heads of gastrocnemius muscle.   Each of them contains in all some 200 afferent fibres.   The pair

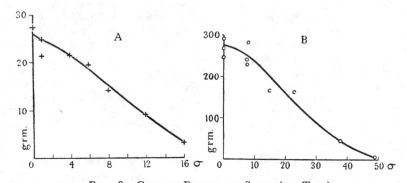

FIG. 78.—CENTRAL EXCITATORY STATE (SEE TEXT)
A, Ipsilateral Flexion Reflex; B, Crossed Extension Reflex.   (Eccles and Sherrington)

are sufficiently similar in length to make negligible any conduction time difference for the afferent path.   Each afferent has been stimulated by a single break induced-current from a coreless coil at subliminal or just liminal strength.   Central reflex reverberation by repercussion from the proprioceptives of the test muscle itself has thus been guarded against in double measure.

The accompanying chart (Fig. 78, A) shows a sample of the results in this way reached.   The central excitement though of subliminal or just liminal degree persists in detectable amount for some 16 σ.[2]   Its highest point falls very early and its decline thence is rapid.   The results observed are not always so simple as in the above sample.   Their upshot for the present argument is that the excitation due to the second afferent finds at the central convergence-point and throughout an interval extending to

---

[1] See Eccles and Sherrington, *J. Physiol.*, 1930, **69**, 1, and *Proc. roy. Soc.*, 1930, **106B**, 326; 1931, **107B**, 511; and also Creed, Denny-Brown, Eccles, Liddell and Sherrington, *Reflex Activity of the Spinal Cord*, Oxford, 1932.

[2] 1 σ = one-thousandth of a second.

much longer than the duration of an ordinary nerve-impulse a state of excitement with which itself can sum. Evidence is thus given of a central reaction which can sum and is therefore unlike the nerve-impulse of nerve-trunks. This "central excitatory state" (c.e.s.)—it needs a specific name but has none—is also more prolonged than the nerve-trunk "impulse"; and in another type-reflex, the "crossed extension," it is again longer still.

In the flexion-reflex we may note in passing that the time-relations of its c.e.s. (central excitatory state) accord with certain features already known for the reflex which had presented difficulty of explanation. The c.e.s. when supraliminal having a higher intensity than when subliminal must, it is fair to suppose, take longer to subside—*i.e.*, endure longer than, *e.g.*, the 16 σ of the above example which is sub-liminal. This relieves from diffi-culty the observation that a single-shock stimulus of fair supraliminal strength applied to the afferent nerve can evoke reflexly a response which as regards some of the activated motor units is, though brief, tetanic[1] (see Fig. 79). If the nerve-impulse generated in the afferent nerve by the single-shock stimulus passed through the central region unmodified on into the motor - unit, a repetitive response on part of the motor-unit was hardly to be expected. But if interposed between afferent conductor and efferent conductor is a central process of wider-range intensity,

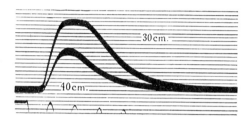

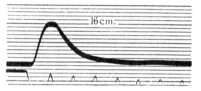

FIG. 79, A AND B

Comparison of single-shock reflexes, A, from isolated ankle-flexor, *tibialis anticus* (cat, spinal 6 days), with, B, response (twitch) of same muscle to similar but stronger single shock stimulus of its motor nerve. For the reflexes the afferent nerve is internal saphenous, and the stimuli at 40 cm. and 30 cm. coil distance. B, the motor response at 16 cm. coil—*i.e.*, maximal. Optical myograph, shadow pattern. Stimulus signal below. Time, 0.04 sec.= 10 mm.

enduring longer than the nerve-trunk impulse, we have a new element in accounting for repetitive response to a single-shock stimulus. There is thus reflex grading by number of units and also by tetanic grading within the unit itself. Even a nerve-trunk fibre under a supraliminal stimulus of not too brief duration can reply repetitively.

In the accompanying myogram (Fig. 80) from the ankle-flexor, *tibialis anticus*, comparison is made between a brief maximal tetanus evoked direct from motor nerve by break-shocks at 40 per second and a brief reflex evoked by stimuli of similar strength and frequency applied to a large

[1] Sassa and Sherrington, *Proc. roy. Soc.*, 1921, **92B**, 108; and Sherrington, *ibid.*, 1921, **92B**, 245, *Arch. int. Physiol.*, 1921, **18**, 620. Also illustrated by electromyograms in original paper.

afferent nerve. Both are tension-curves taken isometrically at short interval. The reflex response departs strikingly from the direct motor response in three main ways: (1) The height of the first contraction-step relatively to the total tension height shows that in the reflex the tension reached in response to the first break-shock stimulus is greater than for the corresponding stimulus in the maximal motor-nerve tetanus. In this latter the first contraction-step is a maximal twitch-contraction. Although the reflex does not activate the whole muscle the first contraction-step of the reflex is in despite of that greater than the entire muscle's maximal twitch-contraction. The first step of the reflex response must therefore be in part

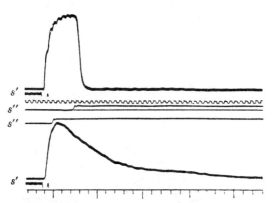

at least—*i.e.*, in some at least of the motor-units activated — tetanic.[1] (2) The tension-increment due to the second break-shock stimulus is under-sized, relatively both to first step and total tension height when standardised by the motor-nerve tetanus. In the reflex those muscle-fibres iteratively excited by the c.e.s. of the initial break-shock stimulus have already developed a tension which excludes the further full amount of increment which as the control shows would normally be due had they been fired but once. The smallness of the second

FIG. 80.—SPINAL REFLEX SHOWING TETANIC RESPONSES TO INDIVIDUAL BREAK SHOCKS OF THE TETANIC SERIES AT 42 PER SEC. MUSCLE, *tibialis anticus*, AFFERENT NERVE, *popliteal*. UPPER RESPONSE MOTOR NERVE ; LOWER REFLEX

Explanation in text. *s'*, short circuiting key for stimulating circuit is recorded as it unshorts circuits; *s''*, record of reclosing of short-circuit cutting off stimulus. Stim. at 14 cm. (coreless coil) for both (max. for motor nerve); 7 bk. sks. for motor stim. series; 3 for reflex. Cat

step confirms therefore that in the first step some of the motor-units fired tetanically at a frequency above that of the external stimulus. (3) The slow gradual subsidence of the reflex contraction after lapse of the external stimulus proves that the tetanic discharge outlasts considerably in some of the units any simple twitch response to the final break-shock stimulus. The myogram shows therefore that the tetanic discharge occurs in some of the motor-units, and that in some others it occurs scarcely or not at all.

This and other related evidence that the reflex response to a single-shock stimulus can be tetanic in character has been known for some time past from observations with the isometric myograph, and its importance for interpreting the central reflex mechanism has been stressed. In the same reflex (ankle-flexion in cat) a beautiful record by Adrian and Bronk[2]

[1] Sherrington, *loc. cit.*, and Liddell and Sherrington, *Proc. roy. Soc.*, 1923, **95B**, 299.
[2] *J. Physiol.*, 1929, **67**, 119.

has recently registered in the actual motor-unit an instance of this tetanic response to single stimuli. The myograph—*e.g.*, Fig. 80 above—had indicated the initial frequency of the autogenous tetanus to be considerably over 50 per second; Adrian and Bronk's instance of it gives 85 per second.

The crossed extension reflex (Fig. 75B) furnishes a somewhat similar sample of the time-intensity relations of the c.e.s. examined by the same method as with the flexion-reflex. Duration and intensity scale larger than in the simpler reflex. This helps understanding of certain features of behaviour of the crossed reflex. Thus, that the rhythm of the external stimulus tends, far more than in the flexion-reflex, to be "smothered" centrally.[1] Also, that a gap in the serial stimuli externally applied occasions relatively little lapse of the reflex contraction even when the succession of stimuli is as slow as 28 per second and when the omission includes two consecutive members of the series. The ample c.e.s. tends to maintain discharge in some motor-units over intervals between widely spaced afferent stimuli (Fig. 81). But the discharge filling in the intervals is the more readily inhibitable.[2] Mild inhibition causes the stimulus rhythm to be therefore more marked in the myogram, "like the ribs of a starved child." In this crossed reflex, more than in the simple flexion-reflex, the motor-units exhibit autonomous rates of firing.[3] The prominent rôle taken by "addition latente" and "recruitment" in this reflex accords with its c.e.s. In those phenomena, however, the summation is

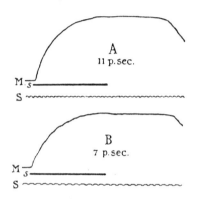

FIG. 81, A AND B.—REFLEX CONTRACTION OF *vastocrureus* FROM CONTRALATERAL POPLITEAL N.; DECEREBRATE PREPARATION

In A stimulation rate 11 per sec.; in B stimulation rate 7 per sec.; in each case prolonged terminal after discharge at plateau level. S, the rate of delivery of the break-shock stimuli; *s*, the duration of the stimulus. Long plateau after discharge. (Liddell and Sherrington, *Proc. roy. Soc.*, 1923, **95B**, 407)

by iteration at the *same* afferent terminals. When further, and in addition, there occurs summation via convergent paths the combination of the two forms of summation becomes strikingly potent. Subliminal, or barely supraliminal, components give summation-results[4] on a scale rarely known for the flexion-reflex. The large c.e.s. thus agrees with the wide subliminal fringe observed by Eccles and Granit.

[1] Liddell and Sherrington, *Proc. roy. Soc.*, 1923, **95B**, 407.
[2] Liddell and Sherrington, *Proc. roy. Soc.*, 1925, **97B**, 488; and Fulton and Liddell, *ibid.*, 1925, **98B**, 214.
[3] Illustrated by electromyograms in original paper.
[4] Eccles and Granit, *J. Physiol.*, 1929, **67**, 97.

Subliminal Fringe as Liaison for Co-operative Reinforcement

Clearly, in subliminal fringe and in summation of subliminal c.e.s. the central nervous system possesses a main means of conjunction of excitatory effects, or, in other words, its main functional liaison between co-operative influences of separate origin. These subliminal factors, arising from sources widely apart and arriving via long convergence paths, interact at the place (or places) of confluence. Subliminal fringe at the convergence place forms the " catch-on " for labyrinthine and other reinforcements, and, if we include inhibitory reductions, in their effects of grading and adjusting the local limb and neck reflexes, etc., for posture and for locomotion. An example furnished by Denny-Brown[1] illustrates it with employment of natural stimuli instead of electrical to bared nerve. Light pressure against the sole of the foot, in itself of barely supraliminal value, was combined with a stretch-reflex in itself barely supraliminal, the reflex muscle being the ankle-extensor soleus. Individually the two stimuli evoked hardly perceptible effect; in concurrence they evoked a contraction developing 1,300-gramme tension. The cerebellum again furnishes instances. Areas of cerebellar surface which under faradisation cannot of themselves initiate movement of the limbs, yet modify concurrent movements otherwise (reflexly) produced (Denny-Brown, Eccles and Liddell).[2] Further, with the progressive serial reflexes called chain-reflexes, each phase by means of its subliminal fringe lowers the threshold for the next phase. So likewise with alternating reflexes. The operations of the nervous system would be impossible without summation of subliminal states.

II.—Confluence of Excitatory with Inhibitory Path

Any treatment, however brief, of problems attaching to convergence must include something of that great class in which the upshot of inter-action is inhibition. Reflex inhibition is central. It has its seat at convergence points. There a clash occurs between central excitation and a process which opposes it. A difficulty in studying this is that the sole test agent for the inhibition is " central excitation " about which in its turn we know barely more than that it excites. If knowledge of the c.e.s. is slight, still more so therefore is that of c.i.s.

A first question is how far the opposition between the two is quantitative. Much goes to show that broadly it is so. There is the oft-attested observation that stronger afferent stimulation of the inhibiting nerve evokes more extensive relaxation of reflex contraction than does weaker. There are the refined experiments of Graham Brown[3] dealing with total balance of the two antagonistic influences, and showing that the remainders can sum to unity for muscles operating at one and the same joint. There is further

[1] *Proc. roy. Soc.*, 1929, **104B**, 252.
[2] *Ibid.*, 1929, **104B**, 418.
[3] *Proc. roy. Soc.*, 1927, **102B**, 143.

the longer lapse of active contraction when interrupted by a stronger single-shock inhibition than by a weaker.

To get at close grips with the antagonism it seems specially needful to know more of the quantitative opposition between inhibition and excitation in respect of the individual motoneurone. The familiar observation that, with successive increases of stimulation of the inhibitory afferent, the relaxation cuts deeper and deeper into the reflex contraction leaves a dilemma. The result may mean that motor-units whose activity resisted a certain degree of inhibition suffered arrest of that activity on intensifying the inhibition. Or it may mean that the stronger stimulation of the inhibitory afferent—*i.e.*, the bringing into play of more of the inhibitory afferent's fibres—merely extends the field of distribution of the inhibitory influence to fresh units in the motoneurone pool so that it reaches a large number of the activated motor-units, and those which it reaches it inhibits, irrespective of quantitative grading. The observation of itself does not decide whether, for instance, any of the motoneurones inhibited under the stronger inhibitory stimulus were, under the weaker stimulus, exposed to a lesser grade of inhibitory influence which grade their activity successfully resisted, though unable to withstand an intenser inhibitory influence developed by completer stimulation of the inhibitory afferent. In short, such an experiment leaves open whether the reflex inhibition possesses various quantitative grades which antagonise corresponding grades of central excitation.

Results of Antagonism on the Individual Motor-unit

From this dilemma escape is afforded by observations[1] such as instanced by the accompanying figure 82. The reflex chosen is one in which sufficient frequency in the stimulus rate ensures that the reflexly activated motor-units react with a complete tetanus. Under increasing stimulation of the excitatory afferent the number of motor-units reflexly activated successively increases. Against each of the three intensities an intercurrent inhibition " *i* " of the same moderate strength in all is tested. The number of units inhibited is greater when " *i* " is exercised within the less numerous field of activated units than when it is exercised within the more numerous. The units activated by the completer (stronger) stimulation of the excitatory afferent must include all those activated by the less complete (weaker). Therefore in this case the same individual motoneurones which under activation by a weaker excitatory stimulus are overcome by the inhibitory influence, when activated by a stronger excitatory stimulus, withstand that same inhibitory influence. There are therefore grades of supraliminal excitation activating the motor-units; and a given grade of inhibitory influence while able to reduce to subliminal a supraliminal excitation of lower grade may yet fail to reduce below threshold a supraliminal excitation of higher grade. As to how a heightening of the intensity of stimulation of the afferent nerve can intensify further the central excitation at moto-

[1] *Ibid.*, 1909, **81B**, 249.

neurones it is already activating, the additional afferent fibres brought in by the stronger stimulus will, having terminals as they must, at some of the motoneurones already activated, contribute c.e.s. to the c.e.s. already there operating. The corresponding motor-units being all-or-none reagents and already completely tetanised will not reveal by the myograph the further heightening of their already supraliminal excitation. That the c.i.s. reveals it indicates that this latter deals with the c.e.s. directly and therefore only indirectly with the motor-unit. That the increase of supraliminal excitation is due to double-firing in the afferent fibres under the increase in stimulus strength is a contingency, but hardly likely unless the external stimulus be very strong.

Inferences are (1) that the activity of the individual motor-unit in these cases is controlled by quantitative interaction between c.e.s. and c.i.s.;

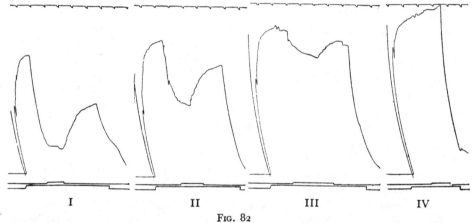

I   II   III   IV

FIG. 82

The activated motor-unit inactivated by centripetal inhibition is then, against the inhibition, reactivated by further increase of centripetal excitation. Knee-flexor decerebrate, reflexly excited from ipsilateral peroneal, with increasing strengths of stimulation: I, 17 cm.; II, 16 cm.; III, 15 cm.; IV, 13·8 cm. During each excitation an intercurrent stimulation of the crossed popliteal afferent (inhibitory) at the one constant strength, 14·5 cm. Time in seconds. (*Proc. roy. Soc.*, 1909, **81B**, 249)

(2) that the tilt of the balance—*i.e.*, the excess—of one process over the other can differ greatly in different individual units despite the muscle-fibres of these all being activated together or quiescent together; and (3) that graded inhibition exercised upon an aggregate of activated motor-units supplies an index for detecting which among them are operated by high and which by low c.e.s. respectively.

Inhibition Selectivity arrests those Activated Motor-units which are under Weaker Central Excitation

The last inference can be tested in several ways. I. The crossed extension reflex under tetanic stimulation opens after a variable latency (due to " addition latente ") with a period of " recruitment " during which the serial stimulus by serial summation activates progressively increasing numbers of motor-units. Hence the slow climbing ascent of the myogram due mainly to the accession of fresh motor-units as the threshold value of central excitation (*i.e.*, the value of c.e.s liminal for making the motor-unit discharge) is attained in succession by motoneurone after motoneurone. Any point in the ascent represents a moment when there are certain moto-neurones in which the summating c.e.s. is about to become liminal—*i.e.*, about to begin activating the motor-units, and is about to add those units' contraction to that of those already contracting. A moderate single-shock stimulus thrown into the inhibitory afferent in the course of this recruiting ascent produces a characteristic effect. No dip in the ascent is produced, but the ascent is " deviated."[1] The entry into contraction of fresh muscle-fibres is checked for, *e.g.*, 0·02 second; recruitment is held up for a moment. It is therefore the motor-units of those motoneurones in which c.e.s. though subliminal is only just so which reveal this slight puff of inhibition, and it is they alone. If the single-shock inhibitory stimulus be strengthened there is added to the arrest of the ascent an actual fall in contraction tension; units already in contraction drop out of contraction under the inhibition. Units just recently activated even if inhibited will not as regards their muscle-fibre contraction reveal a brief inhibition unless the inhibitory effect in them outlast the duration of the contraction-remainder due from their last preceding stimulus. The set-back in the attainment of threshold excitation by units just about to attain it is thus a specially delicate myo-graphic index for inhibition. The galvanometer will not necessarily detect it.

II. A single-shock inhibition applied during the after-discharge con-traction bites characteristically into the declining contraction. It cuts in it a steep drop to a lower contraction-tension which is then maintained level for a time until the after-discharge contraction resumes its previous rate of decline subject, it may be, also to some equable " eclipse."[2] The main point is that the transient inhibition forecloses the activity of just those motor-units whose lease of activity has least long to run.

III. Again, if the single-shock inhibition be applied while the plateau of the reflex-contraction is still in course under the tetanic stimulus, the effect on contraction is selectively restricted to those motor-units whose after-discharge will, on withdrawal of the excitatory stimulus, persist least long.[2] The central supraliminal excitation for the activated motor-units differs greatly in height above threshold for different units, hence differences from individual unit to unit in duration of after-discharge. Those motor-units activated by c.e.s. which though supraliminal is least so, and therefore terminally sinks earliest below threshold, are by inhibition arrested most easily; they require less inhibition to reduce to subliminal the c.e.s. acting on them. It is not, of course, meant that the inhibition affects only those central units the lapse of contraction of whose muscle-fibres reveals it.

[1] Liddell and Sherrington, *Proc. roy. Soc.*, 1925, **97B**, 488.   [2] Liddell and Sherrington, *loc. cit.*

The phenomenon of " eclipse " shows the contrary. Even within the field of overlap of the excitatory and inhibitory afferents there must be central units whose supraliminal c.e.s. though reduced is not reduced low or long enough to interrupt the mechanical contraction. There will be others where the c.e.s. is subliminal so that further reduction is not detectable in the muscle or its nerve by myograph or galvanometer, except through such a circumstance as delay of recruitment (*v.s.*) or prolongation of latency. For example, a brief tetanic stimulus provokes the reflex contraction after a latency of some 40 σ. When preceded by the single-shock inhibitory stimulus the latency of the contraction is increased; the rise of central excitation to threshold value takes longer. The contraction itself is also smaller, fewer units are lifted above threshold.

Fatigue favours Inhibition

Central " fatigue " favours reflex inhibition.[1] Thus, a given inhibitory stimulus pitted against a given contraction background will act more powerfully—*i.e.*, will arrest more active units—when employed late in the

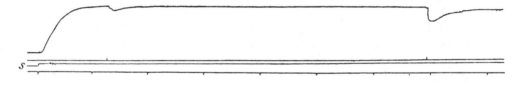

Fig. 83.—Fatigue favours Inhibition

Decerebrate vastocrureus; deafferented; reflexly activated by contralateral plantar nerve at 30 double shocks per sec. coil at 19 cm. Inhibition by single-break current to ipsilateral plantar nerve at 16 cm. of coil. Five seconds interval between the two inhibitory reflexes. Tension of plateau, 1·8 kil.

course of the tetanic plateau than when employed early (Fig. 83). A condition for this sensitisation to inhibition is that the tetanus plateau must be declining, even if only slightly; it is not, in my experience, evident if the plateau be rising ever so slightly; a rising of plateau is a denial of fatigue. If, as presumable, fatigue corresponds with diminution in c.e.s. and a sinking toward threshold of supraliminal c.e.s. the coalition between fatigue and central inhibition is intelligible. On the other hand, a precurrent inhibition if of some strength and duration favours after its withdrawal the development of central excitation at the previously inhibited units.

Central Inhibition exhibits Grades Subliminal and Supraliminal and it exhibits Summation

Clearly the central confluence-place is the field of play of two antagonistic processes, and of these one at least—namely, central excitation—can at one and the same motoneurone develop different grades of strength. Thus,

[1] Sherrington and Sowton, *Proc. roy. Soc.*, 1911, **84B**, 203.

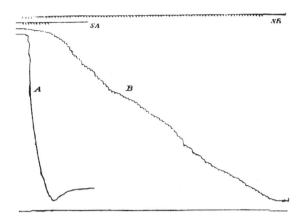

FIG. 84.—VASTOCRUREUS, DECEREBRATE

Inhibition by break-shocks at 4 per sec. to central end of ipsilateral musculocutaneous nerve, in B the stimuli were very weak, 20 K-units; in A less weak, 100 K-units. In both observations the inhibitory relaxation proceeded to the full resting length of the muscle, in A this was reached in eight repetitions of the stimulus; in B in eighty-six repetitions. (*Proc. roy. Soc.*, 1909, **81B**, 249)

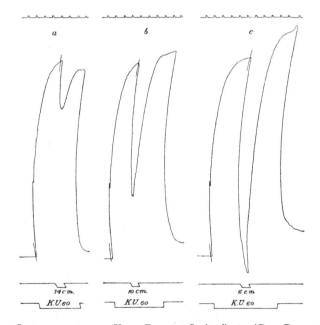

FIG. 85.—INHIBITIONS OF THE KNEE FLEXOR, *Semitendinosus* (CAT, DECEREBRATE)

Lower signal marks stimulation (faradic) of ipsilateral afferent (peroneal+popliteal) exciting reflex contraction of the muscle. This stimulus remains of the same intensity, namely, 60 units of the scale of the Kronecker inductorium, in all three of the successive observations *a, b* and *c*. Upper signal marks stimulation (faradic) of the contralateral afferent (peroneal× popliteal); this intercurrent stimulus is stronger in *b* than in *a*, and in *c* than in *b*, the secondary coil being at 14 cm. in *a*, at 10 in *b*, and at 6 in *c*. Time in seconds, above. (Sherrington and Sowton, 1911) calling " strength " intensity, it can develop an intensity to withstand an inhibition which at lower intensities it could not withstand.

For evidence that central inhibition also exhibits various grades of intensity at the individual unit we have to turn to observations with temporal—*i.e.*, iterative—summation. Mere repetition, at not long interval, of the same weak unvarying stimulus to the same afferent nerve effects a progressive increase of central inhibition upon a motor-unit field activated by a given equally driven central excitation (Fig. 84). The units which withstand earlier grades of the c.i.s. are as the inhibitory stimulus proceeds overpowered by the later grades cumulatively developed. The inhibitory effect thus ultimately reached equals that effected more speedily—*i.e.*, by fewer repetitions—of a stronger stimulus—*i.e.*, one employing more fibres of the inhibitory afferent nerve. Such observations indicate that central inhibitory action can sum and can, in addition to simple extension of central field, exhibit grades of influence upon the individual unit, ranging over different subliminal as well as different supraliminal degrees.

This puts us in a better position for dealing with observations such as instanced by Fig. 85. Since reflex inhibition can develop different grades of intensity in acting on the individual motoneurone, we can fairly infer that some of those motoneurones which are not inhibited by the weaker inhibitory stimulus in *a* (Fig. 85) are none the less exposed to subliminal inhibitory influence then, and that they are inhibited when the inhibitory influence becomes stronger under the stronger stimuli in *b* and *c*—in fact, that just as subliminal central excitation can be converted into supraliminal by increasing the stimulus, so likewise can subliminal central inhibition as tested against a given excitation of not too powerful type.

Inhibition v. Excitation can for a Time maintain a Steady Balance on the Motor-unit Group and Individual

Under tetanic stimulation of two afferent nerves, one inhibitory and one excitatory, the corresponding summations of the central inhibition on the one hand, and of the c.e.s. on the other, can strike a steady balance on the individual motoneurone. Thus a steady fraction of the motor-unit pool can be maintained in inhibition alongside a steady fraction maintained active. Very commonly, however, the poise swings over in one direction or the other and then reversely, so that a slowly rhythmic alternation of dominant excitation and inhibition ensues.[1]

An example of a prolonged muscular act maintained by adjustment between concurrent reflex excitation and inhibition playing at the convergence-point upon the motor-unit is reflex posture, as in standing. Denny-Brown[2] in his recent experimental analysis of this has traced in some detail the sources of the two concurrent proprioceptive streams, excitatory and

---

[1] See Chap. VII, p. 302, and Graham Brown, *Proc. roy. Soc.*, 1912, **85B**, 278; A. Forbes, *ibid.*, 1912, **85B**, 289.   [2] *Proc. roy. Soc.*, 1929, **104B**, 252.

inhibitory respectively, which are the main factors in this balance and its adjustment. "The proprioceptive inhibition is summing at the central units all through the response and opposing there the afferent excitation arriving from the tendon-organs, also summing at each unit." Reflex stepping "consists, in the decerebrate and spinal animals, of a rhythmical waxing and waning of reflex standing,"[1] interpretable "as the rhythmical appearance of a supplementary excitation over the whole 'stretch-reflex' field."[2]

The Discharging Nerve-cell in the Hands of Central Excitation and Inhibition

The motoneurone, specialised nerve-cell though it be, may yet typify for us the reactions of nerve-cells in general. In several ways it offers the best physiological chance of studying the reactions of the unit nerve-cell. Its only access of approach is natural and not artificial. It may be non-typical in exhibiting high resistance to fatigue. An afferent playing upon it in succession to another which has evinced fatigued response obtains from the motoneurone still practically unimpaired response.[3] The motor-unit, subject to the outcome of the two opposed central processes excitation and inhibition at the confluence-structure upstream, is their instrument. But it is an instrument with ways of its own. In so far as it is nerve-fibre its characteristic functional reaction is the nerve-impulse, and, concomitant with and outlasting that, a phase of refractoriness to re-excitation. This reaction when prolonged is simply a series of impulses and corresponding refractory phases. The reflex c.e.s. when above subliminal therefore expresses itself in the nerve-fibre of the motor-unit simply by impulse and refractory state. It commonly generates trains of them.

Rhythm of Centrifugal Discharge : its Degree of Independence of Centripetal Excitatory Rhythm

The serial correspondence between the more or less rhythmic centrifugal trains descending the motor-unit and the centripetal trains of the afferent nerve is close in some reflexes, much less close in others.[4] Between the two sets of trains is interposed the c.e.s. with time-relations and summating powers proper to itself. The centrifugal impulses generated by it tend to be redistributed in time, partly independently of the rhythm of incidence of the centripetal train. In some cases the departure from correspondence of frequency between the two is extreme. The rhythm of action of the responding unit may be quite other than that of the rhythmic excitation applied—e.g., 3.4 per second in response to 50 per second excitation; also the response rhythm may vary actually while the excitatory rhythm is keeping constant.[5]

---

[1] Cf. Chap. VIII, p. 371.   [2] Denny-Brown, loc. cit.   [3] Integrative Action, 1906.
[4] Liddell and Sherrington, Proc. roy. Soc., 1923, 95B, 142.
[5] Illustrated in original paper. See also Adrian and Bronk, J. Physiol., 1929, 67, 119.

Stronger Excitation produces cæteris paribus *Higher Rate of Centrifugal Discharge and Conversely*

The frequency of impulse-discharge in the individual motoneurone increases, within limits, with increase of the central excitation. Thus, in the opening period of the recruiting reflexes the salient feature is gradual intensification of the central excitation. The " addition latente " of the latent period passes over into and becomes apparent as recruitment of the ascending contraction period. This continued increase of reflex result, traceable wholly to temporal—*i.e.*, iterative—summation, bears witness to continued intensification of the c.e.s. at work in the individual motoneurone. The successive surmounting of the threshold by unit after unit through the whole opening period shows the c.e.s. mounting steadily from various grades of subliminal strength to various heights of supraliminal. Adrian and Bronk[1] have shown that in this period of these reflexes the rate of discharge increases in individual units. Since this then goes along with increase of excitation in the individual units, we may infer that the increase of excitation gives the increased rate of discharge.

Conversely, the contraction of decerebrate rigidity, a postural reflex, is a contraction especially readily inhibited—*e.g.*, inhibitable by exceptionally weak stimulation of inhibitory afferents. It instances, therefore, a weak intensity of reflex excitation, and here the rate of discharge in the motor-units engaged has been shown to be quite low; so likewise in the weak, easily inhibitable stretch-reflexes (Denny-Brown[2]).

In respect to the relation between rate of discharge and intensity of excitation we have, besides the reflex observations, the argument of analogy from the reactions of the receptor organ and afferent fibre, now that these have been elucidated and with such brilliant advance of method by Adrian[3] and his successive collaborators. In remarking this similarity we have to remember that the essential excitation obtains expression both for receptor and for motoneurone in a nerve-trunk fibre, a mechanism of characteristic reaction which must impress its own character on both.

Discharge of the Individual Motor-unit can be suppressed altogether or merely slowed in Rate by Reflex Inhibition

Central inhibition acting at a convergence-point can preclude, interrupt, or arrest altogether the train of centrifugal impulses of an individual motor-unit, or it may merely lessen the frequency of succession of the impulses— *i.e.*, slow the discharge without arresting it altogether—just as the vagus nerve may stop or slow the heart. Thus in the record furnished by Denny-Brown[4] from the completely de-afferented soleus muscle, its motor supply being largely cut down, a motor-unit is driven at 20 per second discharge-rate by a crossed stimulus series at 50 per second. Weak stimulation at

[1] *Loc. cit.*   [2] *Loc. cit.*
[3] *J. Physiol.*, 1926, **61.** 49, and *The Basis of Sensation*, London, 1928.   [4] *Loc. cit.*

65 per second applied to an inhibitory afferent then reduces the firing frequency of the motor-unit to about 7 per second during continuance of the inhibitory stimulus. This is followed by a short-lasting post-inhibitory rise in firing-rate motor (rebound). There is thus reflex grading by number of units and, within limits, by (Adrian, Denny-Brown) rate of firing in the unit itself; our point here is that reflex inhibition deals with *both* these means of grading.

Inhibition may be the stabilising of a surface-film; a question which has been raised and offers difficulty is whether the central inhibitory process requires as pre-condition an excitatory state. Certain it is that at present the only test for central inhibition is excitation. A difficulty thus besets the study of reflex inhibition. The test for it is excitation, and almost the sole criterion of central excitation is the centrifugal impulse generated by it. But before central excitation generates an impulse it has to rise to threshold value. And as shown above, there are various subliminal degrees of c.e.s., through which the rise may pass at various rates. The duration of an inhibition as measured by a given excitatory effect is a measurement which, although possessing value and interest, may include more than the period of the actual inhibitory process itself. It may include a variable after-period required for the recovery of excitation and its development to threshold. This, though a consequence of the inhibition, would be different for the same inhibition operating against different grades of excitation, and must tend to obscure the time-limits of the inhibition-process itself.

III

There remains for mention a third class of cases attaching as a problem to convergence. This is the interaction of two concurrently exerted inhibitions, the converse of that of the set of cases taken first above, the concurrent excitations. In light of the afferent overlap at central end of the individual motor-unit revealed by the muscular occlusion in that converse case, it is obvious that there must be similarly a central overlap on the inhibitory side. That there are degrees of that overlap has been shown by Creed and Eccles.[1] A concurrence of the inhibitions may be expected to give a reinforcement of the inhibitory effect, and there is already some evidence of that. The problem has not, however, as yet been systematically proceeded with, and we must leave it there.

In conclusion, one thing which, from even the foregoing summary discussion, emerges, I think clearly, is this: though trains of impulses are the sole reactions which enter and leave the central nervous system, nervous impulses are not the sole reactions functioning within that system. States of excitement which can sum together, and states of inhibition which can sum together, and states which represent the algebraical summation of these two, are among the central reactions. The motoneurone lies at a focus

[1] *J. Physiol.*, 1928, **66**, 109.

of interplay of these reactions and its motor-unit gives their net upshot, always expressed in terms of motor impulses and contraction.   The central reactions can be much longer lasting than the nerve impulse of nerve-trunks.   Further, these central states and reactions are, as compared with the processes of nerve-trunk conductions, relatively very sensitive to physiological conditions, and are delicately responsive to fatigue, blood supply, drugs, etc.   The specific cell units, the neurones, far from behaving merely as passive recipients and transmitters of impulses, modify as well as transmit what they receive.   They can develop rhythm of their own, and their rate of discharge can rise and fall with intensity of central excitation and inhibition respectively.

Finally, if we have dealt less than they deserve with some collateral problems not far removed from those we have been considering, it is that to have embraced them would have been to risk confusing both them and the single succinct set of problems we have had before us.

4. FURTHER REMARKS WITH REFERENCE TO THE DETAILED FLUCTUATIONS IN LATENCY AND INTENSITY OF TRANSMISSION OF SINGLE VOLLEY REFLEXES.   C.E.S. AND C.I.S.

[*The tibialis anticus muscle, which responds actively in reflex flexion, is excited by single break-shock stimulation of an afferent nerve potent in evoking the reflex (spinal cat).   The single shock sets up a single impulse in many afferent nerve-fibres (a " centripetal volley," Proc. roy. Soc., 1931, 107B, 513).   The effect of this volley on the centre was studied by testing it in various strengths and at various time intervals in relationship to another single volley of known effect also activating that centre.   It was also tested against the effect of a single volley sent up the motor fibres supplying the muscle (" antidromic volley "), which was known to exert a transient depression on the motor centre.   In this way it was possible to demonstrate the behaviour and duration of any influence on the centre which did not cause it to discharge.   This influence, which in sufficient intensity causes and is responsible for the discharge of a motoneurone, is defined, and named " central excitatory state."   Thus the nervous condition long recognised to be responsible for facilitation and other subliminal effects is approached and defined, as well as the problem of the general nature of transmission at the synapse.—ED.*]

[1] The experiments described in the preceding four papers bear on various problems presented by reflex activity.   Their results confirm some of the inferences already drawn elsewhere from other experimental work, and they allow certain further inferences.   A brief prefatory statement of all

[1] J. C. Eccles and C. S. Sherrington, *Proc. roy. Soc.*, 1931, 107B, 597-605.   This paper is the fifth of a series entitled " Studies on the Flexor Reflex."   They are: I. Latent Period, *ibid.*, p. 511; II. The Reflex Response Evoked by Two Centripetal Volleys, *ibid.*, p. 535; III. The Central Effects Produced by an Antidromic Volley (by J. C. Eccles alone), *ibid.*, p. 557; IV. After-Discharge, *ibid.*, p. 586; V. General Conclusions (here reprinted).   See also Sherrington, C. S., *Proc. roy. Soc.*, 1921, 92B, 245; *Arch. int. Physiol.*, 1921, 18, 620, and Eccles, J. C., and Sherrington, C. S., *J. Physiol.*, 1930, 69, 1.

these inferences and of the experimental evidence which allows them will advantageously introduce the description of the processes set up in the ipsilateral flexor centres of the spinal cord by a single centripetal volley and by a single antidromic volley. Then, finally, discussion of the theories of reflex excitation can be undertaken in the light of the present experimental observations. The statement treats of the subject in its present phase only; the references to relevant papers are therefore restricted in the main to the more recent ones.

Inferences from Experimental Observations

1. *The Convergence of Different Afferent Paths on the same Motoneurones*

The following evidence shows that this occurs:

(*a*) *Histological.*—Each motoneurone receives its "*boutons terminaux*" from many individual afferent terminals (Cajal[1]).

(*b*) *Physiological.*—Centripetal volleys set up in *different* afferent nerves excite the same motoneurones (Camis[2]; Cooper, Denny-Brown, and Sherrington;[3] Sherrington;[4] Cooper and Denny-Brown;[5] Eccles and Sherrington[6]).

2. *The Central Excitatory State*

This is the name given to an enduring excitatory condition set up by a centripetal volley in the reflex "centre." The experimental evidence for its existence is as follows:

(*a*) When separated by certain intervals (usually not longer than 20 σ), two centripetal volleys (either in the same or different afferent nerves) evoke a reflex discharge from motoneurones which do not respond to either volley alone (Sherrington;[7] Bremer;[8] Eccles and Sherrington[7]).

(*b*) When two centripetal volleys are separated by certain intervals (usually not longer than 20 σ), the central reflex-time of the response to the second volley is greatly shortened (even to less than 0·5 σ) (Eccles and Sherrington).[7]

Both these experiments show that an excitatory condition set up by the first centripetal volley in the reflex "centre" persists until the arrival of the second volley. On account of this property of existing for some time, this central excitatory condition is called the central state, c.e.s. The experimental observations (*a*) and (*b*) also show that for some motoneurones the c.e.s. produced by one centripetal volley sums with that produced by another volley.[9] Since this happens under the most varied conditions, it can be concluded that in any motoneurones there is a summation of the

[1] *Trab. Lab. Invest. biol. Univ. Madr.*, 1903, **2,** 129.   [2] *J. Physiol.*, 1909, **39,** 228.
[3] *Proc. roy. Soc.*, 1926, **100B,** 448, and 1927, **101B,** 262.
[4] *Proc. roy. Soc.*, 1929, **105B,** 332 (p. 464 this vol.).   [5] *Proc. roy. Soc.*, 1929, **105B,** 365.
[6] *J. Physiol.*, 1930, **69,** 1, and *Proc. roy. Soc.*, 1931, **107B,** 511, 535.
[7] *Loc. cit. supra.*   [8] *C. R. Soc. Biol. Paris*, 1930, **103,** 509.
[9] The argument in the case of (*b*) depends on sections 3 and 5 below.

c.e.s. produced by *individual* centripetal impulses which are separated by a sufficiently short interval.   The duration of the c.e.s. set up by a centripetal volley is due partly to the temporal dispersion of the incident excitatory impulses (see section 5 below), and partly to the persistence of the c.e.s. produced by any particular excitatory impulse (Eccles[1]).

3. *Neurone-threshold*

Since the size of the two centripetal volleys can be chosen so that summation of the c.e.s. produced by both is necessary to set up a reflex discharge from motoneurones, it follows that the c.e.s. produced by either volley is alone inadequate to evoke such a discharge.   Therefore in order to set up a reflex discharge of a motoneurone the c.e.s. must reach a certain intensity. This intensity is called the *neurone-threshold* (*cf.* Goldschneider[2]).

4. *Subliminal Fringe*

When a centripetal volley is made large enough to evoke a reflex discharge from some motoneurones—*i.e.*, to produce a c.e.s. of threshold intensity in them—it also produces in other motoneurones a c.e.s. of subliminal intensity (Denny-Brown and Sherrington,[3] Eccles and Sherrington[4]). These latter motoneurones are said to be in the subliminal fringe produced by that centripetal volley.

5. *Temporal Dispersion[5] of Centripetal Impulses incident on a Motoneurone as the Result of a Single Centripetal Volley*

The following experimental observations are difficult to interpret in any other way:

(*a*) The central reflex-time of the response to a centripetal volley is greatly shortened if another volley precedes it by certain intervals.   When the volleys are in different afferent nerves, the central reflex-time usually reaches a minimum when the interval between them is 6 σ to 8 σ (Eccles and Sherrington[6]).

(*b*) The central reflex-time is shortened when the centripetal volley is increased in size.[7]

(*c*) There is a temporal dispersion of the reflex discharge evoked by a centripetal volley (Forbes and Gregg,[8] Eccles and Sherrington[9]).

(*d*) A centripetal volley evokes a reflex discharge after an antidromic volley which latter reaches the motoneurones *after* the foremost impulses of the centripetal volley.   In order to set up such a reflex discharge some

---

[1] *Proc. roy. Soc.*, 1931, **107B**, see p. 580.
[2] *Die Bedeutung der Reize in Lichte der Neuronlehre*, Leipzig, 1898.
[3] *J. Physiol.*, 1928, **66**, 175.
[4] *Proc. roy. Soc.*, 1931, **107B**, see p. 539.
[5] By " temporal dispersion " is meant the scattered arrival of afferent nerve impulses reaching the synapse.   The delay of those arriving late is thought to be due to their having possibly taken a longer route in the grey matter—*e.g.*, via internuncial neurones, called sometimes " delay paths." —ED.   [6] *Proc. roy. Soc.*, 1931, **107B**, 527.   [7] *Ibid.*, p. 517.
[8] *Amer. J. Physiol.*, 1915, **37**, 118.   [9] *Proc. roy. Soc.*, 1931, **107B**, 511.

excitatory impulses must have been incident on the motoneurones *after* the antidromic volley (Eccles).[1]

(*e*) When a centripetal volley reaches the reflex " centre " immediately after an antidromic volley, it evokes a reflex response with a central reflex-time longer than normal.[2]

(*f*) When an antidromic volley reaches the reflex " centre " after the foremost impulses of a centripetal volley, very little or no c.e.s. can be detected for several sigmata, but in some cases this period is followed by a considerable increase in the c.e.s.[3]

(*g*) An antidromic volley set up during an after-discharge produces a complete cessation of all after-discharge for a period varying from 15 σ to 60 σ (Denny-Brown,[4] Eccles and Sherrington[5]).

6. *Refractory Period following an Antidromic Volley*

(*a*) After an antidromic impulse reaches a motoneurone, the neurone-threshold is raised so that for a period of 5 σ to 6 σ no reflex discharge can be set up. The neurone-threshold does not fall to normal for a further period of about 5 σ (Eccles[6]).

(*b*) The period of raised threshold following an antidromic volley is not altered by a preceding antidromic volley except in so far as the second volley is delayed owing to the refractory period following the first volley.[6]

(*c*) Two antidromic volleys can be set up at such a short interval apart that the second reaches the reflex " centre " only 2·4 σ after the first. The absolutely refractory period following an antidromic volley must be less than this.[7]

7. *Refractory Period following a Reflex Discharge*

After a centripetal volley evokes a reflex discharge from a motoneurone there is a period during which the neurone-threshold is raised.[8] In some motoneurones this period is less than 16 σ, and probably is identical in duration with the refractory period following an antidromic volley (Eccles and Sherrington[9]). When the period is longer than 30 σ it can be shown that its long duration is due, not to a refractory period, but to an inhibition set up by inhibitory impulses in the centripetal volley.[10] In those cases where the duration of raised threshold lies between 16 σ and 30 σ experimental evidence does not distinguish between inhibition and refractory period as causes of this duration of the unresponsiveness.

8. *An Antidromic Impulse removes Preformed c.e.s. from a Motoneurone which it reaches*

An antidromic volley reaching the reflex " centre " between two centripetal volleys greatly reduces the facilitation of the second volley by the

[1] *Proc. roy. Soc.*, 1931, **107B**, see p. 569. [2] *Ibid.*, p. 565. [3] *Ibid.*, p. 579.
[4] *Proc. roy. Soc.*, 1929, **104B**, see p. 273. [5] *Loc. cit.*, see p. 586.
[6] *Loc. cit.*, p. 567. [7] Eccles, *loc. cit.*, p. 568. [8] *Cf.* Bremer, *C. R. Soc. Biol. Paris*, 1930, **103**, 513.
[9] *Proc. roy. Soc.*, 1931, **107B**, 553. [10] *Idem*, p. 550.

first. This is not due to the raised neurone-threshold (refractory period) produced by the antidromic volley (Eccles[1]).

9. *When a Reflex Discharge is set up in a Motoneurone there is a Removal of Preformed c.e.s.*

(*a*) An antidromic volley set up during an after-discharge produces a *complete* cessation of all after-discharge for a period varying from 15 σ to 60 σ. This duration is too long to be explained as a refractory period set up by the antidromic volley (Denny-Brown,[2] Eccles and Sherrington[3]). Since some motoneurones are protected from the antidromic volley by impulses which they have just discharged, the complete absence of after-discharge during the period of quiescence suggests that a motoneurone is affected in a similar way by a reflex discharge and by an antidromic volley.

(*b*) An antidromic impulse reaching a rhythmically discharging moto-neurone affects that motoneurone in the same way as a reflex discharge (Eccles and Hoff[4]).

Central Processes set up by a Single Centripetal Volley or by a Single Antidromic Volley

On the basis of the inferences which have just been considered it is now possible to sketch in the outlines of some of the processes set up in the ipsi-lateral flexor centres of the spinal cord both by a single centripetal volley and by a single antidromic volley.

1. *The Central Effects of a Centripetal Volley (provided that it contains no Inhibitory Impulses)*

According to the intensity of the effects which they produce it is possible to divide centripetal volleys into three classes.

(*a*) *A Centripetal Volley which does not give rise to a Reflex Discharge.*—The excitatory impulses incident on a motoneurone have a considerable tem-poral dispersion, and each produces its quantum of c.e.s. so that the maxi-mum intensity of c.e.s. is usually reached in about 6 σ to 8 σ.[5] Thereafter the intensity of c.e.s. declines until a zero value is reached about 20 σ after the initial rise. The maximum intensity of c.e.s. varies in different moto-neurones according to the number of incident excitatory impulses, but in none does it reach neurone-threshold.

(*b*) *A Centripetal Volley which evokes a Reflex Twitch.*—As in the previous instance the excitatory impulses incident on a motoneurone have a con-siderable temporal dispersion, but now the intensity of the c.e.s. of some motoneurones reaches threshold with the result that a reflex discharge is instantly set up—*i.e.*, an impulse passes down the axon (motor nerve fibre) of each of these motoneurones. The interval between the incidence of the

---

[1] *Loc. cit.*, p. 575.
[2] *Proc. roy. Soc.*, 1929, **104B**, see p. 273.
[3] *Loc. cit.*, p. 589.
[4] *Proc. roy. Soc.*, 1932, **110B**, 483.
[5] *Cf.* Eccles and Sherrington, *Proc. roy. Soc.*, 1931, **107B**, 511, Fig. 6.

foremost impulses of the centripetal volley and the setting up of the reflex discharge may be as short as $2 \cdot 5$ σ in some motoneurones or as long as 6 σ to 8 σ in others; hence there is often a considerable temporal dispersion of the individual impulses of the reflex discharge.

The reflex discharge of any motoneurone is accompanied by a reduction in the intensity of its c.e.s., and by an absolutely refractory period lasting not longer than $2 \cdot 4$ σ. The neurone-threshold does not, however, reach a normal value for about another 8 σ (duration of relatively refractory period). Excitatory impulses incident on motoneurones after the reflex discharge build up c.e.s., but not to a threshold intensity, for the response is a reflex twitch (cf. Eccles and Sherrington[1]).

Besides thus evoking a reflex discharge from some motoneurones the centripetal volley also gives rise to a subliminal c.e.s. in other motoneurones (the subliminal fringe). The condition in these is identical with that considered in the previous section.

(c) A Centripetal Volley which evokes a Repetitive Discharge (after-discharge) from some Motoneurones.—When the centripetal volley is still larger than that employed in evoking a reflex twitch, the initial reflex discharge of many motoneurones is set up as in the previous section, but excitatory impulses incident on some motoneurones after this initial discharge are sufficient to raise the c.e.s. to threshold again and so set up a second discharge. In some motoneurones this may be repeated several times. Following a large centripetal volley there may be a bombardment of some motoneurones by excitatory impulses for as long as 50 σ or even 500 σ. Only some moto-neurones of the reflex centre will respond repetitively; others will respond only once as in the previous section; others will be in the subliminal fringe.

2. The Central Effects of an Antidromic Volley

An antidromic impulse reaching any motoneurone removes preformed c.e.s., and is followed by an absolutely refractory period lasting for not longer than about $2 \cdot 4$ σ. A single centripetal volley, however, cannot set up a reflex discharge until about 5 σ after the antidromic volley has reached the motoneurone. The additional interval is due to the time consumed in building up the c.e.s. to threshold value. Neurone-threshold does not fall to a normal value until about $10 \cdot 5$ σ after an antidromic volley (end of the relatively refractory period).

Theoretical Discussion

From the considerations on p. 487 it is clear that the central excitatory state is a convenient term for expressing the experimental facts of summation of the central excitatory conditions set up by centripetal volleys. Since it is now generally agreed that this summation occurs[2] (cf. Fulton, Adrian

[1] Loc. cit., p. 522.
[2] Fulton, J. F., Muscular Contraction and Reflex Control of Movement, Baltimore, 1926, p. 350; Adrian and Bronk, J. Physiol., 1929, 67, 146; Sherrington, p. 443 this volume; Bremer, C. R. Soc. Biol., 1930, 103, 509; Forbes, Davis and Lambert, Amer. J. Physiol., 1930, 95, see p. 165.

and Bronk, Sherrington, Bremer, Eccles and Sherrington, Forbes Davis, and Lambert), the theoretical discussion need only be concerned with ideas on the nature and location of the central excitatory state.

The ideas expressed in the papers quoted above show a considerable difference of opinion between different observers. Thus Fulton favours the view that each excitatory nerve impulse produces a quantum of exciting agent, a chemical substance, which sums with other quanta formed at the same or neighbouring points by other impulses. This summation is pictured as centring about the axon hillock.[1] Forbes, Davis and Lambert,[2] on the other hand, suggest that the electrical responses of successive nerve impulses summate by a process allied to that observed in the " retention of action-current " of crustacean nerve (Levin[3]), or the negative after-potential of vertebrate nerve (Amberson and Downing,[4] Gasser and Erlanger[5]). The position of Adrian and Bronk[6] is not so clearly defined. They suggest that there may be two different mechanisms involved in the spinal flexor reflex. (a) Direct transmission of centripetal impulses to motoneurones by a process not differing greatly from that involved in the conduction of an impulse from one section of a nerve fibre to the next. (b) A more lasting excitatory state (? chemical substance) produced in the synaptic region as a result of the passage of each impulse. Bremer[6] emphasises the undoubted similarity existing between summation in the reflex arc (*addition latente centrale*) and in the partly curarised nerve muscle preparation (*addition latente périphérique*). Sherrington[7] and Eccles and Sherrington[8] are non-committal with regard both to the nature and the location of the c.e.s.

The removal of the c.e.s. of a motoneurone by an antidromic impulse indicates that c.e.s. is restricted to those parts of the motoneurone accessible to such an impulse. It is generally agreed that a nerve impulse in peripheral nerve traverses the surface membrane of the axis cylinder, so it may be assumed that an antidromic impulse also traverses the surface membrane of the motoneurone and its dendrites. It is therefore likely that c.e.s. is confined to this surface membrane. It does not seem possible that a chemical substance, such as is postulated by Fulton, would be restricted to the surface membrane of the motoneurone, or, further, that it would be removed by an antidromic impulse or a reflex discharge.

The hypothesis of Forbes, Davis, and Lambert is also difficult to reconcile with the effect of an antidromic impulse in removing c.e.s. If c.e.s. resembled negative after-potential, one would expect that an antidromic impulse would add to that already existing. Moreover, negative after-potential seems to be an abnormal condition present in excised nerve, for immediately after excision of a nerve it is comparatively small, but then it proceeds to increase in extent and duration. Also it is closely related to

[1] *Loc. cit.*, p. 359.
[2] *Loc. cit.*
[3] *J. Physiol.*, 1927, **63**, 113.
[4] *Ibid.*, 1929, **68**, 19.
[5] *Amer. J. Physiol.*, 1930, **94**, 247.
[6] *Loc. cit.*
[7] This volume, pp. 443-460.
[8] *J. Physiol.*, 1930, **69**, see p. 25.

the supernormal phase (Gasser and Erlanger[1]) which itself is an abnormal condition of nerve (Adrian[2]). For these reasons it does not seem likely that central summation depends on a process allied to the negative after-potential of peripheral nerve.

There is, however, another process in peripheral nerve which may give a clue to the nature of the c.e.s.—namely, the " local excitatory state " (Lucas[3]). It is an excitatory process localised at the stimulated region of the excitable tissue, and it is capable of summation. Though very short in duration in peripheral nerve (about 1 σ at most), it is longer in other excitable tissues—e.g., it has a duration of at least 8 σ in the heart. Moreover, the removal of local excitatory state by a nerve impulse is analogous to the removal of c.e.s. by an antidromic volley, and, again, the disappearance of local excitatory state resulting from the setting up of a propagated disturbance (nerve impulse) is analogous to the disappearance of c.e.s. resulting from the setting up of a reflex discharge.

Thus it seems likely the c.e.s. is a specialised manifestation of the local excitatory state.[4] According to the membrane theory,[5] the latter is a partial depolarisation of the polarised membrane surrounding the axis cylinders of nerve fibres, so on analogy c.e.s. is probably a depolarisation of those parts of the surface membranes of motoneurones on which the excitatory impulses impinge—i.e., the synaptic membranes.

This hypothesis as it stands does not explain the well established fact that there is a summation of the c.e.s. produced by excitatory impulses reaching different synapses of the same motoneurone. In addition to this summation the " synaptic " delay of the response to a centripetal volley can be almost reduced to vanishing point by a suitably timed centripetal volley in another afferent nerve (Eccles and Sherrington[6]). In order to reconcile the hypothesis with these facts it must be assumed that the changes produced at any synapse are not restricted on the surface membrane of the motoneurone to the actual locus of that synapse, but that the changes affect at least the immediately adjacent synapses. The profusion of " boutons terminaux "[7] belonging to the endings of a single afferent fibre on a motoneurone would serve to give opportunity for immediately adjacent synapses (boutons) to be excited by impulses in any two afferent fibres having endings on the same motoneurone.

The parallel which Adrian and Bronk[8] draw between the discharges of receptor organs and of motoneurones, and the similarity which Bremer[8] draws attention to between addition latente centrale and addition latente péri-phérique are both in harmony with the above hypothesis, and it is to be

---

[1] Amer. J. Physiol., 1930, **94**, 247.   [2] J. Physiol., 1920, **54**, 1.
[3] J. Physiol., 1910, **39**, 461, and Proc. roy. Soc., 1912, **85B**, 495.
[4] Cf. Sherrington, Arch. int. Physiol., 1921, **18**, 620.
[5] Bernstein, J., Electrobiologie, Braunschweig, 1912, vi, and Lillie, Phys. Rev., 1922, **2**, 1.
[6] Proc. roy. Soc., 1931, **107B**, see p. 527.
[7] See Cajal, Histologie du Système Nerveux, Paris, 1909, p. 311, Fig. 110.
[8] Loc. cit. supra.

noted that it attempts to explain the facts of excitation in the central nervous system by assuming no properties which are unknown in peripheral nerve.[1]

[*In much the same manner as the problem of the central excitatory state was approached above, inhibition in a flexor centre was analysed. A single inhibitory afferent volley was pitted against a single excitatory volley of known strength, at different intervals of time and in different strengths. Its effect was also analysed in relation to an antidromic volley. The reflex tested was the flexion induced by stimulation of an afferent nerve in the same limb, inhibited by stimulation of the corresponding afferent in the opposite limb (spinal cat). The inhibitory influence on the motoneurone is called the central inhibitory state (" c.i.s."). Only the discussion of the experimental results is reprinted here.*—ED.]*

[2] The inhibition of flexor motoneurones by a single contralateral volley has been investigated by observing the reflex response evoked by a single ipsilateral volley set up at various times after the contralateral volley (*cf.* Samojloff and Kisseleff[3]). A reduction in the size of the reflex response— *i.e.*, inhibition—is not usually observed until the excitatory volley follows the inhibitory by 8 σ or more. After its first appearance the amount of the inhibition increases for 25 σ to 70 σ and then progressively decreases, but is still usually observable at 200 σ.

In some experiments a given inhibitory volley has inhibited a weaker reflex more than a stronger. Consequently it is concluded that with motoneurones the prevention of reflex discharge by inhibition depends on the intensity of the excitation.

Two similar inhibitory volleys in the same afferent nerve produce a greater inhibition than either volley alone, even when the interval between them is as long as 60 σ. Further, a repetitive series of inhibitory volleys produces a gradually increasing inhibition. Both these results show that there is summation of the inhibitory effects of successive afferent volleys.

A volley passing antidromically up motor nerve fibres to inhibited motoneurones has no effect on that inhibition.

Excitatory impulses incident on inhibited motoneurones diminish the inhibition of a reflex evoked by a subsequent excitatory volley. Hence it is concluded that inhibition is a long-lasting state, called a central inhibitory state (c.i.s.), and that it is inactivated by excitatory impulses. In order to explain the results it must further be assumed that the inhibitory impulses from a single inhibitory volley are incident on motoneurones during a considerable period. This temporal dispersion, often at least 100 σ in duration, is attributed to delay paths.

[1] *Cf.* Lucas, K., *Conduction of the Nervous Impulse*, London, 1917, p. 2.
[2] From " Studies on the Flexor Reflex. VI. Inhibition," with J C. Eccles, *Proc. roy. Soc.*, 1931, **109B**, 91. (Only extracts from discussion reprinted here.)
[3] *Pflüg. Archiv. ges. Physiol.*, 1927, **215**, 699.

At first thought it is difficult to imagine the upstream mechanism responsible for converting a single volley of impulses into these prolonged bombardments. However, such is the intricacy of the fibre system of the grey matter, as revealed by microscopic examination, that it would seem to be difficult to over-estimate its potentiality for providing " delay paths " (Forbes[1]) adequate for the most prolonged of bombardments. The rate of conduction along the fine nerve fibres of the grey matter is probably even slower than the slowest rate found by Erlanger and Gasser[2] in the non-medullated fibres of a cat's peripheral nerve—0·25 metres a second or 250 μ a sigma.

The time occupied by the various " synaptic " delays (Eccles and Sherrington[3]) must be added to the total conduction time of the pathway. The shortest " synaptic " delay for the single synapse in the reflex arc of the ipsilateral flexor reflex averages about 4 σ in duration, but " synaptic " delays of twice this duration are common. Thus, if there is only one synapse in the shortest inhibitory pathway, a considerable part of the time (about 12 σ, see above) occupied in this pathway is likely to be due to " synaptic " delay. This is also probably the case with more complicated inhibitory pathways, for in them there will be several synapses.

The rate of production of c.e.s. by incident excitatory impulses controls the reflex discharge of reflex impulses from a motoneurone (Eccles and Sherrington[4]). Inhibition modifies this response of the motoneurone to excitation, not by any direct action on the motoneurone itself (*cf.* Sherrington,[5] 1929), but by inactivating c.e.s. with the result that the rate of increase of c.e.s. is slowed down or stopped altogether.

The locus of the motoneurone from which reflex discharge is set up (probably the synapse, see Eccles and Sherrington[6]) is open to approach from three different types of impulse: the excitatory impulse, the inhibitory impulse, and the antidromic impulse. Each of these is followed by a characteristic condition: c.e.s., c.i.s., and refractory period, respectively. In addition it has already been shown that an antidromic impulse inactivates c.e.s. (Eccles[7]), and in the present series of experiments an excitatory impulse, or the c.e.s. it gives rise to, has been shown to inactivate c.i.s. And finally c.i.s. and therefore the inhibitory impulse probably inactivates c.e.s. Yet in spite of this interaction which exists between two pairs of the three types of impulses, an antidromic impulse has no action whatever on c.i.s.

In many respects c.e.s. and c.i.s. are analogous states, but they differ fundamentally in certain features. In the following respects c.e.s. and c.i.s. are analogous:

[1] Forbes, A., *Physiol. Rev.*, 1922, **2**, 361.
[2] Erlanger, J., and Gasser, H. S., *Amer. J. Physiol.*, 1930, **92**, 43.
[3] Eccles, J. C., and Sherrington, C. S., *Proc. roy. Soc.*, 1931, **107B**, 511.
[4] *Proc. roy. Soc.*, 1931, **107B**, 586.   [5] *Proc. roy. Soc.*, 1929, **105B**, 332.
[6] *Ibid.*, 1931, **101B**, 597.   [7] *Ibid.*, 1931, **107B**, 557.

1. c.e.s. and c.i.s. are only produced when nerve impulses in the terminal branches of one neurone are incident on a neurone next in series—*i.e.*, at synapses. However, there is yet no experimental evidence for the existence of inhibition with neurones other than motoneurones.

2. The c.e.s. or c.i.s. produced by a single impulse undergoes a gradual subsidence. With flexor motoneurones the rate of subsidence for c.e.s. (Eccles and Sherrington[1]) is several times more rapid than the rate for c.i.s.

3. The c.e.s. or c.i.s. produced by one impulse sums respectively with the c.e.s. or c.i.s. produced by other impulses arriving by either the same or other nerve fibres ending on that same motoneurone. It may be that there is only summation between the c.e.s. or c.i.s. produced at immediately adjacent synapses.

4. As a consequence of summation many grades of intensity of either c.e.s. or c.i.s. may be produced on a motoneurone.

5. When c.e.s. and c.i.s. are opposed to each other, there is an inactivation of certain quantities of each. This mutual inactivation is likely to be quantitative, in which case there is a true algebraic summation between the c.e.s. and the c.i.s. of a motoneurone. It follows that c.e.s. and c.i.s. cannot coexist in the same place for any appreciable time. It may be that there is a quantitative interaction between the c.e.s. produced by one excitatory impulse and the c.i.s. produced by one inhibitory impulse, but such a relationship is at present pure hypothesis.

In the following respects c.e.s. and c.i.s. differ fundamentally:

1. If the c.e.s. of a motoneurone reaches a sufficient intensity, then it gives rise to the discharge of an impulse from that motoneurone. No corresponding action is known for c.i.s. It has no direct effect on the motoneurone—it merely inactivates c.e.s.

2. An impulse passing antidromically up a motor nerve fibre to a motoneurone inactivates the c.e.s. of that motoneurone, but does not affect the c.i.s.

The above two differences between c.e.s. and c.i.s. have in all probability a common basis. *Thus it may well be that c.e.s. acts as the sole intermediary between c.i.s. and the motoneurone, c.i.s. having no direct action on this latter.*

None of the experimental evidence bears on the actual nature of c.i.s. Ballif, Fulton and Liddell,[2] Fulton,[3] and Samojloff and Kisseleff[4] have suggested that it is a chemical substance. It may, however, receive its ultimate explanation in terms of physical chemistry—*e.g.*, as the stabilising of a surface membrane (Sherrington[5]). Certain it is that it can exist independently of excitation.

[1] *J. Physiol.*, 1930, **69**, 1.   [2] *Proc. roy. Soc.*, 1925, **98B**, 589.
[3] *Muscular Contraction and the Reflex Control of Movement*, Baltimore, 1926.
[4] *Pflüg. Arch. ges. Physiol.*, 1927, **215**, 699.   [5] *Proc. rov. Soc.*, 1929, **105B**, 332.

XI

FINAL CONSPECTUS: QUANTITATIVE MANAGEMENT OF CONTRACTION IN LOWEST LEVEL CO-ORDINATION[1]

COMPACT in Hughlings Jackson was a fine vein of pithy thought and phrase. Among its memorable examples stands that figure[2] of the nerve centres as rising in three tiers or levels. It gained common usage, and is witness to its author not least in the tacit and complete assurance that neural organisation and co-ordination are inseparably one. Of it I think had he been with us today he would have judged no illustrations happier than the notable studies of asynergia, rigidity and tremor, and the modern advance in knowledge of their nature, which are our debt pre-eminently to clinicians of our own country. The nervous system is indeed both a form and a series of events. These have to be confronted together even for inquiry which concerns itself with function as its chief aim.

Hughlings Jackson describes " dissolution," his great analyst of the nervous system, as pulling to pieces from the top downwards to descend variously far. So likewise physiological experiment, but, for simplicity, starts lower. A rump of mechanism, a stump of spinal cord, these it interrogates through perhaps a single afferent for answer by a single efferent. Such virtuosity has of course its defects; one of them is the mutilation entailed. But its hope is, since bottom is basal, to reach bottom; though even there the elemental may not prove to be the simple.

MOTOR UNITS

Of Jackson's three levels, simplicity's field of choice will lie in the lowest, the Jacksonian third. There, and at its simplest, is that old-fashioned if time-honoured entity, the motor centre. I hesitate to invite recontemplation of such oft-worn ground; yet in light of some fresh detail it seems to accrete endowment. With it, an initial problem, and nowhere more essential, is quantitative adjustment. Sampled by afferent stimulation the motor centre soon reveals that every reflex fractionates its muscle. The fractionation is not pushed so far as to run to the single muscle-fibre. Soleus (cat) has some 30,000 muscle-fibres and the long extensor of the digits

---

[1] The Hughlings Jackson Lecture, 1931, *Brain*, 1931, **54**, 1.
[2] Hughlings Jackson, Croonian Lectures, *Brit. Med. J.*, 1884, **1**, 591.

some 40,000;[1] but nervous co-ordination, as Hughlings Jackson said, is
" based on the anterior horn-cell." That cell by its motor nerve-fibre
innervates a whole packet of muscle-fibres, 150 and more. This packet
of muscle-fibres together with its motor nerve-fibre constitutes what may
be called for short a " motor unit." It is into these packets that the reflex
fractionates its muscle. They give numbers not unmanageable—*soleus*
(cat) consists of some 200, *extensor longus digitorum* 330, medial *gastroc-nemius* 450.[2]

Such motor units yield a contraction-wave of some 2·5 grammes, and
even 9 grammes contraction-tension[2]—a coarse unit, it would seem, to
grade with. The more since its contraction runs on the " all or nothing "
plan, so that to grade the strength of the stimulus, however carefully, does
not arrive at grading the strength of the contraction-wave itself, the con-traction-wave being in so far a fixed quantity independent of the strength
of its stimulus. In reflex action, however, we know that the single con-traction-wave as an isolated event scarcely happens. These the contraction
waves overlap to form tetanus. This tetanus when once the mechanical
fusion of the component waves is *complete* yields in its turn a tension value,
fixed, in so far that no increase of strength or of rate of stimulus will
change it further. This full tetanic tension value for the average unit is
10 grammes in *soleus* (cat) and reaches 35 grammes in gastrocnemius.[2]

Such fixity of value for the tetanised motor unit allows reflexes which
can ensure it to be tested for their share of a given muscle.[3] In this way
it is found that in the limb practically no afferent nerve possesses the whole
of any one muscle, and that every afferent nerve has some reflex share in
practically every muscle.

The motor units which make up tibialis anticus (cat) number some 380;
its spinal motor horn-cells are in effect the expanded receptive central
ends of these motor units. Some of the motor units are larger than others,
and to these attach doubtless the larger motor horn-cells. The overlap of
central terminals of these large cells, if their density on the cell surface is
as elsewhere, must be specially extensive, so that the large motor units will
be the more widely at call and the more often in play.

Of the 380 motor units thus making *tibialis anticus*, the internal saphenous
nerve under faradisation can tetanise some 120, the popliteal 290, a dorsal
digital 135, and so on. We may suppose the central terminals of these
afferent nerves to play largely directly upon the motoneurones, since in
the case of this relatively simple reflex recent work discounts the invariable
mediation of an internuncial neurone between afferent root and ventral
horn-cell.

[1] Clark, D. A., *J. Physiol.*, 1930, **70**, 18.
[2] Eccles and Sherrington, *Proc. roy. Soc.*, 1930, **106B**, 326.
[3] Cooper, Denny-Brown, and Sherrington, *Proc. roy. Soc.*, 1926, **100B**, 448.

Grades of Excitement in the Motor Centre

That many or most of these last are fully tetanised is shown by submitting them to additional excitation and their then yielding no additional contraction.[1] Motor units thus fully tetanised can be classed as *maximally* excited.

When we find in an experiment that full tetanic stimulation, say, of a plantar nerve, tetanises 190 of the 380 motor units and stops at that, may we suppose that the anatomical limit of the number of motoneurones reachable by the afferent has been attained? Hardly, for the number thus found, within limits, can fluctuate quite rapidly during the course of an experiment.[2] A slight subconvulsive dose of strychnine, accelerating reflex recruitment, and shortening, as Bremer and Rylant showed, the reflex latency,[3] will strengthen the response perhaps 25 per cent. Conversely, with spinal shock it shrinks.

The temporary upper limit represents, therefore, not the anatomical total which the nerve can reach, but some, often a large, proportion of that total, a proportion circumscribed by functional condition. And there is abundant evidence that besides those motoneurones which the afferent nerve thus excites, there are others, a subliminal fringe, on which it acts but fails to bring to discharge. The proof of this is that an excitation similarly subliminal from another source when brought to bear concurrently on this subliminal fringe does bring it to discharge.[1,4] Explanation of the variation in the number of motor units a given afferent nerve at different times will excite may lie partly in subliminal excitation from some other reflex or central source being in or out of action on some of the motoneurones at the time.

At the opposite extreme from the subliminal fringe there obtains what we may term " supra-maximal " excitement. By combining tetanising excitations say via two separate afferent nerves, the excitement of some motoneurones can be brought to " supra-maximal " in the sense of more than sufficient for full tetanic contraction of the muscle-fibres of their units. This is detectable by " occlusion " of contraction,[1,5] and it commonly happens under faradic stimulation of even a single afferent nerve because of central overlap between that nerve's own constituent fibres.

Therefore among the reflexly excited units of the motoneurone pool there will obtain, and often at the same time, the different grades of excitement, subliminal, maximal, and supra-maximal. Altogether, since some of the motoneurones are *not* excited, there are *four* states of the motoneurones, *zero*, *subliminal*, *maximal*, and *supra-maximal*.

What then of the gap between maximal and subliminal? Three years

---

[1] Cooper, Denny-Brown, and Sherrington, *Proc. roy. Soc.*, 1927, **101B**, 262.
[2] *Idem, ibid.*, 1926, **100B**, 448.   [3] *C. R. Soc. Biol.*, Paris, 1925, **92**, 199, 1329, 1331.
[4] Denny-Brown and Sherrington, *J. Physiol.*, 1928, **66**, 175; and Eccles and Granit, *ibid.*, 1929, **67**, 97.   [5] Camis, *J. Physiol.*, 1909, **39**, 228.

ago Adrian and Bronk[1] on the one hand, and on the other Denny-Brown,[2] by different methods and independently, succeeded in observing reflex firing in individual motor units. They found rates ranging down to 6 per second and 7·5 per second in slow extensor muscles, and down to 15 per second in the motor phrenic. Now, these rates are not sufficient to secure in their muscle-fibres a complete tetanus; they are not of maximal grade. They are *subtetanic* in the sense of being not sufficient for full tetanus. Different rates, faster and slower, within *subtetanus* grade were observed to occur concurrently among motor units firing in the same muscle.[2] The rates did not correspond with the rate of the break-shock series applied to the afferent nerve.[2, 3] These examples were taken from crossed reflexes; in such there exists of course the internuncial neurone which mediates between the afferent nerve-fibre and the ventral horn-cell. In the simple flexion-reflex the central connection is more direct, and there the rate of firing of the motor unit shows much closer correspondence with that of the repetitive stimulus,[4] at least in some of the motor units and if the repetitive stimulus be not too quick and strong. But even there the motor unit is prone to fire more than once in response to a single centripetal volley.[5] This repetitive after-discharge from a single centripetal volley is still greater in some crossed reflexes and may reach extraordinary proportions. The point here is that often the firing of the motor unit does not agree closely with impulse volleys entering from the afferent nerve. The firing of the motoneurone exhibits a quasi-independence of the rate of volleying of the afferent nerve. This may seem a contradiction of the close correspondence observable in the spinal flexion-reflex under moderate faradic stimulation, but even then the main rhythm tends to be complicated by secondary discharges. Reconciliation of these facts lies in the motor centre being a " summation-mechanism " which takes various summation-times to reach discharging point, and in the neurone-threshold itself varying, and with individuality of duration of refractory phase.

Turning from artificial stimulation to natural, we know now, thanks to the discoveries of Adrian and his collaborators, that natural stimulation —for instance, pressure on the foot[6]—will no less than does faradic develop its reflex by means of impulse-showers, but these are for the former far more diversely arranged. The trains of centripetal impulses engendered by such " natural " stimulations are not only of different rates among themselves, but vary in regularity, and differ in different fibres with heights of frequency related to intensity of the stimulation at different sense organs, and with different periods of crescendo and of adaptation and fatigue. The centripetal stream will resemble less a noise than a musical note.

[1] *J. Physiol.*, 1928, **66**, 51.   [2] *Proc. roy. Soc.*, 1929, **104B**, 252.
[3] Adrian and Bronk, *J. Physiol.*, 1929, **67**, 119.
[4] Liddell and Sherrington, *Proc. roy. Soc.*, 1923, **95B**, 142; and Adrian and Cooper, *ibid.*, 1924, **96B**, 243.
[5] Sherrington, *ibid.*, 1921, **92B**, 245; *Arch. int. Physiol.*, 1921, **18**, 620; and Eccles and Sherrington, *J. Physiol.*, 1930, **69**, 1.   [6] Adrian and Umrath, *J. Physiol.*, 1929, **68**, 294.

This complex inrush, pouring upon internuncial neurones, or directly upon the motoneurone pool, proceeds, however, from a truly functionally related set of receptors. As compared with the centripetal stream sent in under faradic stimulation of the bared nerve, this natural one will have its impulses less synchronised and in more dissimilar individual trains. It will display consequently richer inequality of excitation on the motoneurone pool. In general correspondence with this (though, since the firing of the individual motor unit may not closely agree with that of the afferent fibre, particular correspondence there need not be) there will result still greater diversity between the firing of individual motor units, inasmuch as the grade of excitement of the motoneurone governs the rate of firing of the motor unit.

The rate of firing of the muscle-fibre can be taken as guide to the amount of excitation of the motoneurone. Though there is an intrinsic factor in the rate of response, the quicker the firing the greater the rate of excitation. Thus in the phrenic nerve the individual motor-fibre fires more rapidly the stronger the inspiratory action;[1] again, in the extensor motor unit firing steadily, weak inhibition by an inhibitory afferent slackens the firing until withdrawal of the inhibition, when the former quicker rate returns.[2]

Degrees of Engagement of the Motor Centre

Clearly there obtain under reflex action, and especially with the more natural and less simple, a whole gamut of excitements in the motoneurone pool. Besides the " maximal " (including " supra-maximal ") and " subliminal " grades of motoneurone excitement earlier referred to, there will be grades intermediate between those. These intermediate grades, since they produce in their muscle-fibres only imperfect tetani—i.e., " subtetani "—may be termed subtetanic.

It seems useful to attempt a generalised scheme for the state of a " lowest-level " motor centre of a muscle under reflex excitation. We have to distinguish in it the above broad classes of excitement of the motor units. We may group together as one the maximal and what were styled above the " supra-maximal," and embrace them under one heading—namely, " maximal "—because of their like effect in respect of contraction tension. The broad classes are then three, " subliminal," " subtetanic," and " maximal." There will be in addition a zero class where the excitation is nil. The rate of excitement is greatest where in the centre the successive arrival of converging impulses is quickest and thickest.[3]

First, as regards weak reflexes: since a central excitation field reduced

[1] Adrian and Bronk, J. Physiol., 1928, **66,** 51.
[2] Denny-Brown, Proc. roy. Soc., 1929, **104B,** 252.
[3] Illustrated by a diagrammatic chart in the original paper. See also Reflex Activity of the Spinal Cord, 1932.

to its minimum is entirely subliminal,[1, 2] clearly in weak reflexes the sub-liminal fringe will constitute a larger proportion of the excited field. This has been often observed.

As regards strong reflexes: in them excitement of the " maximal " class embraces in certain exceptional examples the motor units of a whole muscle.[2] Often in strong reflexes " maximal " motor units are plentiful enough to include all of the motor units engaged by a weaker reflex;[2] this latter's contraction tension can then be entirely concealed by that of the former.

ADJUSTMENT TO CHANGES OF EXCITATION

Reduction of the stimulation of the afferent nerve means excitation of fewer fibres in it. The field and density of the exciting central terminals is thus reduced. This reduction may fall heavier on one class than on another. But let us suppose it more general and more equable. Let us suppose, on a diagrammatic scale of the reflexly excited motoneurone pool of a muscle, a general withdrawal of excitation such as to reduce existing excitements by a given, say the just subliminal, amount. We may sample this withdrawal for its effect motor unit by motor unit along the scale of excitation. The total result is a decrease of contraction which is traceable to several factors. Some units, though still excited, now cease to discharge, and the total excited field somewhat shrinks. The old subliminal fringe drops out of action altogether to be replaced by another, in this case not less plentiful, supplied from former " subtetanics." All along the firing line the fire, as examined motoneurone by motoneurone, somewhat slackens. Units well up in the " maximal " class continue to give the same contraction-tension as before ; other " maximals " lower down degrade into the subtetanic class and yield less tension. In the subtetanic class all slip lower, yielding individually less tension, and some cease to discharge, entering the subliminal fringe. In records where two motor units are firing, one somewhat faster than the other, it can be seen that when the faster slackens somewhat its slower companion may disappear altogether—i.e., will cease firing. An excitation causing the remaining one to quicken again restarts the companion which had stopped. The waning and waxing affects the two and in the same direction, and what will slow one will stop the other. Sometimes, however, one unit will persist unaltered although another stops.

On occasion some units are increased in excitement while others are reduced. This happens under conditions, however, which do not preclude inco-ordination—namely, the stimulation of an afferent nerve which tends to produce some ipsilateral extension and some ipsilateral flexion mixed. A likelier field for search might be higher level co-ordination, such as

[1] Sherrington, *Proc. roy. Soc.*, 1929, **105B**, 332; Eccles and Sherrington, *J. Physiol.*, 1930, **69**, 1; Eccles and Granit, *ibid.*, 1929, **67**, 97.
[2] Cooper, Denny-Brown, and Sherrington, *Proc. roy. Soc.*, 1927, **101B**, 262.

Dr. Blake Pritchard[1] has been investigating, though even here there can be quite fractional inhibition.

But the outstanding instance of shift of the individual unit along successive grades of excitement in the course of a single reflex is the instance of which, thanks to Adrian and his co-workers, most is known—namely, that which as they have shown characterises the opening phase[2] even in these " lowest level " reflexes, especially, we may suppose, when evoked by " natural " stimuli. The firing of an engaged motor unit then opens at slow rate and runs a gradually, though it may be rapidly, ascending course to reach a climax frequency. The reflex, in short, even as regards the excitation of the individual neurone, develops gradually. This contrasts with the spinal flexion-reflex as exhibited under faradisation of the bared afferent nerve. The latter with characteristic abruptness develops its full tetanus at once. This d'emblée opening[3] is but in agreement with the form possessed by the stimulus which excites it; that stimulus tetanises at once and at its full rate all the afferent fibres it is going to tetanise. More remarkable is that the crossed extension reflex under similar stimulation does not so respond but opens gradually,[3] showing both " recruitment " and acceleration of individual firing,[2] often after a marked period of *addition latente*.[4] The rate of recruitment is accelerated by strychnine, for as shown by Bremer and Rylant (1926) strychnine shortens the fundamental reflex latency.[5]

Doubtless these features have relation to intermediation by a relay neurone. But the d'emblée opening may be regarded as " artificial," in the sense that few " natural " stimulations are likely to produce it. Cutaneous or proprioceptive stimuli are not easily imagined which will develop their height " rectangularly " and with the suddenness of a faradic current on an afferent nerve-trunk. In the flexion-reflex excited by the " natural " stimulus of pinching the foot, Adrian and Bronk[2] show the rate of firing of an individual motor-fibre to begin at a low rate, gradually reach its climax and gradually decline. Their instance slowly ascended the subtetanic scale during the course of some 4 seconds and never acquired " maximal " grade. With the crossed extension reflex evoked by mechanical stimulation of the opposite foot, they traced a sample individual unit opening firing at a rate low down in the subtetanic scale and rising steadily in rate to enter the " maximals " group (60 per second) in about 5 seconds. Adrian and his co-workers furnish many examples which show that one and the same motor unit climbs through successive grades of excitement in the opening phase of reflex response. In our generalised scheme of the grades of excitement in a motor centre and their distribution, we

[1] *Brain*, 1930, **53**, 344.
[2] Adrian and Bronk, *J. Physiol.*, 1929, **67**, 119.
[3] Liddell and Sherrington, *Proc. roy. Soc.*, 1923, **95B**, 299.
[4] Sherrington, *Arch. Sci. biol.*, 1928, **12**, 1.
[5] Bremer and Rylant, *C. R. Soc. Biol., Paris*, 1925, **92**, 199, 1329, 1331.

may picture the individual unit at beginning of a natural reflex as starting somewhere low down in the subtetanic grade and then climbing to take a more settled place in, if the reflex be strong, the maximals.

The terminal phase of the reflex, when caused by simple withdrawal of the exciting stimulus without complication by inhibition, we may picture as an extension of that weakening already dealt with above, and again with its abruptness softened, especially for strong reflexes, by the protraction of individual after-discharge.

The important and fascinating discoveries of Adrian and his collaborators seem thus to supply a paradigm of the course of discharge of rhythmic reflexes in general. If a natural reflex act exhibits gradual development of its drive of the motor unit, and if similarly the subsidence of that drive be likewise gradual, as we know from after-discharge it is, each alternating phase of a rhythmic train of action (respiratory ventilation, stepping) will in effect be just a waxing and waning of the frequency of discharge of certain individual motor units periodically repeated. The observations of Adrian and Bronk indicate that the grading of contraction of the rabbit's diaphragm in inspiration is effected mainly by grading the frequency of the firing of the motor unit with little " recruitment " at all. The deeper inspiration means in that case quicker and more prolonged firing of many of just those same motor units which in shallow inspiration fire less rapidly and less long. The resemblance between spinal " stepping " and respiration is close in many respects.[1] The tetanic outburst rhythmically repeated in the spinal scratch-reflex is more abrupt and more brief—e.g., one-ninth second—and is less amenable to grading in rate.

Adjustment by Subliminals, Subtetanics, and Maximals Respectively

Thus, then, each of the broad grades of excitement of the motor centre contributes to active adjustment of the reflex contraction, and contributes somewhat in its own way.

Subliminal fringe adjusts mainly on the basis of extensity, increasing or diminishing the total number of motoneurones engaged. It, so to say, mediates between excitation and the quiescent pool outside. That this is so is shown by the *addition latente*[2] and recruiting opening of the crossed extensor reflex, and is to be inferred also from the gradual course of the development of excitement shown by Adrian and Bronk for the individual unit at commencement of various reflexes. The fringe recruits from the quiescent pool; back into that pool it sheds. It also, of course, feeds the supraliminal field. Its relation to this latter is sometimes illustrated under conditions strikingly simple. Thus, to take a particular case:[3]

---

[1] Sherrington, *J. Physiol.*, 1910, **40**, 28, and Graham Brown, *ibid.*, 1914, **48**, 18.
[2] Sherrington, *Livre à Charles Richet*, Paris, 1926, and *Arch. Sci. biol.*, 1928, **12**, 1.
[3] Eccles and Sherrington, *Proc. roy. Soc.*, 1931, **107B**, 535.

Two similar volleys are fired into a flexion centre in quick succession. The first excites a reflex twitch in 70 motor units. The second, following quickly, finds those 70 motoneurones refractory because they have just fired. But in 45 other motoneurones which the first volley excited, though not to the extent of firing them, the second volley finds still some subliminal excitement left by the first, and, itself subliminal for them, yet adds an increment of excitement sufficient for their firing; the myograph gauges their number from their contraction. The exciting volleys are then strengthened, so as each singly to fire 180 motor units instead of 70. But these two stronger volleys in sequence discover little fringe. Therefore evidently the 45 subliminals of the weaker reflex must have become some of the 180 supraliminals of the stronger. In such an experiment, the summation being confined to two stimuli, opportunity for revealing the whole fringe is small. Temporal summation by its mere iteration possesses powers less limited than spatial summation can attain alone.

Subliminal fringe is absent in some strong reflexes, at least as concerns a particular muscle. That is not to say it is absent *altogether*, for a reflex employs concurrently several synergic muscles each with opportunity for fringe.[1]

The large fringes of weak reflexes are an effective factor for co-ordinative liaison and combination between such reflexes, and between them and others. Thus nothing is more frequent than in the course of an experiment with, for instance, the ankle extensor attached to the myograph, to see, if head and neck be passively turned into the so-called favourable position, the same limb stimulus evoke a much greater reflex than before, even although the new posture of the head and neck evoked itself no reflex from the muscle.[2] An individual motor unit, sampled for observation, then beats faster than before; on replacing the head and neck in the less favourable position the motor units fire less quickly again. The facilitation from above is largely, and may be entirely, subliminal and upon it summation builds when the local reflex is repeated. Subliminal reflexes impinging with allied effect on the muscle can produce large quantities of contraction.[3]

Thus again with Rademaker's[4] supporting reaction from the sole of the foot and the soleus postural stretch-reflex. Also with Bremer's[5] cerebellar influences upon the extensor reflex of the limb; and these remind us that there can be inhibitory fringe as well as excitatory, and that its withdrawal can give Hughlings Jackson's " release," as luminously expounded by Sir Henry Head. It is mainly by subliminal fringes of excitation that the higher nervous centres exert the postural adaptations which are as necessary to the animal as is posture itself. Destruction of the rostral cerebellar cortex (Bremer,[5] Rademaker[6]) suggests itself as accounting, by

[1] Creed and Sherrington, *Proc. roy. Soc.*, 1926, **100B**, 258.
[2] Beritoff, *Quart. J. exp. Physiol.*, 1916, **9**, 199.   [3] Eccles and Granit, *J. Physiol.*, 1929, **67**, 97.
[4] *Proc. Akad. Wetensch. Amsterdam*, 1926, **30**,
[5] Bremer, *Arch. int. Physiol.*, 1922, **19**, 189; and Bremer and Ley, *Bull. Acad. Med. Belg.*, 1927, **7**, 60.   [6] *Arch. néerl. Physiol.*, 1927, **11**, 445.

removal of reciprocal—and especially inhibitory—fringe from limb antagonists, for the dysmetria—and hypermetria—observed as a cerebellar symptom.

The Subtetanics Group.—An important attribute of these is their power to grade contraction. Rate of firing of the motor unit grades contraction by so spacing the successive contraction-waves that the integrated tension falls variously short of full tetanic. The shortage is of course greater the slower the wave-succession, and the scale of grading becomes progressively less open as full tetanus is approached. A given increment of frequency of firing of the motor unit represents less increment of contraction-tension in proportion as the frequency of firing in the motor unit is already high, until at last it represents no increment at all (occlusion).[1]

The subtetanic contraction of the individual motor unit is of course tremulous. I suppose, therefore, the weak reflex will contain more tremor, but I do not know that myographically. With a power-unit like that of gastrocnemius, which averages a contraction-wave of some 9 grammes,[2] its tremulous contraction must threaten the steadiness of the whole muscle. But lessening such defect is the circumstance that the various subtetanised units are out of phase one with another. Individual differences of rate of summation of excitation and of duration of refractory phase will tend to keep them so. If a number fall into step tremor must become gross.

Denny-Brown has brought forward,[3] and supported from his experiments, an interpretation on this basis of the clonus readily induced in the decerebrate preparation of the laboratory. There, he says, clonus arises simply from the tonic normally asynchronous discharge of the units becoming synchronised. The tonic stretch-reflex of the laboratory can exhibit in the firing of its units all shades of transition between asynchronism and complete synchronism, and it can be made to pass from one to the other reversibly by suitable conditions of initial pose (Viets[4]), and, as Pritchard[5] has particularly shown, of tension. Conducive to the position taken by Denny-Brown[6] is his interpretation of the " silent period " of the galvanometer string following a knee jerk as an inhibition, derived from the proprioceptives of the muscle itself and evoked by the jerk itself from its own muscle. This inhibition damps the discharge of the jerk down in effect to one centrifugal impulse. Fulton[7] argues the pause a lapse of excitation. In clonus the motor units get into step as regards contraction, and their keeping in step is accentuated by their pauses keeping step likewise. Their beats in the clonus are punctuated by their proprioceptive pauses forming a vicious circle keeping them in step.

Inherent in the operation of the subtetanic motor units is, besides tremor, some waste work, an uneconomy which has been dealt with by Bronk.[8]

[1] Cooper, Denny-Brown, and Sherrington, *Proc. roy. Soc.,* 1927, **101B,** 262.
[2] Eccles and Sherrington, *Proc. roy. Soc.,* 1930, **106B,** 326.
[3] *Proc. roy. Soc.,* 1929, **104B,** 252.   [4] *Brain,* 1920, **43,** 269.   [5] *Brain,* 1929, **52,** 510.
[6] *Proc. roy. Soc.,* 1928, **103B,** 321.   [7] *Amer. J. Physiol.,* 1928, **83,** 554.
[8] *J. Physiol.,* 1930, **69,** 306.

Can we be sure that nature is in love with economy? In this instance the uneconomy seems more than offset by the advantage gained in delicacy and range of means of grading reflex contraction strength.

The " Maximals " Group.—In weak reflexes—for instance, in weak postural reflexes—there may be no " maximals " at all. A weak tonic postural reflex of *soleus* (cat), favourable to isolated examination of single motor units, not rarely fails to exhibit a single unit firing in other than subtetanus. On the other hand, in strong reflexes there may be none but " maximals " in the entire motoneurone pool of a whole muscle,[1] as driven in laboratory experiment, though this is quite exceptional. In the " maximals " group each unit yields its maximal contraction. Motor units added mean added contraction, and removed mean contraction lessened. All additional excitement received here lays aside its mechanical equivalent. That is to say, " occlusion " occurs here and is therefore prominent in strong reflexes. It is the " maximals " group which by its growth limits more and more the further increase of the reflex muscular response. It brings into the relation between increase of reflex contraction and increase of reflex stimulation some resemblance to the approximately logarithmic ratio holding between increment of sensation and increment of stimulus. The maximals are economical in a sense, because contraction-tension is maintained at a smaller expenditure of energy in a stronger contraction than a weaker.

I would not pursue this subject to tiresome length. We arrive at this: that the motor centre—old but expressive term—is not a mere passive relay on the path out to its muscle, nor merely a place of passive assembly of impulses converging upon the muscle. The motor centre grades the excitation of the individual motor unit, causing its faster or its slower firing. The motor centre is a central instrument which adjusts *actively* the contraction-strength of its reflexes; it works on the basis of the " central excitatory state."[2] Driven and fed by centripetal impulses, it deals with them on the summation basis. It is in short a " summation-mechanism." It operates on the individual motoneurone by excitation-summation; in that way it can exert a whole scale of degrees of excitement upon one and the same individual motor unit, firing it faster and so obtaining nearer full tetanic value of contraction, or slower with greater defect from full tetanic contraction. It also shows changes in extensity with variation in the number of motoneurones. Yet, since central impulses in order to excite a motor unit must be summated, the central mechanism is ultimately wholly a summation apparatus. One secret of its co-ordinative power lies in its power of summating with almost negligible time-lag shifting fringes and mobile shades of excitation that meet and overlap upon it. These join and disjoin, expand and shrink, as afferent channels leading from

---

[1] Cooper, Denny-Brown, and Sherrington, *loc. cit.*

[2] Sherrington, *Proc. roy. Soc.*, 1929, **105B**, 332 (see pp, 473 and 487); and Eccles and Sherrington, *J. Physiol.*, 1930, **69**, 1.

various sources come into or drop out of action; and each and every time the central apparatus subjects them to or releases them from its summation.

The motoneurone which this central summation drives reacts in several respects as Adrian has shown a receptor to react. A difference is, however, its more prolonged maintenance of the rate of firing under persistent stimulation—*i.e.*, its greater resistance[1] to fatigue and " adaptation." It does not run down so quickly as do most receptors. Moreover, the central summation mechanism develops a greater range of intensities both upward and downward than the muscle-fibres which it operates can with their tension follow. If this seem wasteful of central activity, we may remember that additional excitation exerted on a motor unit, already driven " maximally " for tetanic contraction, is not necessarily wasted. That surplus remains still a contribution to co-ordination, because further excitation offers a further resistance to inhibition.[2] Just as an added inhibition in the case of an already quiescent neurone although in one sense wasted is a further protection, which co-ordination may need, against excitation. In time of crisis the dilemma lies between strong actions, and the very strength of the action taken may serve to safeguard it from extrinsic interruption.

Concealed Reflexes

Quantitative adjustment of amount of contraction seems to first thought of purely quantitative significance. Yet, since strengths of contraction may affect and shift the scope of an act, contraction-strength can acquire qualitative value. The laboratory plan of obtaining reflexes by direct stimulation of bared afferent nerve is for some purposes essential. It is, however, artificial and certain reflex artefacts derive from it, among them this, that each large afferent nerve presents a dominant reflex which may conceal other reflexes. This dominance is itself a compromise, although often an overwhelming one, between conflicting reactions. To display natural reflexes thus submerged we have to turn to localised stimuli natural for them. In this way can be traced the otherwise concealed ipsilateral extension reflex of the limb. Its broad quantitative course seems rather different from that just considered.

It activates the great extensors of the limbs. It is a reflex included in that complex which works the limb as tool for locomotion and for standing. When, in reflex life, the animal reacting to the geotropic organ in the head (the labyrinth) has been set on its feet, its limbs are by that very fact saddled with its weight. The extensor reflex of the limb becomes then an anti-gravity reaction. *Per se*, it is not so. Just as the hind-limbs of the spinal dog when passively put upright " stand "[3] by reason of the superincumbent

---

[1] Sherrington, *Proc. roy. Soc.*, 1929, **105B**, 332 (reprinted here, Chapter X, p. 464).

[2] Sherrington and Sowton, *Proc. roy. Soc.*, 1911, **84B**, 203; Creed and Eccles, *J. Physiol.*, 1928, **66**, 109; Forbes Davis and Lambert, *Amer. J. Physiol.*, 1930, **95**, 142.

[3] *J. Physiol.*, 1910, **40**, 28 (see also Chapter VIII, p. 364 this vol.).

weight then eliciting the postural extensor stretch-reflex, so in like manner
the ipsilateral extensor reflex, although not itself specifically geotropic,
becomes then an " upstanding " reflex adjuvant to geotropism. This
upstanding reflex in dealing with its habitual burden, the body-weight,
exhibits several grades of strength. Each grade is adapted to a particular
form of the " upstanding " act and behaviour. The weakest is that adapted
to " standing "; there all that is wanted of the great extensors is to support
their load to the extent of preventing their limb from sinking under it.
This grade of the reflex is postural. It is as regards the great extensors at
knee and ankle essentially the static stretch-reflex, with, preparation per-
mitting, some fringes of support from neck and labyrinth. The motor
units it employs in the great extensors are, conformably with its mild
contraction-strength, a small proportion only of the total aggregate composing these muscles. But this small percentage is not a diffused and
scattered population, it is a segregated set which forms at the ankle the
soleus part of the great calf muscle, trespassing little into the gastrocnemius.[1]
At knee it forms similarly the *crureus* and adjoining *vasti* and spreads little
into *rectus*.

Turning to the stronger forms of this same " upstanding " reflex, these
extend its scope from mere static support of the limb to propulsion of the
body; they are locomotor. The extension of the limb then takes the form
of the extensor phase of the step. With increasing grades of strength and
speed this reflex transcends walking and running and becomes the gallop.
All of these several forms are represented spinally.[2] The spinal gallop is
well observable in the dog, when after a cervical spinal section the " shock "
period is over. Harmless pressure applied to the plantar pads, even of a
single hind-foot, will then evoke the extensor thrust in all four of the limbs
together.[2] The brief backward thrust of the hind-limbs is accompanied
by a similarly timed outreaching thrust of both fore-limbs forward. The
picture presented by the reaction even as the animal lies on its side in the
stall is unmistakably the extension phase of the gallop. It is followed in
all four of the limbs by brief active flexion of each limb. In this " extensor
thrust " of the gallop the gastrocnemius can be felt and seen to be actively
involved, and at the knee the contraction, quite differently from the postural
reflex, spreads far beyond crureus.

In short, this ipsilateral extension reflex, which the labyrinth system
impresses into geotropic service for an " upstanding " limb, exhibits a
quantitative grading somewhat different from that of the prototype muscle-
centre we envisaged earlier. In these great extensor muscles the " upstanding " reflex as it grows in strength and changes its functional scope
passes over from the restricted field of slow red-muscle motor units to
large reserves of quick pale-muscle motor units which are in fact the
main masses of these large extensor muscles. These latter motor units

[1] Denny-Brown, *Proc. roy. Soc.*, 1929, **104B**, 252.
[2] *J. Physiol.*, 1910, **40**, 28 (see also Chapter V, p. 178 *et seq.* this vol.).

are, to judge from gastrocnemius, individually more powerful than those of the red kernel muscle *soleus*, thrice as powerful[1] and nearly thrice as rapid.[2]

Thus the majority of the extensor units at ankle and knee appear as antigravity units held in reserve for such work as the run, the gallop, and the jump. At ankle, in the cat, some 1,100 stronger units held in reserve behind 230 weaker ones. In contraction power the reserve is very high. Thus, isometrically measured at the ankle in a 3·5 kg. cat, 35 kg. of reserve contraction; at ankle and knee together and for both hind-limbs an isometric contraction-tension of some 170 kg. for a 3·5 kg. cat.[3] In its quantitative grading the reflex seems to extend its grasp from slow-contracting, less powerful, and in a sense more economical motor units to more rapidly-contracting, more powerful, in a sense less economical units for more occasional use.

We are fortified in tracing the " upstanding " reflex through its graded scale, from weak to strong, as a single functional entity, since there is no ground now for regarding the postural contraction or tonus as a contraction essentially different from that of other forms. It is the same rhythmic process but at slower rate. This slowness may account for a difference which has sometimes been thought qualitative between postural or tonic and other contraction—namely, relative exemption from fatigue. The relative slowness of firing may of itself account for that. Slow firing of the motor nerve, as experiments by Lady Briscoe[4] demonstrate, avoids and even allows recovery from fatigue, which faster firing induces rapidly.

The importance of posture is emphasised sometimes by saying that it is the starting-point and the end-point for every movement. But posture, as Ramsay Hunt remarks, accompanies " movement like a shadow."[5] Stanley Cobb writes[6] that " they coalesce and often cannot be separated." An apt illustration, familiar in the laboratory, is the posturing of the spinal scratch-reflex. The artificial flea in the form of a faint faradic current is applied, for instance, to the skin behind the ear. This electric tickling excites the reflex, probably through the superficial nerve-endings round the hairs, for after shaving the skin the reflex is difficult to get.[7] The same-side hind-foot breaks out into its scratching, a rhythmic movement which involves digits, ankle, knee and hip. Alongside this movement and just as much a part of the reflex, is posture,[8] a maintenance of flexion of the limb as a whole, along with a steady incurvation of the body toward the stimulus side, the neck deviated and the head partly turned back, so

---

[1] Eccles and Sherrington, *Proc. roy. Soc.*, 1930, **106B**, 326.
[2] Denny-Brown, *Proc. roy. Soc.*, 1929, **104B**, 371; and Cooper and Eccles, *J. Physiol.*, 1930, **69, 377**
[3] Sherrington, *J. Physiol.*, 1930, **70**, 101.
[4] *Ibid.*, 1931, **71**, 292.
[5] *Arch. Neurol. Psychiat., Chicago*, 1922, **10**, 37.
[6] *Physiol. Rev.*, 1925, **5**, 518.
[7] Sherrington, *J. Physiol.*, 1906, **34**, 1.
[8] *Idem, Quart. J. exp. Physiol.*, 1910, **3**, 213.

that the foot more readily may reach it. All these are quite steady reflex postures. *Some* of the muscles actually engaged in the rhythmic movement seem engaged in posture as well as in movement, posture and rhythmic contraction together in the same muscle. The posture not merely alternates with the movement but accompanies it and dovetails in with it. Our earlier schema of a reflexly excited motor centre pictured the motoneurone pool as that of a single muscle; but even the simplest flexion-reflex excites several muscles, and from threshold up. Lorente de Nó,[1] recording graphically the contractions of the individual eye muscles, shows that every labyrinthine reflex acting on the eyes employs all twelve muscles together. With the flexion-reflex of the limb excited from any afferent nerve of the limb, the flexion is plurimuscular from the very outset.[2] Thus with a small digital nerve at minimal stimulus the muscular response starts simultaneously in ankle-flexors and knee-flexors and hip-flexors together, and so on. Thus, from the point of view of the spinal reflex, a motor unit in say *tibialis anticus* has closer functional alliance to some in *semitendinosus* and *tensor fasciæ femoris* than to many of the fellow motor units in its own muscle. The simplest spinal reflex, as Hughlings Jackson was wont to insist,[3] " thinks," so to say, in movements, not in muscles.

The tiny skin spot stimulated in the spinal scratch-reflex brings into action a whole array of muscles. In the spinal cat, a wholly insentient preparation, they can be freely laid bare and examined in their activity. Without exhaustive search we soon reach thirty-six:[4] nineteen in rhythmic action at five beats a second, seventeen in steady—*i.e.*, postural-action. The rhythmic beat is a brief tetanus lasting about one-ninth second, followed by a quiescence sometimes long enough for complete relaxation from the tetanic beat. The rhythm is not generated in the cutaneous nerve-ending —the hair-endings—for it occurs on faradising at other rhythms the afferent nerve itself, and indeed quite easily by electrical stimulation applied to the cut cross-surface of the top of the spinal cord itself.[5] Nor is it a rhythm developed, as was suggested above for clonus, by a retropulsive effect from the operating muscles themselves; that is clear, because the reflex persists after the whole of the scratching limb has been desensitised by severance of its posterior nerve-roots. The rhythm is clearly of central origin, with its seat in the hind-limb region of the cord. It is not easy to say what tunes such a rhythm, since it is *not* timed by the periphery as in a *clonus*.

The scratch-reflex does not stand alone in this unexpected independence of actual local peripheral reflex guidance. It is noteworthy that " scratching," " stepping," the " pinna reflex," the " shake reflex " are not elicitable seemingly by any stimulation of the cerebral cortex. They are, however, exaggerated after destruction of the cortical " motor area."

[1] *Trab. Lab. Invest. Biol. Univ. Madr.*, 1928. **23,** 259.
[2] Creed and Sherrington, *Proc. roy. Soc.*, 1926, **100B,** 258.
[3] *Neurological Fragments*, edited by James Taylor, London, 1928.
[4] Sherrington, *Quart. J. exp. Physiol.*, 1910, **3,** 313.
[5] Roaf and Sherrington, *Quart. J. exp. Physiol.*, 1910, **3,** 210.

It is surprising to find the movements evoked by stimulating the motor area of the cerebral cortex not obviously impaired by complete desensitisation of the limb itself. Willed movements are upset in the extreme. In the monkey the desensitised limb is practically useless, for prehension quite so. The animal soon treats it as useless and as an encumbrance worse than useless; it attacks it and would tear it away. Yet, when the motor cortex is examined by electric stimulation, not only does it evoke in the de-afferented arm and hand the customary movements just as readily as usual, but those movements reveal no obvious departure from their usual co-ordination. They can be compared with the movements evoked by corresponding cortical stimulation in the normal fellow-limb and reveal no abnormality. It seemed so to Mott and myself[1] in our observations now long since. It has seemed so again to Dr. Denny-Brown and myself, applying recent myographic and galvanometric technique to sample muscles. Wild inco-ordination under willed action; little or no abnormality under the action of the directly stimulated motor cortex—a striking contrast. One may relate it to the probably very direct play of the pyramidal tract upon the motoneurones.[2] It is a *caveat* against accepting the movement excited electrically at the motor cortex as any close homologue of a willed one. It seems as unimpaired by desensitising its limb as is the spinal scratch-reflex itself. Thus, too, an elemental difference is revealed between the clonus of rigidity—*e.g.*, decerebrate rigidity—and the cortical post-stimulation clonus, the Jacksonian epileptiform. The latter is not affected by de-afferenting the muscles or indeed the whole limb; the former is of course entirely annulled. The intact proprioceptive " circle," which is a factor essential for the one, is quite inessential for the other.

A somewhat similar state of things exists in respect of the stepping reflex; so much so that Graham Brown[3] argues, from many observations, that the stepping is a centrally initiated and executed cyclic reflex essentially independent of—although modifiable by—peripheral stimuli. It certainly often occurs quite in absence of all plantar or foot stimuli—for instance, in the air or with all four feet wholly desensitised (*cf.* p. 181, Chapter V).

FARADISATION OF SPINAL TRACTS

As with scratching so with stepping, the reflex can be excited by weak stigmatic unipolar faradisation from the cut transverse face of the spinal cord[4] at a tiny area in the lateral column, the stepping being, for instance, in the hind-limb and the point stimulated at the top of the cord, the preparation a decapitated cat. The scratch-reflex will not alter its rhythm under either peripheral or central stimulation—*i.e.*, from cut face of cord.

[1] *Proc. roy. Soc.*, 1895, **57**, 481, and this volume, p. 115. Illustrated in *Brain*, 1934, **54**, 1.

[2] Leyton and Sherrington, *Quart. J. exp. Physiol.*, 1917, **11**, 135; Cooper and Denny-Brown, *Proc. roy. Soc.*, 1927, **102B**, 222.

[3] *J. Physiol.*, 1914, **48**, 18.

[4] Roaf and Sherrington, *Quart. J. exp. Physiol.*, 1910, **3**, 210.

But with stepping the weak faradic stimulus excites in the hind-limb of the same side stepping which from walking becomes running as the stimulus is made slightly stronger. It tends to be accompanied by feebler stepping of the opposite hind-limb, agreeing in rate with that of the fellow-limb but oppositely timed so that it alternates in phase with it, as in natural loco-motion. By arranging two electric circuits two stigmatic electrodes can be used with separately adjustable strength of stimulation. If then the right and left points are stimulated concurrently on the cut face of the top of the cord, a subliminal stimulation of one is found to become effective on applying a subliminal stimulus to the other. Galloping can be obtained by stimulating the two points concurrently with somewhat stronger stimuli. This stepping point lies in the deep dorsal part of the lateral column. If, while the stepping is in progress under excitation of this point, a weak stigmatic faradisation be applied to the ventral part of the ventrolateral column (probably vestibulo-spinal tract) of the same side, the stepping at once slows down or stops. Stimulation at this point when the dorsolateral point is not being stimulated gives extension of the same-side hind-limb. The dorsal point I mentioned as the " stepping " point; the ventral point might be called the " standing " point. As yet I have examined it only at the above-mentioned level. The right and left ventral column points when concurrently stimulated reinforce each other. The observations occur equally well with the stepping limbs suspended—that is, with the proprio-ceptive stimuli in the stepping limbs quite otherwise than when the limbs are bearing superincumbent weight, also quite without plantar stimuli, the feet being in the air. The complex cyclic act, with the various timings of is sequence as initiated and maintained by excitation of a slender channel descending into a spinal lumbar region from above, seems strangely inde-pendent, for guidance rhythm or support, of local centripetal factors in the limb itself. Stimulation at the stepping point in the lateral column starts the limb stepping and keeps it going practically at what pace it likes. Stimulation of the antagonistic descending path slows the stepping, and if stronger stops it and changes it into standing. With stepping and standing as incompatible opposites this instance where the reaction deals with the limb on large lines, and suppresses one of two incompatible reactions in order to bring in the other, offers analogy to reciprocal innervation. It further illustrates a feature of co-ordination which I have insisted on else-where—namely, that for a muscle or a muscle group to be contracting does not exclude its being under inhibition. Let us glance back, for instance, at our generalised picture of the excited motor centre, and take it a stage further by inserting some inhibition. We see at once that the inhibition, counter-acting according to its degree less or more of the excitation, can slacken or stop the firing of some or all of the discharging motoneurones. Only in the extreme grade which stops all the motor units will the inhibition reveal itself as a complete absence of contraction of the muscle or muscle group.

Concluding Remarks

I must not detain you longer. I would only remark that the present time seems of unusual promise for neurological investigation, both in the clinic and the laboratory. I think the same feeling informed the penetrating and suggestive lectures given not so long since by Dr. Walshe.[1] The advent of possibilities of sampling the individual nerve and motor unit opens out opportunity for advance. The centre's activity, which for too long has been only a statistical quantity, can yield up some secrets of its precise individual activities.

I have dealt very imperfectly with a small bit of a large problem. I have kept much within the purely experimental laboratory. The smallness of the fragment is disappointing. The problem itself has the interest that, large as it is, it yet—to speak *more Hibernico*—is larger still. Hughlings Jackson, in his writings, turns back and forth between muscular co-ordination and mental experience, as if for him they were but aspects of a single theme. It may be that to decipher how nerve manages muscle is to decipher how nerve manages itself. If so, not without significance should be what we have just glimpsed, that there are in the nervous system heights of excitation and depths of inhibition higher and deeper and with grades of adjustment ampler than muscle with all its subtleties can commensurately express.

[1] *Lancet*, 1929, 1, 963.

EPILOGUE

How a limited set of agents of the outside world working through the nerve and brain of the animal can produce from its muscles the thousand and one dexterous acts of normal behaviour is itself a problem for which the following answer can be attempted. Its motor instrument is essentially separable into a great number of small units which it can use individually and in a great number of different combinations. Each unit has a single nerve-thread, which springs from a wide nerve-net. In the nerve-nets there occur at the nodal points two kinds of nerve-action, one which fires the nerve-thread (and so the motor unit), the other which impedes or prevents the firing of the nerve-thread. On any one of these nerve-threads one or the other of these two opposed nerve-influences can be exerted. Conjointly they quantitatively neutralise one the other. The variety and delicacy of the motor activity of the animal are largely due to the conjoint use of the two opposed processes upon the units of the motor system. The brain with its nerve-nets additional to and superimposed on the other nerve-nets exerts through them a management of supreme delicacy and width over the whole complex of motor units. The animal's motor behaviour where the brain-nets are large excels in variety and nicety. But it fails to offer anything radically different from that of reflex action elsewhere.

I may seem to stress the preoccupation of the brain with muscle. Can we stress too much that preoccupation when any path we trace in the brain leads directly or indirectly to muscle? The brain seems a thoroughfare for nerve-action passing on its way to the motor animal. It has been remarked that Life's aim is an act, not a thought. To-day the dictum must be modified to admit that, often, to refrain from an act is no less an act than to commit one, because inhibition is coequally with excitation a nervous activity.

From *The Brain and its Mechanism*, The Rede Lecture, Cambridge, 1933.

BIBLIOGRAPHY
1884–1938

[*The abbreviations used in the citations of scientific periodicals in this bibliography are in accordance with "The World List of Scientific Periodicals 1900-1933," Oxford University Press, 1934. The "World List" was enthusiastically reviewed and analysed by Sir Charles in "Nature" (see below under 1934). When papers were written in collaboration, the co-authors are given in parentheses after the title, and when Sherrington was not the first author the order of names has been indicated by arabic numerals enclosed in square brackets.—J. F. F., D. D-B.*]

1884

On sections of the right half of the medulla oblongata and of the spinal cord of the dog which was exhibited by Prof. Goltz at the International Medical Congress of 1881 (with J. N. Langley [1]). *Proc. Physiol. Soc., J. Physiol.*, 1884 (Jan.), **5**, vi.

Secondary degeneration of nerve tracts following removal of the cortex of the cerebrum in the dog (with J. N. Langley [1]). *J. Physiol.*, 1884 (June), **5**, 49-65, pl. 1-2.

1885

On secondary and tertiary degenerations in the spinal cord of the dog. *J. Physiol.*, 1885 (Apr.), **6**, 177-191, pl. 4-5.

1886

Preliminary report on the pathology of cholera Asiatica (as observed in Spain, 1885) (with C. S. Roy [1] and J. Graham Brown [2]). *Proc. roy. Soc.*, 1886 (June 10), **41**, 173-181.

Effect of ligature of the optic nerve in a rabbit. *Proc. Physiol. Soc., J. Physiol.*, 1886 (May), **7**, xvi-xvii.

On a case of bilateral degeneration in the spinal cord, fifty-two days after hæmorrhage in one cerebral hemisphere (with W. B. Hadden [1]). *Brain*, 1886 (Jan.), **8**, 502-511, pl. 1.

Note on two newly described tracts in the human spinal cord. *Brain*, 1886 (Oct.), **9**, 342-351, pl. 1.

1887

Note on the anatomy of Asiatic cholera as exemplified in cases occurring in Italy in 1886. *Proc. roy. Soc.*, 1887 (June 16), **42**, 474-477.

1888

The pathological anatomy of a case of locomotor ataxy, with special reference to ascending degenerations in the spinal cord and medulla oblongata (with W. B. Hadden [1]). *Brain*, 1888 (Oct.), **11**, 325-335, pl. 1.

1889

On nerve-tracts degenerating secondarily to lesions of the cortex cerebri (Preliminary). *J. Physiol.*, 1889, **10**, 429-432.

On formation of scar-tissue (with C. A. Ballance). *J. Physiol.*, 1889 (Oct.), **10**, 550-576, pl. 31-33.

1890

Note on bilateral degeneration in the pyramidal tracts resulting from unilateral cortical lesion. *Brit. med. J.*, 1890 (Jan. 4), **1**, 14.

On outlying nerve-cells in the mammalian spinal cord (Preliminary note). *Proc. roy. Soc.*, 1890, **47**, 144-146.

On the regulation of the blood-supply of the brain (with C. S. Roy [1]). *J. Physiol.*, 1890, **11**, 85-108, pl. 2-4.

Addendum to note on tracts degenerating secondarily to lesions of the cortex cerebri. *J. Physiol.*, 1890, **11**, 121-122.

Über die Entstehung des Narbengewebes, das Schicksal der Leucocyten und die Rolle der Bindegewebskörperchen (with C. A. Ballance). *Zbl. allg. Path. path. Anat.*, 1890 (Oct.), **1**, 697-703.

A method to determine the quantity of blood in a living animal (with S. M. Copeman [1]). *Proc. Physiol. Soc.*, *J. Physiol.*, 1890 (May), **11**, viii-ix.

The effect of movements of the human body on the size of the spinal canal (with R. W. Reid [1]). *Brain*, 1890, **13**, 449-455.

Further note on degenerations following lesions of the cerebral cortex. *J. Physiol.*, 1890, **11**, 399-400.

Demonstration of ganglion cells in the mammalian spinal cord. *Proc. Physiol. Soc. J. Physiol.*, 1890 (Dec.), **12**, xxxiv.

1891

On pilo-motor nerves (with J. N. Langley [1]). *J. Physiol.*, 1891, **12**, 278-291.

Note on Cheyne-Stokes breathing in the frog. *J. Physiol.*, 1891, **12**, 292-298, pl. 7.

Note on some functions of the cervical sympathetic in the monkey. *Brit. med. J.*, 1891 (Mar. 21), **1**, 635.

Note on the nerve supply of the bladder and anus. *Brit. med. J.*, 1891 (May 9), **1**, 1016.

Note on the knee-jerk. *St. Thom. Hosp. Rep.*, 1891, **21**, 145-147.

On outlying nerve-cells in the mammalian spinal cord. *Philos. Trans.* (1890), 1891, **181B**, 33-48, pl. 3-4.

1892

The nuclei in the lumbar cord for the muscles of the pelvic limb. *Proc. Physiol. Soc.*, *J. Physiol.*, 1892 (Feb. 15), **13**, viii-x.

Note toward the localisation of the knee-jerk. *Brit. med. J.*, 1892, **1**, 545; Addendum to note on the knee-jerk. *Ibid.* (Mar. 26), 654.

Geminal nerve-fibres. Dichotomous branching of medullated fibres in the brain and spinal cord. *Proc. Physiol. Soc.*, *J. Physiol.*, 1892, **13**, xxi-xxii.

Notes on the arrangement of some motor fibres in the lumbo-sacral plexus. *J. Physiol.*, 1892, **13**, 621-772, pl. 20-23. (Preliminary note in *Proc. roy. Soc.*, 1892 (Mar. 14), **51**, 67-78.) [*Extracts here*, pp. 1-17.]

On varieties of leucocytes. *Zbl. Physiol.*, 1892, **6**, 399.

Sulla localizzazione del riflesso rotuleo. *G. Accad. Med. Torino*, 1892 (Dec.), **40**, 951-959.

In memoriam W. B. Hadden, M.D. (Lond.), F.R.C.P. *St. Thom. Hosp. Rep.*, 1892, **22**, xix-xxi (unsigned).

Experiments in examination of the peripheral distribution of the fibres of the posterior roots of some spinal nerves (Preliminary note). *Proc. roy. Soc.*, 1892 (Dec. 2), **52**, 333-337 (full report 1894).

Experiments on animals (concerning the sensitiveness of the peritoneum; a polemic with Lawson Tait). *Lancet*, 1892 (Dec. 17), **2**, 1416-1417; Experiments on living animals. *Ibid.* (Dec. 31), 1533; third letter *Ibid.*, 1893 (Jan. 28), **1**, 221.

1893

Variations experimentally produced in the specific gravity of the blood. *J. Physiol.*, 1893 (Jan.), **14**, 52-96, pl. 4. (with S. M. Copeman).

Note on the knee-jerk and the correlation of action of antagonistic muscles. *Proc. roy. Soc.*, 1893 (Feb.), **52**, 556-564. [*Reprinted here*, pp. 237-244.]

Further experimental note on the correlation of action of antagonistic muscles. *Proc. roy. Soc.*, 1893 (Apr. 15), **53,** 407-420. Abstr. bearing same title *Brit. med. J.*, 1893 (June 10), **1,** 1218. [*Reprinted here*, pp. 244-256.]

Experimental note on the knee-jerk. *Brit. med. J.*, 1893 (Sept. 23), **2,** 685; also *St. Thom. Hosp. Rep.* (1891), 1893, **21,** 145-147.

Note on the spinal portion of some ascending degenerations. *J. Physiol.*, 1893 (Sept.), **14,** 255-302, pl. 13-18.

Remarks on L. A. Bidwell's paper " Focal epilepsy; trephining and removal of small hæmorrhagic focus; no improvement; removal of part of leg centre after electrical stimulation; improvement." *Brit. med. J.*, 1893 (Nov. 4), **2,** 989.

Note on some changes in the blood of the general circulation consequent upon certain inflammations of an acute local character. *Proc. roy. Soc.*, 1893 (Dec. 11), **54,** 487-488 (full report, 1894).

Experiments on the escape of bacteria with the secretions. *J. Path. Bact.*, 1893 (Jan.), **1,** 258-278.

Sur une action inhibitrice de l'écorce cérébrale. *Rev. neurol.*, 1893, **1,** 318-319.

1894

Note on experimental degeneration of the pyramidal tract. *Lancet*, 1894 (Feb. 3), **1,** 265. [Polemic reply by Horsley (Feb. 10), 370-371]; Second note by C. S. S. (Feb. 17), 439; Third note by C. S. S. (Mar. 3), 571.

Experimental note on two movements of the eye. *J. Physiol.*, 1894 (July 19), **17,** 27-29.

On the anatomical constitution of the nerves of muscles. *Proc. Physiol. Soc., J. Physiol.*, 1894 (June 23), **17,** xix-xx.

On the anatomical constitution of nerves of skeletal muscles; with remarks on recurrent fibres in the ventral spinal nerve-root. *J. Physiol.*, 1894, **17,** 211-258, pl. 5-7. [*Extract here*, pp. 99 and 100.]

Note on some changes in the blood of the general circulation consequent upon certain inflammations of an acute local character. *Proc. roy. Soc.*, 1894, **55,** 161-207.

Experiments in examination of the peripheral distribution of the fibres of the posterior roots of some spinal nerves. (I) *Philos. Trans.* (1893), 1894, **184B,** 641-763, pl. 42-52. [*Extracts here*, pp. 31-56.]

1895

Experiments upon the influence of sensory nerves upon movement and nutrition of the limbs (with F. W. Mott [1]). Preliminary communication. *Proc. roy. Soc.*, 1895 (Mar. 7), **57,** 481-488. [*Extract here*, pp. 115-119.]

Varieties of leucocytes. *Sci. Progr. Twent. Cent.*, 1895 (Feb.), **2,** 415-430.

1896

A note on the physiology of the spinal cord. *St. Thom. Hosp. Rep.* (1894), 1896, **23,** 69-76.

Influence of simultaneous contrast on " flicker " of visual sensation. *Proc. Physiol. Soc., J. Physiol.*, 1896 (Nov. 14), **20,** xviii-xix.

Committee report on the life condition and infectivity of the oyster (with W. A. Herdman and others). *Brit. Ass. Rep.*, 1896, 663; 1897, 363; 1898, 559-562.

1897

Cataleptoid reflexes in the monkey. *Proc. roy. Soc.*, 1897 (Jan. 21), **60,** 411-414; also *Lancet*, 1897 (Feb. 6), **1,** 373-374.

Experiments in examination of the peripheral distribution of the fibres of the posterior roots of some spinal nerves. (Preliminary abstract.) *Proc. roy. Soc.*, 1897 (Jan. 21), **60,** 408-411 (full report 1898).

On reciprocal innervation of antagonistic muscles. Third note. *Proc. roy. Soc.*, 1897 (Jan. 21), **60,** 414-417. [*Reprinted here*, pp. 256-259.]

On reciprocal action in the retina as studied by means of some rotating discs. *J. Physiol.*, 1897 (Feb. 5), **21,** 33-54.

Double (antidrome) conduction in the central nervous system. *Proc. roy. Soc.*, 1897 (Apr. 8), **61**, 243-246. [*Reprinted here*, pp. 225-228.]

Further note on the sensory nerves of muscles. *Proc. roy. Soc.*, 1897 (Apr. 8), **61**, 247-249. [*Reprinted here*, pp. 102 and 103.]

On the question whether any fibres of the mammalian dorsal (afferent) spinal root are of intraspinal origin. *J. Physiol.*, 1897 (Mar.), **21**, 209-212. [*Extract here*, p. 101.]

The central nervous system, vol. 3 (with M. Foster [1]). Sir Michael FOSTER's *A Text Book of Physiology*, 7th ed., London, 1897. (In the 5th ed., 1890, " Mr. Langley " and " Dr. Sherrington " " largely assisted " Foster in the preparation of the volume.)

The mammalian spinal cord as an organ of reflex action. Croonian Lecture. *Proc. roy. Soc.*, 1897, **61**, 220-221. (Abstract. Published *in extenso* as Section IV of Experiments in examination, etc., *Philos. Trans.*, 1898, **190B**, 45-186.)

Über Hemmung der Contraction willkürlicher Muskeln bei elektrischer Reizung der Grosshirnrinde (with H. E. Hering [1]). *Pflüg. Arch. ges. Physiol.*, 1897, **68**, 221-228.

Antagonistic muscles and reciprocal innervation (with H. E. Hering). Fourth note. *Proc. roy. Soc.*, 1897 (Nov. 18), **62**, 183-187. [*Reprinted here*, pp. 259-262.]

The activity of the nervous centres which correlate antagonistic muscles in the limbs. *Rep. Brit. Ass.*, 1897, 516-518.

Observations on visual contrast. *Rep. Brit. Ass.*, 1897, 824-826.

Committee report on the physiological effects of peptone and its precursors when introduced into the circulation (with E. A. Schäfer and others). *Brit. Ass. Rep.*, 1897, 531; 1898, 720; 1899, 605; 1900, 457; 1904, 342.

Committee report on the functional activity of nerve cells (with W. H. Gaskell and others). *Brit. Ass. Rep.*, 1897, 512; 1898, 714-715.

1898

Experiments in examination of the peripheral distribution of the fibres of the posterior roots of some spinal nerves. (II) *Philos. Trans.*, 1898, **190B**, 45-186, pl. 3-6 (rec. Nov. 12, 1896; read Jan. 21, 1897). Also *Thomp. Yates Lab. Rep.*, 1898, **1**, 45-173. [*Extracts here*, pp. 17-28, 56-84, 94-99, 120-125, 127-154, 372-373.]

Decerebrate rigidity, and reflex co-ordination of movements. *J. Physiol.*, 1898 (Feb. 17), **22**, 319-332. [*Reprinted here*, pp. 314-325.]

Cardiac physics. In ALLBUTT, *System of Medicine*, New York and London, 1898, **5**, 464-479 (2nd ed. revised by J. Mackenzie, 1909, **6**, 3-25).

Further note on the sensory nerves of the eye-muscles. *Proc. roy. Soc.*, 1898 (Nov. 17), **64**, 120-121. [*Reprinted here*, pp. 103-105.]

On the reciprocal innervation of antagonistic muscles. Fifth note. *Proc. roy. Soc.*, 1898 (Dec. 15), **64**, 179-181. [*Reprinted here*, pp. 263-264.]

1899

The teaching of physiology and histology. *Brit. med. J.*, 1899 (Apr. 8), **1**, 878.

On the spinal animal (Marshall Hall Lecture). *Med.-chir. Trans.*, 1899 (May 23), **82**, 449-477, pl. 13-17. Abstract, *Brit. med. J.*, 1899 (May 27), **1**, 1276; *Lancet*, 1899 (May 27), **1**, 1433; *Thomp. Yates Lab. Rep.*, 1898, **1**, 27-44. [*Extracts here*, pp. 29, 30, 123, 126, 134, 136.]

Tremor, " tendon-phenomenon," and spasm. In ALLBUTT, *System of Medicine*, 1899, **6**, 511-524 (2nd ed., 1910, **7**, 290-309).

On the relation between structure and function as examined in the arm. (Inaugural address.) *Trans. Lpool. biol. Soc.*, 1899, **13**, 1-20. [*Extract here*, p. xiv.]

Inhibition of the contraction of voluntary muscles by electrical excitation of the cortex cerebri (with H. E. Hering [1]). *J. Physiol.*, 1899, **23** (Suppl. Rep. Internat. Congress), 31.

Inhibition of the tonus of a voluntary muscle by excitation of its antagonist. *J. Physiol.*, 1899, **23** (Suppl. Rep. Internat. Congress), 26.

1900

On the innervation of antagonistic muscles. Sixth note. *Proc. roy. Soc.*, 1900 (Jan. 18), **66**, 66-67. (*Thomp. Yates Lab. Rep.*, 1899, **1**, 175-176.) [*Reprinted here*, pp. 155 and 156.]

Experiments on the value of vascular and visceral factors for the genesis of emotion. *Proc. roy. Soc.*, 1900 (May 10), **66**, 390-403; Abstract, *Brit. med. J.*, 1900 (July 14), **2**, 110.

The spinal cord. In *Text-book of Physiology*. Edited by E. A. SCHÄFER, Edinburgh and London, 1900, **2**, 783-883.

The parts of the brain below cerebral cortex, viz. medulla oblongata, pons, cerebellum, corpora quadrigemina, and region of thalamus. In *Text-book of Physiology*. Edited by E. A. SCHÄFER, Edinburgh and London, 1900, **2**, 884-919.

Cutaneous sensations. In *Text-book of Physiology*. Edited by E. A. SCHÄFER, Edinburgh and London, 1900, **2**, 920-1001.

The muscular sense. In *Text-book of Physiology*. Edited by E. A. SCHÄFER, Edinburgh and London, 1900, **2**, 1002-1025.

Nature of tendon reflexes—a discussion of E. Jendrassik's paper before 13th Int. Congr. Med., *Lancet*, 1900 (Aug. 18), **2**, 530-531. Sur la nature des reflexes tendineux. *Res. Rap. Paris. Sect. Neurol.*, 25-26; *C.R. XIII Int. Congr. Med.*, 1900, Sect. Neurol., 149-155. Also *St. Louis med. surg. J.*, 1900, **79**, 197-198.

Lecture on Physiology for Teachers (Nov. 29, 1900). Printed privately (1901) by The Childhood Society for the scientific study of the mental and physical conditions of children, 15 pp.

1901

The general anatomy and physiology of the nervous system. In ALLCHIN, *Manual of Medicine*, 1901, **3** (*Diseases of the Nervous System*), 1-33.

The name of the red corpuscle: A suggestion. *Brit. med. J.*, 1901 (Mar. 23), **1**, 742.

Über einige Hemmungserscheinungen im Zustande der sog. Enthirnungsstarre (decerebrate rigidity). *Wien. klin. Rsch.*, 1901, **15**, 774-775. (Nothnagel *Festschrift*) (with A. Fröhlich).

The spinal roots and dissociative anæsthesia in the monkey. *J. Physiol.*, 1901 (Dec. 23), **27**, 360-371, pl. 10. [*Reprinted here*, pp. 84-93.]

Observations on the physiology of the cerebral cortex of some of the higher apes (with A. S. F. Grünbaum [1]). *Proc. roy. Soc.*, 1901 (Nov. 23), **69**, 206-209. Also *Thomp. Yates Lab. Rep.*, 1902, **4**, pt. 2.

An address on localization in the "motor" cerebral cortex (with A. S. F. Grünbaum). *Brit. med. J.*, 1901 (Dec. 28), **2**, 1857-1859. (Read before the Pathological Society, London, Dec. 17, 1901; also read before Vth Internat. Congress, Turin, abstract *Brit. med. J.*, 1901 (Oct. 12), **2**, 1091-1093.)

1902

Path of impulses for inhibition under decerebrate rigidity (with A. Fröhlich [1]). *J. Physiol.*, 1902, **28**, 14-19. [*Reprinted here*, pp. 228-232.]

Observations on "flicker" in binocular vision. *Proc. roy. Soc.*, 1902 (July 30), **71**, 71-76.

A discussion on the motor cortex as exemplified in the anthropoid apes (with A. S. F. Grünbaum). *Brit. med. J.*, 1902 (Sept. 13), **2**, 784, 785.

Committee report on the conditions of health essential to carrying on the work of instruction in schools (with E. W. Wallis and others). *Brit. Ass. Rep.*, 1902, 483-496; 1903, 455; 1904, 348; 1906, 433; 1907, 421; 1908, 458.

Committee reports of special chloroform committee of the British Medical Association (with Dr. Barr and others). *Brit. med. J.*, 1902, **2**, 116-118; *ibid.*, 1903, **2**, cxli-cxlii; 1904, **2**, 161-162; 1905, **2**, 180-181; 1906, **2**, 78-79.

Fatigue. A lecture to the Froebel Society, Owens College, Manchester. Abstract only, *Brit. med. J.*, 1902 (Oct. 25), **2**, 1371.

Address to the Conference on the Hygiene of Social Life. *J. R. sanit. Inst.*, 1902, **23**, 311-317; abstract, *Brit. med. J.*, 1902 (Sept. 20), **2**, 885-886, 991.

C. S. Roy, 1854-1897. *Year Book of the Royal Society*, 1902, 231-235.

Note on the arterial supply of the brain in anthropoid apes (with A. S. F. Grünbaum [1]). *Brain*, 1902, **25**, 270-273.

Remarks at discussion on pathology of nerve degeneration. *Brit. med. J.*, 1902 (Sept. 27), **2**, 928.

Note upon descending intrinsic spinal tracts in the mammalian cord (with E. E. Laslett). *Proc. roy. Soc.*, 1902, **71**, 115-121.

1903

The history of the discovery of trypanosomes in man. *Lancet*, 1903 (Feb. 21), **1**, 509-513 (with R. Boyce [1] and R. Ross [2]). Preliminary letter, *Lancet*, 1902 (Nov. 22), **2**, 1426; also *Brit. med. J.*, 1902 (Nov. 22), **2**, 1680.

Observations on some spinal reflexes and the interconnection of spinal segments (with E. E. Laslett). *J. Physiol.*, 1903 (Feb.), **29**, 58-96. [*Extracts here*, pp. 201-225.]

Remarks on the dorsal spino-cerebellar tract (with E. E. Laslett). *J. Physiol.*, 1903 (Mar.), **29**, 188-194.

Physiology and nervous diseases. An address delivered to " Doctorate Graduates," University of Chicago, October, 1903.

An address on science and medicine in the modern university (delivered at the opening of the new medical school, Toronto, 1903). *Brit. med. J.*, 1903 (Nov. 7), **2**, 1193-1196; also *Lancet*, 1903 (Nov. 7), **2**, 1273-1276; *Science*, 1903 (Nov. 27), **18**, 675-684.

Observations on the physiology of the cerebral cortex of the anthropoid apes (with A. S. F. Grünbaum [1]). *Proc. roy. Soc.*, 1903 (June 11), **72**, 152-155. (Also *Thomp. Yates Lab. Rep.*, 1903, **5**, 55-58.)

Qualitative difference of spinal reflex corresponding with qualitative difference of cutaneous stimulus. *J. Physiol.*, 1903 (Aug.), **30**, 39-46. [*Reprinted here*, pp. 157-162.]

Address on medical science. *Canad. J. Med. Surg.*, 1903, **14**, 321-332; *Dom. med. Mon.*, 1903, **21**, 203-215.

On the dosage of the mammalian heart by chloroform (I) (with S. C. M. Sowton). *Brit. med. J.*, 1903 (suppl.), cxlvii-clxi; *Thomp. Yates Lab. Rep.*, 1903, **5**, 69-104.

Opening of discussion on applied hygiene for school teachers. *J. R. sanit. Inst.*, 1903, **24**, 27-31.

1904

On binocular flicker and the correlation of activity of " corresponding " retinal points. *Brit. J. Psychol.*, 1904 (Jan.), **1**, 26-60.

On certain spinal reflexes in the dog. *Proc. Physiol. Soc.*, *J. Physiol.*, 1904 (Mar. 19), **31**, xvii-xix.

A pseudaffective reflex and its spinal path (with R. S. Woodworth [1]). *J. Physiol.*, 1904 (June), **31**, 234-243. [*Extract here*, pp. 232-236.]

On the dosage of the isolated mammalian heart by chloroform (II) (with S. C. M. Sowton). Appendix I to the Third Report of Special Chloroform Committee. *Brit. med. J.*, 1904 (July 23), **2**, 162-168, 721; *Brit. Ass. Rep.*, 1904, 761-762; and *Arch. Fisiol.*, 1904 (Nov.), **2**, 140-141.

The correlation of reflexes and the principle of the common path. *Brit. Ass. Rep.*, 1904 (Aug. 18), **74**, 728-741; also abstract *Brit. med. J.*, 1904 (Aug. 27), **2**, 443; *Nature*, 1904, **70**, 460-466; *Pop. Sci. Mon.*, 1904, **65**, 549-552. [*Extracts here*, pp. 441-443.]

Committee report on madreporaria of the Bermuda Islands (with S. J. Hickson and others). *Brit. Ass. Rep.*, 1904, 299; 1905, 186; 1906, 325.

On the mode of functional conjunction of twin (corresponding) retinal points. *Arch. Fisiol.*, 1904 (Nov.), **2**, 154-155.

1905

On reciprocal innervation of antagonistic muscles. Seventh note. *Proc. roy. Soc.*, 1905 (Apr. 6), **76B**, 160-163.

On reciprocal innervation of antagonistic muscles. Eighth note. *Proc. roy. Soc.*, 1905 (May 18), **76B**, 269-297.

Über das Zusammenwirken der Rückenmarksreflexe und das Prinzip der gemeinsamen Strecke. *Ergebn. Physiol.*, 1905, **4**, 797-850.

On the relative effects of chloroform upon the heart and upon other muscular organs. *Brit. med. J.*, 1905 (July 22), **2**, 181-187. (Appendix I of Fourth Report of Special Chloroform Committee, see 1902.)

Physiology: its scope and method. From Oxford Lectures on *Methods of Science*, 1905, chap. 3, pp. 59-80.

The importance of longer hours of sleep at public schools. *Brit. med. J.*, 1905 (Dec. 2), **2**, 1469-1471 (unsigned).

Obituary. Sir John Burdon-Sanderson. *Brit. med. J.*, 1905 (Dec. 2), **2**, 1491-1492.

Training in hygiene for teachers. *J. R. sanit. Inst.*, 1905, **26**, 132-138.

1906

Integrative Action of the Nervous System. New Haven and London, Yale University Press, 1906, xvi +411 pp.

On the innervation of antagonistic muscles. Ninth note. Successive spinal induction. *Proc. roy. Soc.*, 1906 (Feb. 15), **77B**, 478-497.

On the proprioceptive system, especially in its reflex aspect. *Brain*, 1906, **29** (Hughlings Jackson Number), 467-482. [*Extract here*, pp. 236-239.]

Observations on the scratch-reflex in the spinal dog. *J. Physiol.*, 1906, **34**, 1-50.

On the effect of chloroform in conjunction with carbonic dioxide on cardiac and other muscle (with S. C. M. Sowton [1]). Appendix III of Fifth Report of Special Chloroform Committee, see 1902, 1905. *Brit. med. J.*, 1906 (July 14), **2**, 85-87.

Experiments in examination of the locked-jaw induced by tetanus-toxin (with H. E. Roaf [1]). *J. Physiol.*, 1906 (Aug.), **34**, 315-331; abstract, *Lancet*, 1906 (Sept. 22), **2**, 810; *Brit. med. J.*, 1906, **2**, 9.

The mechanism of " locked jaw " produced by tetanus toxin (with H. E. Roaf [1]). *Brit. med. J.*, 1906, **2**, 1805.

1907

Appreciation of Sir Michael Foster. *Brit. med. J.*, 1907, **1**, 351.

The Association and medical research. (Commenting on Mott's Review of the *Integrative Action of the Nervous System*), *Brit. med. J.*, 1907 (Mar. 16), **1**, 657.

On reciprocal innervation of antagonistic muscles. Tenth note. *Proc. roy. Soc.*, 1907 (Apr. 18), **79B**, 337-349.

Nerve as a master of muscle. *Not. Proc. roy. Instn.*, 1907 (Apr. 19), **18**, 609-618, and *Sci. Amer. Suppl.*, 1908, **65**, 378.

Strychnine and reflex inhibition of skeletal muscle. *J. Physiol.*, 1907 (Nov.), **36**, 185-204.

On reciprocal innervation of antagonistic muscles. Eleventh note. Further observations on successive induction. *Proc. roy. Soc.*, 1907 (Dec. 5), **80B**, 53-71; reprinted *Folia neuro-biol.*, 1908 (Mar.), **1**, 365-383.

Spinal reflexes. *Brit. Ass. Rep.*, 1907, 667.

1908

A discussion on the scientific education of the medical student. (Meeting of the British Medical Association.) *Brit. med. J.*, 1908 (Aug. 15), **2**, 380; also *Lancet*, 1908 (Aug. 15), **2**, 480-481.

On reciprocal innervation of antagonistic muscles. Twelfth note. Proprioceptive reflexes. *Proc. roy. Soc.*, 1908 (Dec. 10), **80B**, 552-564; reprinted *Folia neurobiol.*, 1909, **2**, 578-588. Abstr. *Nature*, 1908, **78**, 592.

On reciprocal innervation of antagonistic muscles. Thirteenth note. On the antagonism between reflex inhibition and reflex excitation. *Proc. roy. Soc.*, 1908 (Dec. 10), **80B**, 565-578; reprinted *Folia Neurobiol.*, 1909, **2**, 589-602. [*Extract here*, pp. 265-269.]

Committee report on body metabolism in cancer (with S. M. Copeman). *Brit. Ass. Rep.*, 1908, 489-492; 1910, 297-300; 1911, 171.

Some comparisons between reflex inhibition and reflex excitation. *Quart. J. exp. Physiol.*, 1908, **1**, 67-78.

1909

On plastic tonus and proprioceptive reflexes. *Quart. J. exp. Physiol.*, 1909, **2**, 109-156. (*Reprinted here*, pp. 329-363.]

Reciprocal innervation of antagonistic muscles. Fourteenth note. On double reciprocal innervation. *Proc. roy. Soc.*, 1909, **81B**, 249-268; reprinted *Folia neuro-biol.*, 1910, **3**, 477-496.

Discussion on the deep afferents; their function and distribution (Meeting of the British Medical Association). *Brit. med. J.*, 1909 (Sept. 11), **2**, 679-690; also *Lancet*, 1909 (Sept. 11), **2**, 791-792.

A mammalian spinal preparation. *J. Physiol.*, 1909, **38**, 375-383.

1910

Obituary. W. Page May. *Brit. med. J.*, 1910 (Jan. 29), **1**, 298.

Flexion-reflex of the limb, crossed extension-reflex, and reflex stepping and standing. *J. Physiol.*, 1910 (Apr.), **40**, 28-121. [*Extracts here*, pp. 163-188, 364-372.]

Remarks on the reflex mechanism of the step. *Brain*, 1910 (June), **33**, 1-25.

Receptors and afferents of the third, fourth and sixth cranial nerves (with F. M. Tozer [1]). *Proc. roy. Soc.*, 1910 (June 6), **82B**, 450-457; reprinted *Folia neuro-biol.*, 1910, **4**, 626-633.

Further remarks on the mammalian spinal preparation (with H. E. Roaf [1]). *Quart. J. exp. Physiol.*, 1910 (Mar.), **3**, 209-211.

Notes on the scratch reflex of the cat. *Quart. J. exp. Physiol.*, 1910 (Mar.), **3**, 213-220.

Brain, physiology of. In *Encyclopædia Britannica*, London and New York, 11th ed., 1910, **4**, 403-413.

Note on certain reflex actions connected with the mouth. *Brit. dent. J.*, 1910, **31**, 785-790.

Committee report on mental and muscular fatigue (with W. MacDougall and others). *Brit. Ass. Rep.*, 1910, 292; 1911, 174.

1911

On reflex rebound (with S. C. M. Sowton). *Proc. Physiol. Soc.*, printed but unpublished, 1911, 5 pp.

Reversal of the reflex effect of an afferent nerve by altering the character of the electrical stimulus applied (with S. C. M. Sowton). *Proc. roy. Soc.*, 1911 (Mar. 22), **83B**, 435-446; reprinted *Z. allg. Physiol.*, 1911, **12**, 485-498.

Motor localization in the brain of the gibbon, correlated with a histological examination (with F. W. Mott [1] and E. Schuster [2]). *Proc. roy. Soc.*, 1911 (May 4), **84B**, 67-74; reprinted *Folia neuro-biol.*, 1911, **5**, 699-707.

Notes on the pilomotor system (with T. Graham Brown [1]). *Quart. J. exp. Physiol.*, 1911 (June), **4**, 193-205.

Muscle and nerve. In *Encyclopædia Britannica*, 11th ed., 1911, **19**, 44-50.

Spinal cord, physiology of. In *Encyclopædia Britannica*, 11th ed., 1911, **25**, 672-684.

Sympathetic system. In *Encyclopædia Britannica*, 11th ed., 1911, **26**, 287-289.

On reflex inhibition of the knee flexor (with S. C. M. Sowton). *Proc. roy. Soc.*, 1911 (June 29), **84B**, 201-214.

The rôle of reflex inhibition. *Sci. Prog. Twent. Cent.*, 1911 (No. 20), 584-610; trans. in *Scientia, Riv. Scienza*, 1911, **9**, 226-246; abstract *Brit. med. J.*, 1911 (Mar. 25), **1**, 690-691, and *Lancet*, 1911 (Mar. 11), **1**, 666.

Chloroform and reversal of reflex effect (with S. C. M. Sowton). *J. Physiol.*, 1911 (July), **42**, 383-388.

Sir Rupert Boyce, 1863-1911. *Proc. roy. Soc.*, 1911 (Sept.), **84B**, 1-6.

Observations on the localization in the motor cortex of the baboon (*Papio anubis*) (with T. Graham Brown [1]). *J. Physiol.*, 1911, **43**, 209-218.

Observations on strychnine reversal (with A. G. W. Owen [1]). *J. Physiol.*, 1911 (Nov.), **43**, 232-241.

1912

Note on present problems of nervous function. In *Mélanges biologiques*, 1912, *dédié à Charles Richet*, pp. 371-379.

On the instability of a cortical point (with T. Graham Brown [1]). *Proc. roy. Soc.*, 1912 (Mar.), **85B**, 250-277.

Bewegung und Leben. Address to the students at Utrecht, 1912 (May).

The rule of reflex response in the limb reflexes of the mammal and its exceptions (with T. Graham Brown [1]). *J. Physiol.*, 1912 (May), **44**, 125-130.

Some instances of uncertainty in reflex reactions. Delivered to British Medical Association, July 26. Abstract, *Lancet*, 1912 (Aug. 24), **2**, 537.

Report of Departmental Committee on Sight Tests, Board of Trade, 1912 (May 10).

1913

Six chapters on physiology " briefly explaining the principles which underlie the precepts and practice described in the other chapters of the book " (pp. 224-307). *A Manual of School Hygiene*, by E. W. Hope, E. A. Brown, and C. S. S. (new edition, Cambridge University Press, 1913, xii+311 pp.).

Reciprocal innervation and symmetrical muscles. *Proc. roy. Soc.*, 1913 (Jan. 13), **86B,** 219-232.

Nervous rhythm arising from rivalry of antagonistic reflexes: reflex stepping as outcome of double reciprocal innervation. *Proc. roy. Soc.*, 1913 (Feb. 20), **86B,** 233-261.

Note on the functions of the cortex cerebri (with T. Graham Brown [1]). *Proc. Physiol. Soc., J. Physiol.*, 1913, **46,** xxii.

Reflex inhibition as a factor in the co-ordination of movements and postures. *Quart. J. exp. Physiol.*, 1913 (June), **6,** 251-310. [*Reprinted here,* pp. 269-313.]

The sight tests of the Board of Trade (Polemic with F. W. Edridge-Green). *Lancet*, 1913 (June 14), **1,** 1691; (Edridge-Green's letters, *ibid.*, 1557, 1752-1754, 1764).

Reciprocal innervation. Seventeenth Int. Congr. Med. *Brit. med. J.*, 1913 (Aug. 23), **2,** 458-459.

An address on the provincial school of medicine and the provincial university. Delivered at the Prize distribution in the School of Medicine, University of Leeds. *Brit. med. J.*, 1913 (Oct. 4), **2,** 844-846.

Rhythmic reflex produced by antagonizing reflex excitation by reflex inhibition. Ninth International Congress of Physiology. *Arch. int. Physiol.*, 1913, **14,** 74.

Further observations on the production of reflex stepping by combination of reflex excitation with reflex inhibition. *J. Physiol.*, 1913 (Nov.), **47,** 196-214.

Reversal in cortical reactions (with T. Graham Brown [1]). *Arch. int. Physiol.*, 1913, **14,** 72-73.

1914

Report on reciprocal innervation. *Trans. Int. Congr. Med.* 1913 (Sect. II, Physiol.), 1914, 85-93.

Acoustic reflexes in the decerebrate cat (with A. Forbes [1]). *Amer. J. Physiol.*, 1914 (Nov.), **35,** 367-376.

1915

Observations on reflex responses to single break-shocks (with S. C. M. Sowton). *J. Physiol.*, 1915 (July), **49,** 331-348.

Some observations on the bucco-pharyngeal stage of reflex deglutition in the cat (with F. R. Miller [1]). *Quart. J. exp. Physiol.*, 1915 (Oct.), **9,** 147-186.

Postural activity of muscle and nerve. *Brain*, 1915, **38,** 191-234. [*Extracts here,* pp. 374-385.]

Simple apparatus for obtaining a decerebrate preparation of the cat. *Proc. Physiol. Soc., J. Physiol.*, 1915 (July 3), **49,** lii-liv.

Committee report on the structure and function of the mammalian heart (with S. Kent). *Brit. Ass. Rep.*, 1915, 226-229; 1916, 304; 1917, 122.

1916

A simple apparatus for illustrating the Listing-Donders law. *Proc. Physiol. Soc., J. Physiol.*, 1916 (July 15), **50,** xlvi-xlix.

1917

Observations on the excitable cortex of the chimpanzee, orang-utan and gorilla (with A. S. F. Leyton [1]). *Quart. J. exp. Physiol.*, 1917, **11,** 135-222. [*Extracts here,* pp. 397-439.]

Reflexes elicitable in the cat from pinna vibrissæ and jaws. *J. Physiol.*, 1917 (Dec.), **51,** 404-431. [*Extracts here,* pp. 189-200.]

Observations with antitetanus serum in the monkey. *Lancet*, 1917 (Dec. 29), **2,** 964-966.

Recent physiology and the war. *Not. Proc. roy. Instn.*, 1917, **22,** 1-3, and *Science*, 1917, **46,** 502-504.

1918

Stimulation of the motor cortex in a monkey subject to epileptiform seizures. *Brain*, 1918 (Mar.), **41,** 48-49.

Brevity, frequency of rhythm and amount of reflex nervous discharge, as indicated by reflex contraction (with N. B. Dreyer [1]). *Proc. roy. Soc.*, 1918 (Oct.), **90B,** 270-282.

Observations on the sensual rôle of the proprioceptive nerve-supply of the extrinsic ocular muscles. *Brain*, 1918 (Dec.), **41,** 332-343. [*Reprinted here,* pp. 105-115.]

1919

Mammalian Physiology. A Course of Practical Exercises. Oxford, Clarendon Press, 1919, xii+156 pp.

Note on the history of the word "tonus" as a physiological term. Contribution to *Medical and Biological Research Dedicated to Sir William Osler*, New York, 1919, **1**, 261-268.

1920

Sir William Osler. Obituary. *Brit. med. J.*, 1920 (Jan. 10), **1**, 65.

Postural activity of muscle. Cavendish Lecture, West London Medico-chirurgical Society. *Brit. med. J.*, 1920 (Aug. 21), **2**, 288. (Apparently never printed *in extenso*.)

Gateways of sense. Huxley Lecture, Birmingham University, November 26, 1919. *Brit. med. J.*, 1920 (Dec. 4), **2**, 875. (Apparently never printed *in extenso*.)

1921

On the myogram of the flexor-reflex evoked by a single break-shock (with K. Sassa [1]). *Proc. roy. Soc.*, 1921 (May), **92B**, 108-117.

Break-shock reflexes and "supramaximal" contraction-response of mammalian nerve-muscle to single shock stimuli. *Proc. roy. Soc.*, 1921 (May), **92B**, 245-258.

Albert Sidney Leyton—Obituary. *Brit. med. J.*, 1921 (Oct. 8), **2**, 579.

Anniversary address delivered before the Royal Society of London, November 30, 1921. *Proc. roy. Soc.*, 1922 (Jan.), **100A**, 353-366; *ibid.*, **93B**, 1-14, extract bearing title: The maintenance of scientific research. *Nature*, 1921 (Dec. 8), **108**, 470-471.

Sur la production d'influx nerveux dans l'arc nerveux réflexe. *Arch. int. Physiol.*, 1921 (Dec.), **18**, 620-627. (Volume dedicated to Léon Fredericq.)

1922

Note on the after-discharge of reflex centres. In *Libro en honor de Santiago Ramón y Cajal*, Madrid, 1922, pp. 97-101.

Some points regarding present-day views of reflex action. Address to Royal Society, Edinburgh, March 20, 1922. Abstract, *Nature*, 1922 (Apr. 8), **109**, 463.

Some aspects of animal mechanism. Presidential Address, British Association for the Advancement of Science, Hull. *Brit. Ass. Rep.*, 1922 (Sept.), 1-15; *Brit. med. J.*, 1922 (Sept. 9), **2**, 485-486. Also *Nature*, 1922, **110**, 346-352; *Vet. Rec.*, 1922, **2**, 762-766; *J. Ment. Hygiene*, 1923, **17**, 1-19.

Inaugural address delivered at the opening of the Biological Building, McGill University, Montreal, October 5, 1922. Printed privately, Murray Printing Co., Ltd., Toronto, 1922, 8 pp.

Anniversary address delivered before the Royal Society of London, November 30, 1922. *Proc. roy. Soc.*, 1923, **102A**, 373-388, and **94B**, i-xvi. Extract under title: The use of a pancreatic extract in diabetes. *Nature*, 1922 (Dec. 9), **110**, 774; also *Brit. med. J.*, 1922 (Dec. 9), **2**, 1139-1140.

1923

The position of psychology. Address to National Institute of Industrial Psychology, March 20, 1923. Abstract, *Nature*, 1923 (March 31), **111**, 439. (Apparently never printed *in extenso*.)

Stimulus rhythm in reflex contraction (with E. G. T. Liddell [1]). *Proc. roy. Soc.*, 1923 (May), **95B**, 142-156. Appendix on separation key by C.S.S.

A comparison between certain features of the spinal flexor reflex and of the decerebrate extensor reflex respectively (with E. G. T. Liddell [1]). *Proc. roy. Soc.*, 1923 (July), **95B**, 299-339.

Recruitment type of reflexes (with E. G. T. Liddell [1]). *Proc. roy. Soc.*, 1923 (Oct.), **95B**, 407-412.

Anniversary address delivered before the Royal Society of London, November 30, 1923. *Proc. Roy. Soc.*, 1924 (Jan.), **105A**, 1-16; *ibid.*, **95B**, 485-499; *Nature*, 1923 (Dec. 8), **112**, 845-848; *Brit. med. J.*, 1923 (Dec. 8), **2**, 1113-1114.

1924

Reflexes in response to stretch (myotatic reflexes) (with E. G. T. Liddell [1]). *Proc. roy. Soc.*, 1924 (Mar.), **96B**, 212-242.

Problems of muscular receptivity. *Nature*, 1924 (June 21 and 28), **113**, 732, 892-894, 929-932. [*Extract here*, pp. 385-396.]

Notes on temperature after spinal transection, with some observations on shivering. *J. Physiol.*, 1924 (May), **58**, 405-424. [*Extract here*, p. 133.]

Anniversary address delivered before the Royal Society of London, December 1, 1924. *Proc. roy. Soc.*, 1925 (Jan.), **107A**, 1-14; *ibid.*, **97B**, 254-267; *Nature*, 1924 (Dec. 6), **113**, 840-841.

1925

Recruitment and some other features of reflex inhibition (with E. G. T. Liddell [1]). *Proc. roy. Soc.*, 1925 (Feb.), **97B**, 488-518.

Remarks on some aspects of reflex inhibition. *Proc. roy. Soc.*, 1925 (Feb.), **97B**, 519-545. [*Extract here*, pp. 443-460.]

The late Sir Clifford Allbutt—Obituary. *Brit. med. J.*, 1925 (Mar. 7), **1**, 495.

Further observations on myotatic reflexes (with E. G. T. Liddell [1]). *Proc. roy. Soc.*, 1925 (Oct.), **97B**, 267-283.

An address on avenues in medicine. Delivered at the opening of the winter session of the London (Royal Free Hospital) School of Medicine. *Mag. Lond.* (Roy. Free Hosp.) *School Med. for Women*, 1925, **20**, 133-141; *Lancet*, 1925 (Oct. 10), **2**, 741-743. Abstract under title: Medicine as a career for women. *Brit. med. J.*, 1925 (Oct. 19), **2**, 667-668.

Address at the unveiling of the Wheatstone Memorial at Gloucester, October 19, 1925. *Nature*, 1925 (Oct. 31), **116**, 659.

J. N. Langley—Obituary. *Brit. med. J.*, 1925 (Nov. 14), **2**, 925.

Anniversary address delivered before the Royal Society of London, November 30, 1925. *Proc. roy. Soc.*, 1926, **110A**, 1-15; *ibid.*, 1926, **99B**, 107-121; *Nature*, 1925 (Dec. 5), **116**, 833-835.

The Assaying of Brabantius and Other Verse. Oxford University Press, 67 pp.

1926

Addition latente and recruitment in reflex contraction and inhibition. *Livre à Charles Richet*. Paris, 1926, 3 pp.

Observations on concurrent contraction of flexor muscles in the flexion reflex (with R. S. Creed [1]). *Proc. roy. Soc.*, 1926 (June), **100B**, 258-267. Appendix on double mirror myograph by C.S.S. [*Extract here*, p. 461.]

Reflex fractionation of a muscle (with S. Cooper [1] and D. E Denny-Brown [2]). *Proc. roy. Soc.*, 1926 (Nov.), **100B**, 448-462. [*Extract here*, p. 462.]

1927

Interaction between ipsilateral spinal reflexes acting on the flexor muscles of the hind-limb (with S. Cooper [1] and D. E. Denny-Brown [2]). *Proc. roy. Soc.*, 1927 (Feb.), **101B**, 262-303. [*Extract here*, pp. 463, 464.]

Whither ?—A footnote. *Nature*, 1927 (Feb. 5), **119**, 205.

Lister and physiology. *Nature*, 1927 (Apr. 23), **119**, 606-608; *Brit. med. J.*, 1927 (Apr. 9), **1**, 653-654; *Lancet*, 1927 (Apr. 9), **1**, 743-744.

Ernest Henry Starling—Obituary. *Brit. med. J.*, 1927 (May 14), **2**, 905.

Second Listerian Oration. *Canad. med. Ass. J.*, 1927 (June 18), 17, **2**, 1255-1263.

Dunham Lectures, 1927 (Harvard Medical School); October 10, Observations on stretch reflexes; October 13, Modes of interaction between reflexes; Octobe.· 17, Some factors of co-ordination in muscular acts. Abstract: *Bost. med. surg. J.*, 1927, **197**, 812 (not published *in extenso*).

Keith Lucas (1879-1916). *Dictionary of National Biography*, 1912-1921. [Supplement III], Oxford University Press, 1927.

Committee report on colour vision, with particular reference to classification of colour blindness (with H. E. Roaf and others). *Brit. Ass. Rep.*, 1927, 307-308.

1928

Foreword [p. v] to L. J. J. MUSKENS, *Epilepsy, Comparative Pathogenesis, Symptoms, Treatment.* London, Baillière, Tindall and Cox, 1928. xiv +435 pp.

Sir Dawson Williams—Obituary. *Brit. med. J.*, 1928 (Mar. 10), **1**, 418.

Eulogy of Harvey. The Harvey Tercentenary Celebrations, Royal College of Physicians, May 14, 1928. *Brit. med. J.*, 1928 (May 19), **1**, 866-868; *Lancet*, 1928 (May 19), **1**, 1034-1035.

Some physiological data toward functional analysis of a simple reflex centre. *Arch. Sci. biol.*, 1928 (June), **12**, 1-7. Bottazzi Birthday Volume.

Introduction [pp. xi-xiii] to F. MASON, *Creation by Evolution. A Consensus of Present-day Knowledge as set forth by Leading Authorities in Non-technical Language that all may understand.* New York, Macmillan, 1928, xxii +392 pp.

A mammalian myograph. *Proc. Physiol. Soc., J. Physiol.*, 1928, **66**, iii-v.

The instability of a single vortex-row. *Nature*, 1928 (Sept. 1), **122**, 314.

Subliminal fringe in spinal flexion (with D. E. Denny-Brown [1]). *J. Physiol.*, 1928, **66**, 175-180.

Sir David Ferrier. *Proc. roy. Soc.*, 1928 (Nov.), **103B**, viii-xvi.

1929

Life in upper Canada in 1827. By B. Aldren. Remarks on foregoing letter by C. S. S., *Canad. med. Ass. J.*, 1929 (Jan.), **20**, 65-67.

Some functional problems attaching to convergence. Ferrier Lecture. *Proc. roy. Soc.*, 1929 (Sept.), **105B**, 332-362; and *Brit. med. J.*, 1929, **1**, 1136-1137. [*Reprinted here*, pp. 464-486.]

Mammalian Physiology. A Course of Practical Exercises (with E. G. T. Liddell [1]). 2nd ed. Oxford, Clarendon Press, 1929, xii +162 pp.

Improved bearing for the torsion myograph (with J. C. Eccles [1]). *Proc. Physiol. Soc., J. Physiol.*, 1929 (Dec.), **69**, i.

Brain, physiology of. *Encyclopædia Britannica*, London and New York, 1929, 14th ed., **4**, 1-9. Rewritten; see also 1910.

The spinal cord—physiology. *Encyclopædia Britannica*, London and New York, 1929, 14th ed., **21**, 220-228. Rewritten; see also 1911.

The sympathetic system. *Encyclopædia Britannica*, London and New York, 1929, 14th ed., **21**, 702-704. Rewritten; see also 1911.

1930

Reflex summation in the ipsilateral spinal flexion reflex (with J. C. Eccles [1]). *J. Physiol.*, 1920 (Mar.), **69**, 1-28.

Numbers and contraction-values of individual motor-units examined in some muscles of the limb (with J. C. Eccles [1]). *Proc. roy. Soc.*, 1930 (June), **106B**, 326-357.

Flexor reflex responses to successive afferent volleys (with J. C. Eccles [1]). *Proc. Physiol. Soc., J. Physiol.*, 1930 (July), **70**, xxv-xxvii.

Notes on the knee extensor and the mirror myograph. *J. Physiol.*, 1930 (Aug.), **70**, 101-107.

Nervous integrations in man. In COWDRY, *Human Biology and Racial Welfare* (with J. F. Fulton [1]), New York: Paul B. Hoeber, 1930 (pp. 246-265).

1931

Studies on the flexor reflex:

    I. Latent period (with J. C. Eccles [1]). *Proc. roy. Soc.*, 1931 (Mar.), **107B**, 511-534.

    II. The reflex response evoked by two centripetal volleys (with J. C. Eccles [1]). *Ibid.*, 535-556.

    III. The central effects produced by an antidromic volley (by J. C. Eccles alone). *Ibid.*, 557-585.

IV. After-discharge (with J. C. Eccles [1]). *Ibid.*, 586-596.

V. General conclusions (with J. C. Eccles [1]). *Ibid.*, 597-605. *[Reprinted here, pp. 486-494.]*

VI. Inhibition (with J. C. Eccles [1]). *Ibid.*, 1931, **109B**, 91-113. *[Extracts here, pp. 494-496.]*

Quantitative management of contraction in lowest level co-ordination. Hughlings Jackson Lecture. *Brain*, 1931 (Apr.), **54**, 1-28. Also abstr. *Brit. med. J.*, 1931, **1**, 207-211. *[Reprinted here, pp. 497-514.]*

1932

State of the flexor reflex in paraplegic dog and monkey respectively (with J. F. Fulton [1]). *J. Physiol.*, 1932 (May), **75**, 17-22.

Concluding remarks to discussion on tonus of skeletal muscle. Internat. Neurol. Congress, Berne, 1931. *Arch. Neurol. Psychiat., Chicago*, 1932 (Sept.), **28**, 676-678.

Chromatolysis of motor-horn cells. *Proc. Physiol. Soc., J. Physiol.*, 1932 (May), **12**, 11-12P.

Reflex Activity of the Spinal Cord (with R. S. Creed, D. Denny-Brown, J. C. Eccles, E. G. T. Liddell [1]). Oxford, Clarendon Press, 1932, viii + 184 pp.

Degeneration of peripheral nerves after spinal transection in the monkey (with S. Cooper [1]). *Proc. Physiol. Soc., J. Physiol.*, 1932 (Nov.), **77**, 18P.

Inhibition as a co-ordinative factor. Nobel Lecture delivered at Stockholm, December 12, 1932. Stockholm, P. A. Norstedt, 1933, 12 pp.

1933

The Brain and its Mechanism. The Rede Lecture delivered before the University of Cambridge, December 5, 1933. Cambridge University Press, 1933, 36 pp. 2nd issue, November, 1937. *[Extract here, p. 515.]*

1934

Reflex inhibition as a factor in co-ordination of muscular acts. *Rev. Soc. argent. Biol.*, 1934 (Nov.), **10**, 510-513.

Review of HALLOWES, K. D. *The Poetry of Geology.* In *Sci. Progr.*, 1934 (July), **29**, 165.

Periodicals and reference. [Review of *World List.*] *Nature*, 1934 (Sept. 22), **134**, 435-437.

Language distribution of scientific periodicals. [Analysis of *World List.*] *Nature*, 1934 (Oct. 9), **134**, 871-872.

1935

Sir Edward Sharpey-Schafer and his contributions to neurology (Sharpey-Schafer Memorial Lecture). *Edinb. med. J.*, 1935 (Aug.), **42**, 393-406.

Functional problems of convergence of nerves. *Orv. Hetil.*, 1935 (Sept.), **79**, 1050-1051.

Santiago Ramón y Cajal, For. Mem. R.S.—Obituary. *Obit. Notes Roy. Soc.*, 1935 (Dec.), No. 4, 425-441.

1936

The chastening. *Cornhill Magazine*, 1936 (Aug.), **154**, 140.

1937

The wise Ulysses. *Cornhill Magazine*, 1937 (Jan.), **155**, 38.

Community. *Cornhill Magazine*, 1937 (May), **155**, 701.

Sir Squire Sprigge. *Lancet*, 1937 (June 26), **1**, 1554.

Review of HORTON and ALDREDGE, *Johannes de Mirfeld of St. Bartholomew's Smithfield: His Life and Works.* In *Medium Ævum*, 1936, **3**, 236-240.

Scientific endeavour and inferiority complex. Review of RAMÓN Y CAJAL, *Recollections of My Life.* In *Nature*, 1937 (Oct. 9), **140**, 617-619.

Preface to *Le tonus des muscles striés* by G. MARINESCO, N. JONESCO-SISESTI, O. SAGER and
A. KREINDLER. Académie Roumaine, *Etudes et Recherches*, Bucarest, 1937 [pp. vii-
viii].

Langley, John Newport.   In *Dictionary of National Biography*, 1922-1930   [Supplement IV],
Oxford University Press, 1937, 479-481.

Ferrier, Sir David.   In *Dictionary of National Biography*, 1922-1930 [Supplement IV],
Oxford University Press, 1937, 302-304.

Paget, Stephen.   In *Dictionary of National Biography*, 1922-1930 [Supplement IV], Oxford
University Press, 1937, 649-651.

1938

The Society's Library.   *Notes Rec.* [Roy. Soc., Lond.], 1938, **1**, 21-27.

INDEX